Nelson

ESSENTIALS
OF
VETERINARY HEMATOLOGY

ESSENTIALS
OF
VETERINARY HEMATOLOGY

Nemi C. Jain, BVSc and AH, MVSc, Phd

Professor of Clinical Pathology
Department of Clinical Pathology
School of Veterinary Medicine
University of California
Davis, California

Lea & Febiger   Philadelphia   1993

Williams & Wilkins
Rose Tree Corporate Center, Building II
1400 North Providence Road, Suite 5025
Media, PA 19063-2043 USA
U.S.A.
(215) 251-2230

Executive Editor—George H. Mundorff
Project Editor—Lisa Stead
Production Manager—Michael DeNardo

Library of Congress Cataloging-in-Publication Data

Jain, Nemi C. (Nemi Chand), 1936–
      Essentials of veterinary hematology / Nemi C. Jain.
            p.   cm.
      Includes index.
      ISBN 0-8121-1437-X
      1. Veterinary hematology.   I. Title.
SF769.5.J35   1993
636.089′615—dc20   92-18138
                                              CIP

PRINTED IN THE UNITED STATES OF AMERICA

Print number: 5   4   3

Dedicated to
my spiritual Sād-Guru,
Shri Sai Sham,
and
in memory of Dr. Oscar W. Schalm,
the Father of Veterinary Clinical Hematology

PREFACE

Essentials of Veterinary Hematology is a concise text on the subject of veterinary hematology. It has been written to provide a ready source of current and fundamental information necessary to the understanding of basic concepts in hematology as a discipline and veterinary hematology as a specialty.

The formulation of this book evolved from the need for a concise text for teaching veterinary hematology. The book is aimed at undergraduate veterinary students, veterinary medical technologists, animal technicians, and all those interested in an abridged text in comparative hematology. Graduate veterinary students can use it as a ready source for reviewing the fundamentals of veterinary hematology. Veterinary practitioners can find it useful for reviewing the pathophysiology of blood as it relates to clinical veterinary medicine. A generalized approach to the interpretation of various hematologic abnormalities is presented throughout the text, along with comments on species-specific hematologic attributes and hematologic abnormalities encountered in various species. I feel that *Essentials of Veterinary Hematology* can be used to build a broad yet sound foundation in veterinary hematology that can be subsequently expanded ad libitum by reading current literature on hematology, immunology, and other relevant disciplines.

Although *Essentials of Veterinary Hematology* essentially evolved from *Schalm's Veterinary Hematology*, there are several important differences. Basically it follows the same format, but the text has been extensively condensed and reorganized to improve readability and comprehension. The information presented has been revised and updated as much as possible. The number of color plates has been increased from 25 to 27 plates, with 230 individual figures. There are 343 black and white illustrations, including many new ones. Most of these illustrations have been rearranged to improve organization and comprehension. Reference citation has been deliberately kept to a minimum for smoother reading. Interested readers can find further details in references listed at the end of each chapter and in *Schalm's Veterinary Hematology*.

The increasing use of commercial diagnostic laboratories by veterinary practitioners has reduced the need to perform in-house hematologic analyses. In view of this trend, and to keep the text concise, a chapter on hematologic techniques has not been included. However, such information can be readily found in *Schalm's Veterinary Hematology* and other standard hematology books.

Essentials of Veterinary Hematology is organized into 22 chapters. Chapter 1 gives general information about the examination of blood and bone marrow, and is a prelude to the clinical usefulness of hematologic examination. Chapter 2 presents the important comparative morphologic features of blood cells and normal hematologic values for common domestic animals (dogs, cats, cattle, horses, sheep, goats, and pigs). It also includes comments on species differences in response to disease. Chapter 3 is a similar presentation of comparative hematology of avian and other mammalian species, including laboratory and zoo animals. Basic concepts of hematopoiesis and its regulation by recently discovered cytokines and growth factors are presented in Chapter 4. Chapter 5 is concerned with the pathophysiologic aspects of coagulation and hemostasis, and Chapter 6 discusses platelet production, structure, function, and abnormalities. The pathophysiology of red cells, including hemoglobin metabolism and the significance of morphologic abnormalities, is discussed in Chapter 7. A general approach to the evaluation of anemias and polycythemias is presented in Chapter 8 and various types of anemias are discussed separately in Chapters 10 to 12. Chapters 13 through 17 provide information about various leukocyte types and their abnormalities and response to disease, and Chapter 18 is concerned with the interpretation of qualitative and quantitative changes in leukocytes. General aspects of leukemias are discussed in Chapter 19, and comparative features of leukemias in common domestic animals are presented in Chapter 20. Various plasma proteins and their abnormalities, particularly those involving immunoglobulins, are discussed in Chapter 21. Chapter 22 presents various aspects of immunohematology that pertain to various animal species, including a discussion of blood groups, blood transfusion, and immune-mediated hematologic disorders.

I am deeply indebted to all those who have been instrumental in expanding our knowledge in medical and veterinary hematology, and whose contributions have served as a source of material for developing this text without formal reference citation. I greatly appreciate the contributions of investigators and colleagues who have provided photographs of their published and unpublished work for inclusion in this book. The skillful word processing assistance provided by Rosanna Ullrich is sincerely appreciated. I also thank the staff of Lea & Febiger for their expertise and efforts in the publication of this book. Indeed, it has been my pleasure to work with George Mundorff and the late Christian C. Febiger Spahr (Kit).

Finally, my deepest gratitude is to my family, whose continual encouragement and moral support have made this work possible. I am highly thankful to my youngest son, Anant, who has willingly given his valuable time for literature searches and manuscript preparation. I am especially grateful to my wife, Javitri, who has been extremely gracious and unselfish in relieving me from household responsibilities so that I could have the time necessary to complete this endeavor.

Davis, California   *Nemi C. Jain*

CONTENTS

Examination of the Blood and Bone Marrow

Blood is a fluid tissue that circulates through vascular channels, carrying the necessities of life for all cells of the body and receiving the waste products of metabolism for transport to the organs of excretion. Blood examination is performed for several reasons: as a screening procedure to assess general health; as an adjunct to patient evaluation or diagnosis; to assess the body's ability to fight infection; and to evaluate the progress of certain disease states. A thorough history and physical examination are essential for a meaningful interpretation of hematologic data and other laboratory tests concerning the subject under investigation.

Abnormal findings in a hemogram are often nonspecific, in that they can be associated with various diseases or conditions that provoke a similar response. Infrequently, however, they may be diagnostic, as when leukemic cells or hemoparasites are found in blood. A single hemogram may be adequate for a general physical examination, but sequential hemograms must be developed to follow recovery from the disease state. A blood examination may also provide clues as to the necessity of bone marrow examination and other laboratory tests.

This chapter presents a general approach to the examination of blood and bone marrow in different animal species. Many of the topics discussed here are covered more fully in other chapters and additional information can be found in other hematology and clinical pathology texts (Duncan and Prasse, 1986, Jain, 1986; Meyer et al., 1992; Williams et al., 1990).

EXAMINATION OF THE PERIPHERAL BLOOD

Collection of Blood

Blood is readily drawn from large vessels, but several alternate sites have been found to be suitable for blood collection from various species (Table 1–1). Blood clots on removal from the body; later the clot retracts, releasing the serum commonly used in biochemical analysis. A hematologic examination requires blood to be in liquid form. For this purpose, blood is collected into a vial containing an appropriate anticoagulant. EDTA (ethylenediaminetetra-acetic acid), which prevents coagulation by complexing Ca^{2+}, is the anticoagulant of choice for most hematologic and biochemical analyses. However, morphologic changes, such as slight vacuolation of cytoplasm, uneven distribution of cytoplasmic granules, irregular cell membrane, or pyknosis, may occur with time in canine neutrophils in EDTA-anticoagulated blood (Gossett and Carakostas, 1984). Thus, blood smears should be prepared immediately after blood collection or, at the most, within 1 hour. Blood collected with heparin, unless processed immediately, results in poor staining of blood cells. Heparin is the anticoagulant of choice for avian and reptile species. Sodium citrate is recommended for blood platelet studies. Oxalate salts (sodium or potassium) should be avoided, because they cause crenation of red cells, bizarre nuclear changes in leukocytes, and gross distortions in platelet morphology.

Blood should be drawn from the animal at rest and under conditions of least excitement to minimize physiologic variations in cell counts. Immobilization of animals with anesthetics makes it easier to obtain blood samples, but may affect values of various blood parameters. For example, RBC counts and lymphocyte numbers in rhesus monkeys decreased significantly 15 minutes after intramuscular injection of ketamine hydrochloride from redistribution of these cells from the circulating blood to the spleen and extravascular sites, respectively (Bennett et al., 1992). Total serum proteins and albumin concentrations also decreased, probably from hemodilution. Vacutainers are best for collecting blood; they must be filled to capacity to yield the desired blood-to-anticoagulant ratio. When a sy-

Table 1–1. Sites and Needle Sizes Commonly Used for Collection of Blood from Various Animals

Animal	Site	Needle Size	
		Gauge	Length (in.)
Horse	Jugular vein	16–19	1½–2
Cow	Jugular vein, tail vein	16–19	1½–2
Sheep and goat	Jugular vein	18–20	1½–2
Pig	Anterior vena cava	20	1½–4
Dog	Cephalic, jugular, or saphenous vein	20–22	1½
Cat	Cephalic, jugular, or saphenous vein	22–25	1
Rabbit and guinea pig	Heart, marginal ear vein	18	3,1
Small primate	Femoral artery	22–26	⅝–1
Rat and mouse	Orbital sinus	Micro blood-collecting tube	
Pet birds	Wing vein, cutaneous ulnar anterior brachial vein	22–26	⅝–1

ringe and needle are used, the needle should be removed from the syringe before transferring blood to the vial containing the anticoagulant to prevent hemolysis. The blood and the anticoagulant should be mixed adequately by inverting the vial a dozen times. A clean venipuncture should be attempted to avoid the formation of blood clots because of contamination with tissue juice. Blood sample from a fasting animal is preferred to obviate any processing problems associated with postprandial lipemia.

Handling the Blood Sample

The blood sample should be processed as soon as possible after collection. If a delay is anticipated, it should be refrigerated at 4° C and tested within 12 to 24 hours. The blood sample should be mixed several times before a portion is removed for a test procedure, but prolonged mixing should be avoided to prevent physical trauma to various blood cells, especially erythrocytes. Blood films should be made immediately after blood collection, either directly from fresh blood or after anticoagulation. Blood films can be made on glass slides or coverslips and should be dried quickly. Leukocytes may degenerate in blood that is several hours old or that was exposed to a high ambient temperature before the blood films were made.

Developing a Hemogram

Various hematologic parameters, their units of measurement, and techniques commonly used to obtain their values are outlined in Table 1–2. The following discussion consists mainly of interpretive aspects of various hematologic tests, along with brief comments about hematologic techniques. Essential hematologic techniques have been described in detail (Jain, 1986) and can also be found in other hematology texts (Brown, 1988; Williams et al., 1990; Willard et al., 1989).

The veterinarian benefits most by establishing a set of tests for initial screening, followed by a more detailed hematologic examination. The choice of tests varies according to the purpose of the patient evaluation, and further laboratory investigation may be required. Initial screening should include at least one

Table 1–2. Common Hematologic Techniques and Units for Hematologic Data

Blood Entity	Common Techniques	Expressed in
Erythrocytes (RBC)	Electronic, hemocytometric	Millions per μl of blood
RBC diameter	Microscopic, electronic	Micrometers (μm)
Hemoglobin (Hb)	Colorimetric, spectrophotometric	Grams per deciliter (g/dl)
Packed cell volume (PCV)	Microhematocrit, electronic	Volume percent
Mean corpuscular volume (MCV)	Manual (arithmetic), electronic	Femtoliters (fl)
Mean corpuscular hemoglobin (MCH)	Manual (arithmetic), electronic	Picograms (pg)
Mean corpuscular hemoglobin concentration (MCHC)	Manual (arithmetic), electronic	Percent (%) or g/dl of red cells
Erythrocyte sedimentation rate (ESR)	Wintrobe method	Fall in mm in 1 hour
Reticulocytes	Vital stains (New methylene blue)	Percent (number per 100 red cells) or number per μl of blood
Nucleated erythrocytes (Nuc RBC)	Microscopic	Number per 100 leukocytes
Erythrocyte resistance to hypotonic saline (also called red cell osmotic fragility test)	Spectrophotometric	Percent saline in solution producing initial and complete hemolysis
Leukocytes, total count (WBC)	Electronic, hemocytometric	Number per μl of blood
Leukocytes, differential count	Microscopic	Percent
Leukocytes, differential absolute count	Arithmetic	Number per μl of blood
Bone marrow, differential cell count	Microscopic	Percent
Thrombocytes (platelets)	Hemocytometric, electronic	Number per μl of blood
Icterus index	Visual	Units of color as compared to standards prepared from potassium dichromate
Plasma protein, total	Refractometric, chemical	Grams per deciliter (g/dl)
Plasma fibrinogen	Refractometric, chemical	Grams per deciliter (g/dl) or milligrams per deciliter (mg/dl)

of the red blood cell (RBC) parameters, preferably packed cell volume (PCV) or hemoglobin (Hb) determination, total plasma protein and fibrinogen concentrations, total white blood cell (WBC) count, and a 200-cell differential leukocyte count. Morphologic evaluation of the various blood cells should be made from Wright-stained blood films, and observed abnormalities should be described briefly (Table 1–3). A subjective evaluation of platelet numbers—above,

Table 1–3. Outline for Examination of a Wright-Stained Blood Smear*

I. Platelets
  1. Distribution
  2. Estimated number
  3. Morphologic abnormalities, (e.g., hypogranulation, basophilia, vacuolation, and megathrombocytes)
II. Erythrocytes
  1. Size
    a. Anisocytosis
    b. Normocytic
    c. Macrocytic
    d. Microcytic
  2. Shape
    a. Poikilocytes
    b. Leptocytes
    c. Target cells
    d. Acanthocytes
    e. Spherocytes
    f. Schistocytes
    g. Other forms (for additional terminology, see Chap. 7)
  3. Distribution
    a. Single
    b. Rouleau formation
    c. Agglutination
  4. Color
    a. Normochromic
    b. Hypochromic
    c. Polychromasia
  5. Abnormal structures
    a. Howell-Jolly bodies
    b. Heinz bodies
    c. Pappenheimer bodies
    d. Basophilic stippling
    e. Nucleated red cells
    f. Parasites
    g. Inclusion bodies (e.g., distemper inclusions)
    h. Nuclear fragmentation and other structures
III. Leukocytes
  1. Estimated number
  2. Differential leukocyte count
  3. Morphologic abnormalities
    a. Toxic changes, such as azurophilic granules, vacuolation, foaminess, basophilia, and Döhle bodies in neutrophils
    b. Nuclear degeneration
    c. Hypersegmentation of neutrophil nucleus
    d. Hyposegmentation of neutrophil nucleus (Pelger-Huët anomaly)
    e. Giant bizarre forms
    f. Other abnormal findings
  4. Cytoplasmic inclusions, e.g., Ehrlichia organisms, distemper inclusions, phagocytosed red cells and bacteria, etc.
IV. Other findings
  1. Various cells, including mast cells, plasma cells, macrophages, megakaryocytes, and tumor cells
  2. Hemoparasites (e.g., trypanosomes)
  3. Microfilariae of heart worm

* Various subjective findings may be graded from slight to marked (e.g., slight polychromasia) or rare to many (e.g., many Heinz bodies).

below, or within normal range for the species—can be made from their distribution on the stained blood film. The platelet count can then be determined when thrombocytopenia is suspected. Similarly, the extent of polychromasia can provide a clue as to the necessity of a reticulocyte count in an anemic animal.

RBC and WBC counts in modern laboratories are performed using an electronic counter (Davies and Fisher, 1991; Tvedten and Wilkins, 1988b; Weiser, 1987). Platelet counts are commonly performed by the hemocytometer method, but they are increasingly being done using an automated method. Cell counts obtained by the use of calibrated electronic particle counters are highly accurate compared to those obtained with the hemocytometer method. Because of species variations in erythrocyte number and morphology, appropriate adjustments are necessary in the dilution of blood and in the calibration of cell-counting equipment to obtain accurate RBC counts. Similarly, automated instruments may also require calibration for counting leukocytes because of species variation in leukocyte size. Feline platelets are larger than those of many species, and have a tendency to clump. Pseudoleukocytosis due to EDTA-induced platelet clumping in human blood has been reported as a significant analytical error in automated WBC counts (Savage, 1984). Platelet clumping in some of these cases involved an IgM or IgG antibody to an unidentified platelet antigen. Thus, such platelets may be counted as leukocytes by an automated method. Leukocyte cytoplasmic fragmentation associated with lymphoid leukemia in cattle and sheep can interfere with the electronic determination of platelet counts and yield erroneous platelet counts (Weiser et al., 1989).

Leukocyte and platelet counts may be estimated indirectly from a stained blood film by determining cell distribution per microscopic field, but such counts are relatively less accurate. An average of 8 to 29 platelets per oil immersion field (100×) and 18 to 51 leukocytes per 10× objective field on canine blood films indicate normal counts (Tvedten et al., 1988a). Roughly, one platelet or leukocyte corresponds to 20,000 platelets or 330 leukocytes/μl of blood.

A reticulocyte count is performed by counting at least 1,000 erythrocytes in smears prepared from a mixture of a few drops of blood and an equal to double volume of 0.5% new methylene blue in physiologic saline. The reticulocyte count is essential for assessing the erythropoietic response to anemia in various species, the horse being an exception. In the latter species, a reticulocyte count performed on a bone marrow sample yields similar information. A "corrected" blood reticulocyte count, or reticulocyte production index, is calculated for a more meaningful assessment of the erythropoietic response to anemia in dogs and cats (see Chap. 8).

The PCV should be determined by a microhematocrit method, rather than by the Wintrobe method. Adequate centrifugal force and time are essential to minimize trapped plasma and to obtain accurate PCV values. Even with the microhematocrit method, goat and sheep bloods require longer centrifugation times (10 to 20 minutes), whereas 5 minutes is sufficient for other species' blood. The PCV obtained by the use of electronic cell counters is computed from the electronically measured cell mean corpuscular volume (MCV). Because the MCV varies widely among animal species, such PCV values may be erroneous unless the instruments have been properly calibrated for the species in question.

Gross examination of the hematocrit tube provides a rough evaluation of both compartments of the blood—the plasma and the formed elements. Centrifugation separates blood into three layers: the plasma at the top, the buffy coat in the middle, and the red cell mass at the bottom. The plasma color suggests the presence of hemolysis, lactescence, lipemia, and bilirubin. The icterus index, which is a measure of the amount of bilirubin in the blood, is determined by comparing the plasma color with standards prepared from 1.0% potassium dichromate solution. The presence of hemolysis, lactescence, or lipemia interferes with the estimation of the icterus index. The buffy coat is an off-white layer composed of platelets above and leukocytes below. Generally, the platelet layer is whitish and should not be mistaken for the leukocyte layer, which is tinged reddish because of the admixture of erythrocytes of low specific gravity (e.g., reticulocytes and leptocytes). The platelet layer is most noticeable and is clearly distinguishable from the leukocyte layer in cat blood.

A quantitative buffy coat (QBC) technique has been developed as a rapid hematologic screening procedure (Levine et al., 1986). The method involves centrifugal separation of anticoagulated blood into layers in a special capillary tube and then reading lengths of RBC, granulocyte, nongranulocyte, and platelet layers. This method can also be used as a screening test for detection of *Dirofilaria immitis* microfilarae in canine blood (Brown and Barsanti, 1988).

Hemoglobin determination is best performed by the cyanmethemoglobin method, which measures almost all types of circulating hemoglobin. The oxyhemoglobin method measures functional hemoglobin; therefore, it generally provides somewhat lower values than the cyanmethemoglobin method and yields significantly lower values in animals with methemoglobinemia. The spectrophotometric measurement of hemoglobin is not accurate when blood is lipemic or contains Heinz bodies in large numbers. The Sahli hemoglobinometer method is less accurate because of variations caused by sampling error and the subjective evaluation of color.

The erythrocyte indices—the MCV, MCHC (mean corpuscular hemoglobin concentration), and MCH (mean corpuscular hemoglobin)—are necessary for the evaluation of an anemic patient and can be used as a guide to the accuracy of various erythrocyte parameters (RBC, Hb, and PCV). For the evaluation of anemias, these indices are more applicable to the dog (as they are to humans) than to other animals. They have limited application to the cat and cow and

are of little practical use in the horse. As a guide to the accuracy of erythrocyte parameters, these indices are applicable to the blood of all species. Their accuracy is only as good as that of the parameters used in their derivation. Therefore, errors in the RBC, Hb, and PCV can become compounded. The erythrocytic indices should be interpreted in conjunction with an assessment of erythrocyte morphology in Wright-stained blood films (Table 1–3). For example, a sample with distinct dimorphic erythrocyte morphology may yield normal erythrocyte indices, and slight changes in red cell size and hemoglobin may not be reflected in corresponding indices.

The total plasma protein concentration can be estimated using a refractometer. The plasma present in a 75-mm long hematocrit tube used for the determination of the PCV is usually sufficient for this purpose. Plasma can also be obtained after the centrifugation of some blood in a Wintrobe hematocrit tube (15 minutes at 2000 G). Hemolysis, lactescence, and lipemia interfere with the refractometer reading, giving falsely higher values. Similarly, higher values have been obtained from samples having increased blood sugar and cholesterol levels. Postprandial lactescence and lipemia can be avoided if blood samples are collected before the animal is fed in the morning. The fibrinogen content of plasma can be readily estimated by the heat precipitation method and by using a refractometer. It is an important procedure in the evaluation of inflammatory responses and disseminated intravascular coagulation (DIC). In cattle, the fibrinogen determination is of considerable value in the diagnosis of internal inflammatory lesions.

The erythrocyte sedimentation rate (ESR) is a nonspecific test that can suggest an organic abnormality. It has occasionally been found useful in the dog and cat. The test is usually set up in a Wintrobe hematocrit tube and read at the end of 1 hour. The test can also be done using a 75-mm capillary tube. The observed ESR value must be corrected for the PCV of the blood before it is interpreted.

The differential leukocyte count on a routinely stained blood film should be performed on a minimum of 200 cells unless the blood sample contains a subnormal number of leukocytes. Standard procedure should be followed to perform the differential count. Simultaneously, any abnormality in the morphologic appearance of various cell types should be recorded. Smears prepared on slides or coverslips can be used. Smears should be prepared to provide a monolayer of cells, and the staining method used should produce quality results that yield discernible cellular details. The necessity for optimal staining of blood and bone marrow films for satisfactory cytologic cellular examination cannot be overemphasized. Precipitates and other staining artifacts should be avoided because they could be mistaken for certain blood cell features, such as erythrocyte parasites or toxic changes in leukocytes. Platelets, particularly in equine blood, and basophils, particularly in canine and feline bloods, could be overlooked in poorly stained films. Erythrocyte morphology may appear defective in poorly fixed blood films.

Automated differential leukocyte counts are performed in many human hospitals to reduce time and improve accuracy compared to the manual method. Differences in the cytochemical reactions of various leukocytes form the basis of cell identification by such instruments. Because the cytochemical reactions of the leukocytes of different animal species vary considerably, particularly neutrophil peroxidase activity, serious inaccuracies may arise in counts obtained by the use of an automated method. Accurate automated differential leukocyte counts, however, have been obtained for blood samples from dogs and rodents (Davies and Fisher, 1991).

Species Variation in Blood Morphology

Wright or any other Romanowsky stain provides the best available means for the morphologic evaluation of blood and bone marrow. Supravital staining, as with new methylene blue, may be performed to demonstrate the presence of reticulocytes and Heinz bodies. Blood films must be examined under 90 to 100× oil immersion lens so that necessary details can be observed and leukocyte differential counts performed. Mechanical trauma to blood cells, from smear making and contact of blood with the glass surface, creates artifacts of morphology. For example, the following might occur: red cells may appear highly crenated and acquire a teardrop form; lymphocytes may become deformed because of compression from red cells; or granules of neutrophils, eosinophils, and, rarely, basophils, may be found scattered from ruptured cells. Veterinarians are knowledgeable about the patient under investigation and can benefit most by examining blood and bone marrow films themselves rather than by relying on the results provided by the laboratory technician.

Mammalian platelets and erythrocytes are non-nucleated, whereas both are nucleated in birds, reptiles, and fish. Mammalian platelets appear as small, roundish, or oblong structures with a cluster of reddish-purple (azurophilic) granules in a pale blue matrix enclosed by a delicate membrane. Their morphology is generally similar in different species. A slight variation in size is apparent, with an occasional platelet being about twice as large as an average platelet, but rarely as large as the red blood cell. Equine platelets generally stain lightly and some may appear elongated or filamentous. Platelet activation occurs on the slightest injury to their surface membrane and some platelet aggregation is therefore common in blood films. Increased platelet clumping results in their irregular distribution and yields a false impression of thrombocytopenia.

Normal mammalian erythrocytes are generally biconcave disks with a light center and a small rim of hemoglobin. A slight variation in size (anisocytosis) is common among erythrocytes of various species. A variation in shape may be artifactual (such as crenation), a natural occurrence (sickle cells in the deer and fusiform and spindle-shaped red cells in Angora goats), or a pathologic abnormality (schistocytes). Porcine erythrocytes have a marked tendency to crenate. Elliptic erythrocytes are characteristic of the family Camelidae (see Chap. 3).

Rouleau formation (rolls of red blood cells, similar to a pile of coins) is prominent in the horse, and some rouleau is apparent in dog and cat blood. Increased rouleau formation in the dog and cat suggests an increase in total plasma protein concentration, globulins, or fibrinogen. Bovine erythrocytes normally do not form rouleaux. Red cell agglutination is certainly an abnormality and must be distinguished from rouleaux. Erythrocytes coated with antierythrocyte IgM tend to aggregate and form macroscopic and/or microscopic clumps. Erythrocytes from horses given heparin therapy may agglutinate in vitro and erroneously decrease the RBC count and increase the MCV (Mahaffey and Moore, 1986). The agglutinating factor appears to be proteinic because red cell suspensions exposed to trypsin reversed the agglutination (Moore et al., 1987).

Young polychromatic erythrocytes (reticulocytes) are normally found in small numbers in the dog and cat, but not in the horse and cow. Howell-Jolly bodies are occasionally seen in the erythrocytes of the cat and horse. Nucleated erythrocytes are usually absent, but an occasional one may be encountered in the dog and cat. They are found in the peripheral blood under various circumstances (Chap. 2). Splenectomy or reduced splenic function is commonly associated with increased numbers of erythrocytes containing Howell-Jolly bodies and nucleated red cells. Heinz bodies can occur naturally in the cat. Red blood cell inclusions such as basophilic stippling (aggregation of ribosomal material) and Pappenheimer bodies (iron particles) are abnormal findings.

Leukocyte morphology, except for some minor differences, is generally similar among various species. Neutrophils, eosinophils, and basophils are collectively referred to as granulocytes, and neutrophils are often called polymorphonuclear leukocytes or segmenters. Similarly, lymphocytes and monocytes are referred to as agranulocytes and also as mononuclear leukocytes. Species differences occur not only with regard to the WBC count, but also in the proportion of different leukocytes (Tables 1–4, 1–5, and 1–6). For example, neutrophils predominate in the human, dog, and cat, but in the horse they slightly exceed lymphocytes, and in ruminants and laboratory animals, such as rats and mice, neutrophils are outnumbered by lymphocytes. Nuclear segmentation in neutrophils of common domestic animals is not as prominent as in human neutrophils. The cytoplasm presents fine pinkish or pale granules. In some animals (e.g., rabbit and guinea pig), the granules are conspicuous and reddish; the cells are then designated as heterophils. The eosinophil and basophil usually have a less segmented nucleus than the neutrophil. Their cytoplasm contains large

Table 1–4. Some Differential Characteristics in Blood Morphology of Domestic Animals

Animal	*Erythrocytes*					*Leukocytes*	
	Rouleaux	*Central Pallor*	*Mean Diameter (μm)*	*Reticulocytes in Peripheral Blood in Health (%)*	*Special Features*	*Approximate Neutrophil: Lymphocyte Ratio*	*Special Features*
Dog	+	+ +	7.0	0–1.5	Essentially uniform in size	70:20	Basophils rare; eosinophil granules do not fill cell; granules variable in size and stain lightly; monocytes have blue ground glass cytoplasm compared to neutrophils.
Cat	+ +	+	5.8	0.2–1.6	Crenation with few blunt processes; slight anisocytosis; eccentric Howell-Jolly body in 1% of cells; occasional to frequent Heinz bodies.	59:32	Basophils rare; basophil granules are round and stain dull gray; eosinophil granules rod-like and stain dull grayish-orange; most lymphocytes of small size; few band neutrophils are normally present
Cow	–	+	5.8	0	Anisocytosis common; giant forms may occur	28:58	Eosinophil granules small, round, intensely stained, and fill cell; azurophil granules of large size may occur in some lymphocytes; vacuoles common in monocytes
Sheep	±	+	4.5	0	Regular in size and shape, with small central pale spot	30:62	Neutrophil nucleus usually multilobed; eosinophil granules well-stained, ovoid and fill cell; frequent large azurophil granules in lymphocytes; monocyte nucleus amoeboid
Horse	+ + +	±	5.5	0	Marked rouleaux, a consistent finding; cells uniform in size; occasional Howell-Jolly body; immature RBC almost never found in peripheral blood	Cold-blooded, 54:35; hot-blooded, 53:39	Eosinophil characteristic, granules large and fill cell; most lymphocytes are small; monocytes usually have kidney bean nucleus
Pig	+ +	±	6.0	0–1.0	Crenation with sharp points characteristic feature; slight anisocytosis; occasional polychromatophilia	37:53	Eosinophil granules ovoid, pale pink-orange, fill cell; band neutrophils occur in health (average, 1%); lymphocytes vary from small to large

and distinctive granules—reddish-orange in the eosinophil and purplish-red in the basophil. Some animals have a characteristic eosinophil (e.g., the horse has large, round granules and the cat has rod-shaped granules). Basophils are rare in normal blood and exhibit some species variation. Canine basophils have few granules and granules of feline basophils lack metachromasia and stain pale gray. An immature feline basophil may exhibit both darkly stained and lightly stained granules. The lymphocyte is the most prominent leukocyte in the cow, sheep, goat, mouse, and rat. The size, shape, and staining features of lymphocytes vary from blood to blood within a species. The most common form has a roundish nucleus and a small amount of light to deep blue cytoplasm. An occasional lymphocyte, especially in the cow, may contain some small to large azurophilic granules in the cytoplasm. Large lymphocytes are seen more often in the cow than in the dog and cat and some of them may be difficult to distinguish from monocytes. The monocyte is generally the largest of the leukocytes in blood. Its nucleus tends to be ameboid; therefore, it assumes a varied morphology. The cytoplasm stains grayish-blue and may present some vacuoles and/or

Table 1–5. Normal Ranges and Means (in parenthesis) for Blood Values in Domestic Animals*

Animal	RBC ($\times 10^6/\mu l$)	Hb (g/dl)	PCV† (%)	MCV (fl)	MCHC (%)	MCH (%)	WBC ($\times 10^3/\mu l$)	Differential Leukocyte Count (%)					
								Neutrophils					
								Band	Mature	Lymphocytes	Monocytes	Eosinophils	Basophils
Dog	5.5–8.5 (6.8)	12–18 (15.0)	37–55 (45.0)	60–77 (70.0)	32–36 (34.0)	19.5–24.5 (22.8)	6.0–17.0 (11.5)	0–3 (0.8)	60–77 (70.0)	12–30 (20.0)	3–10 (5.0)	2–10 (4.0)	Rare
Cat	5.0–10.0 (7.5)	8–15 (12.0)	24–45 (37.0)	39–55 (45.0)	30–36 (33.0)	12.5–17.5 (15.5)	5.5–19.5 (12.5)	0–3 (0.5)	35–75 (59.0)	20–55 (32.0)	1–4 (3.0)	2–12 (5.0)	Rare
Cow	5.0–10.0 (7.0)	8–15 (11.0)	24–46 (35.0)	40–60 (52.0)	30–36 (33.0)	11.0–17.0 (14.0)	4.0–12.0 (8.0)	0–2 (0.5)	15–45 (28.0)	45–75 (58.0)	2–7 (4.0)	0–20 (9.0)	0–2 (0.5)
Sheep	9.0–15.0 (12.0)	9–15 (11.5)	27–45 (35.0)	28–40 (34.0)	31–34 (32.5)	8.0–12.0 (10.0)	4.0–12.0 (8.0)	Rare	10–50 (30.0)	40–75 (62.0)	0–6 (2.5)	0–10 (5.0)	0–3 (0.5)
Goat	8.0–18.0 (13.0)	8–12 (10.0)	22–38 (28.0)	16–25 (19.5)	30–36 (33.0)	5.2–8.0 (6.5)	4.0–13.0 (9.0)	Rare	30–48 (36.0)	50–70 (56.0)	0–4 (2.5)	1–8 (5.0)	0–1 (0.5)
Horse (hot-blooded)	6.8–12.9 (9.0)	11–19 (14.4)	32–53 (41.0)	37–59 (45.5)	31–37 (35.0)	12.3–19.7 (9.0)	5.5–14.3 (9.0)	0–2 (0.5)	22–72 (53.0)	17–68 (39.0)	0–7 (4.3)	0–10 (3.4)	0–4 (0.5)
Pig	5.0–8.0 (6.5)	10–16 (13.0)	32–50 (42.0)	50–56 (63.0)	30–34 (32.0)	17.0–21.0 (19.0)	11.0–22.0 (16.0)	0–4 (1.0)	28–47 (37.0)	39–62 (53.0)	2–10 (5.0)	1–11 (3.5)	0–2 (0.5)

* For influence of age on the total and differential leukocyte counts in the cow, see Table 2–15; for the horse, see Table 2–12.

† PCV obtained at 14,000 G for 2 minutes for dog, cat, cow, sheep, and horse bloods and for 12 minutes for goat blood. Pig blood PCV based on Wintrobe method at 2,260 G for 30 minutes.

fine azurophilic granules. The presence of broken or degenerated cells in stained films suggests mechanical damage during smear making or increased cell fragility. The latter is common in old blood or in blood containing abnormal cells, as in leukemia. Some free nuclei may swell from hydration and present separated chromatin, giving the appearance of "basket cells."

See Chapters 2 and 3 for further comments on the cellular morphology of various animal species.

Physiologic Considerations in the Interpretation of Blood Values

Some blood values are significantly influenced by age and, to a lesser extent, by sex and breed. Emotional disturbance, excitement, and strenuous exercise, which contract the spleen and force stored cells into the circulation, influence certain blood parameters, such as erythrocyte and platelet numbers. Neutrophils in-

crease in numbers because of the mobilization of cells from the marginal pool in the microvasculature. Lymphocyte numbers, particularly in young animals, are similarly elevated by emotional disturbances and exercise because of increased input from the thoracic duct. Dehydration leads to loss of water from the plasma, resulting in hemoconcentration and a subsequent increase in erythrocyte parameters and in total plasma protein and blood urea nitrogen concentrations. Increases in total plasma protein concentrations, however, appear to be a more consistent indicator of hydration status than increases in PCV (Genetzky et al., 1987; Hardy and Osborne, 1979).

General Considerations Regarding Normal Values in Blood

The student can find it helpful to think of the normal blood standards as reflecting certain charac-

Table 1–6. Ranges and Means (in parenthesis) for the Normal Differential Absolute Leukocyte Number per μl of Blood*

Animal	Total Leukocyte Count	Band Neutrophils	Mature Neutrophils	Lymphocytes	Monocytes	Eosinophils	Basophils
Dog	6,000–17,000 (11,500)	0–300 (70)	3,000–11,500 (7,000)	1,000–4,800 (2,800)	150–1,350 (750)	100–1,250 (550)	Rare
Cat	5,500–19,500 (12,500)	0–300 (100)	2,500–12,500 (7,500)	1,500–7,000 (4,000)	0–850 (350)	0–1,500 (650)	Rare
Cow	4,000–12,000 (8,000)	0–120 (20)	600–4,000 (2,000)	2,500–7,500 (4,500)	25–840 (400)	0–2,400 (700)	0–200 (50)
Sheep	4,000–12,000 (8,000)	Rare	700–6,000 (2,400)	2,000–9,000 (5,000)	0–750 (200)	0–1,000 (400)	0–300 (50)
Goat	4,000–13,000 (9,000)	Rare	1,200–7,200 (3,250)	2,000–9,000 (5,000)	0–550 (250)	50–650 (450)	0–120 (50)
Horse (hot-blooded)	5,500–14,300 (9,050)	0–100 (26)	2,260–8,580 (4,745)	1,500–7,700 (3,500)	0–1,000 (388)	0–1,000 (305)	0–290 (45)
Pig	11,000–22,000 (16,000)	0–800 (150)	3,200–10,000 (5,500)	4,500–13,000 (8,000)	250–2,000 (800)	50–2,000 (500)	0–400 (80)

* Ranges for the dog, cat, cow, and horse represent two standard deviations from the mean, with slight modification with respect to minimum numbers of lymphocytes for the dog and cat. Ranges for the sheep, goat, and pig represent estimates from raw data.

teristics of the animal in question (Tables 1–4, 1–5, and 1–6). Hemoglobin is a respiratory pigment and its concentration in the blood, in health, is proportional to the propensity of the animal for sustained muscular activity or ability to meet demands for sudden bursts of speed. The dog, horse, and human represent more active types and their hemoglobin needs and values are greater than those of the more lethargic animals, such as the cow, sheep, goat, and cat.

The size and number of erythrocytes vary among animal species. The smaller the red cell, the greater the number per unit of blood. The distribution of the hemoglobin in a greater number of smaller units results in an increase in the surface area of the erythrocytic mass, thereby enhancing the exchange of gases. Because of this feature, certain breeds of horses are better suited for racing and other active sports. The Arabian horse and all breeds that have stemmed from it, the "hot-blooded" horses, are unique in having erythrocytes that are smaller and are present in greater number than in the "cold-blooded" breeds.

The goat has the smallest red cell among the domestic animals and also the greatest number, with the sheep being a close second. The ancestors of the sheep and goat lived in the rarefied atmosphere of mountaintops. In this environment efficient respiration was required, and this may partly explain why domestic sheep and goats have an arrangement for more efficient respiration than that needed for life under domestication.

The total leukocyte number and differential distribution in peripheral blood are influenced by the stress hormone secreted by the adrenal cortex. The dog and cat respond well to stress, as is reflected in significant changes in their leukocyte picture in disease. The cow, sheep, and goat respond less dramatically to the stress of disease insofar as their total and differential leukocyte counts are concerned. These latter animals, in health, tend to have lower total leukocyte counts and more lymphocytes than neutrophils.

The sedimentation of erythrocytes in plasma depends largely on the tendency of the erythrocytes to form rouleaux. Rouleaux are especially prominent in drawn equine blood, and rapid sedimentation is a normal characteristic feature. The red cells of the dog, cat, and pig are intermediate in tendency toward rouleau formation, so the influence of disease on the sedimentation rate can be best studied in these animals. Red cells of the cow, sheep, and goat show little or no rouleaux, and erythrocyte sedimentation is therefore minimal in these animals.

Lipemia or lactescence of blood plasma occurs principally in dog blood as a physiologic effect following a meal high in lipids (Plate II–4). This is called postprandial lipemia because it generally occurs between 2 and 12 hours after a meal. When blood is taken from dogs at random, cloudy plasmas are common. Lipemia interferes with the accuracy of some laboratory test results (e.g., icterus index and hemoglobin and plasma protein concentrations). Lipemia can generally be avoided by taking blood 12 hours after the last meal.

EXAMINATION OF THE BONE MARROW

A bone marrow examination provides information about the hematopoietic status of the individual. It is a necessary adjunct to blood examination, but must not be performed indiscriminately. Various indications of marrow examination include the following: nonresponsive anemias, megaloblastic or microcytic anemias, persistent neutropenia, thrombocytopenia, pancytopenia, drug toxicities, irradiation, lymphoproliferative disorders, including multiple myeloma, myeloproliferative disorders, and infiltrative diseases. Marrow examination is unnecessary in regenerative anemias unless the response is inadequate. At present, marrow examination is the principal means of evaluating a response to anemia in the horse. Sometimes, marrow examination may be rewarding in parasitic diseases such as leishmaniasis, because parasitized macrophages can be found in marrow aspirates but not in the peripheral blood. A blood examination provides clues as to the necessity for a bone marrow examination. It is imperative that a blood sample always be collected along with the bone marrow specimen for proper comparative evaluation. Iron staining of marrow smears provides information about iron stores and helps differentiate iron deficiency anemias from anemias of chronic inflammatory disease. Marrow smears can also be processed to demonstrate direct immunofluorescence of antibody-coated megakaryocytes in patients suspected of having immune-mediated thrombocytopenia. Similarly, nucleated erythrocytes and neutrophils may exhibit cytoplasmic immunofluorescence in patients with immune-mediated hemolytic anemia and immune-mediated neutropenia, respectively.

Characteristics and Classification of Cells in Marrow Aspirates

The following is a brief description of various morphologically recognizable bone marrow cells (Jain, 1986).

MATURATION OF THE ERYTHROCYTE

Rubriblast (proerythroblast, pronormoblast)	Round cell presenting a narrow rim of dark blue cytoplasm. The nucleus occupies most of the cell, is usually centrally located but may be eccentric. The chromatin is finely stippled and of reddish tinge. Nucleoli or nucleolar rings are present.	Plates IV–1, IV–3 (dog); Plate IV–5 (cat); Plates V–1, VI–4, VI–6 (horse)
Prorubricyte (basophilic or early erythroblast or normoblast)	Similar in appearance to the rubriblast, except that the nuclear chromatin may have minimal condensation and nucleoli or rings are absent.	Plate IV–2 (dog); Plate VI–5 (horse)
Basophilic rubricyte (basophilic erythroblast or normoblast)	The cell is smaller than the prorubricyte. It retains the narrow rim of deep blue cytoplasm. The nuclear chromatin is condensed and separated by light streaks, giving the so-called cartwheel appearance.	Plates V–1, VI–5 (horse); Plate IV–3 (dog); Plate V–2 (cat)
Polychromatophilic rubricyte (early polychromatic erythroblast or normoblast)	Synthesis of hemoglobin is well under way, and this produces a change in color of the cytoplasm to light blue or gray. Condensation of nuclear chromatin has continued, so that the appearance is one of dark blobs separated by light streaks.	Plates IV–1, IV–2, IV–3 (dog); Plates IV–5, V–2 (cat); Plates VI–2, VI–5, VI–6 (horse)
Normochromic (orthochromatic) rubricyte	This stage is most commonly encountered in the cat and horse. The nucleus remains viable, and the cytoplasm stains similarly to the mature erythrocyte.	Plate VI–6 (horse)
Metarubricyte (late polychromatic erythroblast or normoblast)	This stage is recognized by the presence of a non-viable nucleus. The nucleus is solidly black or pyknotic. It may be fragmented, partially extruded, or partially autolyzed. The cytoplasm may be polychromatic or normochromic, depending on the extent of hemoglobin synthesis.	Plates V–1, VI–6 (horse); Plates IV–5, V–2 (cat); Plates IV–2, XVI–2 (dog)
Reticulocyte	Non-nucleated erythrocyte that, when stained with new methylene blue, presents one or more granules or a diffuse network of fibrils. With Romanowsky stains, the reticulocyte is commonly polychromatophilic and infrequently may contain an eccentrically placed nuclear remnant called a Howell-Jolly body.	Plates IV–3, XVI–3 (dog); Plate IV–6 (cat)
Erythrocyte	Non-nucleated, definitive cell of the series.	

MATURATION OF THE GRANULOCYTES

Myeloblast	Large cell, round to irregular in shape, with finely stippled chromatin containing one or more nucleoli or nucleolar rings. The cytoplasm is blue (basophilic) but generally lighter in color than that of the rubriblast. The cytoplasm of a typical (Type I) myeloblast contains no granules, but <15 reddish granules may be present in a late (Type II) myeloblast.	Plate V–3 (dog); Plates V–5, VI–1 (horse)
Promyelocyte (progranulocyte)	Similar in size to the myeloblast. The nuclear chromatin is finely stippled. Nucleolus or nucleolar ring is absent. The cytoplasm is basophilic and commonly presents many reddish azurophilic granules. No specific granules are present.	Plates V–4, XII–3 (dog); Plate VI–2 (horse)
Myelocyte, neutrophilic	Smaller than the progranulocyte, with beginning condensation of the nuclear chromatin. The cytoplasm is light blue and contains few to numerous neutrophilic granules. These granules, when properly stained, are dust-like and faintly pink.	Plate V–6 (horse); Plate IV–4 (cat)
Myelocyte, eosinophilic	This cell is generally larger than the neutrophilic myelocyte. The cytoplasm is more basophilic and the granules are distinctly reddish orange.	Plate V–5 (horse)
Myelocyte, basophilic	Not a common cell in bone marrow preparations. In the cat, the granules are of two types: numerous small, round, and pinkish and fewer large, round, and reddish purple. In other animals, granules are metachromatic or reddish purple.	Plates V–2, XII–4 (cat); Plate VI–3 (horse)
Metamyelocyte, neutrophilic, eosinophilic, and basophilic	The nucleus is indented to assume a kidney bean shape. This cell is no longer capable of division. The cytoplasm may retain a slight basophilia in the neutrophil, but the other two forms retain a bluish cytoplasm as characteristic of the mature cell of the series. The specific granules identify the cell as neutrophilic, eosinophilic, or basophilic.	Plate V–3 (dog); Plates V–5, V–6, VI–3, VI–4 (horse)

MATURATION OF THE GRANULOCYTES—CONTINUED

Band neutrophil	The nucleus has parallel sides but twists to conform to the space within the cytoplasm. Horseshoe or S forms are common. The nuclear membrane is smooth. Irregularity of the nuclear membrane or beginning indentation indicates that maturity has been attained, requiring classification as a segmenter and not a band form.	Plates V–6, VI–4, VII–8 (horse); Plate IV–4 (cat)
Segmenter or neutrophil (polymorphonuclear leukocyte)	The nucleus may be monolobed, but the nuclear membrane is irregular (moth-eaten) or several lobes are separated by filaments. This cell is called a heterophil in some species.	Plate VII–1 (cow); Plate VII–8 (horse); Plate VII–9 (dog); Plate IX–4 (cat)
Eosinophil	Cytoplasm contains eosinophilic granules that vary in intensity of reddish color among species. Granules vary in size, shape, and number with the species of animal. The cytoplasm is light blue.	Plate VII–4 (cow); Plate VII–7 (horse); Plate XII–1 (dog); Plates VII–6, IX–1 (cat)
Basophil	Cytoplasm is basophilic with few to many metachromatic granules, depending on the species. Granules are round and pale gray or pinkish in the cat, although some basophils may retain a few small, darker staining granules.	Plate VII–5 (cow); Plates VII–6, XII–5 (cat); Plate VII–7 (horse); Plate XII–1 (dog)

MATURATION OF THE MEGAKARYOCYTE

Megakaryoblast	The first recognizable cell of this series is larger than other blast cells of bone marrow. It has one to four distinct reddish nuclei. The cytoplasm is small in amount and takes a deep blue stain. Tiny cytoplasmic blebs are often found on the cell surface.	Plates III–1, III–3 (dog)
Promegakaryocyte	Maturation leads to multiplication of nuclei by mitotic division without division of the cytoplasm (endomitosis). The number of nuclei may be eight or more. In the larger cells, the nuclei are commonly fused into a single irregular mass. The cytoplasm stains deep to moderate blue and is limited to a relatively narrow rim around the nuclear mass.	Plates III–2, III–4 (dog)
Megakaryocyte	The cytoplasm is pale blue and presents pinkish azurophilic granules. The cytoplasm is increased considerably over that of the promegakaryocyte. The formation of granules begins in the perinuclear zone and gradually extends to the periphery of the cell. Cell size is variable and depends on the number of nuclear divisions that had taken place before DNA synthesis was terminated by the beginning maturation of the cytoplasm. In films of aspirated bone marrow, some megakaryocytes may present pseudopod-like extensions and a nuclear mass without cytoplasm, or cytoplasm without a nucleus may be encountered.	Plates III–4, III–5 (dog)
Platelets (thrombocytes)	Individual platelets are cytoplasmic fragments of megakaryocytes. They vary in shape and size and contain reddish granules in a light blue field. In blood, they often form small clumps.	Plates VIII–2, VIII–7 (dog); Plate IX–1 (cat)

OTHER CELLS

Osteoclast	Large cells, irregular in shape and presenting multiple oval nuclei distinctly separated in a pinkish granular cytoplasm. These cells are not to be confused with megakaryocytes.	Plate III–6 (dog)
Mitotic figures	These are not numerous in normal marrow. Cells in mitosis in the erythrocytic series are usually readily identifiable as belonging to that series. Otherwise, they are recorded as "other cells."	
Hematogones	Round, pyknotic free nuclei extruded from metarubricytes.	Plate IV–2 (dog)
Lymphocytes	Small lymphocytes may be encountered in aspirated bone marrow. In the cat, they may contribute 10 to 15% of the total nucleated cells.	Plate XV–8 (cat)
Monocytes	Cells morphologically typical of monocytes may occur in small numbers. Monocytes originate in the bone marrow from monoblasts.	Plates VIII–1 to VIII–9 (dog)

Macrophages	Phagocytic cells are present in bone marrow. They are best recognized as such when they contain phagocytosed iron particles, pyknotic nuclear material, or erythrocytes, and rarely an entire leukocyte.	Plate XI–1 (horse); Plates XV–6, XV–7 (cat)
Plasma cells	Cells of irregulr shape but usually round with a large amount of light blue cytoplasm and round, eccentrically placed nucleus. The nucleus is similar in appearance to the rubricyte nucleus but with greater contrast between chromatin and parachromatin. A pale area of cytoplasm may be present near one side of the nucleus. An infrequently encountered plasma cell is filled with round structures called Russell bodies.	Plates XI–4, XI–5, X–12 (dog)
RE nuclei	Bone marrow aspirations contain pinkish-staining roundish structures presenting one or more blue nucleoli. These are classified as free nuclei of reticuloendothelial cells.	Plate XI–2 (dog)
Unclassified cells	Cells may be present in normal bone marrow that do not fit the description of any of the many stages of hematopoietic cells undergoing maturation.	
Degenerated cells	Cells presenting fragmented, pyknotic nuclei or irregularly roundish, pinkish structures without nucleoli or a net-like pinkish structure, commonly referred to as a basket cell, are degenerating cells. They are included in a bone marrow differential cell count.	Plate V–2 (cat); Plate XI–2 (dog)

General Comments About Bone Marrow Cytology

The following general principles apply to the cytology of bone marrow.

1. Megakaryocytes increase in size by endomitosis. That is, the nucleus undergoes division, but the cell itself does not divide (Plates III–1, III–2). The promegakaryocyte is capable of nuclear division only if the cytoplasm remains basophilic and devoid of azurophilic granules. Once formation of granules has been initiated, nuclear division ceases. Thus, mature megakaryocytes may vary considerably in size and are recognized by the presence of azurophilic granules. In bone marrow films on coverslips, the megakaryocytes are concentrated along the base or long straight border of the film.

2. Cells of the erythrocytic and granulocytic series undergo mitosis and decrease in size with each successive stage of maturation. Cells at the same stage of maturation, however, also vary in size. Classification is based not on size but on cytoplasmic and nuclear characteristics.

3. The earliest blast cells contain nucleoli that stain light blue because of their RNA content. After the first mitotic division the nucleolus loses its blue color but may persist as a ring-like structure (Plate V–3).

4. The cytoplasm is basophilic in the blast cells, prorubricytes, basophilic rubricytes, and promyelocytes. It stains progressively less blue as maturation proceeds. The cytoplasm in immature cells of the erythroid series is highly basophilic compared to that of the granulocytic series.

5. Myeloblasts usually do not contain cytoplasmic granules (type I blasts) and occasionally reveal some (less than 15) fine granules (type II blasts). Distinct azurophilic granules occur commonly in promyelocytes and are not apparent in myelocytes that display the specific granules. When a nucleolar ring and many azurophilic granules are both present in the cell, the latter characteristic takes precedence in classifying the cell as a promyelocyte (Plate V–4).

6. Nuclear chromatin is diffuse and finely stippled in blast cells. Beginning condensation of chromatin occurs in promyelocytes and prorubricytes and becomes more pronounced with each successive stage of the maturation series. The condensing, darker staining basichromatin is separated by lighter staining parachromatin. The nuclear chromatin stains darker in the erythrocytic series than in the granulocytic series because the former has a higher DNA content. The nuclear chromatin pattern of the polychromatic rubricyte somewhat resembles a cartwheel (Plate IV–1). In the granulocytic series, the clumped basichromatin finally becomes concentrated along the nuclear membrane, causing it to become "bumpy" in the mature neutrophil (Plate VII–8).

7. The nucleus and cytoplasm usually mature together. Asynchronous maturation is abnormal. Diseases that depress granulopoiesis may lead to skipped mitotic divisions, resulting in

giant forms with bizarre nuclear patterns. Such forms are frequently seen in diseased cats (Plates IX–3 and IX–4, XV–8). The occurrence in cells of the granulocytic series of double nuclei, bluish and foamy cytoplasm (Plates VIII–11, VIII–12, and IX–3), isolated deep blue granular objects (Döhle bodies; Plates IX–2 and XII–6), and scattered or uniformly distributed azurophilic granules ("toxic" granulation; Plates XI–12 and XV–12) are all indicative of aberrant or abnormal granulopoiesis in disease. Enzymatic abnormalities can also be detected in the granulocytic series because of the asynchrony of cellular maturation during the leukemic process.

8. The cells of the granulocytic series are more susceptible to rupture during preparation of the film than are the cells of the erythrocytic series. Thus, degenerated cells are usually granulocytic in origin. Nuclei containing several prominent blue nucleoli originate from the rupture of marrow reticuloendothelial cells.

9. Mature lymphocytes are present in small numbers in the aspirated marrow of common domestic animals. They are usually more numerous (10 to 15%) in bone marrow preparations of the cat than in other species. The dilution of marrow with blood brings increased numbers of lymphocytes into the sample, particularly from those animals in which lymphocytes normally outnumber neutrophils in the blood (e.g., the cow). The marrow of small laboratory animals such as the mouse, guinea pig, and rat often contains a large number of lymphocytes.

10. Plasma cells are infrequent in normal bone marrow. They appear in increased numbers in the bone marrow in diseases involving continuous antigenic exposure (Plate XI–4) and in plasma cell myeloma. The plasma cell can be distinguished from the polychromatic rubricyte on the basis of greater size, a lower nucleus:cytoplasm ratio, and the hue of its basophilic cytoplasm. Plasma cells with one or more nucleoli may be encountered in marrows with intense plasma cell production.

11. The band neutrophil and the reticulocyte stages immediately precede the mature cell of the respective cell series. Both are classified as immature cells and their occurrence in increased numbers in blood indicates intensification of their production in the bone marrow.

12. Deficiencies of vitamin B_{12} and folic acid lead to reduced replication of nucleoprotein and affect cells of both the granulocytic and erythrocytic series. This is evident by the occurrence of some large metamyelocytes in the bone marrow and of hypersegmented neutrophils in the blood and bone marrow (Plate XI–7). Maturation arrest occurs in the prorubricytic and basophilic rubricytic stages. Such cells tend to have larger than normal nuclei, with a stippled chromatin pattern (Plate XXII–1). Depressed DNA synthesis causes nuclear maturation to be out of step with hemoglobinization of the cytoplasm. When the hemoglobin that is synthesized reaches a certain concentration, the nucleus stops dividing, usually short of normal mitotic divisions, and the cell begins to mature. The extrusion of the nucleus from such cells results in the formation of macrocytic erythrocytes characteristic of the macrocytic anemia of vitamin B_{12} and folate deficiency. The abnormal precursor cells are called megaloblasts or megaloblastoid cells (Plate XXII–1). Somewhat similar cells occur in erythremic myelosis and erythroleukemia of the cat (Plates XV–4, XXII–2, and XXIII–3). In iron deficiency, decreased hemoglobin synthesis leads to the retention of a viable nucleus in erythroid precursors, with the capability of dividing beyond the normal number of cell divisions. Thus, erythroid cells undergo additional mitosis, producing the microcytic erythrocytes typical of iron deficiency anemia (Plates XVI–1 and XVI–2). See Chapter 12 for further details of the mechanisms of anemia in these conditions.

Myeloid:Erythroid Ratio

The myeloid:erythroid (M:E) ratio is obtained by dividing the number of nucleated cells of the erythrocytic series into the number of cells of the granulocytic (G) series; thus, it is also called the G:E ratio. Usually, 500 cells are differentiated. All cells, including degenerated cells, are included in the 500-cell differential, but cells other than those in the erythroid and granulocytic series are excluded from the calculation of the ratio. The M:E ratios in marrows from the rib, femur, tibia, and humerus do not vary significantly. Bone marrow is usually obtained from the iliac crest. Smears for cytologic evaluation are generally prepared to include some marrow spicules. The normal ranges and mean values of M:E ratios for the various domestic animals are given in Table 1–7. The cellular compo-

Table 1–7.   Normal Myeloid:Erythroid Ratios of Some Animal Species

Species	Range	Mean
Dog	0.75–2.53	1.25
Cat	1.21–2.16	1.63
Horse	0.50–1.50	0.93
Cow	0.31–1.85	0.71
Sheep	0.77–1.68	1.09
Goat	—	0.69
Pig	0.73–2.81	1.77

Table 1–8. Representative Differential Cell Counts in Marrow Aspirated from the Iliac Crest of the Dog in Normal and Disease States

	Percentage Distribution (500 Cells Differentiated)				
Cells	Normal	Iron Deficiency Anemia in Remission (Blood + Iron Therapy)	Chronic Ulcerative Colitis (Blood Loss)	End-Stage Kidney Disease	Lymphocyte Leukemia
Erythrocytic cells					
Rubriblasts	0.2	1.3	0.0	0.2	0.0
Prorubricytes	3.9	2.7	2.3	5.2	1.1
Rubricytes	27.0	19.0	29.6	3.0	0.7
Metarubricytes	15.3	43.0	18.2	1.0	0.0
Total erythrocytic cells	46.4	66.0	50.1	9.4	1.8
Granulocytic cells					
Myeloblasts	0.0	0.4	1.7	0.2	0.7
Progranulocytes	1.3	0.5	0.3	1.0	3.8
Neutrophilic myelocyte	9.0	1.1	3.3	0.2	9.8
Eosinophilic myelocyte	0.0	0.1	0.3	0.2	0.0
Neutrophilic metamyelocyte	7.5	2.4	6.0	7.0	25.5
Eosinophilic metamyelocyte	2.4	0.0	1.0	0.4	0.7
Neutrophilic bands	13.6	9.3	12.0	20.4	17.5
Eosinophilic bands	0.9	0.3	0.0	0.0	0.2
Neutrophils	18.4	8.8	23.0	34.4	11.8
Eosinophils	0.3	0.1	0.0	0.4	0.0
Basophils	0.0	0.0	0.0	0.2	0.0
Total granulocytic cells	53.4	23.0	47.6	64.4	70.0
M:E ratio	1.15:1.0	0.35:1.0	0.95:1.0	6.85:1.0	38.8:1.0
Other cells					
Prolymphocytes	0.0	0.0	0.0	0.0	21.6
Lymphocytes	0.2	4.1	1.3	11.6	6.6
Monocytes	0.0	0.2	1.0	10.6	0.0
Unclassified cells	0.0	0.7	0.0	1.4	0.0
Degenerated cells	0.0	6.0	0.0	2.6	0.0
Peripheral blood values					
Total leukocytes/µl	12,000	9,100	19,850	13,500	58,000
PCV (%)	45	29	15.5	22.5	21.3

sition of the bone marrow is presented for normal dogs (Table 1–8), cats (Table 1–9), horses (Table 1–10), cows (Table 1–11), and sheep (Table 1–12). Germ-free animals have lower M:E ratios. A higher proportion of eosinophils may be found in the marrow of some cattle and sheep, probably as a result of parasitic infestation or other, undefined factors.

Developing an M:E ratio based on the differentiation of maturation stages in each cell series is time-consuming and delays reports to clinicians. A satisfactory substitute is a narrative of impressions gained from the examination of the morphology and distribution of sequential developmental stages of various hematopoietic cell lines. Although smears of marrow aspirates are not thought to reflect true marrow cellularity, comments should also be made regarding impressions obtained about the general cellularity of smears, particularly after a search has been made for marrow spicules. The presence of megakaryocytes, plasma cells, mast cells, lymphocytes, mitotic cells, and cells foreign to the bone marrow should be noted specifically. A quick M:E ratio can be obtained by counting the different developmental stages of each series as a group, rather than in various subcategories

(Fig. 1–1). If necessary, erythroid as well as myeloid cells may be classified under mitotic and maturative compartments and granulocytic cells may also be classified under storage compartments to obtain information regarding the relative distribution of cells in these functional pools. Such groupings may be desirable in cases of megaloblastic anemia, microcytic hypochromic anemia, and myeloid leukemias.

Left Shift Index

A left shift index has been devised for both myeloid and erythroid cells as an alternative to the M:E ratio for use in toxicologic studies (Brown, 1991). The myeloid left shift index is determined by dividing the total percentage of myeloblasts through band forms by the total percentage of neutrophils, eosinophils, and basophils. The erythroid left shift index is calculated by dividing the total percentage of rubriblasts through basophilic rubricytes by the total percentage of polychromatic rubricytes through metarubricytes. A total of 200 cells is counted in Wright-stained marrow films. The proposed left shift indices were found to

BONE MARROW EVALUATION TALLY SHEET

Case No._____ Animal_____ Date_____

Cell Type	Total	Cell Type	Total
Rubriblast		Myeloblast	
Prorubricyte		Progranulocyte	
RUBRICYTES Basophilic rubricytes		MYELOCYTES Neutrophilic	
Polychromatic rubricytes		Eosinophilic	
Normochromic rubricytes		Basophilic	
Metarubricyte		METAMYELOCYTE Neutrophilic	
Mitotic		Eosinophilic	
TOTAL CELLS ERYTHROCYTIC =		Basophilic	
Hematogones*		BAND Neutrophilic	
Lymphocytes		Eosinophilic	
Plasma cells		Basophilic	
Monocytes		SEGMENTER Neutrophilic	
Mitotic cells		Eosinophilic	
Megakaryocytes		Basophilic	
Osteoclasts			
Macrophages			
Unclassified cells		TOTAL CELLS GRANULOCYTIC =	
Degenerated cells			
*free metarubricyte nucleus		M:E ratio =	

Fig. 1–1. Example of a bone marrow evaluation tally sheet. (From Jain, N. C.: Schalm's Veterinary Hematology. 4th Ed. Philadelphia, Lea & Febiger, 1986, p. 18.)

have clinical application because the myeloid left shift indices (values in parenthesis) were different for normal foals (0.33 to 1.33), stressed foals (1.00 to 2.14), and foals with infections (3.33 to 9.67).

Bone Marrow Evaluation

An M:E ratio of 1.0:1.0 indicates that nucleated erythrocytes and granulocytes are present in equal numbers. When the ratio is less than 1.0, the usual inference is that erythrocyte production exceeds granulopoiesis and, when the ratio is greater than 1.0, granulopoiesis exceeds erythropoiesis. However, the former could also occur if granulopoiesis were suppressed, and the latter could occur if erythropoiesis were diminished. Therefore, the M:E ratio should be interpreted in view of neutrophil numbers and reticulocyte count in the peripheral blood.

When the differential leukocyte count in blood shows a significant neutrophilia, especially if it is accompanied by a left shift (the presence of excessive numbers of immature neutrophils in blood), intensified granulopoiesis is indicated. An M:E ratio much higher than 1.0 would not then necessarily reflect a depression of erythropoiesis. In this instance, the reduction in nucleated erythrocytes in the bone marrow would be relative rather than absolute. In comparison, when the neutrophil count in blood is within the normal range, the M:E ratio is a valuable indicator of intensified erythropoiesis (decreased M:E ratio) or depressed erythropoiesis (increased M:E ratio). Reticulocytosis in the blood or bone marrow indicates increased erythropoiesis and, in such cases, granulopoiesis must similarly be evaluated relative to the degree of erythropoiesis. In some cases (e.g., chronic inflammatory disease), both the erythrocytic and granulocytic series may be affected simultaneously. Interpretation of the M:E ratio in such cases requires an awareness of the pathogenetic mechanisms involved in the hematopoietic changes associated with such disease processes.

Examples of bone marrow differential counts in selected diseases of dogs, horses, and cows are presented in Tables 1–8, 1–10, and 1–11, respectively. In the dog, in iron deficiency in remission, the intensification of erythrogenesis is indicated by an M:E ratio considerably less than 1.0. In end-stage kidney disease, a depression of erythrogenesis is indicated by a nonresponsive normocytic-normochromic anemia and by an increase in the M:E ratio. The M:E ratio is markedly elevated in hematopoietic neoplasias from depression of erythrogenesis, possibly as a result of the displacement of the erythropoietic cells from massive bone marrow infiltration by neoplastic cells (Plates XXIV–2, XXIV–3, and XXVI–4). Suppression of

Table 1–9. Cellular Composition* of the Bone Marrow of Normal Adult Cats

Parameter	Cat Number							Mean ± SD
	1	2	3	4	5	6	7	
WBC/µl of blood	13,400	12,100	7,500	9,700	6,400	5,700	16,800	10,200 ± 4,000
PCV (%)	32	34	36	42	35	32	41	36 ± 4
Cells								
Rubriblast	0.2	0.0	0.2	0.0	0.8	0.0	0.0	0.17 ± 0.29
Prorubricyte	0.6	1.2	1.0	0.0	1.2	1.6	1.4	1.00 ± 0.54
Basophilic rubricyte	6.2	4.0	5.4	1.6	4.0	2.6	4.4	4.02 ± 1.56
Polychromic rubricyte	17.6	17.0	23.2	8.6	17.8	20.2	18.6	17.57 ± 4.48
Metarubricyte	1.0	7.4	5.2	10.4	7.4	2.8	4.6	5.54 ± 3.15
Mitotic rubricyte	0.8	0.4	0.4	0.0	0.4	0.4	0.6	0.43 ± 0.24
Total erythrocytic cells	26.4	30.0	35.4	20.6	31.6	27.6	29.6	28.74 ± 4.64
Myeloblast	0.4	0.0	0.2	0.0	0.0	0.0	0.0	0.08 ± 0.16
Promyelocyte	3.0	3.0	1.6	0.0	1.2	1.8	1.6	1.74 ± 1.04
Myelocyte, neutrophilic	8.0	3.2	5.2	0.6	2.8	3.8	6.6	4.31 ± 2.49
Myelocyte, eosinophilic	1.4	0.6	0.6	0.0	0.6	0.6	0.4	0.60 ± 0.42
Myelocyte, basophilic	0.2	0.2	0.2	0.0	0.2	0.0	0.0	0.11 ± 0.11
Metamyelocyte, neutrophilic	13.2	10.4	11.0	4.4	7.0	12.4	12.0	10.06 ± 3.20
Metamyelocyte, eosinophilic	1.0	0.8	0.8	0.0	0.2	0.8	0.2	0.54 ± 0.39
Metamyelocyte, basophilic	0.0	0.2	0.0	0.0	0.0	0.0	0.0	0.03 ± 0.07
Band, neutrophilic	13.4	15.0	15.0	16.6	12.8	13.4	14.6	14.4 ± 1.30
Band, eosinophilic	0.2	0.2	1.0	0.4	1.0	0.6	0.0	0.49 ± 0.40
Band, basophilic	0.0	0.0	0.0	0.0	0.0	0.0	0.0	0.0
Neutrophil	9.4	11.0	6.8	22.0	13.6	15.0	12.2	12.86 ± 4.85
Eosinophil	0.6	0.8	0.4	0.4	0.8	0.8	0.4	0.60 ± 0.20
Basophil	0.0	0.0	0.0	0.0	0.0	0.0	0.0	0.0
Total granulocytic cells	50.8	45.4	42.8	44.4	40.2	49.2	48.0	45.86 ± 3.78
Myeloid:erythroid ratio	1.92:1	1.51:1	1.21:1	2.16:1	1.27:1	1.78:1	1.62:1	1.63 ± 0.35:1
Hematogones	0.0	0.8	0.8	0.8	0.6	2.4	0.4	0.83 ± 0.75
Lymphocytes	17.2	14.0	11.6	21.6	17.4	10.6	18.8	16.13 ± 2.92
Plasma cells	1.8	1.4	0.6	0.2	0.2	0.8	0.6	0.80 ± 0.60
Monocytes	0.6	1.2	1.6	0.2	0.4	1.0	0.4	0.77 ± 0.51
Mitotic cells	0.4	0.0	0.6	0.0	0.0	0.4	0.0	0.20 ± 0.26
Macrophage	0.0	0.0	0.0	0.2	0.2	0.0	0.0	0.06 ± 0.10
Unclassified cells	0.4	0.8	0.4	0.6	0.8	0.4	0.0	0.49 ± 0.28
Degenerated cells	2.0	6.4	6.2	11.2	8.6	7.6	2.2	6.31 ± 3.32
Total other cells	22.4	24.6	21.8	34.8	28.2	23.2	22.4	25.40 ± 4.75

* Distribution (%) based on 500 cells.

erythropoiesis by factors elaborated by neoplastic cells may also occur. The M:E ratio is increased in horses and cows with acute inflammatory conditions, primarily because of increased neutrophil production.

The effect of drug administration on bone marrow cytology has been determined in some studies. Adult cats receiving aspirin may develop increased M:E ratios and marrow hypoplasia. Cats given chloramphenicol may similarly show elevated M:E ratios and exhibit degenerative changes in their erythroid and myeloid cells.

The M:E ratio in the normal horse is usually below 1.0 and may decrease further during response to anemia (Table 1–10 and Plate VI–6). Marrow examination of anemic horses, however, has indicated that increased erythroid activity as a result of response to anemia is not always reflected in the M:E ratio. Thus, in the horse, a low M:E ratio by itself does not necessarily indicate effective erythrogenesis. The finding of polychromatic erythrocytes or reticulocytes in

ample numbers (>5%) in bone marrow films is a more certain sign of effective erythropoiesis than an M:E ratio lower than 1.0. In contrast, the M:E ratio is increased in cases of chronic inflammatory disease, leukemias and other malignancies, suppurative inflammation, and heavy infestation by intestinal parasites, usually because of the suppression of erythropoiesis and increased granulopoiesis in response to inflammatory stimuli.

Bone Marrow Biopsy

In most cases, marrow aspirates are sufficient for evaluating response to disease and effects of drug therapy. Marrow biopsy may be desired in some situations, however, particularly when information regarding marrow topography, gross cellularity, and relative distribution of various cells is needed (Jacobs and Valli, 1988). Needle biopsy is preferred in certain

Table 1–10. Bone Marrow Differential Cell Counts* in Normal and Patient Horses

Parameter	Range in Four Normal Horses	Lead Poisoning Horse A	Lead Poisoning Horse B	Phenothiazine Toxicosis	Chronic Bleeding	Hemolytic Anemia and Purpura	Progressive Anemia Pyrexia	Emaciated	Stomach Carcinoma
PCV(%)	29–36	24	21	28	16	23	20	27	24
WBC/μl in blood	8,250–12,500	9,900	13,300	14,100	8,800	10,000	7,300	11,000	9,300
Cell types									
Myeloblast	0.3–1.5	1.2	0.6	0.8	1.8	1.2	1.2	2.4	1.8
Progranulocyte	1.0–1.9	0.0	1.2	2.0	1.0	1.2	1.0	1.6	4.8
Neutrophilic myelocyte	1.9–3.2	1.4	2.0	0.8	3.0	1.6	3.4	2.6	3.0
Eosinophilic myelocyte	0.2–0.8	0.6	0.6	0.2	0.8	0.2	0.0	0.0	1.0
Basophilic myelocyte	0.0–0.1	0.0	0.0	0.0	0.0	0.0	0.0	0.0	0.2
Neutrophilic metamyelocyte	2.1–7.3	1.2	3.2	3.2	5.0	2.6	7.8	3.2	12.4
Eosinophilic metamyelocyte	0.2–1.8	0.4	0.4	0.4	0.0	0.0	0.6	0.0	0.0
Band neutrophil	6.8–14.7	6.8	6.6	4.0	12.8	8.8	8.0	11.2	19.4
Band eosinophil	0.6–1.2	0.2	0.0	0.0	0.2	0.4	0.0	0.0	0.2
Neutrophil	9.6–21.0	4.4	5.2	7.8	6.6	3.8	10.6	19.2	20.0
Eosinophil	1.8–3.0	0.2	0.0	0.6	0.4	0.2	0.0	2.0	0.4
Basophil	0.0–1.4	0.6	0.2	0.2	0.2	0.6	0.4	2.8	0.2
Total myeloid	28.1–48.4	17.0	20.0	20.0	31.8	20.6	33.0	45.2	63.0
Rubriblast	0.6–1.1	0.8	0.0	0.4	2.2	0.4	0.6	0.4	0.4
Prorubricyte	1.0–2.0	1.8	1.0	1.6	2.2	1.2	1.4	1.2	0.6
Rubricyte, basophilic	4.5–11.1	3.4	7.2	17.0	9.4	12.4	5.6	3.6	3.2
Rubricyte, polychromatic	14.7–26.0	36.0	33.8	33.4	28.8	34.0	25.4	14.6	10.4
Rubricyte, normochromic	0.7–4.3	0.0	0.0	0.4	1.0	0.0	0.0	0.0	0.0
Metarubricyte	10.7–15.4	30.8	29.0	13.4	11.4	25.0	15.8	8.2	6.4
Mitotic rubricyte	0.0–1.9	2.0	2.8	1.4	1.2	0.0	0.6	1.0	0.0
Total erythroid	33.2–56.2	74.8	73.8	67.6	56.2	73.0	49.4	29.0	21.0
Lymphocyte	1.8–6.7	2.6	2.2	6.8	2.6	1.4	8.8	19.8	6.2
Plasma cell	0.2–1.8	0.0	0.2	0.2	1.8	0.2	0.8	0.8	1.0
Monocyte	0.0–1.0	0.2	0.2	0.2	0.4	0.0	3.2	2.4	1.0
Mitotic cell	0.0–0.2	0.4	0.0	0.2	0.8	0.8	0.0	0.0	0.2
RE nucleus	0.2–1.6	0.0	0.0	0.0	0.6	0.6	1.4	0.2	2.4
Hematogone	0.2–1.4	1.4	0.2	2.2	2.6	0.0	0.8	0.2	0.6
Unclassified cell	0.2–1.7	0.0	0.0	0.2	0.0	0.4	0.0	0.4	0.0
Degenerated cell	2.3–9.0	3.4	3.4	2.6	3.0	2.0	1.8	2.0	4.2
Macrophage	0.0–0.0	0.2	0.0	0.0	0.0	0.0	0.8	0.0	0.0
Myeloid:erythroid ratio	0.52–1.45:1.0	0.23:1.0	0.27:1.0	0.30:1.0	0.57:1.0	0.28:1.0	0.67:1.0	1.56:1.0	3.00:1.0

* Distribution (%) based on 500 cells.

situations, such as when it is suspected that hypocellularity of marrow smears has resulted from hypoplasia rather than hemodilution. Other indications of marrow biopsy include repeated failure to obtain adequate marrow samples ("dry taps"), pancytopenias, lymphoproliferative disorders, including myelomas, tumor metastasis, granulomatous diseases involving the bone marrow, and myelofibrosis. Marrow biopsies can be taken from the iliac crest using a Jamshidi needle in a manner similar to that described for marrow aspiration (Jain, 1986; Relford, 1991). A marrow aspirate must also be collected for simultaneous cytologic examination. When this is not possible, touch preparations of marrow tissue should be prepared, although they are not as satisfactory as smears of marrow aspirate.

Paraffin-embedded bone marrow biopsy specimens are unreliable for the assessment of various hematopoietic elements, especially the immature stages. This major disadvantage stems from processing artifacts of tissue shrinkage. Other techniques of embedding bone marrow in various plastics, particularly methacrylate and glycol methacrylate, provide superior means of evaluating 1- to 2-mm thin sections for overall cellularity and cell types, with high resolution and minimum artifacts. In addition, cytochemical and immunocytochemical staining techniques can be used for such specimens.

Table 1–11. Bone Marrow Differential Cell Counts in Normal and Mastitic Cows*

Cell Classification	Normal Cows			Mastitic Cows†			
	No. 1	No. 2	No. 3	No. 4	No. 5	No. 6	No. 7
Erythroid series							
Rubriblast	0.2	0	0	0.2	0.2	0	0
Prorubricyte	1.2	0.4	0.8	0.6	0.4	0	1.0
Basophil rubricyte	4.8	5.2	8.4	3.2	3.6	1.4	6.0
Polychromic rubricyte	29.6	36.4	23.0	20.4	16.2	26.4	29.0
Metarubricyte	16.8	9.2	12.6	11.8	14.6	11.0	4.6
Mitotic rubricyte	1.0	0	0.4	1.0	0	0.4	1.0
Total	53.6	51.2	45.2	37.2	35.0	39.2	41.6
Myeloid series							
Myeloblast	0.2	0	0	0.8	0.2	0	0
Promyelocyte	1.4	1.4	0	5.6	1.8	2.2	1.6
Myelocyte, neutrophilic	3.2	3.4	2.8	5.2	2.4	5.2	3.6
Metamyelocyte, neutrophilic	2.8	6.2	3.2	12.2	4.2	5.8	2.0
Band, neutrophilic	6.6	4.6	8.4	10.4	10.0	9.2	7.8
Neutrophil	12.6	11.2	22.6	3.0	14.2	18.0	18.4
Metamyelocyte, eosinophilic	0.4	0.6	0.4	0.6	0.8	1.4	0.6
Band, eosinophilic	1.8	2.6	1.0	1.8	3.2	2.2	2.2
Eosinophil	0.6	0.6	1.6	0.8	0.6	1.2	0.2
Basophil (all)	0.4	1.0	0	0.6	0.6	0.4	0.6
Total	32.6	34.8	44.0	41.8	40.0	50.4	39.2
Other cells							
Hematogone	2.6	2.0	0.2	3.4	1.8	0.8	3.0
Lymphocyte	3.6	4.2	6.0	7.0	13.2	3.0	8.6
Plasma cell	1.2	1.0	0.2	1.2	0.8	1.0	0.6
Monocyte	2.2	1.2	0.4	2.4	3.2	1.6	3.8
Macrophage	0.8	0	0.2	0	0.8	0.2	0
Mitotic cell	0.2	0	0	0	0	0	0
Unclassified cell	0.8	0.2	0	1.6	0.2	0.4	0
Degenerated cell	2.4	5.4	3.8	5.4	5.0	3.4	3.2
Total	13.8	14.0	10.8	21.0	25.0	10.4	19.2
Myeloid:erythroid ratio	0.61:1.0	0.68:1.0	0.97:1.0	1.12:1.0	1.14:1.0	1.28:1.0	0.94:1.0

* Distribution (%) based on 500 cells.

† Cow 4 had naturally acquired *Streptococcus agalactiae* infection of unknown duration in right front (RF), right rear (RR), and left front (LF) quarters, with acute flare-up in RR. Cow 5 had experimentally induced *Staphylococcus aureus* infection of 40 days' duration in RF and LF and naturally acquired *Pseudomonas aeruginosa* infection of 5 months' duration in RR. Cow 6 had naturally acquired *S. aureus* infection of unknown duration (chronic mastitis) in RR, LF, and left rear (LR) quarters. Cow 7 had experimentally induced *S. aureus* infection of 186 and 300 days' duration (mild chronic mastitis), respectively, in LF and RR.

From Schalm, O. W., and Lasmanis, J.: Cytologic features of bone marrow in normal and mastitic cows. Am. J. Vet. Res., 37:359, 1976.

Table 1–12. Bone Marrow Differential Counts in the Sheep

Cell Type	Range (%)	Mean (%)	Cell Type	Range (%)	Mean (%)
Myeloblast	0.1–1.4	0.47	Rubriblast	0.5–1.4	0.96
Promyelocyte	0.0–0.6	0.24	Prorubricyte	1.5–4.9	3.30
Neutrophilic myelocyte	1.5–8.1	4.60	Rubricyte	27.2–37.3	31.86
Neutrophilic metamyelocyte	2.1–6.0	4.33	Metarubricyte	4.9–15.1	9.91
Band	10.6–22.8	16.38	Total erythroid		46.03
Neutrophil	1.4–6.9	4.58	Plasma cell	0.0–1.0	0.35
Eosinophilic myelocyte	3.3–6.2	4.85	Lymphocyte	0.6–3.1	1.73
Eosinophilic metamyelocyte	7.8–15.0	10.84	Monocyte	0.0–0.7	0.26
Eosinophil	0.8–5.1	2.80	Mitotic forms	0.2–1.6	0.84
Basophil	0.3–2.3	1.04	M:E ratio		
Total myeloid		50.13	Mean	1.09:1.0	
			Range	0.77–1.68:1.0	

REFERENCES

Bennett, J.S., Gossett, K.A., McCarthy, M.P., et al.: Effects of ketamine hydrochloride on serum biochemical and hematologic variables in rhesus monkeys (*Macaca mulata*). Vet. Clin. Pathol., 21:15, 1992.

Brown, B.A.: Hematology: Principles and Procedures. 5th Ed. Philadelphia, Lea & Febiger, 1988.

Brown, G.: The left shift index: A useful guide to the interpretation of marrow. Comp. Haematol. Int., 1:106, 1991.

Brown, S.A. and Barsanti, J.A.: Quantitative buffy coat analysis for hematologic measurements of canine, feline, and equine blood samples and for detection of microfilaremia in dogs. Am. J. Vet. Res., 49:321, 1988.

Davies, D.T. and Fisher, G.V.: The validation and application of the Technicon H1 for the complete automated evaluation of laboratory animal haematology. Comp. Haematol. Int., 1:91, 1991.

Duncan, J.R. and Prasse, K.W.: Veterinary laboratory medicine. 2nd Ed. Ames, Iowa, Iowa State University Press, 1986.

Genetzky, R.M., Loparco, F.V., and Ledet, A.E.: Clinical pathologic alterations in horses during a water deprivation test. Am. J. Vet. Res., 48:1007, 1987.

Gossett, K.A. and Carakostas, M.C.: Effect of EDTA on morphology of neutrophils of healthy dogs and dogs with inflammation. Vet. Clin. Pathol., 13:22, 1984.

Hardy, R.M. and Osborne, C.A.: Water deprivation test in the dog: Maximal normal values. J. Am. Vet. Med. Assoc., 174:479, 1979.

Jacobs, R.M. and Valli, V.E.O.: Bone marrow biopsies: principles and perspectives of interpretation. Sem. Vet. Med. Surg., 3: 176, 1988.

Jain, N.C.: Schalm's Veterinary Hematology. 4th Ed. Philadelphia, Lea & Febiger, 1986.

Levine, R.A., Hart, A.H., and Wardlaw, S.C.: Quantitative buffy coat analysis of blood collected from dogs, cats, and horses. J. Am. Vet. Med. Assoc., 189:670, 1986.

Mahaffey, E.A. and Moore, J.N.: Erythrocyte agglutination associated with heparin treatment in three horses. J. Am. Vet. Med. Assoc., 189:1478, 1986.

Meyer, D.T., Coles, E.H. and Rich, L.J.: Veterinary Laboratory Medicine. Interpretation and Diagnosis. Philadelphia, W. B. Saunders Co., 1992.

Moore, J.N., Mahaffey, E.A., and Zboran, M.: Heparin-induced agglutination of erythrocytes in horses. Am. J. Vet. Res., 48:68, 1987.

Relford, R.L.: The steps in performing a bone marrow aspiration and core biopsy. Vet. Med., 86:670, 1991.

Savage, R.A.: Pseudoleukocytosis due to EDTA-induced platelet clumping. Am. J. Clin. Pathol., 81:317, 1984.

Tvedten, H.W. Grabski, S., and Frame, L.: Estimating platelets and leukocytes on canine blood smears. Vet. Clin. Path., 17:4, 1988a.

Tvedten, H.W. and Wilkins, R.J.: Automated blood cell counting systems: A comparison of the Coulter S-plus IV, Ortho ELT-8/DS, Ortho ELT-8/WS, Technicon H-1, and Sysmex E-5,000. Vet. Clin. Pathol., 17:47, 1988b.

Weiser, M.G.: Modifications and evaluation of a multichannel blood cell counting system for blood analysis in veterinary hematology. J. Am. Vet. Med. Assoc., 190:411, 1987.

Weiser, M.G., Cockerell, G.L., Smith, J.A., et al.: Cytoplasmic fragmentation associated with lymphoid leukemia in ruminants: Interference with electronic determination of platelet concentration. Vet. Pathol., 26:177, 1989.

Willard, M.D., Tvedten, H., and Turnwald, G.H.: Small Animal Clinical Diagnosis by Laboratory Methods. Philadelphia, W. B. Saunders Co., 1989.

Williams, W.J., Beutler, E., Erslev, A.J., et al.: Hematology. 4th Ed. New York, McGraw-Hill, 1990.

Chapter 2

Comparative Hematology of Common Domestic Animals

Blood is essential for the survival of multicellular organisms. It is necessary for the transport of oxygen, water, electrolytes, nutrients, and hormones to each cell and for the transport of metabolic wastes to the organs of excretion. Erythrocytes, leukocytes, and platelets or thrombocytes constitute the formed elements of blood, and various coagulation factors and immunoglobulins are important constituents of the total plasma protein. The primary function of erythrocytes is carrying hemoglobin for the transport of oxygen, whereas the leukocytes are chiefly concerned with the body's defense against microbial infection. The platelets (thrombocytes) and coagulation proteins are necessary to maintain hemostasis—that is, to prevent the loss of blood from injured vessels. The immunoglobulins are essential components of the humoral immune response, which develops to protect the individual from infectious agents. Other proteins found in blood have various biologic roles, such as the maintenance of colloidal osmotic pressure and the transport of substances essential to maintain health.

This chapter is primarily concerned about the general properties of blood cells and some plasma com-ponents common to domestic animals. Comparative observations are briefly discussed. Additional information on normal hematologic values in various animal species may be found in other texts (Harvey, 1990; Jain, 1986; Hawkey and Dennett, 1989).

NORMAL BLOOD VALUES

Normal blood values are presented for mature dogs (Table 2–1), cats (Table 2–2), horses (Table 2–3), cattle (Table 2–4), sheep (Table 2–5), goats (Table 2–6), and pigs (Table 2–7). These values were determined at the Veterinary Medical Teaching Hospital, School of Veterinary Medicine, University of California, Davis. Age-related changes in blood values of dogs (Tables 2–8 and 2–9), cats (Table 2–10), horses (Tables 2–11 and 2–12), cattle (Tables 2–13, 2–14, and 2–15), sheep (Table 2–16), and pigs (Table 2–17) have been similarly derived or have been obtained from literature reports.

Various factors may influence the reference or normal blood values of various species. Disagreements

Table 2–1. Normal Blood Values for the Dog

Erythrocytic Series	Range	Av.	Leukocytic Series	Range	Av.
Erythrocytes ($\times 10^6/\mu l$)	5.5–8.5	6.8	Leukocytes/μl	6,000–17,000	11,500
Hemoglobin (g/dl)	12.0–18.0	15.0	Neutrophil (band)	0–300	70
PCV (%)	37.0–55.0	45.0	Neutrophil (mature)	3,000–11,500	7,000
MCV (fl)	60.0–77.0	70.0	Lymphocyte	1,000–4,800	2,800
MCH (pg)	19.5–24.5	22.8	Monocyte	150–1,350	750
MCHC (%)	32.0–36.0	34.0	Eosinophil	100–1,250	550
Reticulocytes (%)	0.0–1.5	0.8	Basophil	Rare	0
ESR (see Table 2–19; varies with PCV)					
RBC diameter (μm)	6.7–7.2	7.0	Percentage distribution		
RBC life span (days)	100–120		Neutrophil (band)	0–3	0.8
Resistance to hypotonic saline (%)			Neutrophil (mature)	60–77	70.0
Minimum	0.40–0.50	0.46	Lymphocyte	12–30	20.0
Maximum	0.32–0.42	0.33	Monocyte	3–10	5.2
Myeloid:erythroid ratio	0.75–2.5:1.0	1.2:1.0	Eosinophil	2–10	4.0
Other data			Basophil	Rare	0.0
Thrombocytes ($\times 10^5/\mu l$)	2–5	3.0			
Icterus index (units)	2–5				
Total plasma proteins (g/dl)	6.0–8.0*				
Plasma fibrinogen (g/dl)	0.2–0.4				

* Varies with age; see Table 2-9.

among normal values obtained by various workers relate mainly to differences in such factors, which include the number, source, age, sex, breed, health, and nutrition of the animals used in the study, as well as the method of blood collection and the hematologic techniques employed. Physiologic differences, such as animal excitement, muscular activity, time of sampling, ambient temperature, water balance, and altitude, may also introduce significant differences. In addition, diurnal and seasonal variations may occur, particularly in the young, and these may be influenced by handling of the animals and husbandry practices. Thus, regional variations may occur in some hematologic values, particularly erythrocyte parameters.

A false diagnosis of anemia, apparently from sequestration of erythrocytes in the spleen, may result when blood is collected from animals under the influence of certain anesthetics. Conversely, anemia may be masked by the release of a splenic mass of erythrocytes into the peripheral blood of animals experiencing emotional disturbance.

Animals at high altitude have a higher red blood cell (RBC) number, hemoglobin concentration, and packed cell volume (PCV) than those at sea level. For

Table 2–2. Normal Blood Values for the Cat

Erythrocytic Series	Range	Av.	Leukocytic Series	Range	Av.
Erythrocytes ($\times 10^6/\mu l$)	5.0–10.0	7.5	Leukocytes/μl	5,500–19,500	12,500
Hemoglobin (g/dl)	8.0–15.0	12.0	Neutrophil (band)	0–300	100
PCV (%)	24.0–45.0	37.0	Neutrophil (mature)	2,500–12,500	7,500
MCV (fl)	39.0–55.0	45.0	Lymphocyte	1,500–7,000	4,000
MCH (pg)	12.5–17.5	15.5	Monocyte	0–850	350
MCHC (%)	30.0–36.0	33.2	Eosinophil	0–1,500	650
Reticulocytes (%)	0.2–1.6	0.6	Basophil	Rare	0
ESR (similar to the dog)					
RBC diameter (μm)	5.5–6.3	5.8	Percentage distribution		
Resistance to hypotonic saline (%)			Neutrophil (band)	0–3	0.5
Minimum	0.66–0.72	0.69	Neutrophil (mature)	35–75	59.0
Maximum	0.46–0.54	0.50	Lymphocyte	20–55	32.0
Myeloid:erythroid ratio	1.2–2.2:1.0	1.6:1.0	Monocyte	1–4	3.0
Other data			Eosinophil	2–12	5.5
Thrombocytes ($\times 10^5/\mu l$)	3–8	4.5	Basophil	Rare	0.0
Icterus index (units)	2–5				
Erythrocyte life span (days)	66–78				
Plasma proteins (g/dl)	6.0–8.0	7.0			
Fibrinogen (g/dl)	0.05–0.30				

Table 2–3. Normal Blood Values for the Horse

Parameter	Hot-Blooded Breeds*		Cold-Blooded Breeds†	
	Range	Mean ± SD	Range	Av.
Erythrocytic series				
Erythrocytes ($\times 10^6/\mu l$)	6.8–12.9	9.0 ± 1.2	5.5–9.5	7.5
Hemoglobin (g/dl)	11.0–19.0	14.4 ± 1.7	8.0–14.0	11.5
PCV (%)	32.0–53.0	41.0 ± 4.5	24.0–44.0	35.0
MCV (fl)	37.0–58.5	45.5 ± 4.3	—	—
MCH (pg)	12.3–19.7	15.9 ± 1.5	—	—
MCHC (%)	31.0–37.0	35.2 ± 1.4	—	—
RBC diameter (μm)	5.0–6.0	5.5 —	—	—
Resistance to hypotonic saline (%)	0.34–0.56	0.45 —	—	—
Leukocytic series				
Total leukocytes/μl	5,400–14,300	9,050 ± 1,800	6,000–12,000	8,500
Neutrophil (band)	0–100	36 ± 104	—	—
Neutrophil (segmenter)	2,260–8,580	4,745 ± 1,235	—	—
Lymphocyte	1,500–7,700	3,500 ± 1,120	—	—
Monocyte	0–1,000	388 ± 288	—	—
Eosinophil	0–1,000	305 ± 244	—	—
Basophil	0–290	45 ± 62	—	—
	(See Table 2-12 for influence of age on total and differential leukocyte counts)			
Percentage distribution				
Neutrophil (band)	0–2.0	0.35 ± 0.97	0–2.0	0.5
Neutrophil (segmenter)	22.0–72.0	52.62 ± 8.73	35–75.0	54.0
Lymphocyte	17.0–68.0	38.73 ± 8.66	15–50.0	35.0
Monocyte	0–7.0	4.32 ± 2.42	2–10.0	5.0
Eosinophil	0–10.0	3.35 ± 2.55	2–12.0	5.0
Basophil	0–4.0	0.49 ± 0.65	0–3.0	0.5
Other data				
Plasma proteins (g/dl)	5.8–8.7	6.9 ± 0.6	—	—
Fibrinogen (g/dl)	0.1–0.4	0.26 ± 0.08	—	—
Icterus index (units)	7.5–20	(influenced by plant pigments and PCV)		
Thrombocytes ($\times 10^5/\mu l$)	1.0–3.5	2.25	—	—
Erythrocyte life span (days)	140–150			
Myeloid:erythroid ratio	0.5–1.5:1.0	0.93:1.0	—	—

* Based on 147 clinically normal horses.
† From the literature.

Table 2–4. Normal Blood Values for Cattle

Erythrocytic Series			Leukocytic Series		
	Range	Av.		Range	Av.
Erythrocytes ($\times 10^6/\mu l$)	5.0–10.0	7.0	Leukocytes/μl	4,000–12,000	8,000
Hemoglobin (g/dl)	8.0–15.0	11.0	Neutrophil (band)	0–120	20
PCV (%)	24.0–46.0	35.0	Neutrophil (mature)	600–4,000	2,000
MCV (fl)	40.0–60.0	52.0	Lymphocyte	2,500–7,500	4,500
MCH (pg)	11.0–17.0	14.0	Monocyte	25–840	400
MCH (%)	30.0–36.0	32.7	Eosinophil	0–2,400	700
Reticulocytes (%)	0	0	Basophil	0–200	50
ESR (mm)					
1 hour	0	0	Percentage Distribution		
8 hours	0–3		Neutrophil (band)	0–2	0.5
RBC diameter (μm)	4.0–8.0	5.8	Neutrophil (mature)	15–45	28.0
Resistance to saline (%)			Lymphocyte	45–75	58.0
Minimum	0.52–0.66		Monocyte	2–7	4.0
Maximum	0.44–0.52		Eosinophil	0–20	9.0
Myeloid:erythroid ratio	0.31–1.85:1.0	0.71:1.0	Basophil	0–2	0.5
Other data					
Thrombocytes ($\times 10^5$)	1.0–8.0	5.0			
Icterus index (units)	2–15	5–10			
Erythrocyte life span (days)	160				
Plasma proteins (g/dl)	7.0–8.5				
Fibrinogen (g/dl)	0.3–0.7				

Table 2–5. Normal Blood Values for the Sheep

Erythrocytic Series	Range	Av.	Leukocytic Series	Range	Av.
Erythrocytes ($\times 10^6/\mu l$)	9–15	12.0	Leukocytes/μl	4,000–12,000	8,000
Hemoglobin (g/dl)	9–15	11.5	Neutrophil (band)	Rare	—
PCV (%)	27.0–45.0	35.0	Neutrophil (mature)	700–6,000	2,400
MCV (fl)	28–40	34.0	Lymphocyte	2,000–9,000	5,000
MCH (pg)	8–12	10.0	Monocyte	0–750	200
MCHC (%)	31–34	32.5	Eosinophil	0–1,000	400
Reticulocytes (%)	0	0	Basophil	0–300	50
ESR (mm)	0	0			
RBC diameter (μm)	3.2–6.0	4.5	Percentage distribution		
Resistance to hypotonic saline (%)			Neutrophil (band)	Rare	—
Minimum	0.58–0.76		Neutrophil (mature)	10–50	30.0
Maximum	0.40–0.55		Lymphocyte	40–75	62.0
Myeloid:erythroid ratio	0.77–1.68:1.0	1.1:1.0	Monocyte	0–6	2.5
			Eosinophil	0–10	5.0
			Basophil	0–3	0.5
Other data					
Thrombocytes ($\times 10^5/\mu l$)	2.5–7.5	4.0			
Icterus index (units)	0–5				
Plasma proteins (g/dl)	6.0–7.5				
Fibrinogen (g/dl)	0.1–0.5				
Erythrocyte life span (days)	140–150				

example, hemoglobin concentrations of sheep on mountain pasture in Peru and Norway were found to be 3.0 to 6.0 g/dl greater than those of sheep maintained at a lower altitude, or at sea level.

Significant seasonal variations in red cell parameters have been reported in sheep, but such variations seem to be primarily related to parasitic infection and nutritional state of the animals. A significant association between lower RBC counts and a rise in worm burden has been found in late winter and early spring. However, in the summer months, the period of nutritional abundance, the RBC counts increased, suggesting that

a high level of nutrition partly offsets the effect of the worm burden. In goats, higher red cell parameters (RBC, hemoglobin, and PCV) were found in the late summer and autumn than in the winter and spring. In cattle, red cell parameters are generally highest during the coolest months and lowest during the warmest months of the year. This decrease is ascribed to hemodilution from increased water intake during periods of high temperatures.

With regard to the horses, it is necessary to know whether they are classed as hot-blooded or cold-blooded, because the former group has higher red cell

Table 2–6. Normal Blood Values for the Goat

Erythrocytic Series	Range	Av.	Leukocytic Series	Range	Av.
Erythrocytes ($\times 10^6/\mu l$)	8.0–18.0	13.0	Leukocytes/μl	4,000–13,000	9,000
Hemoglobin (g/dl)	8.0–12.0	10.0	Neutrophil (band)	Rare	—
PCV (%)			Neutrophil (mature)	1,200–7,200	3,250
Microhematocrit			Lymphocyte	2,000–9,000	5,000
(14,000 G $\times$ 10 min)	22–38	28.0	Monocyte	0–550	250
MCV (fl)	16–25	19.5	Eosinophil	50–650	450
MCHC (%)	30–36	33.0	Basophil	0–120	50
MCH (pg)	5.2–8.0	6.5			
Reticulocytes (%)	None	—	Percentage distribution		
ESR (mm)	None	—	Band	Rare	
RBC diameter (μm)	2.5–3.9	3.2	Neutrophil	30–48	36.0
Resistance to hypotonic saline (%)			Lymphocyte	50–70	56.0
Minimum	0.74	—	Monocyte	0–4	2.5
Maximum	0.44	—	Eosinophil	1–8	5.0
Myeloid:erythroid ratio		0.69:1.0	Basophil	0–1	0.5
Other data					
Thrombocytes ($\times 10^5/\mu l$)	3.0–6.0	4.5			
Icterus index (units)	2–5				
Plasma proteins (g/dl)	6.0–7.5				
Fibrinogen (g/dl)	0.1–0.4				
Erythrocyte life span (days)	125				

Table 2–7. Normal Blood Values for the Pig

Erythrocytic Series	Range	Av.	Leukocytic Series	Range	Av.
Erythrocytes ($\times 10^6/\mu$l)	5.0–8.0	6.5	Leukocytes/μl	11,000–22,000	16,000
Hemoglobin (g/dl)	10.0–16.0	13.0	Percentage distribution		
PCV (%)	32–50	42.0	Neutrophil (band)	0–4	1.0
MCV (fl)	50–68	60	Neutrophil (mature)	28–47	37.0
MCH (pg)	17.0–21	19.0	Lymphocyte	39–62	53.0
MCHC (%)	30.0–34.0	32.0	Monocyte	2–10	5.0
Reticulocytes (%)	0.0–1.0	0.4	Eosinophil	1.0–11	3.5
ESR (mm in 1 hr)	Variable		Basophil	0–2	0.5
RBC diameter (μm)	4.0–8.0	6.0			
RBC life span (days)	86 ± 11.5		Other data		
Resistance to hypotonic saline (%)			Thrombocytes ($\times 10^5/\mu$l)	1–9	5.2
Minimum		0.70	Icterus index (units)	<5	
Maximum		0.45	Plasma proteins (g/dl)	6.0–8.0	
Myeloid:erythroid ratio	0.73–2.81:1.0	1.77:1.0	Fibrinogen (g/dl)	0.1–0.5	

parameters and a lower neutrophil:lymphocyte (N:L) ratio than the latter group. Fright or emotional influences alter the total and differential leukocyte counts, causing the neutrophil and lymphocyte numbers to be elevated considerably. This is particularly true for cats less than 1 year of age and for cats introduced into a strange environment. "Stress-susceptible" pigs have higher total leukocyte and lymphocyte numbers and exhibit greater stress-induced changes in total and differential leukocyte counts than "stress-resistant" pigs. Miniature swine reveal no major differences in hematologic values compared to standard domestic swine.

Differences referable to techniques result mainly from the method of blood collection, sampling site, type and concentration of anticoagulant, and methods employed for the determination of RBC and white blood cell (WBC) counts, hemoglobin concentration, and PCV. Technical problems also include difficulties in obtaining blood, which lead to slow withdrawal of the sample so that platelets begin to clump and present problems in the electronic counting of cells. Collection of a smaller amount of blood than intended for the amount of EDTA present in a collection vial results in the shrinkage of red cells and erroneous PCV and mean corpuscular volume (MCV) values. The small size of caprine, ovine, and even bovine erythrocytes places special demands on centrifugation (increased time) to ensure complete packing of erythrocytes to obtain a valid PCV and minimize plasma trapped within the column of packed red cells.

ERYTHROCYTES

Morphologic and Physiologic Characteristics

ERYTHROCYTE MORPHOLOGY

Most mammalian erythrocytes are typically anucleate, biconcave disks, whereas elliptic nucleated erythrocytes are characteristic of birds, amphibians,

Table 2–8. Blood Values in Normal Beagles to 2 Months of Age

Parameter	Age				
	0–3 days	14–17 days	28–31 days	40–45 days	56–59 days
Number of dogs	46	46	48	44	42
RBC ($\times 10^6/\mu$l)	4.8 ± 0.8	3.5 ± 0.3	3.9 ± 0.4	4.1 ± 0.4	4.7 ± 0.4
Hemoglobin (g/dl)	15.8 ± 2.9	9.9 ± 1.1	9.6 ± 0.9	9.2 ± 0.7	10.3 ± 0.9
PCV (%)	46.3 ± 8.5	28.7 ± 2.9	28.4 ± 2.5	28.3 ± 2.3	31.4 ± 2.4
MCV (fl)	94.2 ± 5.9	81.5 ± 3.3	71.7 ± 3.5	68.2 ± 2.6	65.8 ± 2.3
MCH (pg)	32.7 ± 1.8	28.0 ± 2.0	24.3 ± 1.6	22.4 ± 1.0	21.8 ± 1.2
MCHC (%)	34.6 ± 1.4	34.3 ± 1.6	33.5 ± 1.4	32.4 ± 1.7	32.6 ± 1.8
NucRBC/100 WBC	7.2 ± 6.7	2.4 ± 3.8	1.1 ± 1.5	0.6 ± 0.9	0.1 ± 0.4
Reticulocytes (%)	6.5	6.7	5.8	4.5	3.6
WBC/μl	16,800 ± 5,700	13,600 ± 4,400	13,900 ± 3,300	15,300 ± 3,700	15,700 ± 4,400
Absolute number of WBC/μl					
Band neutrophils	600 ± 500	200 ± 200	100 ± 200	200 ± 200	300 ± 300
Segmenters	9,200 ± 6,600	6,900 ± 3,100	6,800 ± 2,000	7,400 ± 2,400	8,500 ± 2,900
Lymphocytes	3,700 ± 2,300	4,900 ± 1,700	5,400 ± 1,600	6,100 ± 1,900	5,000 ± 1,500
Monocytes	1,400 ± 1,300	1,100 ± 600	1,100 ± 600	1,300 ± 600	1,400 ± 700
Eosinophils	400 ± 400	500 ± 500	400 ± 400	300 ± 300	400 ± 400
Platelets/μl	302,000	290,000	287,000	321,000	411,000
M:E ratio	1.6:1	1.7:1	1.7:1	1.8:1	1.4:1

Table 2–9. **Influence of Age on the Blood Values of Normal Basenji Dogs***

Parameter	Age				
	6–8 weeks	*9–12 weeks*	*4–6 months*	*1–2 years*	*>2 years*
Number of dogs	24	21	9	13	7
RBC (×10⁶/μl)	4.73 ± 0.38	5.45 ± 0.54	6.56 ± 0.46	6.91 ± 0.60	7.19 ± 0.64
Hemoglobin (g/dl)	10.4 ± 0.58	11.8 ± 0.81	14.4 ± 0.82	15.9 ± 1.2	16.6 ± 1.1
PCV (%)	33.1 ± 2.2	37.2 ± 2.9	44.0 ± 2.4	49.3 ± 3.4	49.8 ± 3.4
MCV (fl)	70.1 ± 2.9	68.6 ± 2.9	67.2 ± 2.9	71.1 ± 4.0	69.6 ± 4.1
MCH (pg)	22.1 ± 1.4	21.8 ± 1.5	21.9 ± 0.9	23.0 ± 0.8	23.2 ± 1.8
MCHC (%)	31.5 ± 1.4	31.8 ± 1.3	32.7 ± 0.6	32.3 ± 1.2	33.3 ± 0.41
Icterus index units	1.3 ± 0.9	2.8 ± 1.9	0.66 ± 0.94	2.2 ± 2.3	2.0 ± 2.1
Plasma proteins (g/dl)	5.33 ± 0.29	5.87 ± 0.46	6.6 ± 0.25	7.03 ± 0.33	7.5 ± 0.24
Fibrinogen (g/dl)	0.18 ± 0.07	0.20 ± 0.08	0.22 ± 0.07	0.22 ± 0.08	0.20 ± 0.06
Reticulocytes (%)	3.4 ± 1.0	2.6 ± 1.8	0.24 ± 0.41	0.84 ± 0.9	0.84 ± 1.12
WBC/μl	13,433 ± 2,045	15,033 ± 2,077	13,589 ± 1,751	14,031 ± 2,270	12,157 ± 1,987
Percentage distribution of WBC					
Band neutrophils	0.65 ± 0.77	0.57 ± 1.1	0.61 ± 0.81	0.27 ± 0.42	0.07 ± 0.17
Segmenters	58.8 ± 10.9	56.4 ± 7.8	52.4 ± 5.5	58.1 ± 7.3	66.4 ± 6.7
Lymphocytes	30.1 ± 8.1	33.5 ± 8.1	36.9 ± 5.5	28.6 ± 7.7	23.1 ± 4.8
Monocytes	6.9 ± 2.6	6.7 ± 2.7	6.0 ± 1.8	5.2 ± 2.1	4.0 ± 1.4
Eosinophils	3.3 ± 1.9	2.3 ± 1.6	4.1 ± 1.9	7.3 ± 3.5	6.3 ± 2.3
Basophils	0.08 ± 0.24	0.07 ± 0.23	0.0 ± 0.0	0.12 ± 0.4	0.14 ± 0.22
Absolute numbers of WBC/μl					
Band neutrophils	85 ± 101	94 ± 186	88 ± 117	38 ± 62	8 ± 21
Segmenters	8,015 ± 2,387	8,463 ± 1,638	7,196 ± 1,509	8,169 ± 1,732	8,107 ± 1,864
Lymphocytes	3,965 ± 1,059	5,059 ± 1,555	4,948 ± 510	4,203 ± 1,207	2,805 ± 634
Monocytes	912 ± 325	986 ± 405	818 ± 311	715 ± 266	495 ± 191
Eosinophils	426 ± 239	341 ± 243	538 ± 225	990 ± 455	727 ± 229
Basophils	10 ± 29	10 ± 33	0 ± 0	17 ± 58	15 ± 23

* Means and 1 SD.

reptiles, and fishes. Mammalian erythrocytes range from about 4 to 9 μm in diameter, and, in most species, particularly the dog, exhibit a distinct central pallor and slight anisocytosis. Slight artifactual crenation occurs frequently, but other shape transformations are generally abnormal. Sharp-pointed crenation is a commonly seen artifact in pig blood films. Rouleau formation is common in the horse and pig, occasional in the dog and cat, and absent in some ruminants (cows). The marked natural aggregation of equine erythro-cytes leads to the separation of cells and plasma within minutes. Therefore, equine blood should be mixed repeatedly whenever a portion is to be removed from a sample vial for examination.

An occasional polychromatic erythrocyte may be found in the blood films of some species, but not in others (e.g., the horse). These cells, which are deficient in hemoglobin, appear gray in Wright-stained film and usually appear as reticulocytes in blood stained with new methylene blue. Thus, the number of poly-

Table 2–10. **Some Aspects of Postnatal Changes in the Blood of the Cat**

Age	Number*	RBC (×10⁶/μl)	Hb (g/dl)	PCV (%)	MCV (fl)	MCH (pg)	MCHC (%)	MCD (μm)	WBC (×10³/μl)
0–6 hr	24; 24	4.95	12.2	44.7	90.3	24.6	27.3	6.7	7.55
12–48 hr	23; 26	5.11	11.3	41.7	81.6	22.1	27.1	—	10.18
7 days	21; 21	5.19	10.9	35.7	68.8	21.0	30.5	6.7	7.83
14 days	18; 18	4.76	9.7	31.1	65.3	20.4	31.2	6.5	8.08
21 days	19; 19	4.99	9.3	31.3	62.7	18.6	29.7	6.1	8.82
28 days	20; 20	5.84	8.4	29.9	51.2	14.4	28.1	5.9	8.55
42 days	21; 20	6.75	9.0	35.4	52.4	13.3	25.4	5.9	8.42
56 days	19; 19	7.10	9.4	35.6	50.1	13.2	26.4	5.8	8.42
70 days	22; 22	7.33	9.9	—	—	13.5	—	—	9.18
80 days	21; 21	7.69	10.3	39.0	50.7	13.4	26.4	—	9.12
90 days	21; 21	8.26	10.4	43.1	52.2	12.6	24.1	—	9.01
120 days	21; 21	8.77	10.7	35.7	40.7	12.2	29.9	—	9.36
150 days	7; 7	9.27	11.4	41.5	44.7	12.3	27.7	—	11.66
Adult male	37; 35	9.02	12.2	40.6	45.0	13.5	30.0	5.7	12.4
Adult female	64; 64	8.39	12.0	41.3	49.2	14.3	29.1	5.8	10.5

* Number of cases averaged for RBC (first figure) and Hb (second figure).

Table 2–11. Normal Blood Values of Thoroughbred and Quarter Horse Foals of Both Sexes*

Parameter	1	2–7 (Av., 5)	8–14 (Av., 9)	21–30 (Av., 28)	30–90 (Av., 51)
			Age (days)		
Number of foals	34	16	15	8	14
RBC ($\times 10^6$/μl)	10.5 ± 1.4	9.5 ± 0.8	9.0 ± 0.8	11.2 ± 1.3	11.9 ± 1.3
Hb (g/dl)	14.2 ± 1.3	12.7 ± 0.9	11.8 ± 1.2	13.1 ± 1.1	13.4 ± 1.6
PCV (%)	41.7 ± 3.6	37.1 ± 2.8	34.9 ± 3.7	37.8 ± 3.3	38.3 ± 4.1
MCV (fl)	40.1 ± 3.8	39.2 ± 2.8	39.1 ± 2.2	34.0 ± 2.4	32.4 ± 1.9
MCH (pg)	13.6 ± 1.2	13.4 ± 1.0	13.1 ± 0.8	11.8 ± 0.8	11.2 ± 0.6
MCHC (%)	33.9 ± 1.6	34.2 ± 1.2	33.6 ± 0.9	34.5 ± 1.0	34.9 ± 1.2
Icterus index units	40 ± 30 (30)	29 ± 21	19 ± 6	12.5 ± 5.6	15 ± 5
Plasma protein (g/dl)	6.2 ± 0.9 (32)	6.4 ± 0.5	6.1 ± 0.6	6.2 ± 0.4	6.4 ± 0.4
Fibrinogen (g/dl)	0.27 ± 0.06 (15)	0.33 ± 0.13 (6)	0.30 ± 0.05 (9)	0.40 ± 0.05 (5)	0.46 ± 0.07 (10)
Total leukocytes/μl	9,602 ± 3,372	9,300 ± 2,346	9,483 ± 2,196	9,688 ± 1,940	10,893 ± 2,977
Band neutrophils	138 ± 198	29 ± 37	48 ± 125	19 ± 33	10 ± 28
Mature neutrophils	6,824 ± 2,757	6,448 ± 2,128	6,338 ± 1,849	5,501 ± 1,346	5,315 ± 2,437
Lymphocytes	2,192 ± 891	2,420 ± 739	2,633 ± 933	3,823 ± 863	5,086 ± 1,419
Monocytes	414 ± 373	308 ± 172	302 ± 124	266 ± 192	348 ± 175
Eosinophils	0	30 ± 34	21 ± 38	48 ± 53	115 ± 88
Basophils	14 ± 78	41 ± 44	29 ± 50	11 ± 29	12 ± 26
Leukocytes (%)					
Band neutrophils	1.5 ± 1.8	0.3 ± 0.4	0.5 ± 1.1	0.2 ± 0.3	0.1 ± 0.3
Mature neutrophils	68.9 ± 10.7	68.2 ± 9.4	66.2 ± 9.0	56.8 ± 7.4	46.9 ± 12.1
Lymphocytes	25.1 ± 10.3	27.0 ± 9.8	28.5 ± 9.4	39.6 ± 6.5	48.5 ± 11.5
Monocytes	3.9 ± 2.9	3.4 ± 1.9	3.3 ± 1.5	2.6 ± 2.0	3.3 ± 1.8
Eosinophils	0	0.3 ± 0.4	0.2 ± 0.4	0.4 ± 0.5	1.0 ± 0.8
Basophils	0.02 ± 0.08	0.4 ± 0.4	0.3 ± 0.5	0.1 ± 0.3	0.1 ± 0.3
N:L ratio (mean)	2.8:1.0	2.5:1.0	2.3:1.0	1.4:1.0	1.1:1.0

* Means and 1 SD; numbers in parentheses indicate number of foals when less than total for series.

chromatic erythrocytes generally correlates with the number of reticulocytes in blood. Polychromasia and reticulocyte counts are increased in responsive anemias (Plates IV–6 and XVI–3). A single nucleated erythrocyte and a rare erythrocyte with a Howell-Jolly body may be encountered. The Howell-Jolly body is a nuclear remnant that stains deep purple (Plate XII–9). It must not be mistaken for red cell parasites such as *Haemobartonella felis, H. canis,* or *Anaplasma marginale.* Nucleated erythrocytes (normoblastemia) and Howell-Jolly bodies are commonly found in blood during response to anemia. Increased numbers of erythrocytes with Howell-Jolly bodies (Fig. 2–1) and, less commonly, nucleated erythrocytes, may appear in the blood of animals on continuous corticosteroid therapy. These findings reflect suppressed splenic function. A transient normoblastemia may occur in acutely stressed animals. Cats with myeloproliferative disorders and dogs and horses with chronic lead poisoning exhibit normoblastemia of variable magnitude (Plates XVII–12 and XXII–4). Rarely, hemoglobin crystals may be seen within and outside the red cells in the blood of dogs and cats. Its significance remains unknown.

Variations in red cell shape (poikilocytosis) may be physiologic or pathologic. Elliptic erythrocytes are characteristic of the family Camelidae and sickle cells are found in the oxygenated blood of certain deer. Stomatocytes are seen in Alaskan malamutes and spheroechinocytes may be found in basenji dogs with pyruvate kinase deficiency. Abnormalities of erythrocyte shape during disease are more often encountered

in the dog and cat than in other animal species (see Chap. 7 for a discussion of terminology and descriptions of various red cell shapes).

The red blood cells of the goat are the smallest among the domestic animals. Poikilocytosis is striking in goat kids under 3 months of age and may be

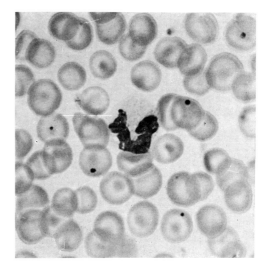

Fig. 2–1. Blood film from a dog receiving corticosteroids and cytotoxic drugs for the treatment of lymphosarcoma. Depression of splenic activity is indicated by the occurrence of numerous Howell-Jolly bodies and also possibly by the presence of target cells, (× 3150). (From Jain, N.C.: Schalm's Veterinary Hematology. 4th Ed. Philadelphia, Lea & Febiger, 1986, p. 378.)

Table 2–12. Influence of Age on Normal Blood Values of Hot-Blooded Horses*

No. of Horses	Age	RBC (×10⁶/μl)	Hb (g/dl)	PCV (%)	MCV (fl)	MCH (pg)	MCHC (%)	Protein (g/dl)	Fibrinogen (g/dl)†	WBC/μl
8	8–18 mo	8.60 ± 0.58	11.8 ± 1.6	34.5 ± 3.8	40.1 ± 2.9	13.7 ± 1.3	34.1 ± 1.4	7.3 ± 0.9	0.29 ± 0.04 (7)	10,812 ± 1,874
27	2 yr	9.88 ± 1.34	14.7 ± 1.6	41.4 ± 4.2	42.7 ± 2.8	14.9 ± 1.1	34.9 ± 1.3	6.8 ± 0.5	0.29 ± 0.07 (14)	9,678 ± 1,883
50	3–4 yr	9.10 ± 1.16	14.3 ± 1.4	40.8 ± 4.3	44.8 ± 3.4	15.7 ± 1.2	35.2 ± 1.5	6.8 ± 0.5	0.24 ± 0.08 (30)	8,666 ± 1,560
62	5+ yr	8.57 ± 0.98	14.4 ± 1.6	40.8 ± 4.1	47.8 ± 4.0	16.8 ± 1.3	35.4 ± 1.4	7.0 ± 0.5	0.26 ± 0.07 (36)	8,822 ± 1,760

* Means and 1 SD.
† Numbers in parentheses indicate number of samples, when less than total for all other values.

Table 2–13. Influence of Age on the Hemogram of Cattle*

Parameter	Fetuses (7–8½ Mo)	Calves (Day of Birth)	Calves (3–16 Weeks)	Yearlings†	Adult Cows†
Number of animals	7	37	15	35	42
Erythrocytes (×10⁶/μl)	5.86 ± 0.63	7.72 ± 1.73	9.5 ± 1.0	8.36 ± 1.05	6.36 ± 0.8
Hemoglobin (g/dl)	8.5 ± 0.05	10.2 ± 1.8	11.2 ± 1.5	11.4 ± 1.7	10.9 ± 1.7
PCV (%)	31.4 ± 1.4	34.5 ± 7.7	35.9 ± 3.8	35.9 ± 4.3	33.6 ± 5.2
MCV (fl)	53.9 ± 5.1	46.2 ± 4.8	37.8 ± 3.2	43.2 ± 7.1	52.8 ± 4.4
MCH (pg)	14.7 ± 1.5	13.3 ± 1.3	11.8 ± 1.6	13.6 ± 1.7	17.0 ± 1.6
MCHC (g/dl)	27.3 ± 0.8	28.7 ± 1.5	31.2 ± 2.8	32.3 ± 1.7	32.5 ± 1.2
Icterus index units	4.8 ± 2.1	7.7 ± 11.7	4.4 ± 2.3	—	—
Plasma proteins (%)	4.4 ± 0.3	5.0 ± 0.8	6.2 ± 0.6	—	—
Fibrinogen (g/dl)	0.10 ± 0.08	0.16 ± 0.13	0.08 ± 0.20	—	—
Total leukocytes/μl	6,743 ± 2,114	9,623 ± 3,453	10,713 ± 3,047	—	—
Band neutrophils	10 ± 25	123 ± 184	24 ± 56	—	—
Mature neutrophils	1,389 ± 646	4,869 ± 3,439	2,872 ± 1,331	—	—
Lymphocytes	4,762 ± 1,364	3,931 ± 1,744	6,861 ± 2,179	—	—
Monocytes	323 ± 209	497 ± 374	794 ± 270	—	—
Eosinophils	227 ± 150	124 ± 167	106 ± 342	—	—
Basophils	31 ± 38	33 ± 53	54 ± 76	—	—
Leukocytes (%)					
Band neutrophils	0.29 ± 0.7	1.2 ± 1.5	0.23 ± 0.5	—	—
Mature neutrophils	19.3 ± 6.9	47.2 ± 18.8	26.2 ± 8.8	—	—
Lymphocytes	72.1 ± 7.9	44.5 ± 19.2	64.1 ± 8.6	—	—
Monocytes	4.7 ± 2.9	4.8 ± 2.8	8.2 ± 4.2	—	—
Eosinophils	3.1 ± 1.9	1.4 ± 1.9	0.7 ± 2.0	—	—
Basophils	0.5 ± 0.6	0.4 ± 0.6	0.5 ± 0.6	—	—
Neutrophil:lymphocyte ratio	0.27:1.0	1.1:1.0	0.41:1.0	—	—

* Means and 1 SD.
† Blood samples from clinical patients whose erythrocyte parameters were within normal ranges.

Table 2–14. Mean Blood Values in Purebred Jersey Female Cattle as Influenced by Age

No. of Animals	Age	RBC (×10⁶/μl)	Hb (g/dl)	PCV (%)	MCV (fl)	MCH (pg)	MCHC* (%)	WBC/μl	Differential Leukocyte Count (%)				
									Neutrophils	Lymphocytes	Monocytes	Eosinophils	Basophils
6	3½–4½ mo	13.10	11.07	36.16	27.6	8.45	30.6	7567	28.2	62.9	8.0	0.8	0.1
5	7½–9 mo	10.65	10.10	30.40	28.5	9.48	33.2	8000	8.8	82.2	8.0	1.0	0.0
8	11–12 mo	8.62	9.60	28.10	32.6	11.13	34.0	8281	12.9	78.4	6.9	1.5	0.3
5	15–19 mo	9.15	10.97	34.80	38.0	11.99	31.5	8840	26.2	63.0	3.4	6.6	0.8
11	20–36 mo	7.50	10.70	34.80	46.4	14.30	30.7	8050	24.0	64.5	5.0	6.0	0.5
7	3–4 yr	8.70	11.30	40.00	46.0	13.00	28.2	7063	25.0	60.5	3.8	9.7	1.0
6	4–6 yr	7.89	11.20	38.70	49.2	14.20	28.8	6950	21.0	64.2	5.0	8.8	1.0
7	6–14 yr	7.47	11.10	37.40	50.0	14.86	29.7	6630	18.5	65.8	3.2	12.0	0.5

* Determined from the PCV of the Wintrobe hematocrit. The microhematocrit PCV gives higher values because of more complete packing of the erythrocytes.

					Differential Leukocyte Count								
Neutrophils													
Band		Segmenter		Lymphocytes		Monocytes		Eosinophils		Basophils			
No.	%	No.	%	No.	%	No.	%	No.	%	No.	%	N:L Ratio	
16 ± 28	0.1 ± 0.2	4,658 ± 745	43.8 ± 7.0	5,210 ± 1,250	47.9 ± 6.0	398 ± 278	3.6 ± 2.0	478 ± 403	4.1 ± 2.9	43 ± 47	0.4 ± 0.5	0.9:1.0	
39 ± 81	0.4 ± 1.1	4,805 ± 1,196	50.1 ± 10.1	4,059 ± 1,456	41.4 ± 10.5	445 ± 255	4.7 ± 2.8	278 ± 232	2.8 ± 2.1	33 ± 58	0.3 ± 0.5	1.2:1.0	
48 ± 153	0.4 ± 1.2	4,568 ± 1,189	52.5 ± 8.0	3,376 ± 787	39.3 ± 7.7	360 ± 176	4.2 ± 2.0	278 ± 218	3.2 ± 2.6	34 ± 46	0.4 ± 0.5	1.3:1.0	
22 ± 57	0.3 ± 0.7	4,877 ± 1,316	55.0 ± 7.7	3,146 ± 826	36.0 ± 7.4	385 ± 240	4.4 ± 2.6	316 ± 231	3.6 ± 2.6	60 ± 72	0.7 ± 0.8	1.5:1.0	

prominent in some mature goats of certain breeds (Fig. 2–2). Erythrocytes of the adult goat may be fairly discoid and slightly biconcave or bluntly triangular. In addition, spindled, fusiform, matchstick form, oblong, triangular, and pear-shaped erythrocytes may be found in varying numbers in some normal goats, particularly Angora goats (Fig. 2–3). Polymerization of hemoglobin in the form of longitudinal tubular filaments confers fusiform and spindle shapes to goat red cells (Fig. 2–4), as is the case with sickle-shaped human and deer erythrocytes. The cell shape is influenced by temperature, pH, oxygen tension and, more importantly, by the formation of hemoglobin C in response to anemia. For example, acute blood loss anemia in an Angora goat was associated with a gradual reduction in the numbers of fusiform and discoid erythrocytes and an increase in poikilocytes (Table 2–18). These changes in erythrocyte morphology gradually reversed with the decrease in synthesis of hemoglobin C during recovery from anemia (Fig. 2–5).

RETICULOCYTES

In general, two types of reticulocytes are recognized based on their morphology in blood stained with vital dyes such as new methylene blue (Plate IV–6). Aggregate reticulocytes have strings and clumps of bluish reticular material resulting from the precipitation of cytoplasmic ribonucleoprotein by the dye. In comparison, punctate reticulocytes contain small granules of

Table 2–15. Normal Absolute Values for Leukocytes/μl in Female Jersey Cattle*

Age	No. of Cattle	Total Leukocyte Count	Band Neutrophils	Mature Neutrophils	Lymphocytes	Monocytes	Eosinophils	Basophils
1–6 mo	16	8,750 ± 2,500	50 ± 75	3,000 ± 1,750	4,650 ± 1,300	680 ± 370	170 ± 520	50 ± 60
6–12 mo	10	7,750 ± 1,800	0	800 ± 450	6,300 ± 1,500	600 ± 170	80 ± 50	0
1–2 yr	14	9,000 ± 2,500	0	2,350 ± 1,400	5,900 ± 1,600	420 ± 170	500 ± 380	60 ± 60
2–3 yr	31	9,400 ± 1,750	25 ± 125	2,150 ± 930	5,300 ± 1,200	475 ± 220	1,300 ± 1,000	70 ± 100
3–4 yr	28	7,700 ± 1,900	0	1,900 ± 950	4,600 ± 1,050	325 ± 150	900 ± 650	50 ± 50
4–6 yr	29	7,500 ± 1,100	15 ± 45	1,800 ± 650	4,000 ± 850	450 ± 200	1,200 ± 700	60 ± 50
>6 yr	21	7,700 ± 2,500	5 ± 30	1,800 ± 900	4,250 ± 2,050	350 ± 200	1,300 ± 700	20 ± 30

* Means and 1 SD.

Table 2–16. Hemograms of Growing Lambs*

Age	RBC (×10⁶/μl)	Hb (g/dl)	PCV (%)	MCV (fl)	MCH (pg)	MCHC (%)	Reticulocytes (%)	WBC (×10⁶/μl)	Neutrophils (%)	Lymphocytes (%)	Monocytes (%)	Eosinophils (%)	Basophils (%)
Birth	11.08 ± 0.20	12.9 ± 0.02	41.9 ± 0.06	36.5 ± 0.7	12.1 ± 0.2	30.9 ± 0.4	0.08 ± 0.1	3,032 ± 207	34.0 ± 3.0	64.0 ± 3.0	0.40 ± 0.13	0.20 ± 0.07	0.05 ± 0.03
12 hr	9.55 ± 0.25	11.4 ± 0.2	35.8 ± 0.08	36.8 ± 0.8	12.2 ± 0.3	32.0 ± 0.5	0.11 ± 0.02	6,129 ± 378	52.0 ± 3.0	46.0 ± 3.0	0.30 ± 0.30	0.40 ± 0.10	0.02 ± 0.02
24 hr	9.93 ± 0.25	11.6 ± 0.2	36.2 ± 0.8	35.9 ± 0.6	11.9 ± 0.2	32.0 ± 0.4	0.08 ± 0.02	3,349 ± 273	48.0 ± 3.0	50.0 ± 3.0	0.40 ± 0.13	0.60 ± 0.13	0.09 ± 0.04
48 hr	9.74 ± 0.25	11.1 ± 0.2	33.4 ± 0.8	33.5 ± 0.6	11.5 ± 0.2	33.6 ± 0.4	0.16 ± 0.03	4,262 ± 219	37.0 ± 2.0	62.0 ± 2.0	0.90 ± 0.16	0.20 ± 0.07	0.16 ± 0.06
5 days	10.04 ± 0.29	10.4 ± 0.3	30.9 ± 0.9	32.0 ± 0.5	11.0 ± 0.2	33.8 ± 0.4	0.33 ± 0.08	6,342 ± 247	36.0 ± 2.0	62.0 ± 2.0	1.30 ± 0.21	0.20 ± 0.07	0.08 ± 0.04
8 days	8.79 ± 0.16	9.6 ± 0.2	29.2 ± 0.3	31.6 ± 0.1	11.1 ± 0.1	33.9 ± 0.3	0.31 ± 0.05	7,809 ± 145	38.0 ± 2.0	60.0 ± 2.0	1.30 ± 0.21	0.20 ± 0.10	0.08 ± 0.04
14 days	8.91 ± 0.03	8.9 ± 0.2	27.2 ± 0.5	30.8 ± 0.4	9.9 ± 0.2	32.2 ± 0.4	0.72 ± 0.10	7,404 ± 366	36.0 ± 2.0	60.0 ± 2.0	1.30 ± 0.17	1.20 ± 0.18	0.09 ± 0.03
1 mo	11.39 ± 0.14	10.4 ± 0.1	31.5 ± 0.3	28.0 ± 0.5	9.1 ± 0.2	33.0 ± 0.4	0.31 ± 0.07	7,892 ± 224	29.0 ± 1.0	68.0 ± 1.0	0.80 ± 0.50	2.00 ± 0.22	0.25 ± 0.05
2 mo	12.43 ± 0.14	11.6 ± 0.1	34.0 ± 0.2	27.6 ± 0.3	9.3 ± 0.1	33.9 ± 0.7	0.02 ± 0.01	9,014 ± 221	22.0 ± 1.0	76.0 ± 1.0	0.50 ± 0.06	1.10 ± 0.11	0.19 ± 0.04
3 mo	12.95 ± 0.17	11.8 ± 0.1	34.2 ± 0.4	26.2 ± 0.3	9.0 ± 0.1	34.6 ± 0.2	0.03 ± 0.02	9,525 ± 186	23.0 ± 1.0	76.0 ± 1.0	0.60 ± 0.07	0.70 ± 0.12	0.30 ± 0.05
5 mo	12.35 ± 0.13	11.3 ± 0.3	31.4 ± 0.7	26.1 ± 0.3	9.0 ± 0.1	34.6 ± 0.2	0.02 ± 0.01	9,097 ± 219	20.0 ± 1.0	78.0 ± 1.0	0.60 ± 0.11	1.40 ± 0.17	0.33 ± 0.07
8 mo	10.96 ± 0.27	10.9 ± 0.2	31.8 ± 0.5	29.2 ± 0.5	10.3 ± 0.2	34.5 ± 0.4	0.03 ± 0.01	6,637 ± 291	25.0 ± 1.0	71.0 ± 1.0	0.80 ± 0.14	2.50 ± 0.33	0.45 ± 0.10
12 mo	11.85 ± 0.23	11.8 ± 0.2	33.8 ± 0.5	26.5 ± 0.5	9.3 ± 0.2	35.0 ± 0.3	0.02 ± 0.01	7,341 ± 552	16.0 ± 1.0	78.0 ± 3.0	1.80 ± 0.53	2.60 ± 0.51	0.16 ± 0.05

* Means ± SE.

Table 2–17.   Influence of Age and Husbandry on the Hematology of Young Duroc-Jersey Pigs*

Age (days)	Value	Wt. (lb)	RBC (×10⁶/μl)	Hb (g/dl)	PCV (%)	MCV (fl)	MCHC (%)	MCH (pg)	Retic. (%)	Nuc. RBC/100 WBC	ESR (1 hr)	WBC (×10³/μl)†	Band	Neutrophil	Lymphocyte	Monocyte	Eosinophil	Basophil
1	Min.	1.7	4.3	8.4	27.0	57	28.9	18.0	4.5	0.5	0	7.6	1.0	64.5	16.0	0.5	0	0
	Max.	3.3	6.4	12.3	42.5	71	31.3	21.0	10.0	4.0	4	15.3	7.0	75.5	31.0	7.5	2.0	1.0
	Av.	2.4	5.3	10.5	35	67	30.5	20	6.7	2	2	11.5	3.6	71	20	4.7	0.9	0.2
3	Min.	2.4	3.3	7.8	26.5	70	29.1	21.0	6.9	7	2	6.3	1.0	38.0	23.5	6.0	0	0
	Max.	4.0	5.2	11.0	36.5	81	30.3	24.0	16.6	57	12	13.4	5.5	61.5	54.0	9.5	1.5	0
	Av.	3.2	4.5	9.8	33	73	29.5	22	12.0	17	5	9.4	3.3	51	37.6	6.8	0.8	0
6	Min.	3.5	3.4	6.4	22.0	60	26.4	17.0	4.5	5	12	7.4	1.0	33.0	32.5	2.0	0	0
	Max.	5.0	4.7	9.4	31.0	74	30.9	23.0	13.0	54	33	10.5	3.3	60.5	55	10.5	1.0	0
	Av.	4.5	4.0	8.0	26.7	67	29.1	20	7.7	14	22.6	8.2	2	45.4	45.3	4.9	0.3	0
10	Min.	5.2	2.1	4.2	15.0	62	29.0	19.0	6.0	3	1	5.6	0	8.0	36.5	1.0	0	0
	Max.	7.1	4.3	8.7	20.0	78	31.0	24.0	12.0	30	35	19.1	2.0	51.0	82.0	10.0	0.5	0.5
	Av.	6.4	3.5	7.0	24	68	29.6	20	10	11	12	10.9	1	27	64	7	0.1	0.05
20	Min.	8.5	4.4	9.0	35.5	70	26.0	19.0	9.0	1	0	6.2	0	13.5	55.0	2.0	0	0
	Max.	11.5	5.3	11.2	40.5	82	29.0	23.0	13.0	25	1	10.5	3.5	39.5	82.0	7.0	2.0	0.5
	Av.	10.5	4.9	10.2	37	76	27.6	21	10.6	11.5	0	7.7	1.4	25.7	66.8	4.3	0.8	0.05
36	Min.	—	5.9	11.3	37.0	62	28.0	18.8	1.6	0	0	12.7	0	28.0	40.0	3.0	3.5	0
	Max.	—	6.8	13.3	44.0	68	32.0	20.0	6.8	1	2	20.9	5.0	43.0	68.0	10.5	14.0	1.5
	Av.	—	6.2	12.1	39.7	64	30.5	19.4	3.0	0.5	0.5	16.3	1.8	33	52	6	7	0.5

* Ranges and means for a single litter of five males and four females; pigs kept on concrete until 10 days of age and then placed on soil.
† Corrected for nucleated red cells.

reticular material dispersed loosely within the cell. Aggregate reticulocytes are characteristic in the dog, and punctate reticulocytes are typical of cats, particularly newborn kittens, although both types of reticulocytes can be found in dogs and cats responding to anemia. In most species, the number of aggregate reticulocytes increases during response to anemia and correlates with the polychromatic red cells seen in Romanowsky-stained blood films. Therefore, the reticulocyte count routinely performed during hematologic examination is mainly comprised of aggregate reticulocytes.

The number of reticulocytes in normal blood generally correlates with the life span of the erythrocyte. Animals with a shorter red cell life span have more reticulocytes in the circulation, and vice versa. Reticulocytes, nucleated erythrocytes, and polychromasia are prominent features of blood in the neonate. The rapid replacement of fetal red cells and an increased need to compensate for growth result in increased

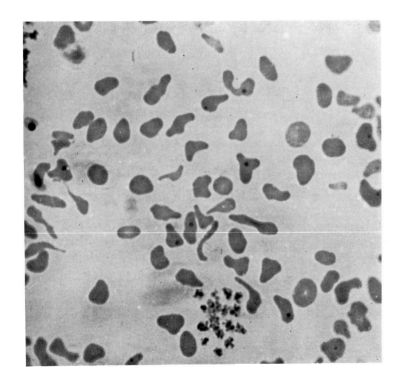

Fig. 2–2. Poikilocytes (irregularly shaped erythrocytes) in the blood of a goat kid 2 months of age. The dark, spherical body in each of several poikilocytes may be a Howell-Jolly body. A cluster of thrombocytes is seen at bottom center (×1800). (From Jain, N.C.: Schalm's Veterinary Hematology. 4th Ed. Philadelphia, Lea & Febiger, 1986, p. 232.)

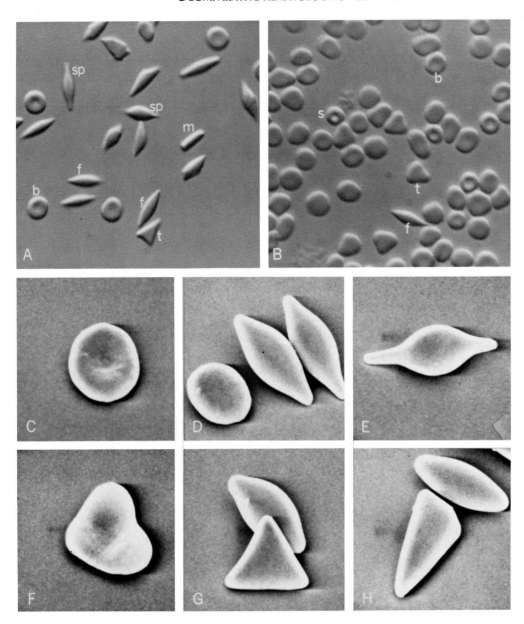

Fig. 2–3. Morphology of erythrocytes from two Angora goats, one with nearly 60% fusiform cells. (A, C–H) and another with only 2% such cells (B). A and B are from wet preparations of fresh blood examined with Nomarski interference-contrast optics; various forms of fusiform (f), spindle-shaped (sp), matchstick (m), and triangular (t) cells are compared with stomatocytes (s) and normal discoid cells (b). Scanning electron photomicrographs (C–H) of glutaraldehyde-fixed cells show their distinctive morphology (A, B, ×1450; C–H, ×4500). (From Jain, N.C., and Kono, C.S.: Fusiform erythrocytes resembling sickle cells in Angora goats: Light and electron microscopic observations. Res. Vet. Sci., 22:169, 1977.)

Table 2–18. Hematologic Changes in an Angora Goat as a Result of Acute Blood Loss Anemia

Week after Start of Bleeding†	RBC (×10⁶/μl)	Hb (g/dl)	PCV (%)	Plasma Proteins (g/dl)	MCV (fl)	MCHC (%)	MCH (pg)	Reticulocytes (%)‡	Erythrocyte Types (%)		
									Fusiform	Other Forms	Discoid
0	17.88	11.75	29.0	7.5	16.2	40.5	6.6	0	50	10	40
3	10.29	7.00	20.0	6.0	19.4	35.0	6.8	1.8	26	13	61
5	8.24	7.25	19.5	6.0	23.7	37.2	8.8	2.5	13	40	47
8	8.10	6.00	16.0	6.1	19.7	37.5	7.4	1.3	4	82	14
13	17.31	11.00	29.0	7.1	16.7	37.9	6.3	3	3	69	28
17	17.43	10.50	28.0	7.1	16.1	37.5	6.0	0	17	24	59
21	17.82	10.50	29.0	7.5	16.3	39.5	6.5	0	27	12	61
25	17.64	10.50	26.0	7.5	14.7	40.4	6.0	0	32	16	52
28	15.45	10.25	26.0	7.7	16.8	39.4	6.6	0	49	14	37

From Jain, N. C., Kono, C. S., Myers, A., et al.: Fusiform erythrocytes resembling sickle cells in Angora goats: Observations on osmotic and mechanical fragilities and reversal of cell shape during anemia. Res. Vet. Sci., 28:25, 1980.

† Bleeding to induce anemia discontinued after the eighth week.

‡ Highest count of 5.7% recorded at the fourth week.

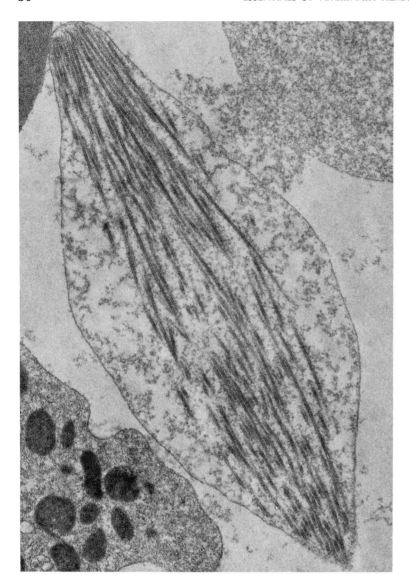

Fig. 2–4. Transmission electron photomicrograph of a partially lysed fusiform erythrocyte having many long tubular filaments of polymerized hemoglobin. Note that the filaments seem to extend throughout the entire cell length even though a filament discontinuity occurs at many places (×4200). (From Jain, N.C., and Kono, C.S.: Fusiform erythrocytes resembling sickle cells in Angora goats: Light and electron microscopic observations. Res. Vet. Sci., 22:169, 1977.)

erythropoietic activity and the release of more reticulocytes. In the adult dog, the circulating reticulocyte count is commonly less than 1%, whereas in puppies the reticulocyte count may be as high as 7%. The reticulocyte count in young dogs (less than 16 months of age) may show sex difference in that the count is lower in females than in males. In the adult dog, reticulocytes are released into the blood with a periodicity of 14 days and their average maturation time in the circulation is about 31 hours (range, 19 to 43 hours). The oscillatory nature of reticulocyte release, the release rate, and the intravascular maturation time may all change considerably during response to anemia. An increased erythropoietic response to anemia is associated with an elevation in reticulocyte numbers in the bone marrow, which precedes increases in the peripheral blood reticulocyte count by about 3 days.

It has been suggested that a corrected reticulocyte count should be calculated before reaching conclusions about the erythropoietic response to anemia. An ab-

solute reticulocyte count may be calculated by multiplying the percentage of reticulocytes by the RBC count (see Chap. 8). Similarly, a reticulocyte production index (RPI) can be calculated by correcting the reticulocyte percentage for the degree of anemia and reticulocyte maturation time (see Chap. 8). In the dog, an absolute reticulocyte count greater than 60,000/μl of blood indicates an erythropoietically more active marrow, a count greater than 100,000/μl indicates slightly more activity, and a moderate to marked erythropoietic activity is indicated by a count greater than 150,000/μl. An RPI greater than 1 indicates some response to anemia, and a value greater than 2 suggests an intense erythropoietic response.

Studies on the erythropoietic response of cats to blood loss anemia have indicated that both aggregate and punctate reticulocytes form an integral part of the reticulocyte count, and that a sustained reticulocytosis occurs during recovery from acute blood loss anemia. It was concluded that both types of reticulocytes must

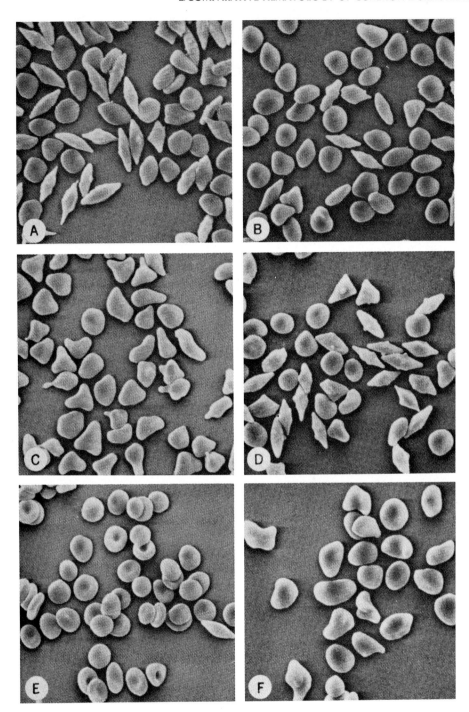

Fig. 2–5. Scanning electron photomicrographs of goat 6773 (*A–D*) and goat 6828 (*E, F*) before, during, and after recovery from experimentally induced blood loss anemia. The former goat had more than 50% fusiform erythrocytes, whereas the latter had nearly 98% discoid cells. (So that the reader can follow the effect of anemia on the erythrocyte morphology, the hemoglobin values for each sampling time are given in parentheses; see Table 2–18 and text for details). *A,* Prebleeding sample (Hb, 11.75 g/dl) containing many fusiform and discoid erythrocytes and a few odd-shaped cells. *B,* Three weeks postbleeding sample (Hb, 7.0 g/dl) showing a decrease in the proportion of fusiform erythrocytes and an increase in the discoid cells. *C,* Eight weeks postbleeding sample (Hb, 6.0 g/dl) depicting a marked poikilocytosis, but the absence of typical fusiform cells. *D,* 28 weeks postbleeding sample (Hb, 10.5 g/dl) showing the return of fusiform erythrocytes and many discoid cells essentially identical to those in *A. E,* Prebleeding sample (Hb, 11.0 g/dl) containing predominantly discoid, slightly concave erythrocytes, a few stomatocytic forms, and a fusiform cell. *F,* Five weeks postbleeding sample (Hb, 7.0 g/dl) depicting a marked poikilocytosis and a few macrocytes; this erythrocyte morphology reverted to prebleeding type by 28 weeks, as in the other goat (× 2000). (From Jain, N.C., et al.: Fusiform erythrocytes resembling sickle cells in Angora goats: Observations on osmotic and mechanical fragilities and reversal of cell shape during anaemia. Res. Vet. Sci., 28:25, 1980.)

be included in the reticulocyte count, but enumerated separately to determine past and present erythropoietic activity accurately. Aggregate reticulocytes appear in large numbers in early response, whereas punctate reticulocytes are seen at a later stage and parallel the increase in the PCV. An increase in primarily punctate reticulocytes in a cat may indicate a response to a previous episode of anemia. This is because punctate reticulocytes have a long circulating half-life (about 2 to 3 weeks) in cats. Furthermore, it has been shown that excitement and struggling during blood sampling can elevate the reticulocyte count in cats markedly, particularly in those with responsive anemia.

In the horse, erythrocytes are released into the peripheral blood in a mature state, so reticulocytes are not present in health. The horse is unique among domestic animals in the response of its erythropoietic tissue to acute blood loss or hemolytic anemia. Reticulocytes or polychromatic erythrocytes are absent or extremely rare in the circulation during anemia in remission. Hence, the reticulocyte count on the peripheral blood of an anemic horse is of little help in assessing erythropoietic response. Consequently, reticulocyte counts are performed on bone marrow aspirates to evaluate the erythropoietic response of an anemic horse; an increase in reticulocyte numbers greater than 5% indicates increased erythropoietic activity.

Reticulocytes are normally rare in the peripheral blood of ruminants and any increase, therefore, reflects stimulated erythropoietic activity. Reticulocytes appear in greater numbers in blood after acute hemorrhage or hemolytic destruction of erythrocytes. In sheep, a few reticulocytes (<1.0%) may be found at birth, but a higher number (up to 9.0%, including punctate reticulocytes) have been found in lambs 2 to 7 days of age. No reticulocytes are found in the peripheral blood of normal goats, but up to 5 to 6% reticulocytes have been found in response to acute blood loss.

BASOPHILIC STIPPLING

In ruminants, particularly cows and sheep, an occasional young erythrocyte may exhibit some basophilic stippling (delicate bluish, dot-like structures) as a species characteristic. Basophilic stippling of immature erythrocytes in these animals becomes more prominent during response to anemia (Plate XVII–10). Basophilic stippling may also occasionally be seen in dogs and cats with intense response to anemia, and is of no special significance insofar as the cause of the anemia is concerned. Basophilic stippling is most prominent in EDTA-anticoagulated blood and in rapidly dried blood films stained with Wright-Leishman stain without prior fixation with alcohol.

Basophilic stippling unassociated with anemias has been found in erythrocytes of dogs with chronic lead poisoning (Plate XVII–11). Because basophilic stippling in ruminants is a normal finding, it should not be taken as definitive evidence for lead poisoning; other tests, such as determination of the serum lead level, should be conducted to diagnose lead toxicity.

HEINZ BODIES

A feature unique to the erythrocyte of the family Felidae is the occurrence in health of a small, eccentric, refractile object called the Heinz body (Plates XVIII–1 to XVIII–4). This structure is rarely visible in blood films stained with Romanowsky stains. It appears as a small, pale area within the red cell or as a dense object along the periphery or slightly protruding from the cell margin. Heinz bodies are readily apparent in air-dried blood films stained with a vital stain such as 0.5% new methylene blue or methyl violet in physiologic saline. Heinz bodies appear as bluish structures or refractile bodies against a clear background of red cells. They are formed by the aggregation of fine granules of precipitated, denatured hemoglobin. The physiologic occurrence of Heinz bodies in the erythrocytes of all members of the family Felidae probably indicates an unusual propensity for hemoglobin denaturation. This has been ascribed to a large number

(eight) of reactive sulfhydryl groups in the feline hemoglobin molecule.

Heinz body formation is generally associated with oxidative damage to erythrocytes and results in hemolytic anemia. The incidence of Heinz bodies varies greatly among cat populations (from <1.0% to >50%), however, without evidence of hemolytic anemia. In healthy cats, Heinz bodies are currently believed to be of dietary origin (see Chap. 11). The Heinz body in the blood of healthy cats is usually 0.5 to 1 μm in diameter, occasionally up to 3.0 μm in diameter. The larger structure may be detected in the routinely stained dry blood film as a round, pale area near the edge of the cell or protruding from its surface. In some cats with large Heinz bodies, evidence indicative of accelerated erythrocyte replacement, such as anisocytosis and polychromasia, may be found.

When Heinz bodies are plentiful, hemoglobin determination by use of the cyanmethemoglobin method becomes inaccurate unless the hemolysate is centrifuged to remove suspended Heinz bodies before the reading is made in the spectrophotometer. Failure to remove the Heinz bodies leads to the reduced transmission of light and to a correspondingly increased value for the hemoglobin concentration. Inaccuracy in the hemoglobin value results in erroneous elevations of mean corpuscular hemoglobin (MCH) and mean corpuscular hemoglobin concentration (MCHC) values.

ERYTHROCYTE SEDIMENTATION RATE

The erythrocyte sedimentation rate (ESR) of canine and feline blood may be determined to obtain some useful information for the clinical evaluation of the patient. The extent of the ESR varies with the method used and is affected by various factors. Most importantly, the ESR varies inversely with the number of red cells. Hence, for proper evaluation of the influence of disease on the ESR, the observed ESR value must be corrected by subtracting from it the anticipated rate of fall caused entirely by the ratio of red cells to plasma. A correction table is available for ESR values of dogs obtained with the Wintrobe method (Table 2–19). The pattern of the ESR in cats is generally similar to that in the dog. A diphasic ESR is obtained when young red cells (reticulocytes) or leptocytes exhibit a propensity to settle slowly and mature, discoid red cells settle at a faster rate. A diphasic ESR is characteristically seen during response to immune-mediated hemolytic anemia, when reticulocytes settle slowly and clumped, mature, red cells coated with cold agglutinins settle more quickly.

The ESR has not been found to be useful in clinical practice with horses because of the natural rapid settling of their erythrocytes in anticoagulated blood. This rapid settling of equine red cells is also evident when they are suspended in sheep or dog plasma. Experimental observations have indicated that, if an ESR were to be determined on horse blood, a 20-minute reading with the Wintrobe method, using

Table 2–19. Relative Anticipated Erythrocyte Sedimentation Rate of Canine Blood

PCV (%)	ESR	PCV (%)	ESR	PCV (%)	ESR
9	82	23	40	37	13
10	79	24	38	38	12
11	76	25	36	39	11
12	73	26	34	40	10
13	70	27	32	41	9
14	67	28	30	42	8
15	64	29	28	43	7
16	61	30	26	44	6
17	58	31	24	45	5
18	55	32	22	46	4
19	52	33	20	47	3
20	49	34	18	48	2
21	46	35	16	49	1
22	43	36	14	50	0

* In mm in 1 hour. For example: (1) PCV 43, observed ESR 45, anticipated ESR 7 (from the table), corrected ESR is 45 − 7 = +38; (2) PCV 24, observed ESR 16, anticipated ESR 38 (from the table), corrected ESR is 16 − 38 = −22.

freshly drawn blood anticoagulated with EDTA, would be the most useful. A correction table for such ESR values for equine blood, analogous to that for canine blood, has been developed (Table 2–20). A 60-minute reading is taken with the Westergren technique.

Limited observations on equine patients have shown that, in disease, the ESR is more often less than anticipated rather than greater, even during inflammatory diseases. In contrast, a marked increase above the anticipated ESR is expected in the blood of dogs, cats, and humans with such conditions. It appears, therefore, that erythrocyte sedimentation is slowed in inflammatory diseases of the horse, rather than increased. The ESR in horses correlates inversely with the hematocrit and directly with fibrinogen level, plasma viscosity, and, to some extent, with serum total

Table 2–20. Anticipated 20-Minute Erythrocyte Sedimentation Rates in Horse Blood (ESR-20) for PCV Increments From 10 to 50%

PCV (%)	Anticipated ESR-20 (mm)	PCV (%)	Anticipated ESR-20 (mm)	PCV (%)	Anticipated ESR-20 (mm)
10	86 ± 1	26	58 ± 4	41	8 ± 4
11	85 ± 1	27	55 ± 4	42	5 ± 4
12	84 ± 1	28	53 ± 4	43	4 ± 4
13	83 ± 1	29	50 ± 4		
14	82 ± 1				
15	80 ± 1	30	47 ± 5	44	3.0 ± 1
16	78 ± 1	31	44 ± 5	45	2.5 ± 1
17	76 ± 1	32	40 ± 5	46	2.0 ± 1
		33	36 ± 5	47	1.5 ± 1
18	74 ± 2			48	1.0 ± 1
19	72 ± 2	34	32 ± 15	49	0.5 ± 1
20	70 ± 2	35	28 ± 15	50	0.0 ± 1
21	68 ± 2	36	24 ± 15		
		37	20 ± 15		
22	66 ± 3				
23	64 ± 3	38	17 ± 8		
24	62 ± 3	39	14 ± 8		
25	60 ± 3	40	11 ± 8		

globulin levels (Allen, 1988). Plasma viscosity is increased in horses following surgery (>1.8 centipoises, compared to the normal range of 1.43 to 1.74 centipoises) and in cases of chronic inflammation, parasitic infections, neoplasia, and paraproteinemia. Similarly, whole blood viscosity, corrected for PCV, is significantly increased in horses with colic, and may be used as a prognostic indicator (Andrews et al., 1990). Whole blood viscosity varies directly with the RBC count and is influenced by other factors, such as concentrations of total plasma protein, fibrinogen, and various globulins, rouleaux formation, red cell shape and deformability, and rate of blood flow in microcirculation (Andrews et al., 1992). It has been shown that increases in blood viscosity induced by increases in PCV may contribute substantially to exercise-induced pulmonary and systemic hypertension in ponies (Davis and Manohar, 1988).

Erythrocyte rouleaux may be found to a limited extent in sheep and, therefore, the red cell sedimentation may be anticipated. Erythrocytes of the pig exhibit a tendency to rouleau formation and sedimentation. A diphasic sedimentation is observed in suckling pigs during the period of most intense erythrogenesis. Bovine erythrocytes do not form rouleaux or sediment in health and these phenomena are rare, even in extremely sick animals.

ERYTHROCYTE OSMOTIC FRAGILITY

Among red cells of common domestic and laboratory animals, the small red cells of the goat appear to be the most sensitive to lysis by hypotonic saline. On the other hand, red cells of the dog are the least susceptible to osmotic changes, but they are more prone to lysis caused by a change in pH as compared to human or sheep red cells. Hence, osmotic fragility determinations should always be made with buffered saline solution. Maximum and minimum values of resistance to hypotonic saline solution have been measured and correlated to red cell diameter (Table 2–21). Apparently, smaller red cells have a limited ability to swell in hypotonic saline compared to larger red cells, so the latter can withstand more hypotonic shock than the former. Mature red cells normally yield a sigmoid osmotic fragility curve (Fig. 2–6), but the pattern may change in disease, particularly in immune-mediated hemolytic anemia (see Fig. 7–15). Reticulocytes are more resistant to osmotic lysis than mature erythrocytes, probably because of their greater surface area and higher metabolic activity for maintaining intracellular ionic balance.

The osmotic fragility of goat red cells may be related to the red cell shape, in that fusiform erythrocytes are more resistant to osmotic lysis than are normal caprine erythrocytes. Breed differences may occur in fragility of caprine red cells in that red cells of Pygmy goats are more susceptible to osmotic lysis and mechanical stress than red cells from Togenburg goats (Fairley et al. 1988). Erythrocyte osmotic fragility is increased in pigs genetically susceptible to malignant hyperthermia (O'Brien et al., 1985).

Table 2–21. Osmotic Fragility of Erythrocytes from Normal Adult Animals as Indicated by Maximum and Minimum Resistance to Hypotonic Saline Solutions

Animal	RBC Diameter (μm)	% of Buffered NaCl Solution (Max.)	(Min.)
Camel	7.5 × 4.4	0.21	0.30
Dog	7.0	0.29	0.50
Pig	6.0	0.29	0.52
Rat	6.3	0.30	0.42
Rabbit	6.7	0.30	0.50
Mouse	6.1	0.30	0.50
Guinea pig	7.5	0.30	0.52
Hamster	6.5	0.30	0.51
Horse	5.8	0.34	0.54
Donkey	6.2	0.35	0.54
Cat	5.8	0.36	0.60
Cow	5.8	0.38	0.59
Sheep	4.5	0.43	0.56
Goat	3.2	0.44	0.66

From Perk, K., Frei, Y. F., and Herz, A.: Osmotic fragility of red blood cells of young and mature domestic and laboratory animals. Am. J. Vet. Res., 25:1241, 1964.

Two populations of red cells were demonstrated in the blood of newborn lambs on the basis of erythrocyte osmotic fragility peaks. In cattle, osmotic resistance of erythrocytes to hypotonic saline is greatest at birth, decreases with growth over the next 3 to 5 months, and then increases to reach adult level by 2 years of age. A correlation is found between the type of hemoglobin and the fragility of the erythrocyte population. At birth, fetal hemoglobin constitutes about 60 to 90% of total hemoglobin. With advancing age fetal hemoglobin diminishes at a fairly steady rate, until it disappears after 8 to 12 weeks. Erythrocytes containing fetal hemoglobin are osmotically more resistant than erythrocytes containing an adult hemoglobin. Thus, the osmotic fragility of bovine erythrocytes increases as the larger fetal erythrocytes are replaced by smaller postnatal erythrocytes.

The natural occurrence of water intoxication associated in some instances with hemoglobinuria is a unique phenomenon occurring in young calves. The condition has been observed in calves 2 to 10 months of age, but most frequently it occurs in calves 3 to 5 months of age. It is during this period that the mean red cell size is lowest. Lysis of the more susceptible small erythrocytes apparently results as the plasma becomes hypotonic coincident with water overloading and the failure of rapid development of diuresis.

The determination of erythrocyte osmotic fragility may be helpful to establish the pathogenesis of a hemolytic anemia. For example, the erythrocyte osmotic fragility is usually increased in autoimmune hemolytic anemia in dogs and cats because of antibody-mediated damage to the red cells and the formation of spherocytes (Plate XVI–4; Fig. 7–15). Similarly, parasitized red cells, as in haemobartonellosis in cats and anaplasmosis in cows, are highly fragile. Dogs with pyruvate kinase deficiency may show increased resistance to osmotic lysis because of highly elevated reticulocyte counts. A marked increase in the osmotic fragility of incubated red cells may be seen, however, because of the reduced ability of their red cells to produce the ATP needed to maintain the intracellular osmotic balance. Mechanical fragility but not the osmotic fragility of canine erythrocytes is increased during postprandial lipemia (Plate II–4).

ERYTHROCYTE LIFE SPAN

The erythrocytes of each species have a characteristic, finite, intravascular life span (see Table 7–2). Species having a mean erythrocyte life span of less than 100 days normally have some reticulocytes in the peripheral blood, but no reticulocytes are normally found in the circulation of species with longer erythrocyte life spans (horse, cow, sheep, and goat). The erythrocyte life span is shorter in newborns than in the adults. The red cell life span of adult sheep is not related to their hemoglobin type or to the presence of the high-K$^+$ (HK) or low-K$^+$ (LK) type of erythrocytes, but it is short for erythrocytes deficient in glutathione. In some species (cats, dogs, sheep, horses, cattle, and Mongolian gerbils), the mean erythrocyte life span may be inversely proportional to the pyrimidine 5′-nucleotidase activity of red cells. The erythrocyte life span is reduced in hemolytic anemias and in anemias of nutritional deficiencies (e.g., iron deficiency anemia).

HEMOGLOBIN TYPES

Embryonic, fetal, and adult hemoglobins have been recognized in various species. Fetal hemoglobin gradually replaces embryonic hemoglobin during gestation, and constitutes approximately 90 to 95% of the hemoglobin present at birth in many mammalian species. Fetal hemoglobin is usually replaced by adult hemoglobin(s) within 4 to 8 weeks after birth, but in some species this may take a few months. One to two adult hemoglobins have been identified in dogs, cats, horses and pigs and one to six in cows, sheep, and goats (see Table 7–6).

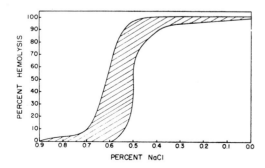

Fig. 2–6. Osmotic fragility curve for erythrocytes of the cat. (From Jain, N.C.: Schalm's Veterinary Hematology. 4th Ed. Philadelphia, Lea & Febiger, 1986, p. 132.)

Common adult hemoglobin types in sheep and goats are A, B, and AB. Hemoglobin C occurs in lambs soon after birth, with a rise to about 10 to 30% followed by a gradual disappearance. Hemoglobin C reappears in response to blood loss anemia in sheep of hemoglobin types A and AB but not in type B sheep. Hemoglobin C has a higher oxygen affinity compared to hemoglobins A and B but releases oxygen more readily than hemoglobins A and B and, therefore, may be advantageous under conditions of tissue hypoxia. The switch from hemoglobin A to C is easier to induce in goats than in sheep. In addition, for comparable degrees of anemia, goats apparently produce more hemoglobin C than do sheep, and the rate of disappearance of hemoglobin C from blood is slower in goats than in sheep. The A to C switching is stimulated by erythropoietin.

Physiologic Variations in Erythrocyte Parameters

INTERRELATIONSHIP OF ERYTHROCYTE PARAMETERS

In a normal animal, the hemoglobin occupies one-third of the volume of the red cell. Therefore, it is possible to predict the hemoglobin concentration by dividing the PCV by 3, or vice versa. A rough estimate of the RBC number in millions/μl of blood can be obtained by dividing the PCV by 6. This relationship does not hold when laboratory errors occur in the determination of various red cell parameters and it may change during disease states. For example, in dwarfism in the Alaskan malamute, the PCV:hemoglobin ratio is regularly 4:1 or 5:1 instead of 3:1. This interrelationship of erythrocyte parameters also does not apply for certain animals, such as camels and other members of the family Camelidae.

FETAL BLOOD VALUES

The fetal blood values of cats, cows, sheep, and pigs have been determined. In general, RBC, hemoglobin, and PCV values in the fetus increase progressively, and are highest at birth. Fetal erythrocytes are larger than those of the adult. The MCV and MCH decrease gradually during fetal life and for a few months after birth before stabilizing, whereas the MCHC fluctuates inconsistently within a narrow range. For example, the MCV in fetal calves decreases throughout gestation from a high of 90 to 100 fl to half that size (about 46 fl) at birth (see Fig. 4–3). Erythrocyte size continues to decrease for the first 3 to 4 months in the neonatal calf, reaching a value of 37.8 ± 3.2 fl. This gradual reduction in the MCV coincides with the disappearance of fetal hemoglobin and its replacement by hemoglobin A. Erythrocyte size gradually increases again after the fourth month, paralleling a gradual decrease in the RBC count (Table 2–14).

Nucleated erythrocytes are prominent during early fetal life, but decrease to small numbers at birth. The reticulocyte count is high in fetal blood and at birth.

Fetal erythrocytes seem to be osmotically more resistant than adult erythrocytes. Plasma protein and fibrinogen concentrations are low during fetal life, except for the last few weeks before birth when an increase may be seen. Plasma protein values at birth, however, are significantly lower than adult values in all species. In comparison, fibrinogen concentration in neonates is generally at the adult level.

AGE DIFFERENCES

As mentioned above, the newborn has large erythrocytes of fetal origin. As fetal erythrocytes are replaced by cells of smaller size, the MCV becomes reduced, so that by 2 to 12 months of age the erythrocyte size is representative of the normal adult of that species (see Table 2–14). Similarly, the MCH is high at birth and decreases to about the normal adult level during the same period, whereas the MCHC varies only slightly with age. Red cell indices attain normal adult values earlier (by 2 to 3 months of age) in the dog than in the horse (by 10 to 12 months of age). Erythrocyte volume distribution curves, obtained by modern automated cell counting machines, depict such changes in erythrocyte size better than the MCV. Aged horses (≥20 years old) consistently showed larger erythrocytes than young horses (≤5 years old), although MCVs in the aged horses were within reference range (Ralston et al., 1988).

Blood values for animals of different age groups have been reported for dogs (Tables 2–8 and 2–9), cats (Table 2–10), horses (Tables 2–11 and 2–12), cattle (Tables 2–13, 2–14, and 2–15), sheep (Table 2–16), and pigs (Table 2–17). In general, RBC, hemoglobin, and PCV values are high at birth, but fall rapidly as the newborn begins to nurse. A reduction in these parameters continues during the first month or so of postnatal life. At about the beginning of the second month of life, a gradual increase in RBC, hemoglobin, and PCV values takes place and continues until adult levels have been attained, at about 1 year of age. Age-related decreases in red cell values may continue to occur steadily for a few years in some species (e.g., the horse). Red cell counts may uncommonly decline with age to anemic levels in some high-producing dairy cows and certain breeds of dogs (e.g., greyhounds). No significant age-related differences were found in hematologic parameters in beagle dogs 3 to 14 years of age (Lowseth et al., 1990).

The decline in red cell values during the first week of life is related to the rapid expansion of plasma volume from colostrum consumption, increased destruction of fetal erythrocytes, and inadequate supply of iron needed for hemoglobin synthesis. The most dramatic changes are seen in piglets, which may experience as much as a 30% reduction in the RBC count (Table 2–17). Colostrum consumption during the first 24 hours of life is also associated with an increase in total plasma protein and globulin levels as a result of absorption of globulins through the gut.

Because of the low iron content of milk, nursing

animals (puppies, kittens, lambs, calves, and piglets) become deficient in iron as their blood volume expands to accommodate the increasing body size. Some calves may be born anemic (PCV < 25%) and have low levels of serum iron, possibly as a result of congenital iron deficiency anemia. Anemic animals and animals with a low PCV respond quickly to iron therapy, such as the administration of iron dextran. Similarly, the injection of iron dextran into newborn animals prevents the decrease in hemoglobin and PCV values observed in untreated animals.

Erythrocyte sedimentation is nil or slight at birth and it is generally negative during the first few weeks of life because of low total plasma protein values during the neonatal period. In some species, a diphasic sedimentation rate may be observed as a reflection of the high number of reticulocytes in blood. The icterus index may be high in the newborns of some species (foals and calves).

BREED DIFFERENCES

Breed differences are found in blood values, particularly in red cell parameters. Certain breeds of dogs tend to have high RBC, hemoglobin, and PCV values, which may sometimes exceed the normal range provided for the species. Dogs most frequently involved have been poodles, German shepherds, boxers, beagles, dachshunds, Chihuahuas, greyhounds, Afghan hounds, salukis, and whippets. It is highly probable that these breeds have a normal PCV, between 50 and 55%, that becomes elevated as a result of apprehension or fear. The animal that becomes apprehensive when being examined by a veterinarian may experience contraction of the spleen, forcing a concentrated mass of erythrocytes into the circulation. Such a change is not seen in splenectomized animals. Other examples of breed differences in blood values of the dog include the Japanese Akita, which generally exhibits MCV values of 55 to 65 fl, and certain poodles, which show macrocytosis in that their MCV is normally over 80 fl, compared to the reference range of 60 to 77 fl for the adult dog.

Among horses, thoroughbreds generally have greater RBC counts, lower MCV values, and higher total blood volume in relation to body weight than other breeds. In comparison with hot-blooded horses, cold-blooded horses have lower RBC counts, hemoglobin and PCV values, and blood volume. The ESR is relatively high in cold-blooded animals (von Hammerl and Kraft, 1983). The mean N:L ratio in a cold-blooded horse is 1.7:1.0, as compared to 1.0:1.0 in thoroughbreds and Arabians. American miniature horses have a lower RBC count, as do donkeys and ponies, and an N:L ratio opposite that of full-sized horses (37:59 versus 53:39) (Harvey and Hambright, 1985).

Statistically significant breed differences have been found in cattle, but the differences are not large enough to cause concern in the clinical interpretation of hemograms. In general, Jersey, Guernsey, and Brown Swiss cattle have a lower RBC count, whereas Charlais have higher RBC, hemoglobin, and PCV values than most other breeds.

SEX DIFFERENCES AND INFLUENCE OF PARTURITION AND LACTATION

Investigators disagree about sex differences in the circulating mass of erythrocytes. Slightly higher mean values for hemoglobin concentration in males than in females have been reported in studies involving dogs, cats, horses, cattle, pigs, and goats. Female horses have higher mean WBC counts than males because they have slightly more neutrophils and lymphocytes. The differences in blood values between the sexes, however, seem to be of little practical value.

Observations on pregnant mares, sows, sheep, and bitches indicate that during gestation red cell parameters become gradually reduced and remain low until a few weeks postpartum. The decline in erythrocyte parameters during the last part of gestation is primarily a hemodilution effect resulting from an increased plasma volume, which may increase by as much as 23% in sheep. The total plasma protein concentration also declines during pregnancy.

Lactation-related changes in cows may be irregular and vary from herd to herd. In general, nonlactating cows have higher RBC, hemoglobin, and PCV values than lactating cows. This decline in red cell values may be related to milk yield; high producers tend to have lower red cell values than low producers, and a few may even develop anemia, particularly during the winter. In bitches, red cell values begin to recover at lactation and normal levels are generally attained after weaning (Allard et al., 1989).

INFLUENCE OF ALTITUDE

It is well known that reduced oxygen tension leads to the increased production and release of erythropoietin, thereby stimulating erythropoiesis. Cattle grazing on high mountain ranges naturally experience an increase in RBC, hemoglobin, and PCV values. When 11 cattle were studied at an elevation of 5000 feet (1524 m) in early summer, their mean RBC count was 8.7 million/μl of blood. These cattle were transferred to an elevation of 9000 feet (2743 m) in late summer; at this time, their mean RBC count was 9.2 million/μl. It was stated that the effect of altitude is much greater than the data indicated at first glance, because the latter counts were made in late summer, when previous experience had shown that the RBC count normally declines.

ROLE OF THE SPLEEN

The spleen serves as a large reservoir of erythrocytes that can be released into the circulation within minutes during periods of excitement or strenuous exercise. The red cell parameters of the horse increase promptly with excitement, twitching, handling, exertion, and racing (Table 2–22). The slight excitement caused by

Table 2–22. Effect of Strenuous Exercise in the Horse on Red Cell Mass and Total Leukocyte Count

Date	Condition	RBC ($\times 10^6/\mu l$)	PCV (%)	Hb (g/dl)	WBC (/μl)
Jan. 13	Rest	7.97	40	13.3	8,050
	Exercise	11.28	52	17.5	10,700
Jan 26	Rest	7.90	36.5	13.5	8,500
	Exercise	10.80	50	17.0	10,200
Feb. 10*	Rest	10.60	53	17.0	9,250
	Exercise	9.43	51.5	16.9	8,650
Feb. 25	Rest	9.42	47	15.8	8,800
	Exercise	11.02	54	17.5	9,550
Mar. 10	Rest	8.32	43	14.5	9,000
	Exercise	11.40	56	18.6	11,450

* Stranger present.

venipuncture by a stranger may result in an increase in the RBC count of 10 to 15%, and greater elevations can occur with increases in the degree and duration of physical stress, although individual variations are found. Similarly, a high normal PCV may reflect the influence of emotional stress found under basal conditions, particularly in females (Martinez et al., 1988). Larger differences may be seen with an increase in age of the horse. The normalization of red cell parameters in an excited animal may take about 40 to 60 minutes or several hours, depending on the extent of excitement. Such effects of splenic contraction on red cell values have also been observed in other species.

The increase in red cell parameters seen after exertion is attributed largely to splenic contraction and partly to reduction in plasma volume. The splenic release of red cells is considered an epinephrine effect. Physical stress or epinephrine injection does not cause an increase in PCV in splenectomized animals. The

relaxing effect of certain anesthetics may cause erythrocytes to become sequestered in the spleen. Thus, anesthetics such as promazine hydrochloride, acetylpromazine, barbiturates, and halothane cause a decrease in the PCV. A concomitant slight decrease in plasma protein concentration may also be seen. In comparison, anesthetics such as ether and nitrous oxide cause an increase in the PCV, presumably because of splenic contraction. Both PCV values and total plasma protein concentrations have been found to increase in horses immediately after a swimming exercise (Garcia and Beech, 1986).

In addition to changes in red cell values, the MCV is increased and the MCHC and MCH are decreased in horses after vigorous exercise (Smith et al., 1989). The red cell shape and deformability are not altered, but cells released from the splenic reservoir are apparently more resistant to osmotic lysis. Whole blood and plasma viscosity are increased (Coyne et al., 1990).

A slight increase in total plasma protein concentration may also occur from a compensatory movement of fluid out of the vessels into the tissues. Platelet counts may also increase because the spleen sequesters about one-third of the circulating platelet mass. Slight to moderate increase in WBC counts may also occur on exertion, primarily because of increases in the numbers of neutrophils and/or lymphocytes from marginal pools (Table 2–23).

INFLUENCE OF TRAINING HORSES

Training race horses was found to increase total blood volume and elevate hemoglobin concentration by as much as 30% within 2 years. In addition, changes also occurred in some other blood values: the ESR, erythrocyte 2,3-diphosphoglycerate, and serum folate

Table 2–23. Effect of Strenuous Muscular Activity and Excitement on Circulating Erythrocyte Volume (PCV), Total Leukocyte Count, and Differential Leukocyte Count in Yearling Horses

Sequence of Being Caught	Sex	Signs of Excitement	PCV (%)	WBC/μl	Differential Leukocyte Count in Absolute Numbers/μl					N:L Ratio
					Neutrophils	Lymphocytes	Monocytes	Eosinophils	Basophils	
1*	F	No comment	37	13,900	6,046	7,158	418	278	0	0.84:1.0
2	F	No comment	42	17,700	6,372	9,205	1,150	796	177	0.69:1.0
3	F	Slight excitement	41	16,100	6,279	8,694	483	644	0	0.72:1.0
4*	F	No comment	37	13,630	5,822	6,918	274	616	0	0.84:1.0
5	F	Slight excitement	43	18,000	7,110	9,720	540	630	0	0.73:1.0
6*	F	No comment	38	11,700	5,148	5,616	468	468	0	0.92:1.0
7	F	No comment	45	19,200	4,920	11,870	770	1,544	96	0.41:1.0
8	XM†	Excited	42	19,100	12,572	5,568	96	864	0	2.26:1.0
9*	F	No comment	39	16,700	6,596	8,100	584	1,420	0	0.81:1.0
10	XM	No comment	40	14,400	4,896	8,712	288	504	0	0.56:1.0
11	XM	Excited	44	22,800	7,296	14,022	570	798	114	0.52:1.0
12	XM	Excited	42	23,200	14,384	7,076	1,160	580	0	2.03:1.0
13	XM	Excited	43	26,300	11,572	13,544	790	394	0	0.85:1.0
14	F	No comment	44	20,300	7,410	11,164	914	812	0	0.66:1.0
15	XM	No comment	44	16,600	3,735	10,956	1,079	830	0	0.34:1.0
16	XM	Excited	40	20,200	6,666	12,625	606	303	0	0.53:1.0

From Schalm, O.W., and Hughes, J.P.: Some observations on physiologic leukocytosis in the cat and horse. Cal. Vet., 18:23, 1964.
* Hemograms approximating normal control values.
† M, gelding

concentrations decreased, whereas serum bilirubin increased significantly. Exercise-induced changes in greyhounds included increases in PCV, RBC, WBC, and hemoglobin values (Snow et al., 1988).

IRON REQUIREMENT OF SUCKLING PIGS

Milk is notoriously low in iron. Nursing puppies, kittens, piglets, lambs, and goat kids rapidly develop iron deficiency if not given supplemental iron during the period of rapid growth. The most dramatic observations in this regard have been made on pigs. Newborn piglets have a mean hemoglobin level of 10 to 12 g/dl of blood, and their mean total body iron content is about 50 mg. Less than 10% of this iron is in reserve and available for new blood formation. Suckling pigs grow rapidly. Their weight is doubled by the end of the first week of life and a gain of four times the birthweight can be expected by the end of the third or fourth week. Unless a source of iron is available, the pigs become severely anemic during the first 2 to 3 weeks of postnatal life, leading to stunting, lowered resistance to disease, and some deaths. Spontaneous recovery begins about the fifth or sixth week of life, when the pigs begin to take nourishment in addition to milk.

Contact with soil early in the life of the pig is important in the prevention of anemia. Soil may contain as much as 1.5% iron, and pigs begin to root and eat dirt about the third or fourth day. Supplementing the ration of the sow with iron during pregnancy and lactation may lead to a slight increase in the iron content of the milk, but this is not sufficient to prevent the development of anemia in the baby pigs. Pigs receiving no added iron develop microcytic-hypochromic anemia within 6 weeks of birth as a result of decreased hemoglobin synthesis. About 125 parts per million (ppm) of oral iron appear to be adequate to maintain the RBC count and hemoglobin concentration at normal levels in growing pigs. Iron may be supplied to suckling pigs by the daily application of a saturated solution of iron sulfate to the teats of the sow or by dosing pigs daily during the second week of life with 30 mg of iron pyrophosphate. A less tedious procedure is to give a single intramuscular injection of 100 mg of an iron-dextran complex on the fourth day of life. Copper-deficient pigs develop microcytic anemia from shortened red cell survival. The red cell life span of iron-deficient pigs is said to be normal.

LEUKOCYTES

Morphologic Characteristics

NEUTROPHILS

In most species, neutrophils are produced in the bone marrow over a period of 3 to 7 days. Their release into the general circulation is regulated by humoral factors as well as by need in body tissues.

Once in blood, neutrophils distribute into the circulating and marginal pools almost equally, or sometimes preferentially into the latter (cats). They leave the circulation randomly, with a half-time of disappearance of about 6 to 14 hours in different species (see Chap. 13 for details).

Mature or Segmented Neutrophils. The nucleus of the mature neutrophil is irregularly lobed (Figs. 2–7A, 2–7B, and 2–7I). Filaments joining two lobes are occasionally seen, but simple narrowing between lobes without true filament formation is the rule among animals, compared to humans. The chromatin is clumped into large, deeply stained masses separated by lighter staining ground substance (Plates VII–1 and VII–8). The nuclear membrane is irregular, or "moth-eaten." The cytoplasm stains faintly and contains diffuse, distinct or indistinct, pinkish or pale granules. Granular staining may be prominent in some species to the extent that the cells may resemble eosinophils. Such cells, with deep pink to reddish purple granules, are known as heterophils or pseudoeosinophils (Fig. 3–1; Plate XXVII–1). Heterophils are common in the blood of laboratory animals, birds, elephants, primates, and reptiles.

Band Neutrophils. Band neutrophils are present in normal blood only in small numbers. The nucleus is a curved band (horseshoe-shaped) having a smooth nuclear membrane and parallel sides to an appreciable length (Fig. 2–7C). The chromatin is somewhat less clumped than in the mature cell. Because of the heavy chromatin plaques at the nuclear membrane, the nuclear outline of the band neutrophil in the horse is more irregular than in other domestic animals (Plate VII–8). The cytoplasmic features are characteristic of the mature neutrophil. Band neutrophils with or without toxic changes in the cytoplasm are common in the blood of patients with bacterial infections and inflammatory diseases (Plates XI–10, XI–11, and XII–6). Neutrophilic metamyelocytes and more immature cells of the neutrophil lineage are normally not found in blood.

Female Sex Chromatin Lobe. The nuclei of some neutrophil leukocytes of the female characteristically reveal a chromatin appendage called the drumstick or Barr body (Fig. 2–7B; Plate XI–7). The typical drumstick may be found in about 1 to 7% of the neutrophils of the female dog and in 4 to 11% of the neutrophils of the female cat. Occasionally, eosinophils in blood and mature and band neutrophils in bone marrow may also reveal a sex chromatin lobe. Neutrophils may occasionally also show minor lobes and sessile nodules in either sex (Fig. 2–7C). Rarely, the drumstick lobe may be found in males.

EOSINOPHILS

Eosinophil granules have a weak to strong affinity for the eosin stain. In Wright-stained blood films, granule color is normally only a little more intense than that of erythrocytes in the same blood film (Figs. 2–7C, 2–7D, and 2–7E). A slightly better staining can be achieved using Wright-Leishman, May-Grünwald,

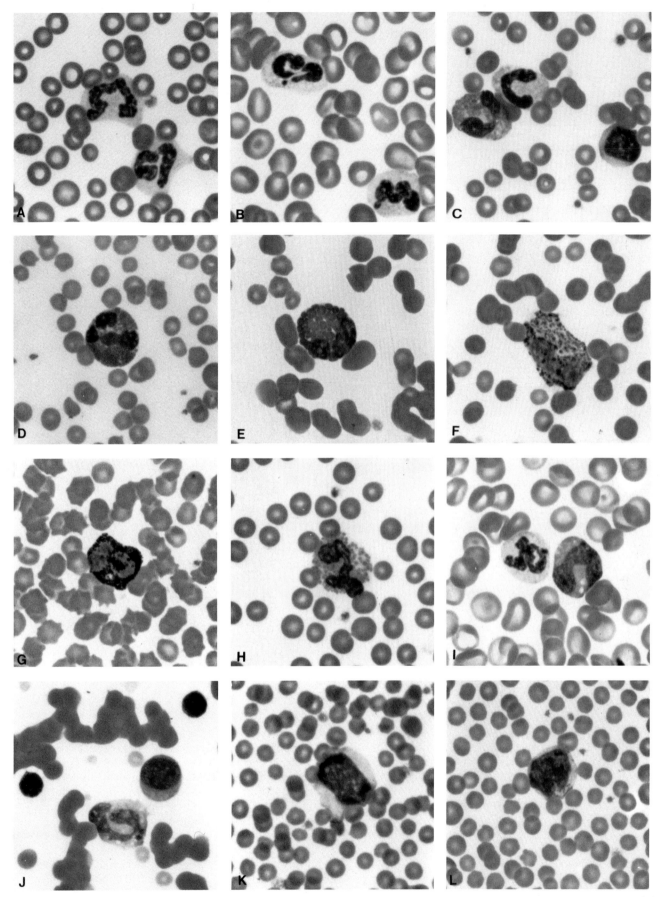

Fig. 2–7. Leukocytes in blood of common domestic animals: A, feline neutrophils. B, canine neutrophils with a sex chromatin lobe (upper left) and a sessile body (lower right). C, feline band neutrophil, mature eosinophil, and small lymphocyte. D, bovine eosinophil. E, equine eosinophil. F, equine basophil. G, porcine basophil. H, feline basophil. I, canine neutrophil and monocyte. J, equine monocyte, two small lymphocytes, and a medium lymphocyte. K, bovine large lymphocyte. L, bovine lymphocyte with indented nucleus and several small azurophilic granules. (×1800).

or Giemsa stain. The nucleus may be segmented or poorly lobed and partially obscured by granules. The granules commonly fill the cytoplasm. The cytoplasm between the granules takes a light blue to pale stain.

Eosinophil granules vary in size and shape among different species. Granule morphology is characteristic of certain species. For example, the cat typically has rod-like granules (Fig. 2–7C and Plate VII–6), and the horse has the largest granules seen in common domestic animals (Fig. 2–7E; Plate VII–7). Granule shape in cat eosinophils is best observed when the granules are less compact in the cytoplasm or when the granules are freely dispersed because of cell rupture. In the horse, eosinophil granules are large, tightly packed, and almost completely fill the cytoplasm. Because of the larger size of the granules, the cell outline conforms to the granule contour, giving the cell a raspberry-like appearance. The eosinophil leukocyte of the cow is readily identifiable by its numerous small, round, jewel-like, intensely red, refractile granules of uniform size (Plate VII–4). The granules in canine eosinophils are generally small and uniform (Plate XII–1). An occasional canine eosinophil may contain a few vacuolated granules and, infrequently, eosinophils with extremely large granules may be found, particularly in dogs with eosinophilias (Plate XII–2). Occasionally, a few small cytoplasmic vacuoles may be seen in canine eosinophils; they correspond to electron-lucent, membrane-bound structures seen on electron microscopy (see Fig. 14–2). The eosinophil of the adult greyhound is highly vacuolated. The ultrastructure of cat and sheep eosinophil granules is distinctive in that they appear crystalloid, whereas equine eosinophil granules are homogeneous (see Figs. 14–3 and 14–4).

BASOPHILS

In methanol-fixed blood films stained with Wright stain, basophil granules stain metachromatically (reddish-purple) in a gray-blue cytoplasm (Figs. 2–7F and 2–7G). The granules vary in number and size. They may pack the cell, as in the cow (Plate VII–5) and horse (Plate VII–7), or they may partially fill the cytoplasm, as in the dog (Plate XII–1). Basophil granules are water-soluble and tend to disappear in unfixed films stained with new methylene blue. In poorly fixed smears, the basophil granules may appear smudged, partially vacuolated or less numerous from dissolution. The nucleus of the mature basophil tends to coil, with a limited tendency toward lobe formation. Basophils rarely occur in normal blood, but tend to appear in appreciable numbers in association with eosinophilia (see Table 14–1). Special stains such as toluidine blue, omega-exonuclease, and naphthol AS-D choloracetate esterase (Plate X–10) may be used to demonstrate basophils in blood.

The cat basophil presents a unique morphology as compared to the basophils of other domestic animals. Generally, the mature basophil contains numerous small, round, lightly stained (pinkish, orangish, or grayish) granules in light gray cytoplasm (Fig. 2–7H;

Plate VII–6). Some basophils may, in addition, contain a few somewhat larger, darkly stained purplish granules (Plate XII–5). These cells are believed to be less mature forms of basophils, because basophil precursors (myelocytes) in the bone marrow of the cat often show the two types of granules (Plates V–2 and XII–4).

LYMPHOCYTES

Lymphocytes vary in size from small to large. Small lymphocytes most commonly occur in the dog and cat, whereas large lymphocytes are frequently seen in the cow. In small lymphocytes the nucleus is generally round and almost fills the cell, leaving only a narrow rim or crescent of cytoplasm (Figs. 2–7C and 2–7J). The nuclear chromatin is clumped and stains deeply. The cytoplasm varies in color, but is usually pale blue. Occasionally, a small lymphocyte with intensely blue stained cytoplasm may be found; the cell is then known as an immunocyte. Medium and large lymphocytes have modest to abundant pale blue cytoplasm and less deeply stained nuclei (Figs. 2–7J and 2–7K; Plate VII–2). An occasional lymphocyte may have a slightly indented nucleus and sometimes the cytoplasm may be more on one side of the cell because of eccentric location of the nucleus. An infrequent lymphocyte may present a cluster of small, reddish-purple (azurophilic) granules in the cytoplasm (Fig. 2–7L; Plate VII–3). Such lymphocytes are more common in cows than in other domestic animals.

In the cow, some large lymphocytes may present a kidney bean or clefted nucleus. A lymphocyte with the latter form of nucleus is called a Reider cell; such cells are more common in animals with lymphocytic leukemia. The finding of an occasional lymphocyte with a nucleolus or faint nucleolar rings in bovine blood should be viewed with extreme caution as a sign of lymphocytic leukemia, because such cells may be found in health. Lymphoblasts are not found in the peripheral blood of other species in health. Some large lymphocytes in cows may be difficult to distinguish from monocytes. It has been shown that cells that appear to be large lymphocytes by light microscopy may have the ultrastructural features of monocytes.

MONOCYTES

The monocyte is generally the largest of the mature leukocytes in the blood. Its characteristic features are a basophilic ground-glass cytoplasm and a pleomorphic nucleus (Figs. 2–7I and 2–7J). The cytoplasm commonly presents vacuoles that vary in size and are frequently clustered at one side of the cell or are found along the cell periphery (Plates VII–3, VII–10, and VIII–9). An occasional vacuole may appear to be within the nucleus. The cytoplasm may also reveal few to many dust-like, pinkish, azurophilic granules. The nucleus is extremely variable and is said to be "amoeboid," in that it can assume any shape (Plate VIII–9). It is often broad, irregular, and without lobulation. The nucleus may at times resemble that of the early band neutrophil or late metamyelocyte (Plates VIII–5 to VIII–8). The ends of the band-like nucleus of the monocyte, however, are enlarged and knob-like. The nuclear chromatin is characteristically streaky, diffuse, or mesh-like. When chromatin clumping or condensation is present, it generally does not assume the uniform pattern that is present in cells of the neutrophilic series. In cells with confusing nuclear shapes, the monocytes can be distinguished by their relatively bluish and denser staining cytoplasm compared to pale cytoplasm of neutrophils (Plates VIII–7 and VIII–8).

Physiologic Variations in Leukocyte Counts

The differential leukocyte count is expressed both in percentage and absolute number of each cell type per microliter of blood. Responses to disease are more critically evaluated from absolute values than from percentages. The normal values of the total leukocyte and differential counts for common domestic animals are given in Tables 2–1 to 2–7. The normal values are lower and the ranges are narrower for animals maintained in colonies developed for research purposes than are similar values for small groups of animals or an animal population at large. Little sex difference occurs, but significant age differences may occur in both the total and differential leukocyte counts (Tables 2–8 and 2–11 to 2–17). Some breed, diurnal, seasonal, and physiologic (as during pregnancy) variations have been noted for dogs. Breed differences in WBC counts have also been found in cattle and horses, but these do not seem to be significant enough to influence the clinical interpretation of leukocyte values in these animals.

The normal range of the WBC count for different animals includes the effects of age and normal activity. The normal range for the WBC count is similar in the cow, sheep, and goat. Lymphocyte numbers in these species generally exceed neutrophil counts, giving a neutrophil:lymphocyte (N:L) ratio of less than one. The WBC count has a wider range in the dog and cat. Neutrophil numbers in these species generally exceed lymphocyte counts, giving an N:L ratio of greater than one. It is interesting to note that the absolute values of neutrophils and lymphocytes are reversed in germ-free cats as compared to conventional laboratory cats. The N:L ratio of germ-free cats changes to that usually seen in conventional cats after recovery from infections such as feline panleukopenia or feline rhinotrachiitis.

INFLUENCE OF AGE AND THE NEUTROPHIL:LYMPHOCYTE RATIO

Leukocytes are usually absent or low in number at early stages of fetal life. Leukocyte numbers gradually increase during gestation and, at birth, are usually above normal adult values. Species variations occur in the predominant leukocyte type seen at birth. For example, neutrophils generally exceed lymphocytes in cattle, sheep, and pigs, whereas the reverse is found in horses and goats. The N:L ratio in newborn calves declines rapidly and may reverse during the first week (Fig. 2–8). The higher N:L ratio at birth is attributed to the stress-induced increased secretion of corticosteroids at birth and their effects on neutrophils and lymphocytes. Calves delivered by cesarean have N:L ratios similar to those in adult cattle, whereas calves delivered after dystocia may show marked stress-induced changes.

With advancing age, the absolute neutrophil count remains essentially unchanged but lymphocyte numbers decline progressively, yielding a high N:L ratio. For example, the N:L ratio in horses changes over the first 3 months from 2.88:1.0 at birth to 1.1:1.0 at an average age of 51 days because of a substantial increase in lymphocyte numbers and some decrease in neutrophil numbers (Table 2–11). Lymphocyte numbers continue to increase, resulting in an N:L ratio below 1.0 between 6 and 8 months and a peak lymphocyte count at 7 months. The lymphocyte numbers then decline to reverse the trend. Thus, the 1.0:1.0 ratio attained during the early life of the foal persists throughout the first 1 to 2 years of life and then the ratio increases as lymphocyte numbers are reduced and neutrophil numbers remain stable. In comparison, the N:L ratio is high (about 2.0:1.0) in race horses with "poor performance" syndrome (Fogarty and Leadon, 1987). The N:L ratio may similarly increase in goats because of an age-related decreasing trend in lymphocyte numbers and an increasing trend in neutrophils (Somvanski et al., 1987). The gradual decrease of lymphocyte numbers in humans with age is attributed to a decline primarily in T lymphocytes because of declining thymic function, but B lymphocyte numbers remain stable. In cattle, the number of null cells also decreases.

Young dogs, cats, and horses have high lymphocyte counts and hence a greater tendency to develop physiologic lymphocytosis than adults. The extent of decrease in lymphocytes with age is useful when interpreting the degree of stress imposed by the disease. Lymphopenia may be said to exist when the absolute lymphocyte count is lower than 2000/μl of blood in dogs 3 to 6 months of age, lower than 1500 in dogs 8 to 24 months of age, and lower than 1000 in dogs over 2 years of age. Similarly, an age-related decrease in lymphocyte numbers in calves should be taken into consideration when screening animals for persistent lymphocytosis, which is considered to be a prodromal sign of impending lymphocytic leukemia in cattle. A high lymphocyte count is characteristic of certain pigs between 4 and 18 weeks of age.

Circulating eosinophil numbers in some animals may also change with age. A mean count of 1.5% in calves during the first 6 months of life increases steadily to 10.0% or more in adult cattle. High eosinophil counts in lactating dairy cows might represent an allergic reaction to their own milk or parasitism. Higher eosinophil and basophil numbers may be found in the adults of most species, probably as a result of changes

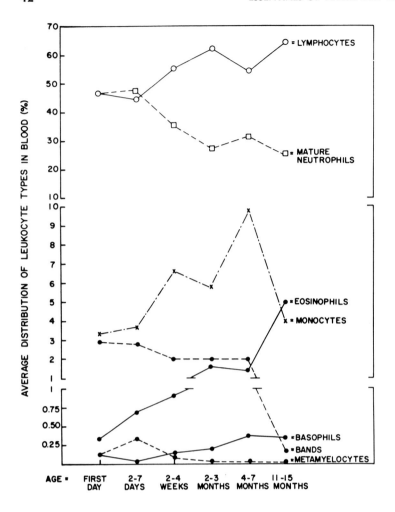

Fig. 2–8. Graphic depiction of the changes occurring in the differential distribution of leukocytes in blood during the first year of life of cattle. (From Straub, O.C.: Über das Blutbild von gesunden kalbern leukosefrier Herkunst in den ersten 3 Lebensmonaten und vergleichende Untersuchungen an gleichaltrigen klinisch gesunden Kalbern aus Leukosebestanden. Inaug. diss., Tierärztl. Hochsch., Hanover, Germany, 1956.

in immunologic experience, particularly after parasitism. The numbers of monocytes do not seem to be greatly influenced by age.

PHYSIOLOGIC LEUKOCYTOSIS

The leukocytosis produced by psychologic and physical activity is called "physiologic leukocytosis" as opposed to the "reactive leukocytosis" seen in response to disease. Physiologic leukocytosis often occurs in acutely stressed animals. The stress may be physical, emotional, or induced by disease. Changes in WBC counts under such circumstances are mediated through the release of epinephrine and corticosteroids. Major differences in the responses mediated by these hormones are the following: (1) a transient leukocytosis is evident within minutes of epinephrine secretion, whereas corticosteroid-induced changes are not seen until few hours later; and (2) neutrophilia and/or lymphocytosis are evident after epinephrine release, whereas neutrophilia with lymphopenia is a consistent feature of a stress response produced by corticosteroids.

Epinephrine Effect. In animals at rest, a considerable number of leukocytes remains sequestered in the capillary beds (marginal pool). The secretion of epinephrine in acutely stressed animals increases the

circulation of blood and lymph. Consequently, leukocytes sequestered in the microvasculature and lymph nodes may be pored into the peripheral blood, causing leukocytosis accompanied by neutrophilia and/or lymphocytosis (Tables 2–23 and 2–24). The effect is transient, lasting only for a short time (usually <30 minutes). An increase in neutrophil numbers resulting from physiologic influences is more pronounced in the cat than in the dog. This is related to differences

Table 2–24. Physiologic Leukocytosis in a Clinically Normal 3-Month-Old Male Beagle

Parameter	At Rest (9 AM)	After Normal Activity (4 PM)
PCV (%)	36	46
Hemoglobin (g/dl)	11.9	15.4
ESR/1 hr (corrected)	−14	−4
Icterus index units	2	5
WBC/μl	13,100	18,900
Neutrophils	8,777	12,096
Lymphocytes	3,668	4,914
Monocytes	393	1,418
Eosinophils	262	472
Plasma proteins (g/dl)	5.6	5.9

* In an outside run.

in the intravascular distribution of neutrophils in these species. The mean marginal pool of neutrophils of clinically normal cats is about three times greater than the circulating pool, whereas in the dog it is about equal to or only slightly greater (see Table 13–3). Thus, the existence of a large marginal pool of neutrophils contributes to the relative ease with which cats can develop a physiologic leukocytosis.

Hemograms of young vigorous horses are likely to be affected by physiologic leukocytosis under conditions requiring restraint, such as the collection of blood (Table 2–23). A WBC count of 18,000 is significantly in excess of normal resting values. An N:L ratio lower than 0.9:1.0 or greater than 1.0:1.0 reflects a significant disturbance in the normal proportion of circulating lymphocytes and neutrophils, respectively. The increase in lymphocyte count is generally proportional to the severity of the muscular activity. A modest leukocytosis is chiefly the result of a rise in neutrophils, whereas a marked leukocytosis may indicate a preponderance of lymphocytes. An increase in blood and lymph flow with strenuous exercise or increased heart action from fright or apprehension leads to the mobilization of neutrophils and lymphocytes into the circulation from vast reserves in the marginal pool and from peripheral lymphoid organs, respectively.

Sustained muscular activity in the horse during an endurance ride causes a marked increase in both PCV and plasma protein levels, primarily because of dehydration from the shifting of intravascular fluid to extravascular fluid compartments and from the loss of water through profuse sweating (Fig. 2–9). A significant portion of the increase in the PCV is also the result of the epinephrine-induced contraction of the smooth muscles of the splenic capsule and trabeculae, forcing stored red cells into the general circulation to increase oxygen transport. The WBC count and changes in the absolute numbers of various leukocyte types are similar to those seen in horses given corticosteroids. Plasma levels of catecholamines and corticosteroids increase after physical activity such as exercise, racing, and endurance rides. Horses in an endurance race may also exhibit clinical dehydration and metabolic alkalosis. Most severely exhausted horses may develop partially compensated acidosis and a slight left shift. Similarly, hematologic changes associated with racing in greyhounds include significant increases in the RBC and WBC counts, hemoglobin

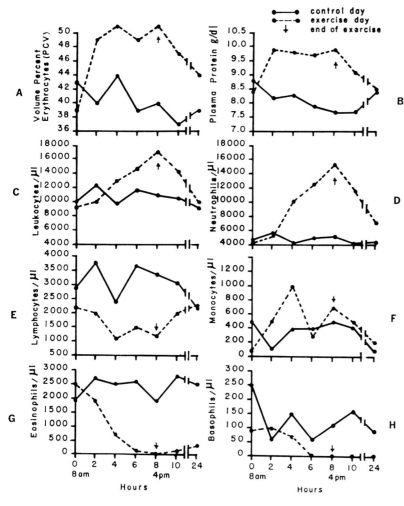

Fig. 2–9. A–H, Sequential hemograms of a 12-year-old mare during no exercise (control day) and during exercise in covering a 32-mile distance. (From Cardinet, G.H., III., et al.: Effects of sustained muscular activity upon blood morphology in the horse. Cal. Vet., 18:31, 1964.)

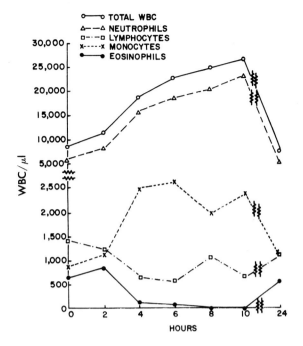

Fig. 2–10.   Effect of 20 mg of oral prednisolone on leukocyte numbers in blood of a dog. (From Jain, N.C.: Schalm's Veterinary Hematology. 4th Ed. Philadelphia, Lea & Febiger, 1986, p. 111.)

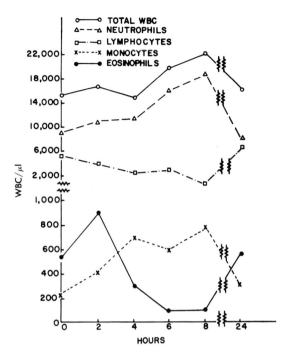

Fig. 2–11.   Blood leukocyte changes in a cat in response to oral administration of prednisolone (5 mg).

and PCV values, plasma protein concentrations, and neutrophil and lymphocyte numbers (Snow et al., 1988; Ilkiw et al., 1989).

Corticosteroid Effect.   The release of corticosteroids from the adrenal cortex in response to physiologic stress or disease produces marked changes in the total and differential leukocyte counts. Similar changes are seen following the administration of exogenous corticosteroids or ACTH. The extent and duration of the changes observed vary with the species and health status of the animal, as well as with the dose and type of corticosteroid preparation administered. A typical response is that of leukocytosis, neutrophilia, lymphopenia, and eosinopenia (Figs. 2–10 and 2–11; Tables 2–25 and 2–26). The neutrophil increase is comprised essentially of mature cells. This is attributed to the release of mature neutrophils from the marrow reserve, a decrease in diapedesis of circulating neutrophils into the tissues, and possibly increased movement of cells from the marginal pool. Lymphopenia results from lympholysis or the preferential sequestration of lymphocytes in lymphoid tissues. The cause of eosinopenia remains speculative (see Chap. 14). A hemogram developed from the blood of an animal on corticosteroid therapy may be misinterpreted when the effects of the corticosteroids are not taken into consideration. The leukocytic response to corticosteroids in the horse may be somewhat age-related, in that adult animals show greater increases in N : L ratios for a longer period than foals.

In the dog, in addition to the triad of neutrophilia, lymphopenia, and eosinopenia, a monocytosis results from exposure to synthetic corticosteroids or the injection of ACTH (Fig. 2–10). The occurrence of monocytosis in the dog is significant in view of the opposite effect (monocytopenia) in humans, mice, and rabbits. Its cause remains unknown. The monocyte response is variable in the cat, horse, and cow (Fig. 2–11). Although monocytosis may occur occasionally in response to exogenous corticosteroids, monocytes commonly disappear initially from the circulation in peracute and acute inflammatory diseases in these animals. In fact, from a clinical viewpoint, the return of monocytes to the blood in the cat, cow, and horse may be considered a sign of chronic disease.

Effect of Parturition.   Changes typical of a stress response are seen in the total and differential leukocyte counts of cows at parturition. WBC counts are significantly elevated, mainly through a marked increase in neutrophils, with or without a left shift. Lymphocyte numbers vary, depending on the degree of stress involved, and numbers of other leukocyte types vary, depending also on the degree of stress and the status of fetal membranes. These changes are evident within 12 to 24 hours postpartum and subside over the next few days. Similarly, RBC, hemoglobin, and PCV values may also change. The retention of fetal membranes is associated with the development of leukopenia, a shift to the left to band and metamyelocyte neutrophils, and monocytosis within 2 to 5 days. The bone marrow of cows with a retained placenta contains a low percentage of mature neutrophils because of the depletion of the neutrophil reserve pool as these cells are drained from the blood and bone marrow into the uterus.

Changes in total and differential leukocyte counts have been reported for sows during the gestation and

Table 2–25. Leukocyte Responses of the Lactating Cow to Intramuscular Administration of 9α-Fluoroprednisolone Acetate*

Cow	Dose (mg)	Elapsed Time (hr)	WBC/μl		Neutrophils	Lymphocytes	Monocytes	Eosinophils	Basophils	Other
					Differential Leukocyte Counts in Absolute Numbers/μl					
44	50	0	6,200		3,069	2,418	372	310	31	0
		12	11,800		8,850	2,065	*885*	*0*	*0*	0
		18	*13,350*		*9,745*	2,737	868	0	0	0
		36	9,000		6,750	1,890	270	45	45	0
		60	7,500		4,950	*1,800*	488	225	37	0
		66	7,200		3,924	2,700	396	114	36	0
		72	7,900		4,187	2,805	710	118	0	80
		78	6,000		2,520	2,520	510	60	90	0
1249	100	0	14,200		4,118	8,662	355	923	142	0
		12	22,800		*12,198*	8,664	*1,710*	228	0	0
		18	19,900		12,239	5,671	1,692	298	0	0
		36	15,100		9,211	*4,530*	1,208	151	0	0
		42	18,500	(Band) 68)	10,175	6,382	1,758	185	0	0
		60	13,600		6,392	6,052	952	*68*	68	0
		66	11,800		6,077	5,074	590	59	0	0
		84	14,400		7,488	5,328	1,440	144	0	0
		90	14,500		6,380	6,815	1,015	290	0	0
2208	500	0	8,400		2,688	4,284	504	840	84	0
		5	11,550		*7,392*	2,945	578	578	57	0
		9	13,900		9,730	3,267	486	*278*	*0*	139
		24	13,600		*10,132*	2,448	952	68	0	0
		30	13,200	(Band) 113	9,768	*2,112*	*1,254*	66	0	0
		35	11,300		7,910	2,260	904	*0*	0	113
		48	*14,600*		10,366	2,336	1,898	0	0	0
		54	14,180		9,784	2,411	1,914	71	0	0
		72	11,100		7,381	2,553	1,166	0	0	0
		78	8,000		5,320	1,680	1,000	0	0	0

* Figures in italics represent a major change in cell numbers.

Table 2–26. Leukocyte Reponses of the Horse to Intravenous Administration of 9α-fluoro-16α-methylprednisolone (Dexamethasone)

Horse	Date	Dose (mg)	Clock Time	Elapsed Time (hr)	PCV (%)	WBC/μl	Band	Mature	Lymphocytes	Monocytes	Eosinophils	Disintegrated Cells
							Neutrophils					
I: mature male	June 10		9 AM (Control)		44	8,700	44	4,959	2,349	392	870	87
quarter horse	June 11	10	9 AM (Control)		42	9,000	0	4,995	2,835	225	900	45
	June 11		11 AM	2	41	*15,200*	152	*10,488*	3,876	304	*304*	76
	June 11		1 PM	4	42	16,700	584	13,193	2,422	418	84	0
	June 11		4:30 PM	7½	46	16,400	82	13,612	2,132	574	*0*	0
	June 11		7:30 PM	10½	43	16,500	330	13,695	*1,980*	412	82	0
	June 12		9 AM	24	40	11,600	0	8,236	2,900	464	0	0
	June 12		3 PM	30	43	10,200	0	7,140	2,601	357	102	0
II: mature	Sept. 14		9 AM (Control)		44	8,800	0	5,324	2,860	308	264	44
thoroughbred	Sept. 14		3:30 PM (Control)		41	10,800	0	6,048	3,456	756	486	54
gelding	Sept. 15	5	7 AM	0	—	—	—	—	—	—	—	—
	Sept. 15		8 AM	1	35	6,600	0	4,191	1,881	198	165	165
	Sept. 15		9 AM	2	41	*17,800*	267	*13,261*	3,115	979	178	0
	Sept. 15		10 AM	3	42	17,000	170	12,920	2,890	510	170	340
	Sept. 15		1 PM	6	41	15,900	398	12,482	2,544	477	0	0
	Sept. 15		4 PM	9	44	19,300	96	15,440	3,184	579	0	0
	Sept. 16	5	8 AM	25	37	12,000	0	7,560	3,180	*1,200*	60	0
	Sept. 16		1 PM	5	41	15,800	237	12,719	*1,738*	*1,106*	0	0
	Sept. 16		4 PM	8	40	18,700	94	14,960	3,179	468	0	0
	Sept. 17	5	9 AM	25	41	10,700	0	6,046	3,852	749	54	0
	Sept. 17		10:30 AM	1½	—	12,200	122	7,442	3,782	732	0	122
	Sept. 17		2:30 PM	5½	40	18,800	376	16,168	*1,598*	658	0	0
	Sept. 17		4 PM	7	*38*	12,500	62	10,875	1,250	312	0	0
	Sept. 18		9 AM	24	*38*	11,000	0	6,875	3,685	275	110	55
	Sept. 18		4 PM	31	*32*	11,900	0	6,069	4,998	536	238	60

peripartum periods. WBC counts and lymphocyte numbers were greater at 30 and 60 days of gestation than on day 90; the reverse was found with regard to immature neutrophils, however, and the numbers of mature neutrophils did not change significantly. Marked neutrophilia and lymphopenia were evident at 1 to 6 hours postpartum. Plasma corticosteroid levels increased at 1 to 24 hours postpartum and were associated with increases in WBC counts and numbers of neutrophils, and decreases in lymphocyte and eosinophil numbers.

Response to Disease

Leukocyte response to disease is discussed in Chapter 18 and additional information about neutrophils is presented in Chapter 13. Brief comments about the most common abnormalities with regard to neutrophil leukocytes, left shift, and toxic changes are made here to help explain the fundamental responses of various species to acute and chronic infections.

SHIFT TO THE LEFT AND TOXIC NEUTROPHILS

An important function of neutrophils is to control microbial infections, particularly those involving suppurative bacteria. Neutrophils from body reserves in the microvasculature and bone marrow are mobilized to combat infection. Neutropenia usually develops as the supply becomes depleted because of an increased need for neutrophil functions, as in early peracute and acute infections. In less severe infections, granulopoiesis in the bone marrow is stimulated to produce increased numbers of neutrophils to sustain increased functional demands. Thus, neutrophilia is common in the later stages of acute infection and in chronic infections. These neutropenic and neutrophilic responses may be accompanied by a shift to the left, which suggests the presence of excessive numbers of immature neutrophils in blood. Immature neutrophils, such as bands and metamyelocytes, occasionally myelocytes, less frequently promyelocytes, and rarely myeloblasts, may appear in the peripheral blood, depending on the severity and duration of infection. The left shift is further categorized as regenerative, degenerative, or transitional (see Chap. 18).

In severe toxemic states, granulopoiesis becomes suppressed and neutrophil morphology is altered because of maturation defects. Changes in cytoplasmic and nuclear characteristics lead to the formation of so-called "toxic" neutrophils (Table 13–7; Figs. 2–12 and 2–13). A common alteration is the inappropriate development of cytoplasmic granules and the persistence of bluish staining cytoplasm. The primary granules retain their azurophilia through various maturative stages and are visible in mature neutrophils as reddish-purple granules. This is generally referred to as toxic granulation (Plates XI–12 and XV–12). In severe toxemia, the cytoplasm stains a deeper blue and may be extensively vacuolated. The bluish color is

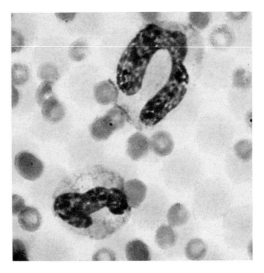

Fig. 2–12. Giant band neutrophil with bizarre nucleus and a somewhat smaller band neutrophil in cat blood. Both leukocytes have retained a bluish staining of the cytoplasm (toxic forms; × 3200). (From Jain, N.C.: Schalm's Veterinary Hematology. 4th Ed. Philadelphia, Lea & Febiger, 1986, p. 135.)

attributed to the presence of ribosomal RNA in the cytoplasm and vacuolation or foaminess is the result of restricted cytolysis caused by intracellular degranulation. Another common abnormality of neutrophils is the occurrence of one or more round or angular, bluish cytoplasmic structures known as Döhle bodies (Plates IX–2 and XII–6). Döhle bodies are remnants of rough endoplasmic reticulum resulting from defective maturation of the cytoplasm. Toxic granulation is a common feature of equine neutrophils and Döhle bodies are common to feline neutrophils. Sometimes, the nucleus of the neutrophil precursors may undergo

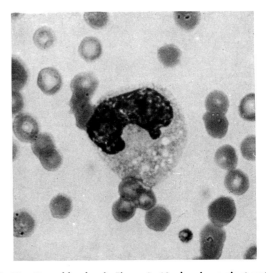

Fig. 2–13. Same blood as in Figure 2–12, showing a giant metamyelocyte with vacuolation of the cytoplasm (toxic form; × 3200). (From Jain, N.C.: Schalm's Veterinary Hematology. 4th Ed. Philadelphia, Lea & Febiger, 1986, p. 136.)

maturation without cell division. This results in the formation of occasional giant band forms and mature neutrophils known as pleokaryocytes, which present large, twisted, and bizarre nuclei (Plate IX–4), or a polyploid cell with double nuclei. Infrequently, nuclear maturation begins with the formation of a central hole, leading to the release of a giant cell with a doughnut-shaped nucleus. Such bizarre neutrophils are common in cats with toxemic diseases (Plates XV–9, XV–10, and XV–11).

The ability to identify immature neutrophils and to recognize toxic cells is a prerequisite to the use of the leukogram as an aid to diagnosis and prognosis in the cow. In the initial stages of an acute inflammatory disease, such as peritonitis, mastitis, or metritis, the mature neutrophils readily leave the blood to enter the lesion. The bone marrow of the cow does not have a large reserve of neutrophils and therefore immature neutrophils quickly make their appearance in the peripheral blood, often exceeding the mature forms and producing a degenerative left shift (Table 2–27). A marked fall in the WBC count is a common finding during the developmental stage of an acute, localizing, inflammatory process. The degree of generalized toxemia is reflected in the morphology and staining characteristics of both mature and immature neutrophils. Convalescence is heralded by the transformation of a degenerative left shift to a regenerative left shift and by increases in neutrophil numbers and WBC counts (Table 2–27).

SHIFT TO THE RIGHT

Five or more lobes of the nucleus in the mature neutrophil constitute hypersegmentation, which generally represents aging of the cell in the circulation. Corticosteroids usually reduce neutrophil diapedesis into tissues; as a result, neutrophils remain longer in the circulation and some may become hypersegmented. Thus, an occasional hypersegmented neutrophil may be observed in animals (particularly dogs and horses) with reactive neutrophilias. Hypersegmenta-

tion of neutrophils is seen in poodles with macrocytosis. It is also a feature of vitamin B_{12} and folate deficiency in humans. In these conditions, reduced cell mitosis leads to larger neutrophils with hypersegmented nuclei (Plate XI–7). Hypersegmentation of leukocytes may occasionally be an artifact in stored blood. Idiopathic hypersegmentation has been reported in a horse.

INFLAMMATORY RESPONSE IN THE COW

The general trend observed during an acute inflammatory response of the cow is briefly discussed here (Fig. 2–14) because it differs remarkably from that in other species. The WBC count in the early stage of inflammatory disease in the cow generally does not reflect the seriousness of the disease. This is because lymphocytes exceed the neutrophils in health and decrease in response to stress-induced release of corticosteroids. Eosinophil numbers are also reduced. Simultaneously, neutrophils and monocytes leave the blood to participate in the developing inflammatory lesion. Although mature neutrophils from the bone marrow pool now enter the circulation, they are also attracted to the site of injury. Thus, the neutrophilic response to corticosteroids is masked by the rapidity of emigration of neutrophils into the inflammatory lesion. The net effect is a precipitous fall in the WBC count to leukopenic levels. As the bone marrow reserve of mature neutrophils becomes depleted, immature neutrophils enter the circulation in increasing numbers during the first 24 to 48 hours, resulting in a degenerative left shift (Fig. 2–14). Subsequently, the stimulation of bone marrow stem cells leads to an intensification of neutrophil production so that, as the disease passes into a more chronic phase, the degenerative left shift disappears and is replaced by a regenerative left shift or neutrophilia primarily comprised of mature forms. Monocytes also increase and may exceed their maximum normal range. The WBC count may now show an increase above normal, with counts of 20,000 to 30,000/µl being representative of an extreme leukocytosis. Thus, transitory leukopenia with a

Table 2–27.   Sequential Leukograms Before and After Introduction of 2.3 Million Enterobacter aerogenes into Three Lactating Quarters of a Cow

Elapsed Time	Temp. (°F)	WBC/ µl of Blood	Myelo-cyte	Meta-myelocyte	Band	Mature	Lympho-cytes	Mono-cytes	Eosino-phils	Baso-phils	Unclassi-fied	Direct Eosinophil Count
–18 hr	—	9,600	0	0	0	4,320	3,360	816	1,008	96	0	—
0 hr	101.5	6,600	0	0	0	2,673	2,904	561	363	99	0	311
+ 3 hr	101.8	6,100	0	0	0	2,257	2,562	854	427	0	0	422
+ 6 hr	106.4	2,900	0	0	58	580	2,059	0	203	0	0	244
+10 hr	105.2	1,850	0	0	55	777	999	0	18	0	0	83
+24 hr	106.0	2,650	0	26	291	424	1,802	79	26	0	0	11
+31 hr	106.2	2,200	22	66	110	198	1,584	154	22	0	44	6
+48 hr	101.4	4,300	215	387	774	387	2,064	129	301	0	43	189
+72 hr	100.8	8,100	81	202	688	3,280	2,065	1,134	567	81	0	266
+96 hr	101.4	8,200	0	82	492	3,280	2,706	1,312	328	0	0	178
+ 6 days	101.6	7,650	0	114	229	3,480	2,830	765	153	76	0	189
+ 9 days	—	8,750	0	0	0	4,812	2,975	612	262	87	0	188

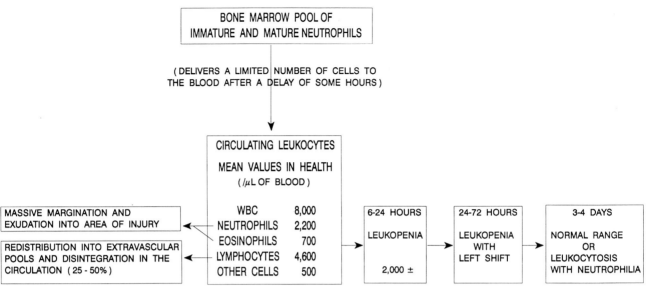

Fig. 2–14. Dynamics of leukocyte responses in localized acute bacterial infection in the bovine.

marked left shift is the common initial response to
severe inflammatory disease in the cow. The persistence of leukopenia beyond the third or fourth day is
a sign of inadequacy of granulopoiesis to meet the
demands for neutrophils. Myeloid hypoplasia may
develop in certain chronic infections and thereby
contribute to a persistent neutropenia or leukopenia.

Observations in 50 cattle with traumatic reticulitis
and in 8 with traumatic pericarditis revealed that the
leukogram is more reliable as an indicator of the
existence of an inflammatory lesion in cows displaying
an elevation in body temperature above 102°F (39°C).
In febrile cases of traumatic reticulitis, neutrophilia
and monocytosis were the most prominent findings
(in > 80% of cases), whereas leukocytosis (62%), left
shift (40%), and lymphopenia (33%) were less common. In traumatic pericarditis, left shift and monocytosis were most common (in 87 to 88% of cases),
whereas neutrophilia (6%), leukocytosis (37%) and
lymphopenia (37%) were less common.

RESPONSE TO ENDOTOXEMIA AND SEPTICEMIA

Leukocytic changes are generally similar in septicemia and endotoxemia except for differences in magnitude, which depend on extensiveness of the lesion
and the amount of toxin in circulation. Experimental
studies in humans and animals have shown that endotoxin given in minute amounts systemically produces a transient neutropenia (hence, leukopenia)
followed by a "rebound" neutrophilia (Table 2–28).
The former is attributed to a shift of circulating
neutrophils into the marginal pool and the latter to
the accelerated release of cells from the bone marrow
reserve. The neutrophil response, as well as changes
in other leukocytes in blood, depend on the amount
and route of endotoxin administration. For example,
neutropenia may not develop at low doses, but neu-

**Table 2–28. Changes in Peripheral Blood Leukocyte
Numbers of Cows Given an Intravenous Injection of
Escherichia coli Endotoxin**

Endo-toxin (μg)	Time (hr)	Leukocyte count	Immature Neutrophils*	Mature Neutrophils	Lymphocytes
5	0	7,200	0	2,376	3,924
	1	6,300	0	1,922	3,348
	2	5,500	0	2,117	3,080
	4	10,500	0	6,247	3,150
	6	10,500	0	5,652	3,780
	8	10,500	0	5,774	3,622
	10	8,100	0	3,888	3,280
	24	7,600	0	2,584	3,914
20	0	7,100	71 B	2,023	4,012
	1	6,000	0	1,920	3,600
	2	5,600	0	2,352	2,968
	4	7,600	0	3,876	2,850
	6	8,500	0	3,995	3,570
	8	8,600	0	3,569	4,042
	10	8,000	40 B	2,920	4,120
	24	6,800	0	1,530	4,352
50	0	8,100	0	3,078	4,212
	1	4,000	0	1,480	2,420
	2	2,300	58 B	402	1,610
	4	2,400	24 B	588	1,584
	6	3,500	70 B	1,015	2,152
	8	4,700	47 B	1,692	2,585
	10	5,300	26 B	1,404	3,418
	24	5,800	29 B	1,218	3,973
100	0	8,900	0	1,691	5,295
	1	1,700	0	68	1,496
	2	2,300	80 Mt	69	1,898
	4	1,600	16 B	80	1,336
	6	1,700	17 B	153	1,317
	8	3,900	468 Mt	643	2,281
	10	6,800	1632 Mt	1,088	3,366
	24	11,600	2088 Mt	3,422	5,104

From Jain, N.C., and Lasmanis, J.: Leucocytic changes in cows
given intravenous injections of Escherichia coli endotoxin. Res. Vet
Sci., 24:386, 1978.
* Left shift involving B, band cells; Mt, metamyelocytes.

tropenia, a slight to marked left shift, and lymphopenia may manifest at relatively higher doses. Nucleated erythrocytes may also appear in blood, and death may follow within a few hours of injection of a large dose. Thrombocytopenia is also a characteristic finding in endotoxic animals. Species variations, however, may occur with respect to the sensitivity to endotoxin.

Endotoxin induces an acute inflammatory reaction in the mammary gland, and causes a massive mobilization of neutrophils into the mammary parenchyma and milk. This, along with the systemic absorption of endotoxin, leads to quantitative changes in the blood and bone marrow myeloid cells (Fig. 2–11). Similar responses may be anticipated from endotoxin absorption from other lesions, such as coliform mastitis and enteritis. For example, leukopenia was evident in terminal cases of septicemia, but a variable degree of leukocytosis was seen in calves with primary coliform enteritis. Leukocytic changes may be evident within hours of infection, as shown by experimental studies on acute salmonellosis in calves. Lymphopenia and neutrophilia were evident with the onset of fever within a few hours of infection before diarrhea was apparent, whereas plasma protein levels decreased with the onset of watery, fibrinous diarrhea.

Endotoxemia may be associated with altered cardiovascular functions because of increases in synthesis of prostacyclin and thromboxane B_2. Treatment of endotoxic ponies with flunixin meglumine, a potent cyclo-oxygenase inhibitor, prevented cardiovascular alterations but not leukopenia associated with neutropenia (Ward et al., 1987).

PLATELETS

Platelets are cytoplasmic fragments of megakaryocytes. They are pleomorphic and exhibit noticeable variations in size and shape. Most commonly, they appear as disk-like roundish or oval structures with diffuse or a central cluster of fine, reddish-purple azurophilic granules in a pale blue matrix enclosed by a delicate membrane (Plate IX–1; Fig. 6–1A). Some platelets may appear agranular or have scanty granules. Equine platelets typically stain lightly, and their shape varies from the more common oval form to an elongated structure (Fig. 6–2A). Round platelets measure about 2.5 μm in diameter and oval forms may be about 3.5 μm in length. Occasionally, large forms equal in size to the red cell may be found, particularly in the cat. Large forms are common in animals recovering from thrombocytopenia. Young platelets are large and granular. They appear in increased numbers following blood loss. Activated platelets show long, thread-like membranous processes projecting from their surface or appear globular, with an uneven surface and irregular pseudopodia (Fig. 2–15). Platelet clumping may occur in blood in which the clotting mechanism may have begun before anticoagulation was complete, causing platelet activation. Platelet clumping and the presence of giant platelets may interfere with the accuracy of WBC counts by the electronic particle counter, particularly in the cat and mouse. Platelets form a distinct whitish layer over leukocytes in the buffy coat of blood centrifuged in a microhematocrit or Wintrobe tube (Plates I–1 and II–2).

The normal range of platelet counts in various species is given in Table 6–3. Among the common domestic animals, the horse has the lowest normal number of platelets and the cow has the highest. Platelet counts in laboratory mice are over 1 million. Platelet counts in the pig seem to be age-dependent, in that they are slightly higher in young animals than in adults. Excitement in normal cats has been found

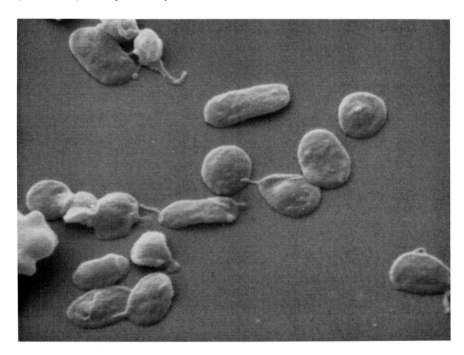

Fig. 2–15. Scanning electron photomicrograph of canine platelets (×5600). (From Jain, N.C.: Schalm's Veterinary Hematology. 4th Ed. Philadelphia, Lea & Febiger, 1986, p. 120.)

to cause a sudden increase in the platelet count (epinephrine effect). Platelet counts in cows may vary during the estrous cycle.

Platelet production from newly formed megakaryocytes takes about 3 to 4 days. Platelet survival time in the blood of different species normally ranges from 3 to 11 days (see Table 6–2). Platelets are important for the maintenance of hemostasis. Marked reductions in platelet numbers (thrombocytopenia) and abnormalities of platelet function (thrombopathia) are associated with bleeding tendencies in humans and animals (see Chap. 6 for details).

PLASMA

Icterus Index

The icterus index is the measure of plasma color. Bilirubin produced from the catabolism of hemoglobin released from the physiologic destruction of senescent red cells and ineffective erythropoiesis contributes most of the yellow color to the plasma. In addition, plant pigments from the feed, carotenoids and xanthophylls, impart a yellow color to the plasma of cattle and horses. The liver plays an important role in the production, conjugation, and excretion of bilirubin into bile. Conjugated bilirubin is excreted into the urine when the kidney threshold for bilirubin diglucuronide is exceeded. Thus, an increase in the icterus index usually suggests increased bilirubin concentration in plasma because of increased hemolysis, liver disease, or bile duct obstruction.

The icterus index of the dog and cat in health seldom exceeds 5 units. A plasma color equal to 7.5 units is considered suspicious because it may occur in severe dehydration, and a reading of 10 units or greater is distinctly abnormal and clinically significant.

The normal icterus index in cattle ranges from 5 to 15 units. Cattle on green feed may have an icterus index as high as 25 units, but cattle on dry feed have an almost colorless plasma as a result of the efficient excretion of bilirubin diglucuronide by the liver. In contrast, the plasma color in sheep and goats is not affected by the yellow pigments of the ration. Thus, the icterus index in these animals normally does not exceed 5 units in health, although in dehydration it may reach 7.5 units.

The icterus index in horses is generally elevated at birth (25 to 100 units), gradually declines over a period of 2 weeks, and attains the normal value of 25 units or less. The plasma of the horse normally contains a greater quantity of bilirubin (0.6 to 1.7 mg/dl) than that of other domestic animals. Breed and individual differences may be found in serum bilirubin values, with thoroughbreds having higher values than draft horses and perhaps as many as 15% of horses having plasma bilirubin levels of 2.0 mg/dl or higher. In fasting horses and ponies, the bilirubin concentration begins to increase rapidly, exceeding baseline values by 15 hours and leveling off by 2 to 3 days. An icterus index of 50 units (rarely, 100) may be seen in anorectic horses. Fasting may result in a clinical icterus in horses with high normal levels of plasma bilirubin. The fasting hyperbilirubinemia in the horse has been shown to be essentially of hepatic origin, because bilirubin synthesis or redistribution did not change but bilirubin excretion decreased by 50 to 80% during fasting, and increased markedly following refeeding. The efficiency of liver in the removal of plasma bilirubin in certain other species also decreases during fasting, resulting in increased plasma bilirubin levels.

Observations on plasma color in horses on a low plant pigment intake have revealed that the icterus index varies indirectly with the PCV (Table 2–29). Thus, a PCV of 25% or lower and an icterus index of 20 units or more should excite suspicion of the existence of a hemolytic process as the possible cause of anemia. Conversely, a marked increase in the icterus index (50 units or more), but without anemia, does not indicate a hemolytic disease. Icterus index scores in horses increase proportionately with increasing amounts of total bilirubin, primarily because of elevations in indirect-acting (unconjugated) bilirubin. Thus, results of the van den Bergh test are interpreted somewhat differently in the horse. Even in complete extrahepatic bile duct obstruction, less than half of the plasma bilirubin is direct-reacting (conjugated). When the direct-reacting bilirubin represents 25 to 35% of the plasma bilirubin, however, regardless of the total concentration, either intrahepatic or extrahepatic cholestasis may be suspected, with good reason.

Although increases in the icterus index usually parallel elevations in the serum bilirubin level, the degree of bilirubinemia cannot be assessed accurately from the subjective reading of the icterus index, particularly when it has reached its maximum (100 units) or when interference in light transmittance (lipemia or hemolysis) is encountered. Total bilirubin and, if possible, direct and indirect bilirubin, should be determined for proper evaluation. Kernicterus (bilirubin encephalopathy) may develop from the persistent accumulation of exceedingly high amounts of bilirubin in the circulation.

Total Plasma Proteins

The plasma protein concentration is lowest during fetal life and is low at birth. It gradually increases to adult levels by 6 months to 1 year of age. Plasma

Table 2–29. Relationship of Icterus Index and Packed Cell Volume In Horses

Icterus Index (Units)	PCV (%)
2.0–5.0	25
5.0–7.5	25–30
7.5–15.0	30–35
10.0–15.0	35–40
15.0–25.0	40–55

protein and globulin concentrations increase precipitously within hours of colostrum consumption because of the absorption of β- and γ-globulins from the gut. This is particularly apparent in foals and calves. A subsequent increase in plasma protein concentration occurs primarily because of the γ-globulin fraction from the antigenic stimulation of the immune system of the young animal as it grows. This is associated with a reduction in the albumin:globulin ratio, particularly between 1 and 6 months of age.

Dogs at birth commonly have a plasma protein concentration below 5.0 g/dl, and it is between 6.0 and 7.0 g/dl in dogs 4 to 6 months in age. Dogs 1 year of age or older commonly have a plasma protein level, between 7.0 and 8.0 g/dl.

The normal range of the total plasma protein concentration in cats is 6.0 to 7.5 g/dl. As with other animals, lower plasma protein values are characteristic of young cats. Some apparently normal cats, particularly aged cats, may have a total plasma protein concentration of 8.0 to 8.5 g/dl as a result of an increase in γ-globulins.

Plasma protein levels in cattle increase early in neonatal life from the low level at birth. In colostrum-deprived calves, mostly taken by cesarean section, the plasma protein concentration is markedly low (4.0 to 5.3 g/dl; mean, 4.7). Colostrum feeding may increase the plasma protein concentration to as high as 7.0 g/dl. Among 15 calves 3 to 16 weeks of age the mean value was 6.2 ± 0.6 g/dl. By 1 year of age, a common range is 6.8 to 7.5 g/dl and, for mature cattle, it is 7.0 to 8.5 g/dl. The plasma protein concentration may exceed 8.5 g/dl in normal cows during periods of high environmental (ambient) temperature. The plasma protein concentration in septicemic calves was lower (5.8 ± 0.69 g/dl) because of hypogammaglobulinemia than in calves with primary enteric infection and clinical evidence of dehydration (8.6 ± 1.5 g/dl). The PCV was similar in both groups of animals. In sick cows, refusal of food and water leads to rapid hemoconcentration, with elevations of plasma proteins to between 10 and 12 g/dl. High total plasma protein levels in sick cows may also be partly the result of an increase in fibrinogen.

The plasma protein concentration is below 6.0 g/dl in foals at birth and increases precipitously to 6.0 to 7.0 g/dl within 3 to 10 hours of colostrum consumption because of increases in β- and γ-globulins. The serum of the newborn foal, with rare exception, is devoid of IgG but contains IgM, which is detectable in fetal serum, at least during the latter part of gestation. In Arabian foals with combined immune deficiency, both IgG and IgM are absent in prenursing serum. After the ingestion of colostrum, normal as well as immune-deficient foals absorb various immunoglobulins. This raises their serum immunoglobulin concentrations to levels seen in their dams. The absorption is usually complete within 24 hours. Subsequently, serum immunoglobulin values decline because of the catabolism of maternal immunoglobulins, but the normal foal begins to synthesize its own immunoglobulins and

gradually attains adult values by 5 months to 1 year of age.

The total plasma protein value of sheep fetuses in late gestation is generally below 4.0 g/dl. It increases to 4.0 to 5.0 g/dl at birth and a slight increase follows the ingestion of colostrum. Total plasma proteins continue to increase gradually, attaining a level of 6.0 g/dl at approximately 3 months of age. The normal level of total plasma proteins for mature sheep commonly ranges from 6.5 to 7.5 g/dl. Similar values are found in adult goats.

Pigs under 1 month of age normally have total plasma proteins lower than 5.5 g/dl, whereas pigs 2 to 6 months of age have 5.5 to 7.0 g/dl, and pigs over 1 year of age have 7.0 to 8.0 g/dl of blood. Plasma protein levels in pigs may be affected by weaning, growth rate, food intake, and hormone action.

Normal plasma protein concentrations in adult common domestic animals are generally 6.0 to 8.5 g/dl (Tables 2–1 to 2–7). In diseases affecting general health, food and water intake is reduced and hemoconcentration develops. The plasma proteins become elevated, attaining levels of 8.0 to 10.0 g/dl or higher. Plasma protein concentration may exceed normal values in cows during periods of high environmental temperatures. An elevation of plasma protein levels should also be anticipated in response to chronic infections as a result of an increase in γ-globulins. High total plasma protein levels in acute and chronic inflammatory diseases may also result in part from increases in fibrinogen concentration. Plasma protein levels are decreased during pregnancy and after splenectomy. Hypoproteinemia is a common finding in diseases of the gastrointestinal system, such as salmonellosis and parasitism, which lead to excessive fluid or blood loss. Renal disease with proteinuria may also be associated with hypoproteinemia. For a further discussion of the influence of dehydration and disease on the plasma protein concentration, see Chapter 21.

Plasma Fibrinogen

Fetuses in late gestation may lack fibrinogen and newborns may have low levels of circulating fibrinogen. Generally, no age-related increase in plasma fibrinogen occurs once the neonatal period has ended. In most animals, the fibrinogen concentration normally ranges between 0.1 and 0.4 to 0.5 g/dl, except in the cow, in which it may be as high as 0.7 g/dl (see Table 21–8).

Fibrinogen is an acute phase protein, so its concentration increases in inflammatory and tissue-destroying diseases. Increases of the plasma fibrinogen level in diseases of the dog and cat are commonly in the range of 0.6 to 0.9 g/dl. An increase in plasma fibrinogen concentration, with total and differential leukocyte counts within the normal range, may be found in diseased animals (Fig. 2–16). In fact, high plasma fibrinogen values are more indicative of a response to disease in the cow than are changes in the differential

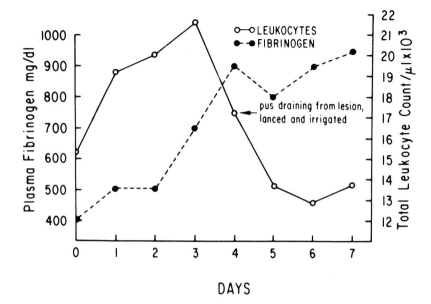

Fig. 2–16. Total leukocyte counts and plasma fibrinogen levels in a 2-year-old pony during development of an acute localized inflammation following inoculation of live *Corynebacterium pseudotuberculosis* into the pectoral muscles. The developing abscess was drained and irrigated daily from day 4 on. (From Schalm, O.W.: Equine hematology. III. Significance of plasma fibrinogen concentration in clinical disorders in horses. Equine Pract., 1:24, 1979.)

counts, particularly neutrophil numbers, during acute and many chronic inflammatory diseases. Cows often show hyperfibrinogenemia in the absence of neutrophilia and it seems to persist longer than the reactive neutrophilia. Plasma fibrinogen values of 1.0 to 1.5 g/dl or more have been recorded in marked inflammatory diseases in the cow, horse, and sheep. The goat is not as responsive as the cow in elevating the plasma fibrinogen level in response to disease. Neonatal calves that develop gastrointestinal disease or pneumonia also show hyperfibrinogenemia.

The plasma protein:fibrinogen ratio is calculated to differentiate an absolute increase in the fibrinogen level caused by disease from that resulting from hemoconcentration, which is associated with an increase in both plasma protein and fibrinogen levels without affecting their ratio. A plasma protein:fibrinogen ratio lower than 10:1 is generally considered indicative of an increase in the fibrinogen level caused by disease (see Chap. 21).

Physiologic factors such as changes in water balance and parturition, as well as vaccination, may temporarily elevate the plasma fibrinogen concentration. A 2- to 3-fold increase in the plasma fibrinogen level may be seen in the pregnant bitch. This may be partly a result of increases in the plasma progesterone level, because its injection has been found to elevate the plasma fibrinogen level.

Lipemia

A slight lactescence of plasma is a common finding in the postprandial blood of dogs and cats, but not in fasting blood samples collected 12 hours or more after the last meal. When lipids are present in the plasma in large amounts, the plasma may appear uniformly lactescent, or a white, opaque layer of chylomicra may

appear at the top of the plasma column (Plates II–3 and II–4). Lactescence and a more intense turbidity known as lipemia interfere with the accurate determination of hemoglobin by spectrophotometry and of the total plasma protein concentration by refractometry. Lipemia interferes with the determination of the icterus index and may also increase the mechanical fragility of erythrocytes and promote hemolysis in vitro. A marked lipemia occurs in dogs shortly (between 2 and 12 hours) after feeding a meal rich in fat. Lipemia in dogs is pronounced in diseases such as hypothyroidism, hepatopathy, Cushing's syndrome, pancreatitis, and diabetes mellitus. Dogs on prolonged corticosteroid therapy may frequently show lipemia. The occurrence of lipemia in equine blood is clinically significant. Lipemia has been observed in horses with severe hepatitis, carcinoma of the stomach, and diabetes mellitus. Lipemia is prominent in the blood of fasted ponies, and ponies appear to be particularly susceptible to lipemia in association with certain disease states.

REFERENCES

Allard, R.L., Carlos, A.D. and Faltin, E.C.: Canine hematological changes during gestation and lactation. Companion. Anim. Prac., 19:3, 1989.

Allen, B.V.: Relationship between the erythrocyte sedimentation rate, plasma proteins and viscosity, and leucocyte counts in thoroughbred racehorses. Vet. Rec. 122:329, 1988.

Andrews, F.M., Hamlin, R.L. and Stalnaker, P.S.: Blood viscosity in horses with colic. J. Vet. Intern. Med., 4:183, 1990.

Andrews, F.M., Korenek, N.L., Sanders, W.L., et al.: Viscosity and rheologic properties of blood from clinically normal horses. Am. J. Vet. Res., 53:966, 1992.

Coyne, C.P., Carlson, G.P., Spensley, M.S., et al.: Preliminary investigation of alterations in blood viscosity, cellular composition, and electrophoresis plasma protein fraction profile after competitive racing activity in Thoroughbred horses. Am. J. Vet. Res., 51:1956, 1990.

Davis, J.L. and Manohar, M.: Effect of splenectomy on exercise-induced pulmonary and systemic hypertension in ponies. Am. J. Vet. Res., 49:1169, 1988.

Fairley, N.M., Price, G.S. and Meuten, D.J.: Evaluation of red cell fragility in Pygmy goats. Am. J. Vet. Res., 49:1598, 1988.

Fogarty, U. and Leadon, D.: Poor performance syndrome: A review of the literature and some data on the haematological and blood biochemical changes in two groups of thoroughbred racehorses performing below expectation. Irish Vet. J., 41:203, 1987.

Garcia, M.C. and Beech, J.: Endocrinologic, hematologic, and heart rate changes in swimming horses. Am. J. Vet. Res., 47:2004, 1986.

von Hammerl, J. and Kraft, W.: Blutkorperchensenkungsreaktion beim Pferd. Berl. Munch. Tierarztl. Wochenschr., 96:145, 1983.

Harvey, J.W.: Neonatal hematologic values. In: Koterba, A.M., Drummond, W.H. Kosch, P.C. (eds.), Equine clinical neonatology, Philadelphia, Lea & Febiger, p. 561, 1990.

Harvey, R.B. and Hambright, M.B.: Normal serum chemistry and hematology values of the American miniature horse. Equine Prac., 7:6, 1985.

Hawkey, C.M. and Dennett, T.B.: Colour atlas of comparative veterinary haematology. London, Wolfe, 1989.

Ilkiw, J.E., Davis, P.E. and Church, D.B.: Hematologic, biochemical, blood-gas, and acid-base values in Greyhounds before and after exercise. Am. J. Vet. Res., 50:583, 1989.

Jain, N.C.: Schalm's Veterinary Hematology. 4th ed. Philadelphia, Lea & Febiger, 1986.

Lowseth, L.A., Gillett, N.A., Gerlach, R.F., et al.: The effects of aging on hematology and serum chemistry values in the beagle dog. Vet. Clin. Pathol., 19:13, 1990.

Martinez, R., Godoy, A., Naretto, E., et al.: Neuroendocrine changes produced by competition stress on the thoroughbred race horse. Comp. Biochem. Physiol. [A], 91:599, 1988.

O'Brien, P., Rooney, M.T., Reik, T.R., et al.: Porcine malignant hyperthermia susceptibility: erythrocytic osmotic fragility. Am. J. Vet. Res., 46:1451, 1985.

Ralston, S.L., Nockels, C.F. and Squires, E.L.: Differences in diagnostic test results and hematologic data between aged and young horses. Am. J. Vet. Res., 49:1387, 1988.

Smith, J.E., Erickson, H.H. and Debowes, R.M.: Changes in circulating equine erythrocytes induced by brief, high-speed exercise. Equine Vet. J., 21:444, 1989.

Snow, D.H., Harris, R.C., and Stuttard, H.E.: Changes in haematology and plasma biochemistry during maximal exercise in greyhounds. Vet. Rec., 123:487, 1988.

Somvanshi, R., Biswas, J.C., Sharma, B., et al.: Haematological studies on Indian pashmina goats. Res. Vet. Sci., 42:124, 1987.

Ward, D.S., Fessler, J.F., Bottoms, G.D., et al.: Equine endotoxemia: cardiovascular, eicosanoid, hematologic, blood chemical, and plasma enzyme alterations. Am. J. Vet. Res., 48:1150, 1987.

Chapter 3

Comparative Hematologic Features of Some Avian and Mammalian Species

Veterinarians are involved in the control of diseases of a great variety of animals other than the common domestic types—namely, chickens and pet birds, laboratory animals used in research, animals in zoos, and certain wild animals. A knowledge of the normal hematology of these animals is essential for the evaluation of their health status (Tables 3–1 to 3–12). Normal values determined by investigators in different laboratories can vary significantly. Many factors influence the composition of drawn blood. These include capillary versus large-vessel or heart blood, time of day, genetic factors (breed, strain), age, sex, anesthesia and type of anesthetic, nutrition, environmental conditions, and physiologic status, including state of excitation of the animal. All factors that might influence blood composition should be recorded when normal blood values are developed.

Many species characteristics have been observed in the erythrocyte, leukocyte, and thrombocyte morphology of birds and mammals. A brief description of the major differences is presented here. Interested readers are referred to other publications for a more detailed discussion of the normal and abnormal hematology of birds and laboratory, wild, and zoo animals (Brandt, 1989; Campbell, 1988; Fowler 1986; Frye, 1991; Hawkey, 1975, 1991; Hawkey and Dennett, 1989; Hawkey and Gulland, 1988; Hawkey and Hart, 1986, 1988; Jain, 1986; Jones et al., 1990; Leonard and Ruben, 1986).

AVIAN SPECIES

The blood of birds and mammals differs primarily in that birds have nucleated erythrocytes, nucleated thrombocytes, and heterophils (the counterpart of mammalian neutrophils). Birds also differ in coagulation, particularly in the intrinsic system, because they appear to lack coagulation factors V, VII, X, XI, and XII. Their fibrinolytic mechanisms seem to be similar to those of mammals.

Hematologic Examination

Blood samples for the hematologic examination of chickens and other pet birds can be obtained by clipping the toenail, nicking the comb or the wing vein, or venipuncture of the ulnar, brachial, medial metatarsal, or jugular vein. Cardiac puncture can be used to obtain large volumes of blood, but it is a dangerous procedure and should not be used unless the bird is to be euthanized after bleeding. Heparin, EDTA, and sodium citrate can be used as anticoagulants for avian blood. Heparin has a destructive effect on erythrocytes because it causes nuclear and cytoplasmic membranes to become permeable to chromatin (Freidlin, 1985).

Several characteristics of avian blood are difficult to evaluate by techniques routinely used to study mam-

Table 3–1. Normal Blood Values for the Chicken (Gallus gallus domesticus)

Erythrocytic Series			Leukocytic Series		
Parameter	Range	Ave.	Parameter	Range	Ave.
Erythrocytes ($\times 10^6$/μl)	2.5–3.5	3.0			
Hemoglobin (g/dl)	7.0–13.0	9.0	Leukocytes/μl	12,000–30,000	12,000
PCV (%)	22.0–35.0	30.0	Heterophil (band)	Rare	—
MCV (fl)	90.0–140.0	115.0	Heterophil (mature)	3,000–6,000	4,500
MCH (pg)	33.0–47.0	41.0	Lymphocyte	7,000–17,500	14,000
MCHC (%)	26.0–35.0	29.0	Monocyte	150–2,000	1,500
Reticulocytes (%)	0–0.6	0.0	Eosinophil	0–1,000	400
ESR (mm)*	3.0–12.0	7.0	Basophil	Rare	—
RBC size (μm)	7.0 $\times$ 12.0				
Other data			Percentage distribution		
Thrombocytes ($\times 10^3$/μl)	20.0–40.0	30.0	Heterophil (band)	Rare	—
Icterus index (units)	2–5	2	Heterophil (mature)	15.0–40.0	28.0
Plasma proteins (g/dl)	4.0–5.5	4.5	Lymphocyte	45.0–70.0	60.0
Fibrinogen (g/dl)	0.1–0.4	0.2	Monocyte	5.0–10.0	8.0
Erythrocyte life span (days)	20–35 days		Eosinophil	1.5–6.0	4.0
			Basophil	Rare	—

* ESR determined after 1 hour at 45° angle.

Table 3–2. Erythrocyte Parameters and Plasma Composition in Normal Rabbits, Guinea Pigs, Rats, and Mice*

Animals	PCV (%)	RBC ($\times 10^6$/μl)	Hb (g/dl)	MCV (fl)	MCHC (%)	MCH (pg)	Reticulo-cytes (%)	Icterus Index (units)	Plasma Proteins (g/dl)	Fibrinogen (g/dl)
New Zealand white rabbits (both sexes, 7–12 mo)	42.0 ± 2.7	5.98 ± 0.39	13.3 ± 0.9	70.4 ± 2.9	31.7 ± 1.1	22.3 ± 1.1	3.7 ± 1.3	2.4 ± 2.6	6.2 ± 0.5	0.21 ± 1.00
Wild jack rabbit (both sexes, <1 yr)	49.08 ± 3.98	7.73 ± 0.78	15.97 ± 1.30	63.62 ± 2.47	32.52 ± 1.04	20.70 ± 1.07	0.3 ± 0.74	2.5 ± 1.1	5.9 ± 0.68	0.28 ± 0.10
Guinea pigs (both sexes, 7–12 mo)	42.1 ± 3.1	5.09 ± 0.47	12.90 ± 1.2	83.0 ± 4.0	30.6 ± 1.2	—	2.3 ± 1.9	—	5.7 ± 0.4	—
Long-Evans rats (both sexes, 7–12 mo)	47.4 ± 2.2	8.26 ± 0.65	15.2 ± 0.8	57.3 ± 5.6	32.0 ± 1.1	18.5 ± 1.3	2.4 ± 1.5	4.3 ± 2.1	7.5 ± 0.5	0.16 ± 0.07
Sprague-Dawley rats (both sexes, 7–12 mo)	46.1 ± 2.5	7.83 ± 0.62	14.8 ± 0.8	59.0 ± 3.2	32.5 ± 1.1	18.9 ± 1.2	2.2 ± 1.2	3.4 ± 2.2	7.7 ± 0.7	0.23 ± 0.09
Mice, regular yellow A^y strain (both sexes, 7–12 mo)	40.4 ± 3.8	8.25 ± 0.90	13.1 ± 1.5	49.1 ± 3.4	32.3 ± 1.4	15.9 ± 1.1	4.7 ± 3.3	1.9 ± 2.3	7.1 ± 0.5	0.22 ± 0.11
Mice, Parkes strain (both sexes, 7–12 mo)	41.8 ± 3.0	8.45 ± 0.62	13.4 ± 1.1	49.0 ± 4.0	31.5 ± 2.9	15.9 ± 1.0	6.7 ± 4.0	1.4 ± 2.8	6.0 ± 0.6	0.17 ± 0.08

* Mean ± 1 SD.

Table 3–3. Total and Differential Leukocyte Counts in Normal Rabbits, Guinea Pigs, Rats, and Mice*

Animals	WBC/μl	Differential Leukocyte Count (%)					
		Neutrophils		Lymphocytes	Monocytes	Eosinophils	Basophils
		Band	Mature				
New Zealand white rabbit (both sexes, 7–12 mo)	8,179 ± 1,882	0	29.2 ± 9.1	62.5 ± 13.9	3.2 ± 2.6	1.1 ± 1.0	2.7 ± 2.2
Wild jack rabbit (both sexes, <1 yr)	4,908 ± 2,193	0.08 ± 0.28	34.6 ± 11.4	54.2 ± 11.6	6.3 ± 3.5	4.5 ± 3.6	0.4 ± 0.6
Guinea pigs (both sexes, 7–12 mo)	11,111 ± 2,891	0.02 ± 0.09	23.4 ± 9.5	71.4 ± 9.6	2.7 ± 1.9	2.4 ± 3.3	0.05 ± 0.15
Long-Evans Rats (both sexes, 7–12 mo)	8,309 ± 2,365	0.08 ± 0.30	24.9 ± 7.6	68.3 ± 9.1	3.0 ± 2.3	3.6 ± 3.1	0.08 ± 0.20
Sprague-Dawley Rats (both sexes, 7–12 mo)	9,975 ± 2,680	0.05 ± 0.18	24.5 ± 8.0	71.1 ± 8.7	2.5 ± 2.0	1.7 ± 1.3	0.08 ± 0.28
Mice, regular yellow A^y strain (both sexes, 7–12 mo)	6,333 ± 3,721	0.09 ± 0.30	21.0 ± 11.5	74.3 ± 13.1	2.4 ± 2.0	1.5 ± 1.6	0.08 ± 0.40
Mice, Parkes strain (both sexes, 7–12 mo)	7,517 ± 3,009	0.04 ± 0.21	20.4 ± 9.7	76.9 ± 10.1	1.6 ± 1.5	1.1 ± 1.3	0.01 ± 0.06

* Mean ± 1 SD.

Table 3–4. **Total and Differential Leukocyte Numbers and Platelet Counts in Normal Rabbits, Guinea Pigs, Rats, and Mice***

Animal	WBC/μl	Neutrophils Band	Neutrophils Mature	Lymphocytes	Monocytes	Eosinophils	Basophils	Platelets (×10³/μl)
New Zealand white rabbit (both sexes, 7–12 mo)	8,179 ± 1,882	0	2,350 ± 858	5,176 ± 1,821	245 ± 195	83 ± 73	211 ± 154	428 ± 178
Wild jack rabbit (both sexes, <1 yr)	4,908 ± 2,193	4 ± 14	1,721 ± 874	2,598 ± 1,202	334 ± 294	229 ± 237	23 ± 35	447 ± 215
Guinea pigs (both sexes, 7–12 mo)	11,111 ± 2,891	2 ± 12	2,501 ± 1,150	8,014 ± 2,541	312 ± 251	274 ± 416	6 ± 18	545 ± 162
Long-Evans Rats (both sexes, 7–12 mo)	8,309 ± 2,365	6 ± 22	2,075 ± 1,041	5,548 ± 1,757	244 ± 219	301 ± 274	6 ± 20	969 ± 185
Sprague-Dawley Rats (both sexes, 7–12 mo)	9,975 ± 2,680	5 ± 21	2,475 ± 1,226	7,070 ± 2,001	247 ± 193	167 ± 128	8 ± 33	1,043 ± 200
Mice, regular yellow A^y strain (both sexes, 7–12 mo)	6,333 ± 3,721	5 ± 17	1,197 ± 799	4,858 ± 3,584	143 ± 148	82 ± 91	3 ± 18	1,163 ± 382
Mice, Parkes strain (both sexes, 7–12 mo)	7,517 ± 3,009	4 ± 23	1,538 ± 1,033	5,800 ± 2,420	118 ± 126	80 ± 85	0 ± 4	1,950 ± 1,022

The header spans: Differential Leukocyte Count in Absolute Numbers/μl

* Mean ± 1 SD.

Table 3–5. **Selected Hematologic Values of Monkeys of the Genus Macaca***

Species	Number (Sex)	RBC (×10⁶/μl)	Hb (g/dl)	PCV (%)	MCV (fl)	MCHC (%)	MCH (pg)	WBC (×10³/μl)	Differential Leukocyte Count (%) Neutrophils	Lymphocytes	Monocytes	Eosinophils	Basophils
Macaca rhesus	45	4.6–7.3	10.7–14.4	—	—	—	—	5.5–19.5 (10.95)	52.3	38.5	4.0	2.0	0.15
Macaca mulatta	200	5.38 ± 0.41	12.2 ± 0.6	42.1 ± 2.2	78.6 ± 4.8	28.9 ± 1.3	22.8 ± 1.7	10.95 ± 2.87	41.1 ± 11.4	55.7 ± 11.5	0	2.7 ± 1.8	0
Macaca aretoides	79 (females)	—	12.0 ± 1.4	40.0 ± 5.2	—	—	—	14.13 ± 5.05	31.4 ± 15.2	61.9 ± 16.9	0.52 ± 1.56	5.2 ± 5.2	0.22 ± 0.57
	76 (males)	—	12.2 ± 1.2	39.3 ± 5.8	—	—	—	14.69 ± 5.46	28.3 ± 15.2	67.3 ± 15.2	0.54 ± 1.39	3.6 ± 3.5	0.20 ± 0.60

* Range or mean ± 1 SD.

Table 3–6. **Selected Hematologic Values of Hamsters and Some Fur-Bearing Animals***

Species	Number Sex, Age	RBC (×10⁶/μl)	Hb (g/dl)	PCV (%)	MCV (fl)	MCHC (%)	MCH (pg)	WBC (×10³/μl)	Differential Leukocyte Count (%) Neutrophils	Lymphocytes	Monocytes	Eosinophils	Basophils
Golden hamster	—	7.5 ± 2.4	16.8 ± 1.2	52.5 ± 2.3	71.2 ± 3.2	—	—	7.62 ± 1.30	29.9 ± 8.0	73.5 ± 9.4	2.5 ± 0.8	1.1 ± 0.02	0
Muskrat	71	6.4 ± 0.8	13.6 ± 2.8	50.0 ± 6.0	80.0 ± 11.0	—	—	7.5 ± 3.0	70.1	24.9	2.84	0.61	1.66
Raccoon	6 adult males	9.6–13.3	11.0–12.0	—	—	—	—	12.2–16.2	19.5–37.5	59.0–78.5	0.0–2.0	1.5–7.0	0
Mink	15	5.7–9.3	13.5–17.5	41.0–57.0	62.0–82.0	—	—	3.2–11.2	45.0–88.0	14.0–50.0	0.0–3.0	0.0–3.0	0
Kit fox	65	8.4 ± 0.8	14.9 ± 1.5	46.9 ± 3.9	56.4 ± 3.6	32.0 ± 2.1	18.2 ± 0.9	6.9 ± 2.1	80.3 ± 8.1	15.6 ± 7.8	2.8 ± 1.9	0.4 ± 0.7	0
Chinchilla lamigera	41 males, 1–8 yr	5.8–10.3 (7.3)	8.0–15.1 (11.7)	27.0–54.0 (38.7)	(53)	—	—	1.6–39.9 (7.6)	9.0–75.0 (42.4)	19.0–86.0 (54.7)	0.0–5.0 (1.3)	0.0–7.0 (0.4)	0.0–10.0 (0.4)
	52 females, 1–8 yr	5.2–9.9 (6.6)	8.8–15.4 (11.7)	25.0–52.0 (38.3)	(58)	—	—	2.2–45.1 (8.0)	1.0–78.0 (44.6)	19.0–98.0 (53.6)	0.0–5.0 (1.2)	0.0–9.0 (0.5)	0.0–11.0 (0.4)

* Range or mean ± 1 SD.

Table 3–7. **Selected Hematologic Values of the Cervidae and Camelidae Families***

Species	Number, Sex, Age	RBC (×10⁶/μl)	Hb (g/dl)	PCV (%)	MCV (fl)	MCHC (%)	MCH (pg)	WBC (×10³/μl)	Differential Leukocyte Count (%) Neutrophils	Lymphocytes	Monocytes	Eosinophils	Basophils
Mule deer	170–175 males and females, 1–162 mo	8.8 ± 0.2	16.4 ± 0.3	46.7 ± 0.6	—	—	—	3.0 ± 0.1	40.6 ± 1.2	43.4 ± 1.1	6.2 ± 0.5	8.3 ± 0.6	0.4 ± 0.1
Whitetail deer	>500 males and females, >1 yr	17.0–20.0	17.0–21.0	55.0–61.0	—	—	—	1.5–3.0	30.0–35.0	55.0–70.0	2.0	2.0–15.0	0.0–2.0
Blacktail deer	9 males, 3–5 mo	10.60 ± 1.39	14.04 ± 1.08	38.7 ± 2.9	36.8 ± 3.6	36.3 ± 0.8	13.4 ± 1.3	2.8 ± 1.1	—	—	—	—	—
Camelus dromedarius	10 males, 10 females	6.7 ± 0.2	11.1 ± 0.3	—	—	—	—	10.6 ± 0.4	44.7 ± 1.4	47.5 ± 1.4	1.2 ± 0.1	7.2 ± 0.4	<0.1
Lama glama	7 young, mature	8.3–12.5	11.6–14.5	—	—	—	—	8.9–22.0	22.0–48.0	15.0–59.0	0.5–2.0	3.5–6.0	0.5–3.0
Lama guanicoe	8 young, mature	8.9–11.7	14.6–19.2	—	—	—	—	6.4–17.0	14.0–35.0	15.0–27.0	0.5–2.5	4.0–16.5	1.0–2.0
Lama pacos	8 young, mature	7.8–10.8	7.5–16.7	—	—	—	—	6.9–15.5	16.0–32.0	14.0–27.0	0.0–0.5	9.0–33.5	0.0–1.5
Lama vicugna	6 young, mature	9.4–11.5	9.4–14.8	—	—	—	—	6.4–19.2	25.0–55.0	11.0–40.0	0.0–0.5	5.5–18.0	0.5–3.0

* Range or mean ± 1 SD.

Table 3–8.　Hematologic Values of Llamas*

Values	Neonate (<1 mo) (n)	Nursing (2 to 6 mo) (n)	Juvenile (6 to 18 mo) (n)	All Young (n)	Adult Female (n)	Adult Male (n)	All Adults (n)	All Llamas (n)
Plasma protein (g/dl)	4.7 to 6.1 (28)	5.2 to 6.9 (30)	4.9 to 7.0 (35)	4.8 to 7.0 (85)	5.4 to 7.2 (54)	5.4 to 7.2 (35)	5.1 to 7.9 (89)	4.9 to 7.9 (174)
Icteric index (units)	2 to 5 (20)	2 to 5 (30)	2 (35)	2 to 5 (85)	2 (54)	2 (35)	2 (89)	2 to 5 (174)
Fibrinogen (mg/dl)	100 to 400 (20)	100 to 400 (30)	100 to 400 (35)	100 to 400 (85)	100 to 500 (54)	100 to 500 (35)	100 to 500 (89)	100 to 400 (174)
Erythrocyte count ($\times 10^6/\mu$l)	9.6 to 15.2 (20)	11.4 to 17.2 (30)	10.0 to 16.1 (35)	10.2 to 17.1 (85)	10.6 to 17.2 (54)	10.5 to 17.1 (35)	10.5 to 17.2 (89)	10.1 to 17.3 (174)
Hb (g/dl)	10.1 to 14.9 (20)	12.7 to 18.1 (30)	11.1 to 16.7 (35)	10.4 to 17.4 (85)	12.5 to 19.2 (54)	11.7 to 19.1 (35)	11.9 to 19.4 (89)	11.3 to 19.0 (174)
PCV (%)	24 to 35 (20)	28 to 42.5 (30)	25.5 to 38.5 (35)	25 to 40 (85)	27.5 to 45 (54)	27 to 45 (35)	27 to 45 (89)	25 to 45 (174)
MCV (fl)	22.2 to 26.1 (20)	21.5 to 29.0 (30)	22.4 to 28.0 (35)	21.9 to 28.1 (85)	22.9 to 30.2 (54)	22.5 to 29.1 (35)	22.8 to 29.9 (89)	22.0 to 29.5 (174)
MCHC (g/dl)	39.4 to 44.1 (20)	39.7 to 44.9 (30)	39.3 to 45.5 (35)	38.9 to 45.3 (85)	40.0 to 46.7 (54)	39.9 to 48.7 (35)	39.3 to 46.8 (89)	38.9 to 46.2 (174)
MCH (pg)	9.0 to 11.1 (20)	9.4 to 11.9 (30)	9.5 to 11.9 (35)	9.2 to 11.9 (85)	10.0 to 12.7 (54)	10.3 to 12.5 (35)	10.1 to 12.7 (89)	9.6 to 12 (174)
Nucleated erythrocytes/ 100 WBC	0 to 26 (20)	0 to 1 (30)	0 to 8 (35)	0 to 8 (85)	0 to 1 (54)	0 to 3 (35)	0 to 2 (89)	0 to 3 (174)
Reticulocytes (% of RBC)	0 to 7.5 (20)	0 to 2.1 (30)	0 to 0.4 (35)	0 to 4.8 (85)	0 to 0.3 (54)	0 to 0.5 (35)	0 to 0.4 (89)	0 to 2.4 (174)
Leukocytes ($\times 10^3/\mu$l)	7.1 to 19.4 (20)	9.1 to 22.9 (30)	10.2 to 23.6 (35)	8.0 to 23.8 (85)	8.3 to 19.2 (54)	7.9 to 23.6 (35)	8.0 to 21.4 (89)	8.0 to 23.3 (174)
Band neutrophils/μl	0 to 487 (19)	0 to 99 (27)	0 to 90 (35)	0 to 91 (81)	0 to 145 (53)	0 to 21 (35)	0 to 147 (88)	0 to 128 (169)
Neutrophils/μl	1,128 to 14,556 (19)	4,295 to 14,267 (27)	4,220 to 12,952 (35)	2,502 to 13,411 (81)	5,107 to 14,145 (53)	4,620 to 16,163 (35)	4,711 to 14,868 (89)	4,182 to 14,868 (169)
Lymphocytes/μl	1,701 to 4,725 (19)	3,049 to 10,670 (27)	1,878 to 7,680 (35)	1,762 to 7,911 (81)	645 to 4,739 (53)	982 to 4,922 (35)	689 to 4,848 (88)	963 to 7,642 (169)
Monocytes/μl	0 to 1,418 (19)	154 to 1,394 (27)	0 to 1,407 (35)	0 to 1,462 (81)	113 to 1,001 (53)	0 to 937 (35)	0 to 1,009 (88)	0 to 1,342 (169)
Eosinophils/μl	0 to 1,090 (19)	82 to 2,819 (27)	301 to 6,940 (35)	0 to 5,934 (81)	614 to 5,514 (53)	794 to 4,205 (35)	647 to 4,867 (88)	72 to 5,825 (169)
Basophils/μl	0 to 150 (19)	0 to 234 (27)	0 to 385 (35)	0 to 383 (81)	0 to 275 (53)	0 to 341 (35)	0 to 298 (88)	0 to 298 (169)

* Reference ranges, 2.5 to 97.5 percentile. From Fowler, M. E., and Zinkl, J. G.: Reference ranges for hematologic and serum biochemical values in llamas (*Lama glama*). Am. J. Vet. Res. 50:2049, 1989.

malian blood. These include the presence of nucleated erythrocytes, nucleated thrombocytes, and intensely red heterophil granules, which resemble those in eosinophils. Special procedures and precautions need to be used to enumerate these elements in avian blood (Campbell, 1988; Jain, 1986; Russo et al., 1986). Hemoglobin (Hb) concentration, determined by the cyanmethemoglobin method, is erroneously high unless the nuclei of the erythrocytes are removed by centrifuging the cyanmethemoglobin reagent-blood mixture before performing spectrophotometric measurement, as is done for mammalian blood containing Heinz bodies.

Normal Blood Values

Normal blood values of the domestic chicken, Gallus gallus domesticus, are presented in Table 3–1. Although the blood of various avian species is similar in many respects, moderate to marked species differences should be expected. For example, the erythrocytes of

Table 3–9.　Selected Hematologic Values of Certain Domesticated and Wild Large Animals*

Species	Number, Sex, Age	RBC ($\times 10^6/\mu$l)	Hb (g/dl)	PCV (%)	MCV (fl)	MCHC (%)	MCH (pg)	WBC ($\times 10^3/\mu$l)	Differential Leukocyte Count (%)				
									Neutrophils	Lymphocytes	Monocytes	Eosinophils	Basophils
Barren ground caribou	7	9.5—11.8	11.5–16.5	—	—	—	—	2.25–5.4	38.0–70.0	26.0–57.0	1.0–4.0	1.0–3.0	0.0–1.0
Asian elephant	42	3.18 ± 1.01	12.1 ± 2.2	33.30 ± 1.99	—	—	—	14.70 ± 6.15	40.3 ± 8.7	52.7 ± 10.9	5.3 ± 3.4	2.4 ± 1.9	0.2
Giraffes	37–38	12.4 ± 3.4	13.5 ± 2.4	38.80 ± 5.80	—	—	—	13.50 ± 4.2	9,400 ± 3,700	3,000 ± 2,500	200 ± 300	300 ± 360	400 ± 600
Springbok	34	6.1–9.9	—	36.0–54.0	—	—	—	3.6–20.1	42.0–76.0	11.0–46.0	1.0–11.0	3.0–30.0	0.0–5.0
Oryx	27–31	10.0 ± 2.4	13.9 ± 2.0	39.8 ± 6.0	—	—	—	7.24 ± 2.89	4,700 ± 2,125	2,420 ± 1,260	180 ± 220	220 ± 420	220 ± 420
Yak	6–7	6.4 ± 0.9	13.7 ± 17	38.4 ± 4.0	—	—	—	6.6 ± 1.2	42.0 ± 12.0	46.0 ± 10.0	0.4	10.7	0.5
Mules	8 males	6.46	13.76	38.87	62.1	22.4	35.5	10.25	47.75	45.38	1.63	4.13	—

* Range or mean ± 1 SD.

Table 3–10. Hematologic Values of Donkeys

Analyte*	All Donkeys Mean ± SD (N)	Miniature Mean ± SD (N)	Standard Mean ± SD (N)	Mammoth Mean ± SD (N)	Miscellaneous Mean ± SD (N)	Adopted Burros Mean ± SD (N)	Saline Valley Burros Mean ± SD (N)	Grand Canyon Burros Mean ± SD (N)
RBC (×10⁶/μl)	6.65 ± 1.05 (166)	6.43 ± 1.16 (27)	5.83 ± 1.21 (23)	6.79 ± 0.73 (12)	6.96 ± 1.27 (12)	6.49 ± 0.62 (34)	7.49 ± 0.81 (39)	6.21 ± 0.64 (19)
Hb (g/dl)	13.1 ± 1.7 (166)	12.8 ± 1.6 (27)	12.2 ± 2.3 (23)	13.2 ± 1.8 (12)	12.8 ± 2.1 (12)	13.8 ± 1.4 (34)	13.8 ± 1.2 (39)	12.2 ± 1.2 (19)
PCV (%)	38 ± 5 (166)	39 ± 5 (27)	35 ± 7 (23)	38 ± 5 (12)	37 ± 6 (12)	40 ± 4 (34)	40 ± 3 (39)	36 ± 4 (19)
MCV (fl)	57.9 ± 5.5 (166)	59.7 ± 6.3 (27)	60.8 ± 3.1 (23)	56.3 ± 4.9 (12)	53.9 ± 4.9 (12)	61.2 ± 3.4 (34)	54.2 ± 5.3 (39)	57.4 ± 4.6 (19)
MCHC (g/dl)	34.3 ± 1.1 (166)	33.9 ± 1.1 (27)	34.4 ± 0.8 (23)	34.8 ± 0.7 (12)	34.3 ± 1.1 (12)	34.7 ± 1.0 (34)	34.1 ± 1.0 (39)	34.5 ± 1.4 (19)
MCH (pg)	19.9 ± 1.9 (166)	20.5 ± 2.2 (27)	20.9 ± 1.2 (23)	19.5 ± 1.8 (12)	18.5 ± 1.7 (12)	21.2 ± 1.0 (34)	18.5 ± 1.8 (39)	19.8 ± 1.3 (19)
Platelets (×10³/μl)	330 ± 110 (89)	370 ± 110 (26)	270 ± 50 (21)	270 ± 60 (9)	351 ± 158 (11)	349 ± 109 (34)	ND	ND
WBC (×10³/μl)	10.3 ± 2.5 (165)	11.4 ± 1.9 (27)	10.2 ± 2.5 (23)	10.0 ± 1.7 (12)	11.3 ± 2.4 (12)	10.4 ± 2.2 (34)	9.7 ± 3.0 (39)	9.0 ± 3.0 (18)
Bands (%)	0.1 ± 0.3 (165)	0.1 ± 0.1 (27)	0.3 ± 0.4 (23)	0.0 ± 0.0 (12)	0.1 ± 0.4 (12)	0.1 ± 0.3 (34)	0.0 ± 0.0 (39)	0.1 ± 0.2 (18)
(×10³/μl)	10 ± 20 (165)	10 ± 10 (27)	20 ± 40 (23)	0 ± 0 (12)	10 ± 30 (12)	10 ± 30 (34)	0 ± 0 (39)	10 ± 20 (18)
Neutrophils (%)	45.5 ± 11.5 (165)	39.3 ± 8.2 (27)	45.3 ± 8.8 (23)	51.2 ± 11.5 (12)	40.4 ± 4.7 (12)	46.9 ± 9.0 (34)	45.3 ± 12.0 (39)	59.7 ± 14.3 (18)
(×10³/μl)	4.7 ± 1.7 (165)	4.0 ± 1.2 (27)	4.6 ± 1.3 (23)	5.1 ± 1.5 (12)	4.6 ± 1.2 (12)	4.9 ± 1.4 (34)	4.5 ± 2.3 (39)	5.4 ± 2.3 (18)
Lymphocytes (%)	42.9 ± 11.8 (165)	48.6 ± 9.2 (27)	41.0 ± 9.8 (23)	36.4 ± 11.5 (12)	50.3 ± 6.7 (12)	42.9 ± 9.5 (34)	45.5 ± 11.8 (39)	30.3 ± 13.1 (18)
(×10³/μl)	4.4 ± 1.7 (165)	5.5 ± 1.2 (27)	4.2 ± 1.7 (23)	3.6 ± 1.3 (12)	5.7 ± 1.4 (12)	4.5 ± 1.5 (34)	4.3 ± 1.5 (39)	2.7 ± 1.5 (18)
Monocytes (%)	5.1 ± 2.9 (165)	3.6 ± 1.6 (27)	5.5 ± 3.3 (23)	3.3 ± 2.0 (12)	3.9 ± 2.2 (12)	4.0 ± 2.0 (34)	6.6 ± 2.7 (39)	7.4 ± 3.3 (18)
(/μl)	510 ± 290 (165)	420 ± 200 (27)	580 ± 400 (23)	300 ± 200 (12)	420 ± 230 (12)	410 ± 230 (34)	630 ± 270 (39)	650 ± 330 (18)
Eosinophils (%)	5.4 ± 4.4 (165)	7.9 ± 4.0 (27)	7.5 ± 5.3 (23)	8.8 ± 5.0 (12)	5.0 ± 2.8 (12)	5.7 ± 3.8 (34)	2.4 ± 2.6† (39)	3.0 ± 2.8† (18)
(/μl)	580 ± 530 (165)	940 ± 560 (27)	800 ± 720 (23)	890 ± 560 (12)	550 ± 330 (12)	580 ± 360 (34)	240 ± 310† (39)	270 ± 270† (18)
Basophils (%)	0.4 ± 0.5 (165)	0.5 ± 0.5 (27)	0.5 ± 0.5 (23)	0.4 ± 0.4 (12)	0.3 ± 0.6 (12)	0.4 ± 0.6 (34)	0.2 ± 0.4 (39)	0.4 ± 0.5 (18)
(/μl)	40 ± 50 (165)	50 ± 60 (27)	40 ± 60 (23)	40 ± 50 (12)	30 ± 40 (12)	50 ± 70 (34)	20 ± 40 (39)	30 ± 40 (18)
N:L ratio	1.3 ± 1.2 (165)	0.9 ± 0.3 (27)	1.2 ± 0.5 (23)	1.6 ± 0.9 (12)	0.8 ± 0.2 (12)	1.2 ± 0.8 (34)	1.2 ± 0.9 (39)	2.9 ± 2.6† (18)
Icteric index	2 ± 2 (151)	2 ± 2 (24)	2 ± 2 (23)	2 ± 2 (12)	2 ± 2 (12)	2 ± 0 (31)	2 ± 2 (36)	2 ± 2 (18)
Plasma protein (g/dl)	7.3 ± 0.6 (166)	7.4 ± 0.6 (27)	7.2 ± 0.4 (23)	7.2 ± 0.7 (12)	6.8 ± 0.5 (12)	7.5 ± 0.3 (34)	7.5 ± 0.7 (39)	6.9 ± 0.6 (19)
Fibrinogen (mg/dl)	300 ± 100 (166)	300 ± 100 (27)	200 ± 100 (23)	200 ± 100 (12)	300 ± 100 (12)	200 ± 100 (34)	400 ± 100 (39)	300 ± 100 (19)

From Zinkl, J. G., Mae, D., Merid, G. P., et al.: Reference ranges and the influence of age and sex on hematologic and serum biochemical values in donkeys (*Equus asinus*). Am. J. Vet. Res., 51:408, 1990.

* Hb, hemoglobin concentration; MCV, mean corpuscular volume; MCH, mean corpuscular hemoglobin; MCHC, mean corpuscular hemoglobin concentration; N:L, neutrophil-to-lymphocyte ratio; N, no. of samples; ND, no data.

† Significantly (p < 0.05) different from value for other groups of donkeys.

Table 3–11. Hematologic Values in 50 Clinically Normal, Lactating Murrah Buffaloes

Parameter	Range	Mean	Standard Deviation
RBC (×10⁶/μl)	5.07–8.27	6.54	0.77
Hb (g/dl)	9–13.5	11.1	0.96
PCV (%)	26–34	31.0	2.0
MCV (fl)	40.6–55.2	48.2	4.60
MCHC (%)	30.5–38.5	35.2	2.34
MCH (pg)	13.5–20.5	17.10	1.85
Icterus index (units)	2–5	2	1.25
ESR (mm at 1 hr)	17–69	53	12.30
Plasma protein (g/dl)	6–9	7.8	0.70
Fibrinogen (g/dl)	0.2–0.8	0.37	0.20
Reticulocytes (%)	0	0	0
WBC (number/μl)	6,250–13,050	9,676	1,789
Bands	0–106	18	40
Neutrophils	1,285–6,893	3,257	1,262
Lymphocytes	2,554–9,637	5,065	1,595
Monocytes	63–1,349	584	301
Eosinophils	170–1,471	592	452
Basophils	0–326	131	98
WBC, percentages			
Bands	0–1	0.2	0.34
Neutrophils	13–54	32.9	8.74
Lymphocytes	26–75	52.7	12.0
Monocytes	1–11.5	5.9	2.63
Eosinophils	2–14.0	6.9	4.64
Basophils	0–3.5	1.4	1.02

Modified from Jain, N. C., Vegad, J. L., Jain, N. K., et al.: Haematological studies on normal lactating Indian water buffaloes. Res. Vet. Sci., 32:52, 1981.

Chilean flamingos and cranes do not sediment (i.e., no erythrocyte sedimentation rate, or ESR), but those of chickens do.

Age- and sex-related differences in blood values are prominent in many species. For example, the red blood cell count (RBC), Hb concentration, and packed cell volume (PCV) are generally lower in young birds compared to those in adults. The ESR is both age- and sex-related in the ostrich (Struthio camelus) in that young birds have a higher ESR than older birds and females have a higher ESR than males (Levi et al., 1989). Undernourished birds of prey have lower hematocrit values and total plasma protein concentrations than well-nourished birds (Ferrer et al., 1987). Breed differences are found in erythrocyte osmotic fragility in domestic fowl (Oyewale and Durotoye, 1988). The total blood volume in white leghorn female chickens is higher (131.9 ± 38.3 ml/kg body weight) than in male chickens (94.9 ± 26.9 ml/kg).

Morphology of Blood Cells

Avian erythrocytes are generally elliptic and large (Plates XXVII–1 to XXVII–12). The nucleus is also elliptic and has condensed chromatin. The cytoplasm appears orange-pink. The mean corpuscular hemoglobin concentration (MCHC) in avian erythrocytes,

Table 3–12. Hematologic Values of Individual Clinically Normal Animals of Various Species

Animal	Age	Sex	RBC (Mill/μl)	Hb (g/dl)	PCV (%)	MCV (fl)	MCH (pg)	MCHC (%)	II (units)	TPP (g/dl)	Fib (g/dl)	WBC (/μl)	Neutro-phils	Lympho-cytes	Mono-cytes	Eosino-phils	Baso-phils	Platelets (/μl)
African Lion (Panthera leo)	8 mo	—	7.85	11.5	36.0	45.9	14.6	31.9	—	—	—	4,500	59.5	31.0	9.0	0.0	0.5	NA
African Lion (Panthera leo)	20 yr	F	8.12	13.9	41.0	50.5	17.1	33.9	2.0	8.0	0.1	20,500	73.0	9.0	17.0	6.0	—	NA
African Lion (Panthera leo)	20 yr	M	7.19	13.1	36.0	50.1	18.2	36.4	2.0	8.3	0.2	13,400	90.0	7.0	2.0	1.0	—	NA
Bear, American Black (Ursus americanus)	15 yr	M	7.32	18.2	55.0	75.1	24.9	33.1	2.0	7.3	0.2	8,900	73.0	13.5	12.0	1.5	0.0	NA
Baboon (Papio sp.)	—	F	5.65	14.6	48.0	85.0	25.8	30.4	2.0	8.3	0.2	8,900	45.0	48.0	5.5	1.5	—	NA
Baboon (Papio sp.)	—	M	6.30	15.4	52.0	82.5	24.4	29.6	5.0	9.2	—	15,700	88.0	8.0	3.5	0.5	—	NA
Baboon (Papio sp.)	18 yr	F	5.19	12.9	39.2	75.5	24.9	32.9	2.0	7.3	0.1	9,600	85.0	6.0	8.0	1.0	0.0	352,000
Barbary Sheep (Ammotragus lervia)	9 yr	M	17.56	17.0	44.0	25.1	9.7	38.6	Hemo	7.8	0.4	9,000	80.0	10.0	9.0	1.0	0.0	NA
Barbary Sheep (Ammotragus lervia)	2.5 yr	M	20.86	16.1	46.0	22.1	7.7	35.0	5.0	7.8	0.3	10,700	65.0	30.0	3.0	2.0	0.0	NA
Bear (Ursus sp.)	?	F	6.49	17.5	47.9	73.8	27.0	36.5	2.0	7.0	0.2	10,500	74.0	14.0	8.0	4.0	0.0	NA
Bengal Tiger (Panthera tigris tigris)	6 mo	M	6.18	9.8	31.0	50.2	15.9	31.6	2.0	6.7	0.2	20,900	69.0	18.5	8.0	4.5	0.0	NA
Bengal Tiger (Panthera tigris tigris)	3 yr	M	6.59	12.1	37.0	56.1	18.4	32.7	—	8.0	0.3	16,600	78.0	17.5	2.5	1.0	1.0	NA
Bengal Tiger (Panthera tigris tigris)	—	F	7.43	14.9	45.0	60.6	20.1	33.1	5.0	7.7	0.2	12,600	73.5	15.0	8.0	3.5	—	NA
Blackbuck (Antilope cervicapra)	1 yr	F	12.92	17.1	48.0	37.2	13.2	35.6	Hemo	7.1	0.3	3,500	34.0	64.0	2.0	0.0	0.0	NA
Blackbuck (Antilope cervicapra)	1 yr	M	14.38	18.0	49.0	34.1	12.5	36.7	Hemo	7.6	0.2	3,900	14.0	82.0	2.0	1.0	1.0	NA
Blackbuck (Antilope cervicapra)	5 yr	M	13.28	17.4	49.0	36.9	13.1	35.5	Hemo	7.8	0.3	5,900	77.0	20.0	3.0	0.0	0.0	NA
Bobcat (Felis rufus)	3 yr	F	9.26	14.4	45.0	48.6	15.6	32.0	—	8.1	0.1	8,300	40.5	54.5	2.5	2.5	—	NA
Camel, Bactrian (Camelus bactrianus)	4 yr	F	14.94	16.7	37.0	24.8	11.2	45.1	2.0	6.3	0.3	15,800	81.0	8.0	4.0	7.0	0.0	279,000
Camel (Camelus dromedarius)	1 dy	—	8.36	12.5	28.0	33.5	15.0	44.6	7.5	4.8	0.3	6,000	61.0	35.0	3.5	0.0	0.5	NA
Capuchin (Cebus capucinus)	7 mo	M	4.96	12.6	37.0	74.6	25.4	34.1	2.0	7.0	0.1	9,500	32.5	61.5	4.0	2.0	—	NA
Capuchin (Cebus capucinus)	9 yr	M	5.49	15.5	45.6	83.1	28.2	34.0	2.0	8.9	0.2	8,400	52.0	42.0	4.0	2.0	0.0	434,000
Caracal (Felis caracal)	—	F	9.89	13.4	40.0	40.4	13.5	33.5	2.0	8.1	0.1	7,900	63.0	16.0	3.0	18.0	0.0	NA
Cat, Black Footed (Felis nigripes)	?	F	6.06	9.8	30.5	50.3	16.2	32.1	2.0	7.7	0.2	9,200	65.0	28.0	7.0	0.0	0.0	734,000
Cat, Jungle (Felis chaus)	8 yr	F	7.46	13.0	41.3	55.4	17.4	31.5	2.0	8.0	0.2	8,800	47.0	47.0	1.0	5.0	0.0	218,000
Cavy, Rock (Kerodon rupestris)	?	M	3.32	15.5	53.0	159.6	46.7	29.2	Hemo	5.0	0.2	8,000	44.0	48.0	8.0	0.0	0.0	Adequate
Cheetah (Acinonyx jubatus)	1.5 yr	F	—	—	46.0	—	—	—	—	6.9	—	11,600	52.0	33.0	2.5	12.5	0.0	NA
Cheetah (Acinonyx jubatus)	10 yr	M	—	—	35.0	—	—	—	—	7.1	—	13,300	74.5	16.0	3.0	6.5	0.0	NA
Chimpanzee (Pan troglodytes)	—	M	5.46	15.0	45.0	82.4	27.5	33.3	2.0	7.2	0.4	9,700	49.0	26.0	4.0	1.0	—	NA
Chimpanzee (Pan troglodytes)	—	F	5.08	13.8	44.0	86.6	27.2	31.4	2.0	7.5	0.3	7,000	44.5	51.0	2.5	1.5	0.5	NA
Chimpanzee (Pan troglodytes)	2 yr	F	5.53	13.7	42.2	76.3	24.8	32.5	2.0	7.7	0.5	7,900	48.0	46.0	4.0	2.0	0.0	378,000
Chimpanzee (Pan troglodytes)	28 yr	F	4.84	12.6	37.7	77.9	26.0	33.4	2.0	7.3	0.3	7,100	78.0	16.0	5.0	1.0	0.0	193,000
Cinchilla (Chinchilla sp.)	5 yr	?	6.46	11.7	38.4	59.4	18.1	30.5	Hemo	7.6	—	6,700	64.0	24.0	5.0	5.0	2.0	838,000
Cougar (Felis concolor)	?	MC	8.07	11.6	36.9	45.7	14.4	31.4	5.0	8.4	0.4	6,800	89.0	5.0	6.0	0.0	0.0	256,000
Deer, Muntjac (Muntiacus sp.)	1 yr	F	18.41	14.0	39.5	21.5	7.6	35.4	2.0	6.2	0.1	6,200	53.0	40.0	5.0	1.0	1.0	479,000
Eland (Taurotragus oryx)	—	M	9.29	12.8	39.8	42.8	13.8	32.2	5.0	6.3	0.2	4,200	44.0	44.0	8.0	4.0	0.0	422,000
Elephant (Elephas maximus)	38 yr	F	2.96	13.3	35.6	120.3	44.9	37.4	2.0	8.4	0.5	10,400	30.0	12.0	57.0	1.0	0.0	548,000
Elephant (Elephas maximus)	8 yr	M	4.08	15.2	48.0	117.6	37.3	31.7	2.0	8.9	0.6	20,800	34.5	18.5	47.0	0.0	0.0	NA
Elephant (Elephas maximus)	6 yr	F	3.08	12.3	34.0	110.4	39.9	36.2	2.0	7.1	0.5	12,700	18.0	29.5	51.5	1.0	0.0	NA
Fox (Vulpes fulva)	?	?	8.90	11.7	49.3	55.4	13.1	23.7	2.0	6.2	0.2	6,300	72.0	22.0	4.0	1.0	1.0	305,000
Fox (Vulpes fulva)	5 mo	—	5.21	9.2	34.0	65.3	17.7	27.1	2.0	6.8	0.2	11,400	44.0	34.0	9.0	10.5	1.0	NA
Gazelle, Adora (Gazella sp.)	6 yr	F	10.24	16.3	48.6	47.5	15.9	33.5	2.0	7.5	0.3	4,700	86.0	11.0	3.0	0.0	0.0	484,000
Gazelle (Gazella subgutturosa)	—	M	9.27	16.0	44.0	47.5	17.3	36.4	5.0	6.3	0.3	4,000	53.0	38.0	8.0	—	1.0	NA
Gibbon (Hylobates sp.)	16 yr	F	6.40	13.7	41.5	64.8	21.4	33.0	2.0	6.9	0.2	8,700	76.0	18.0	5.0	1.0	0.0	325,000
Gibbon (Hylobates sp.)	18 yr	M	6.14	12.6	39.1	63.7	20.5	32.2	2.0	6.2	0.1	6,100	70.0	25.0	3.0	1.0	1.0	296,000
Giraffe (Giraffa camelopardalis)	5 mo	M	18.24	18.1	51.0	28.0	9.9	35.5	5.0	6.7	0.3	10,300	37.5	56.5	2.5	3.0	0.5	NA
Giraffe (Giraffa camelopardalis)	4 yr	F	12.82	15.1	43.0	33.5	11.8	35.1	7.5	9.1	0.1	14,400	65.0	30.5	1.5	2.5	0.5	NA
Giraffe (Giraffa camelopardalis)	Neonate	M	12.52	14.1	44.0	35.1	11.3	32.0	5.0	6.0	0.2	8,700	55.0	38.0	7.0	—	—	NA
Gorilla (Gorilla gorilla)	—	M	5.34	13.1	43.0	80.5	24.5	30.5	10.0	8.1	0.3	5,600	84.0	24.0	10.0	2.0	—	NA
Grison (Grison vittata)	2 yr	M	6.25	14.4	44.0	70.4	23.0	32.7	—	8.5	0.3	5,400	41.0	36.0	13.0	10.0	—	NA
Guenon (Cercopithecus sp.)	11 yr	M	4.41	11.2	33.0	74.8	25.4	33.9	5.0	6.8	0.1	6,400	43.0	54.0	2.0	0.0	1.0	311,000
Guenon (Cercopithecus sp.)	7 yr	F	5.30	13.5	39.4	74.3	25.5	34.3	5.0	8.0	0.3	6,200	12.0	83.0	3.0	2.0	0.0	367,000
Impala (Aepyceros melampus)	5 yr	F	20.25	13.5	40.0	19.8	6.7	33.8	2.0	5.9	0.6	10,100	75.5	23.5	1.0	0.0	0.0	NA
Jaguar (Panthera onca)	15 yr	F	7.76	11.7	36.9	47.6	15.1	31.7	2.0	8.5	0.3	8,900	80.0	10.0	6.0	4.0	0.0	177,000
Jaguar (Panthera onca)	5 yr	M	—	—	44.0	—	—	—	—	8.3	—	12,300	74.0	15.0	1.0	3.0	0.0	NA
Kinkajou (Potos flavus)	—	M	8.42	14.8	45.0	53.4	17.6	32.9	—	8.4	0.1	19,200	15.0	76.0	1.0	7.5	0.5	NA
Kinkajou (Potos flavus)	—	F	8.88	16.8	49.0	55.2	18.9	34.3	—	8.9	0.1	7,100	31.0	66.0	2.0	1.0	—	NA
Langur, Francois (Presbytis francoisi)	4 yr	F	5.98	13.8	40.8	68.2	23.1	33.8	2.0	7.3	0.2	9,000	56.0	38.0	5.0	0.0	1.0	272,000

(continued)

Table 3–12. Hematologic Values of Individual Clinically Normal Animals of Various Species—(Continued)

Animal	Age	Sex	RBC (Mil/μl)	Hb (g/dl)	PCV (%)	MCV (fl)	MCH (pg)	MCHC (%)	II (units)	TPP (g/dl)	Fib (g/dl)	WBC (/μl)	Neutrophils	Lymphocytes	Monocytes	Eosinophils	Basophils	Platelets (/μl)
Langur, Francois (Presbytis francoisi)	8 yr	M	7.05	16.1	48.0	68.1	22.8	33.5	2.0	6.9	0.1	4,800	76.0	14.0	7.0	2.0	1.0	340,000
Lemur, Brown (Lemur fulvus)	15 yr	M	10.34	14.7	46.8	45.3	14.2	31.4	2.0	8.0	0.3	6,600	62.0	27.0	4.0	6.0	1.0	477,000
Lemur, Mongoose (Eulemur mongoz)	23 yr	F	7.83	12.1	36.6	46.7	15.5	33.1	2.0	7.0	0.2	11,000	36.0	51.0	6.0	7.0	0.0	667,000
Lemur, Ringtailed (Lemur catta)	7 yr	M	7.76	14.4	49.7	64.0	18.6	29.0	2.0	8.5	0.2	8,500	63.0	30.0	5.0	2.0	0.0	268,000
Lemur, Ruffed (Varecia variegata)	7 mo	F	7.87	12.6	41.1	52.2	16.0	30.7	2.0	8.2	0.3	7,000	32.0	61.0	4.0	3.0	0.0	386,000
Leopard (Panthera pardus)	11 yr	F	9.62	14.6	49.4	51.4	15.2	29.6	2.0	7.6	0.3	14,500	82.0	9.0	3.0	6.0	0.0	408,000
Leopard (Panthera pardus)	1 yr	M	10.45	14.2	44.5	42.6	13.6	31.9	2.0	7.8	0.2	11,800	82.0	12.0	4.0	2.0	0.0	293,000
Lion (Panthera leo)	10 yr	FS	8.15	13.5	41.4	50.8	16.6	32.6	2.0	8.0	0.1	13,800	81.0	13.0	5.0	1.0	0.0	302,000
Mangabey (Cercocebus sp.)	20 yr	FS	4.94	12.8	39.0	78.9	25.9	32.8	2.0	7.2	0.2	10,800	64.0	32.0	3.0	0.0	1.0	199,000
Mangabey (Cercocebus sp.)	11 yr	M	4.38	11.2	34.3	78.3	25.6	32.7	2.0	7.3	0.1	5,100	53.0	40.0	5.0	1.0	1.0	189,000
Monkey, Green (Cercopithecus sabaeus)	15 yr	M	4.28	10.6	31.4	73.4	24.8	33.8	5.0	5.2	0.2	8,400	64.0	32.0	2.0	2.0	0.0	394,000
Monkey, Grivet (Cercopithecus aethiops)	16 yr	F	5.10	14.1	35.9	70.4	27.6	39.3	5.0	7.2	0.2	6,300	58.0	35.0	5.0	2.0	0.0	257,000
Monkey, Howler (Alouatta sp.)	2 yr	M	3.37	7.7	25.2	74.8	22.8	30.6	2.0	7.8	0.2	5,700	57.0	39.0	3.0	1.0	0.0	421,000
Monkey, spider (Ateles belzebuth)	7 yr	F	5.52	15.3	45.2	81.9	27.7	33.8	5.0	8.4	0.2	7,400	49.0	41.0	2.0	7.0	1.0	418,000
Monkey, Squirrel (Samiri sciureus)	24 yr	F	6.60	11.9	37.7	57.1	18.0	31.6	2.0	8.5	0.3	5,800	22.0	66.0	6.0	6.0	0.0	410,000
Monkey, Vervep (Cercopithecus aethiops)	2 yr	F	4.45	11.6	32.9	73.9	26.1	35.3	5.0	6.6	0.1	6,600	52.0	37.0	2.0	8.0	1.0	297,000
Mountain Lion (Felis concolor)	2 yr	M	10.52	15.4	47.0	44.7	14.6	32.8	2.0	8.8	0.4	22,000	86.0	10.0	4.0	0.0	0.0	NA
Ocelot (Felis pardalis)	10 yr	M	9.36	13.8	45.0	48.1	14.7	30.7	Hemo	9.8	0.2	13,650	60.0	35.0	2.5	2.0	0.5	NA
Okapi (Okapia johnstoni)	2 yr	M	12.36	11.9	36.0	29.1	9.6	33.1	2.0	7.8	0.5	5,500	36.0	60.0	2.0	1.0	1.0	NA
Orangutan (Pongo pygmaeus)	Neonate	M	5.95	16.3	46.0	77.3	27.4	35.4	—	—	—	8,700	50.0	45.0	5.0	—	—	NA
Orangutan (Pongo pygmaeus)	Adult	M	5.70	14.3	44.0	77.2	25.1	32.5	10.0	8.2	0.4	9,300	67.5	26.5	4.5	1.0	0.5	NA
Orangutan (Pongo pygmaeus)	31 yr	F	4.35	12.0	35.3	81.1	27.6	34.0	2.0	7.9	0.5	8,400	50.0	46.0	3.0	1.0	0.0	447,000
Oryx (Oryx sp.)	5 yr	M	15.00	20.4	61.2	40.8	13.6	33.3	5.0	7.6	0.4	7,000	82.0	14.0	4.0	0.0	0.0	332,000
Peccary (Tayassu sp.)	3.5 yr	F	8.17	13.5	43.0	52.6	16.5	31.4	5.0	8.9	0.3	7,400	43.0	53.5	1.5	1.5	0.5	NA
Peccary (Tayassu sp.)	2 yr	F	8.27	14.1	47.0	56.8	17.0	30.0	Hemo	8.9	0.3	7,100	20.0	77.0	2.0	1.0	0.0	NA
Polar Bear (Ursus maritimus)	8.5 yr	F	8.00	18.1	52.0	65.0	22.6	34.8	5.0	9.3	0.2	11,800	71.5	12.5	5.5	10.5	0.0	NA
Polar Bear (Ursus maritimus)	8.5 yr	M	8.67	21.3	57.0	65.7	24.6	37.4	Hemo	9.3	0.3	11,200	82.5	6.0	6.5	5.0	0.0	NA
Reindeer (Rangifer tarandus)	8 yr	M	11.14	16.8	51.0	45.8	15.1	32.9	2.0	7.7	0.2	6,100	57.0	36.0	6.0	1.0	0.0	380,000
Lemur, Ringtailed (Lemur catta)	—	M	8.30	15.0	52.0	62.7	18.1	28.8	Hemo	8.8	0.2	9,200	44.5	48.0	5.0	1.5	1.0	NA
Seal, Harbor (Phoca vitulina)	?	M	4.83	20.2	57.3	118.6	41.8	35.3	2.0	9.4	0.2	9,400	56.0	19.0	10.0	12.0	3.0	491,000
Sealion (Zalophus californianus)	4 yr	MC	3.83	14.8	41.3	107.8	38.6	35.8	5.0	9.0	0.4	8,400	60.0	26.0	7.0	7.0	0.0	313,000
Serval Cat (Felis serval)	4 yr	F	6.83	14.0	50.3	73.6	20.5	27.8	2.0	7.8	0.1	6,200	66.0	29.0	3.0	2.0	0.0	160,000
Serval Cat (Felis serval)	6 yr	F	6.73	13.3	36.0	53.5	19.8	36.9	Hemo	7.9	0.4	22,500	44.0	49.0	5.5	1.5	0.0	NA
Serval Cat (Felis serval)	6 mo	M	5.29	10.3	34.0	64.3	19.5	30.3	2.0	6.4	0.5	13,600	81.5	12.0	4.5	2.0	0.0	NA
Sloth Bear (Ursus ursinus)	8 yr	F	6.31	17.5	49.0	77.7	27.7	35.7	2.0	8.0	0.3	9,500	81.0	17.0	1.0	1.0	0.0	NA
Snow Leopard (Felis uncia)	4 mo	M	9.06	11.1	34.0	37.5	12.3	32.6	2.0	6.7	0.2	12,500	73.0	21.5	4.5	1.0	0.0	NA
Spider Monkey (Ateless sp.)	15 yr	M	5.29	11.4	38.0	71.8	21.6	30.0	—	7.5	0.4	13,000	89.0	11.0	—	—	—	NA
Spotted hyena (Crocuta crocuta)	3 mo	M?	5.65	9.0	28.0	49.6	15.9	32.1	—	6.5	—	17,100	—	—	—	—	—	NA
Striped Hyena (Hyaena hyaena)	6 yr	M	—	—	43.0	—	—	—	—	7.1	—	19,300	72.0	15.0	4.0	4.0	0.0	NA
Tamarin (Saguinus oedipus)	1 yr	F	6.64	17.5	50.9	76.7	26.4	34.4	2.0	8.0	0.4	7,400	64.0	30.0	5.0	1.0	0.0	360,000
Tamarin (Saguinus oedipus)	6 yr	F	6.47	15.2	46.5	71.9	23.5	32.7	5.0	8.3	0.2	11,700	42.0	41.0	11.0	2.0	4.0	326,000
Tiger (Panthera tigris)	14 yr	F	7.19	12.8	40.0	55.6	17.8	32.0	2.0	8.0	0.3	8,100	79.0	14.0	4.0	3.0	0.0	222,000
Tiger (Panthera tigris)	2 yr	F	6.79	13.1	39.6	58.3	19.3	33.1	2.0	7.3	0.1	8,800	82.0	15.0	3.0	0.0	0.0	158,000
Wallaby (Wallabia sp.)	3 yr	M	5.67	15.6	44.5	78.5	27.5	35.1	2.0	7.4	0.3	6,800	66.0	25.0	6.0	3.0	0.0	329,000
Wallaroo (Macropus sp.)	7 mo	M	7.52	20.1	60.4	80.3	26.7	33.3	2.0	7.4	0.4	6,400	84.0	13.0	3.0	0.0	0.0	231,000
Wolf (Canis lupus)	6 yr	M	6.04	13.5	38.7	64.1	22.4	34.9	2.0	5.6	0.1	5,900	77.0	12.0	3.0	8.0	0.0	240,000
Yak (Bos grunniens)	35 yr	M	6.21	12.8	36.0	58.0	20.6	35.6	7.5	7.8	0.7	4,500	67.0	23.0	3.0	7.0	0.0	NA
Yak (Bos grunniens)	40 yr	M	5.81	12.7	36.0	62.0	21.9	35.3	5.0	7.0	0.5	4,000	59.0	30.0	2.0	9.0	—	NA
Zebra (Hippotigris sp.)	1 yr	F	11.47	14.2	44.2	38.5	12.4	32.1	10.0	6.8	0.1	9,800	72.0	25.0	3.0	0.0	0.0	287,000
Zebra (Hippotigris sp.)	1 yr	M	15.10	16.9	53.3	35.3	11.2	31.7	5.0	7.0	0.3	12,600	80.0	18.0	1.0	1.0	0.0	316,000
Zebu (Bos indicus)	3 yr	M	9.04	12.5	40.0	44.2	13.8	31.3	5.0	6.9	0.3	6,600	25.0	62.0	5.0	8.0	0.0	NA
Zebu (Bos indicus)	8 yr	F	5.83	11.6	36.0	61.7	19.9	32.2	5.0	7.8	0.4	3,500	25.0	68.0	0.0	7.0	0.0	NA

Hemo = hemolyzed; FS, female spayed; MC, male castrated.

particularly in juveniles, is lower than in mammalian erythrocytes, probably because of the space occupied by the nucleus (Hawkey, 1991). A few large polychromatic erythrocytes (reticulocytes) may be found. These cells are almost round and have less condensed nuclear chromatin. More immature erythrocytic precursor cells can be seen occasionally in the blood films of anemic birds (Plate XXVII–5). Erythrocyte volume distribution curves in ducks commonly reveal two populations of red cells, with an average mean corpuscular volume

(MCV) of 128.37 fl/cell and 308.50 fl/cell, respectively, with males having a greater (76%) proportion of smaller RBCs than females (58%) (Herbert et al., 1989). Heinz body formation may occur in avian erythrocytes as a primary toxic manifestation of the ingestion of crude oil, which leads to the production of a hemolytic anemia. Lead poisoning in birds may manifest as mild hypochromic anemia with reticulocytosis.

Thrombocytes appear to function in hemostasis in birds analogous to the platelets of mammals. Although the terms "thrombocyte" and "platelet" have become synonymous with regard to their usage in mammalian hematology, only the former term should be used in descriptions pertaining to avian species. Typical thrombocytes are oval and usually have oval nuclei and a moderate amount of pale blue cytoplasm (Plate XXVII–4). They frequently contain a few small, reddish-purple granules in the cytoplasm. Occasionally, small groups of aggregated thrombocytes may be found, more frequently in blood samples that were difficult to obtain. The origin of the avian thrombocyte remains elusive. No megakaryocytes are present in avian bone marrow.

Leukocytes of various types are found in avian blood. The heterophil in birds is the counterpart of the neutrophil in mammalian species. This designation refers to the staining quality of the cell, and does not imply different functional activities. Differentiating heterophils and eosinophils can be difficult and lymphocytes, monocytes, and thrombocytes can cause confusion. Both heterophils and eosinophils are segmented cells with reddish-orange granules. The former cell predominates over the latter. In both cells, the nucleus may be obscured by overlying, intensely stained granules. Heterophils generally have rod-shaped granules, whereas eosinophils have round granules (Plates XXVII–1 and XXVII–2). Such a distinction, however, is not always easily made with light microscopy. Chicken heterophils do not stain for alkaline phosphatase (ALP), peroxidase (PO), Sudan black B (SBB), chloroacetate esterase (CAE), α-naphthyl acetate esterase (NAE), acid phosphatase (ACP), and periodic acid-Schiff (PAS) reaction, whereas eosinophils do react for PO, SBB, and ACP (Andreasen and Latimer, 1990). Chicken and duck eosinophils have a crystalline core in specific granules, similar to that seen in eosinophils of some mammalian species (Maxwell, 1986a). In addition, normal quail eosinophils show cytoplasmic lipid droplets (1–1.5 μm) that are surrounded by profiles of endoplasmic reticulum and stain positive for peroxidase (Maxwell, 1986b). The number of lipid droplets is decreased in eosinophils from stressed birds.

Small, medium, and large lymphocytes may be found in the peripheral blood of birds (Plate XXVII–4). Small lymphocytes have a thin rim of basophilic cytoplasm around an oval nucleus. The deeper staining of the cytoplasm and its sparse amount are usually sufficient criteria to distinguish small lymphocytes from thrombocytes. Medium and large lymphocytes have more cytoplasm that may stain light blue. Some large lymphocytes have a few azurophilic granules in their homogeneous cytoplasm. These granules are larger and less numerous than the tiny azurophilic granules found in some thrombocytes. "Intermediate cells," cells with features of small lymphocytes and thrombocytes, have small round or oval nuclei with coarsely condensed chromatin and moderately abundant blue cytoplasm devoid of granules and vacuoles. These cells should be classified as lymphocytes because they do not fluoresce after gaseous formaldehyde treatment and fail to react with Grimelius or PAS stain, similar to typical lymphocytes and unlike most typical thrombocytes. Gaseous formaldehyde condenses with the serotonin present in thrombocytes to produce a fluorescent product, whereas Grimelius staining is based on the argyrophil reaction, which detects serotonin and other biogenic monoamines in cells (Swayne et al., 1986).

Monocytes are usually the largest of the leukocytes seen in the blood smears of birds. Their nuclei are usually round or oval but may be elongated, with an indentation on one side. Their cytoplasm is usually abundant and frequently vacuolated or foamy (Plate XXVII–3). Azurophilic granules, like those in thrombocytes, are not seen in monocytes. Small, unvacuolated monocytes may resemble large lymphocytes and, similarly, some large lymphocytes may be mistaken for monocytes.

Hematopoietic Features

A unique feature of avian bone marrow is that erythropoiesis and possibly thrombopoiesis occur within the vascular sinuses (intravascular), whereas granulopoiesis takes place outside the vascular sinuses (extravascular). This distribution of hematopoietic cells can be easily recognized in histologic sections of bone marrow. Cells of the erythropoietic and granulocytic series in birds are similar to those of mammals. Lymphocytic progenitor cells probably originate from pluripotent stem cells in the bone marrow, as in mammals. The bursa of Fabricius is a well-known site for processing the B lymphocytes responsible for humoral immunity, and the thymus processes T lymphocytes. Lymphocytes in blood probably arise from the "peripheral" lymphoid tissues, however, including the spleen, cecal tonsils, and other gut-associated lymphoid tissues.

Response to Anemia

Recovery from acute blood loss in most avian species occurs within a shorter period than in mammalian species (Schindler et al., 1987). Chickens (Gallus domesticus) regain normal RBC counts within 7 days of a 35% decrease in hematocrit. Japanese quail (Coturnix coturnix japonica) regain RBC counts within 72 hours of a 30% reduction in blood volume. The recovery period in mammals with a 5 to 15% reduction in blood volume is generally longer: 40 days in humans, 14 to 17 days in rabbits, and 8 to 15 days in rats. RBC counts in birds are restored from rapid stimulation of erythropoiesis in bone marrow and not from splenic reserve, because birds apparently do not store erythrocytes in the spleen (Hawkey, 1991). Similarly, the storage capacity of the spleen is lower in primates, so dramatic changes in red cell values do not occur. In quails, stimulation of erythropoiesis is reflected by increased numbers of reticulocytes in bone marrow between 6 and 24 hours and in circulation by 72 hours after blood loss. Birds also restore plasma volume following hemorrhage more rapidly than mammals. White blood cell (WBC) counts and agranulocytes recover by 72 hours postphlebotomy in quails.

Blood Parasites

Several protozoan parasites occur in the blood of birds. The most important are Plasmodium, Haemoproteus, and Leukocytozoon, but Trypanosoma and Lankersterella (also known as Atoxoplasma) species and Piroplasma organisms (Nuttalia and Aegyptianella species) may also be found. Iron pigment and developing schizonts in erythrocytes are important criteria for differentiating Plasmodium, Haemoproteus, and Leukocytozoon species. Organisms of the first two species have iron pigment in the erythrocytes, but organisms of Leukocytozoon do not (Plates XXVII–8 to XXVII–12).

Plasmodium species cause avian malaria and are transmitted by mosquitos to many species of birds. Clinical signs of malaria are nonspecific and the presence of the malarial organism does not mean a bird has the disease. Birds with malaria may be anorectic, depressed, and weak, and may die suddenly. Intense and severe anemia may occur. Splenomegaly and hepatomegaly are present. Reticuloendothelial hyperplasia with mature schizonts in the cells is found on histopathologic examination. Erythrocytes containing schizonts are found in blood smears. Antimalarial drugs have been used to treat malaria with some success, and transmission might be prevented in domestic and pet birds through isolation from mosquito vectors by housing, screening, and nets.

Haemoproteus and Parahaemoproteus species are apparently nonpathogenic or of low pathogenicity. Unlike Plasmodium species, schizonts are found only in endothelial cells, but erythrocytes contain gametocytes. The gametocytes of *Haemoproteus* sp. are usually halter-shaped compared to those of *Plasmodium* sp. (Plates XXVII–8 and XXVII–9).

Leukocytozoon species can cause severe disease in some birds. They are transmitted by black flies and perhaps by midges. The infection is diagnosed by finding gametocytes in leukocytes. The gametocytes are round or elongated, and may be dark-staining macrogametocytes or light-staining microgametocytes (Plates XXVII–10, XXVII–11, and XXVII–12). Pig-

ment granules are not found. Schizogony does not occur in blood.

Microfilariae (longer than 200 μm), larval forms of filarial roundworms, are frequently seen in the blood of birds, but mostly as an incidental finding (Plate XXVII–6).

Spirochetosis, caused by Borrelia anserina, may occur in many species of birds. In fowl, it is an acute disease characterized by fever, depression, weakness, cyanosis, and diarrhea. Anemia may develop. Hepatomegaly and splenomegaly may be found at necropsy. Surviving birds show a response to anemia, such as reticulocytosis, macrocytosis, and polychromasia. The diagnosis is based on finding organisms in fresh blood by the use of darkfield microscopy or in Giemsa-stained films on light microscopy (Plate XXVII–7).

Leukocyte Response to Disease

The leukocyte response to disease has been summarized (Latimer et al., 1988). White leghorn chickens are similar to ruminants in that the lymphocyte is the major circulating leukocyte, with a heterophil: lymphocyte (H:L) ratio of 0.27 ± 0.07. Like rodents, different avian species vary in having either lymphocytes or heterophils predominate in the circulation. Most chickens and white-naped cranes have a predominance of lymphocytes, whereas California gray chickens, ducks, and many exotic and pet birds usually have more heterophils in blood.

Leukocyte values in birds should be interpreted with caution because the stress of capture, handling, caging, social interactions, and environmental conditions can induce lymphopenia and heterophilia (increase in heterophil numbers in blood), presumably through the endogenous release of corticosteroids. Heterophilia also occurs in birds in response to ACTH administration, similar to neutrophilia in mammals. In contrast, physiologic leukocytosis from epinephrine release may produce a lymphocytosis in association with heterophilia, as seen in other species.

Leukocytosis, predominantly from heterophilia, occurs during acute inflammation in chickens. Infectious diseases such as coccidiosis, Escherichia coli air sacculitis, and schistosomiasis produce a similar pattern in chickens. Mild lymphocytosis has been observed in birds with nonspecific inflammation, as well as bacterial infection, parasitism, chronic viral infections, and leukemia. Hyperfibrinogenemia (63%) was found slightly more frequently than heterophilia (56%) in birds with bacterial infections, but when either finding was taken in account, the diagnosis was confirmed in 77% of cases (Hawkey and Hart, 1988). Monocytosis is usually a consequence of chronic diseases such as granulomatous lesions, bacterial infections, chlamydiosis, parasitism, and zinc deficiency. Monocytosis may also occur in acute inflammatory diseases and may manifest as early as 12 hours after the induction of inflammation. Changes in eosinophil and basophil numbers may vary widely, and should be interpreted with caution.

Detection of left shifts in chicken blood is challenging because heterophils are normally hyposegmented, and their intensely stained reddish granules usually obscure the nuclear morphology. Chicken heterophils generally contain a range of late band-shaped nuclei to three nuclear lobes, with an average of approximately two nuclear lobes. Determination of a heterophil mean nuclear score in hematoxylin-stained blood films is considered a sensitive indicator of left or right shift in heterophils. The inflammatory response in chickens injected intramuscularly with turpentine was associated with heterophil nuclear hyposegmentation during the early stages (12 to 48 hours) and hypersegmentation during convalescence (4 to 7 days). Toxic changes in heterophils are similar to those seen in other species and include variable degrees of cellular swelling, degranulation, vacuolation, and cytoplasmic basophilia. Binucleate heterophils and "toxic" granules (oblong to needle-shaped red granules and variable numbers of chunky, round, purple granules) may occur in chickens with the most intense left shifts and toxic changes. Degranulation occurring as a staining artifact (cells with clear cytoplasm) may create a problem during the differential leukocyte count, but is easily distinguished from that seen in toxic heterophils (cells with blue cytoplasm).

MISCELLANEOUS DOMESTIC, ZOO, AND WILD MAMMALIAN SPECIES

Selected Blood Values

Hematologic values of some normal laboratory animals and miscellaneous domestic, zoo, and wild mammalian species are presented in Tables 3–2 to 3–12. Comparative morphologic features of erythrocytes, leukocytes, and platelets in some of these species are described below. Special hematologic characteristics of some of the species are presented separately.

ERYTHROCYTES

Mammalian erythrocytes are non-nucleated and, with rare exception, discoid, with varying degrees of biconcavity. Erythrocytes of the camel are typically elliptic and devoid of central depression, as are the red blood cells of other members of the family Camelidae. Deer blood often reveals erythrocyte sickling, usually as an in vitro phenomenon. The Malay chevrotain has the smallest erythrocyte (about 1.5 μm in diameter) and the elephant has the largest erythrocyte (about 9.0 to 10.0 μm) among mammals. The guinea pig erythrocyte is the largest among the more common laboratory animals. Nucleated, elliptic erythrocytes characterize the blood of reptiles, amphibians, fish, and birds. Nucleated red blood cells are usually absent or rare in the adult mammal, but 4 to 40% nucleated erythrocytes are normally seen in koala blood. In the newborn golden hamster, 10 to 30% of circulating erythrocytes may be nucleated, although in the adult

hamster they may be either absent or sparse (<2.0%). The red blood cell life span of some reptiles may be as long as 3 years, and appears to be temperature-dependent. The peccary is a pig-like animal that is classified separately from swine. Its erythrocytes are not crenated, as is common with pig blood.

The reticulocyte percentage is higher in rodents, reflecting a rapid erythrocyte turnover because of shorter life span as compared to that of common domestic animals. Rats at birth have nearly 99% reticulocytes, which decline to approximately 25% at weaning (21 days of age), to 3.0% at 70 days of age, and to less than 3.0% in older rats. This decline in reticulocyte numbers in rats correlates with an age-related decrease in the erythrocytic delta-aminolevulinic acid dehydratase activity (Davis and Avram, 1978). Basophilic stippling is common in gerbils; fetal and newborn gerbils may have up to 40% of red cells exhibiting basophilic stippling, compared to approximately 5% in the adult gerbil. Heinz bodies are common in the Felidae, white rhinoceroses and marmosets (Hawkey and Dennett, 1989; Omorphos et al., 1989a). Cabot rings (remnants of mitotic spindle) are occasionally found in normal Bactrian camel blood films stained with new methylene blue. Howell-Jolly bodies, also called micronuclei, are rare in rat and mouse blood, but increased numbers are found during response to anemia (George et al., 1990).

In general, RBC counts among different species vary inversely with erythrocyte size (MCV), but Hb, PCV, and MCHC values are remarkably constant (Hawkey, 1991). Thus, a species has either many small or fewer larger erythrocytes. An inverse relationship is also found between erythrocyte dimensions (MCV and mean cell diameter) and osmotic resistance of red cells (Peinado et al., 1992). The MCHC is over 40% in the camel, but in other mammals it fluctuates around a mean value of 33%. The RBC counts of mules and donkeys are similar to those of the cold-blooded horses, but their MCV is somewhat higher. The ESR in the burro is high as in the horse. In wild Felidae (adult pumas, lions, tigers, leopards, jaguars, and cheetahs), the ESR varies widely and is inversely related to the RBC count, and the MCV is directly related to average body weight, except in cheetahs (Hawkey and Hart, 1986). The serum bilirubin concentration is much lower (0.4 mg/dl) and the serum lipid level higher (1.0 mg/dl) in the donkey than in the horse. Red cell parameters of Mexican wolves (Canis lupus baileyi) (>24 weeks old) are comparable to those of the adult dog (Drag 1991).

THROMBOCYTES

Thrombocytes are nucleated structures in species that exhibit nucleated erythrocytes, but they are non-nucleated in mammals. Platelet numbers are high in laboratory animals, often exceeding 1 million/μl of blood. High platelet counts relative to the small blood volume in rodents probably reflect a physiologic adaptation to contain the smallest possible blood loss crucial to survival. The platelet shape varies from round, oval, oblong, or cigar-shaped to elongated forms. Spiny anteaters present elongated platelets in addition to regular forms. Species variations have been demonstrated in platelet aggregation and blood clotting factors. As mentioned above, birds lack coagulation factors V, VII, X, XI, and XII.

LEUKOCYTES

Leukocyte count and morphology vary among various species. WBC counts are highest in the tail blood of rats and mice compared to heart blood. Neutrophils vary with regard to granule color, shape, size, and nuclear morphology. The neutrophil in the peripheral blood of common laboratory animals (e.g., the rabbit, guinea pig, rat, and mouse) is often referred to as a heterophil because its granules do not display a neutral staining reaction in blood films stained with a Romanowsky stain. The granules often stain a strong pink and are similar in color to eosinophil granules, so the cell is sometimes also called a pseudoeosinophil (Figs. 3–1 and 3–2). For all practical purposes, the heterophils of laboratory animals are equivalent to the neutrophils seen in common domestic animals and humans. Heterophils are also observed in other animal species, such as birds and elephants. Their staining properties are similar to basophils, but the granules are much smaller. Heterophils of the ring-tailed lemur are unique in that their granules stain dark-purple to almost black. Nuclear segmentation also varies in different species. Most nonhuman primates have well segmented neutrophils, whereas rodents often display U-shaped, doughnut-shaped, or distorted nuclei. Chinchilla neutrophils may have hyposegmented nuclei similar to those of the rabbit and dog with Pelger-Huët anomaly. Pelger-Huet neutrophils may be occasionally found in camel blood. Alkaline phosphatase activity of neutrophils of laboratory animals varies from no activity in mice to moderate to marked activity in rats, rabbits, gerbils, hamsters, and guinea pigs (Tamburlin and Glomski, 1988).

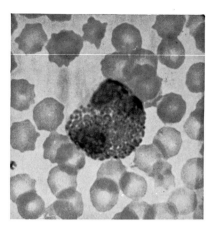

Fig. 3–2. Rabbit eosinophil (× 1400). (From Jain, N.C.: Schalm's Veterinary Hematology. 4th Ed. Philadelphia, Lea & Febiger, 1986, p. 281.)

Eosinophil granules are generally round but may sometimes be rod-shaped (guinea pig), as in the cat. Similar rod-like eosinophil granules are seen in the cheetah, but round granules are characteristic of eosinophils of the lion, mountain lion, tiger, and leopard. The eosinophil number is high in the normal owl monkey, and the granules are cigar-shaped. The eosinophil of the hyena presents distinct round vacuoles in the place of granules in a gray cytoplasm (Fig. 3–3). In this respect, the eosinophil of the hyena resembles the vacuolated eosinophil of the greyhound. Vacuolated eosinophils may also be found in an occasional bear. The neutrophil sex chromatin lobe may be helpful in distinguishing male and female spotted hyena, especially at a young age, when gender is difficult to determine from the external genitalia (Fig. 3–4). Sex chromatin and sessile lobes may be found in neutrophils of other wild and zoo animals.

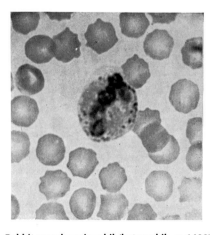

Fig. 3–1. Rabbit pseudoeosinophil (heterophil; × 1400). (From Jain, N.C.: Schalm's Veterinary Hematology. 4th Ed. Philadelphia, Lea & Febiger, 1986, p. 281.)

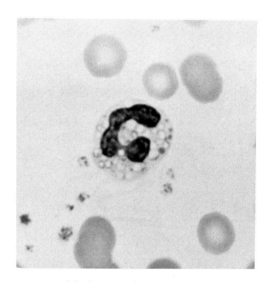

Fig. 3–3. Eosinophil of Hyaena hyaena (× 4500). (From Jain, N.C.: Schalm's Veterinary Hematology. 4th Ed. Philadelphia, Lea & Febiger, 1986, p. 341.)

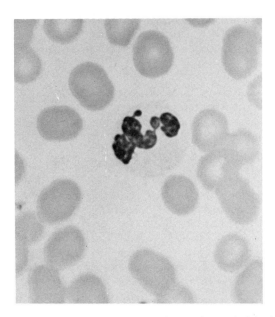

Fig. 3–4. Neutrophil with typical female sex chromatin lobe in the blood of a 3-month-old spotted hyena that was considered to be a male from the appearance of the external genitalia, (× 3600). (From Jain, N.C.: Schalm's Veterinary Hematology. 4th Ed. Philadelphia, Lea & Febiger, 1986, p. 342.)

The basophil number in blood generally is inversely proportional to the number of tissue mast cells. Lymphocytes and monocytes do not present any unusual features. Lymphocytes with some small azurophil granules can be found occasionally along with small to large lymphocytes in various animal species. In rats, the neutrophil:lymphocyte ratio varies widely in health

and disease and is influenced by the age and sex of the animals.

Leukocyte response to disease in most mammalian species in the wild and in zoos is similar: neutropenia to neutrophilia with or without left shift and toxic changes may occur in response to inflammation and infection. Stress-related changes similarly include neutrophilia, lymphopenia, and eosinopenia. Rarely, leukemia may be diagnosed; a case of myelomonocytic leukemia was encountered in a jaguar at the Veterinary Medical Teaching Hospital, University of California, Davis. Criteria for differentiation of myeloid hyperplasia from granulocytic leukemia in mice have been reviewed (Long et al., 1986).

Unique Blood Features of Certain Species

CAMELIDS

The ruminant family Camelidae includes camels, guanacos, llamas, alpacas, and vicunas. The erythrocytes of these animals are elliptic (Fig. 3–5) compared to reticulocytes and nucleated red cells, which appear to be round. The red cells lack a central depression and are thin (Figs. 7–10E and 7–10F). The MCHC is generally over 40%, which is considerably in excess of the range of 30 to 36% common to animals with discoid erythrocytes. The high MCHC of camel erythrocytes is a species characteristic and not a technical artifact. Camels, like humans, seem to lack a splenic reserve of red cells, as indicated by a minimal increase in Hb and PCV after maximal exercise over 4 or 5 km (Snow et al., 1988). The small increase in red cell values is seen in association with a similar increase in total plasma proteins and is therefore attributed to a

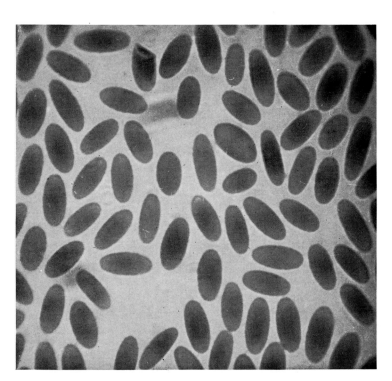

Fig. 3–5. Elliptic erythrocytes (from Lama guanicoe) typical of the family Camellidae (× 1600). (From Jain, N.C.: Schalm's Veterinary Hematology. 4th Ed. Philadelphia, Lea & Febiger, 1986, p. 336.)

slight decrease in plasma volume (dehydration). The absence of splenic reserve of red cells in normal camels is unlike that in other species, such as dogs, cats, horses, cows, and sheep.

Among mammals, camel erythrocytes are the most resistant to hemolysis in hypotonic saline solution as a result of their high water-binding capability. Initial hemolysis may be observed in 0.30% saline solution and complete hemolysis in 0.21% solution. This unique property of the camel erythrocyte may be related to its membrane structure and is of physiologic significance. Their red cell membranes have a high protein:lipid ratio, lack ankyrin (band 2.1), contain pre-band 1 high-molecular-weight protein bands, have a spectrin band 1:2 ratio of 0.7 compared to 1.3 in humans (Hawkey and Gulland, 1988; Omorphos et al., 1989b). Camel erythrocytes are relatively nondeformable in that they are highly resistant to drugs that cause echinocytic and stomatocytic changes in discocytic erythrocytes of humans (Omorphos et al., 1989b). Erythrocytic glutathione peroxidase activity correlates significantly with red cell selenium concentration.

Hematologic values of 174 llamas (Lama glama) from ranches in California and Nevada are presented in Table 3–8 (Fowler and Zinkl, 1989). Compared with hematologic values for horses and cattle, llamas have more RBCs but a lower PCV because the smaller elliptic cells pack tighter. Their MCV is about half that of horses and cattle, the MCHC is higher, and the MCH slightly lower. The neutrophil:lymphocyte ratio is similar to that of horses, with most of the cells being neutrophils. Red cell values are lower in neonates less than 1 month old than in adults. Eosinophil counts are low in neonates and crias, but high in adults.

A study of the blood counts of healthy juvenile and adult llamas and guanacos showed that guanacos have higher RBC counts and Hb and PCV values (Hawkey and Gulland, 1988). In both species, absolute lymphocyte counts and platelet numbers were higher in juveniles than in adults. Neutrophilia, hyperfibrinogenemia, and a tendency to develop regenerative hypochromic anemia were observed in many animals with acute and chronic inflammatory diseases. Macrocytic hypochromic anemia occurred in animals with

parasitic infections. Eosinophilia was the only abnormal hematologic finding in many animals suspected of having subclinical intestinal parasitic infection. An eperythrozoon-like parasite was found to infect llamas and cause a mild to moderate anemia. The organisms were coccoid or ring-shaped, measured about 0.5 to 1.0 μm in diameter, and epicellular. The serologic antibody titer to Eperythrozoon suis was positive (McLaughlin et al., 1990). A syndrome characterized by anemia, erythrocyte dyscrasia, low body weight, and hypothyroidism was observed in eight llamas (Smith et al., 1991). The PCV in two of the llamas decreased to less than 10%. Erythrocyte abnormalities included severe poikilocytosis, anisocytosis, asymmetric distribution of hemoglobin, and cytoplasmic extensions from one or both poles. Five of the llamas had hypophosphatemia and seven had low serum iron levels. Hypochromic red cells may be found in blood films of camelids with iron deficiency anemia (Plates XVIII-5 and XVIII-7). Rarely, hemoglobin crystals may be seen as a nonspecific finding in erthyrocytes of a sick animal (Plate XVIII-6).

DEER

The erythrocytes of deer belonging to the family Cervidae are of special interest because of a sickling phenomenon first described by Gulliver in 1840 (Figs. 3–6 and 3–7). The erythrocytes circulate as round cells and are similar in size to the erythrocytes of cattle. The normal deer erythrocyte is not sickled when first removed from the body, but sickling occurs as the sample stands at room or refrigerator temperature. Sickling can be prevented by acidifying the blood—a relatively sharp transition from normal to sickle shape occurs between pH 7.0 and 7.5, with almost all cells sickling at pH 7.4. Sickling can be enhanced by passing oxygen gas through the blood. Similarly, transient alkalosis and oxygenation of blood in vivo have enhanced sickling.

Sickling results from the formation of insoluble tactoids of variant hemoglobin in the oxygenated state. Deer blood contains several hemoglobins with different electrophoretic properties. Sickling does not occur

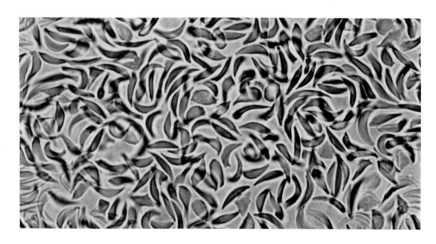

Fig. 3–6. Classic sickle-shaped deer erythrocytes. (From Kitchen, H., Putnam, F.W., and Taylor, W.J.: Hemoglobin polymorphism: Its relation to sickling of erythrocytes in white-tailed deer. Science, 144: 1237, 1964.)

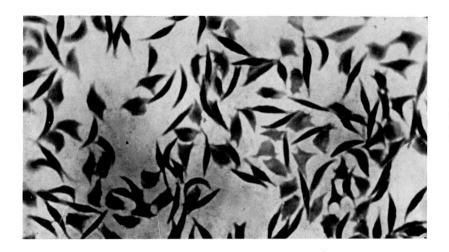

Fig. 3–7. Crescent and holly leaf forms of sickled deer erythrocytes. (From Jain, N.C.: Schalm's Veterinary Hematology. 4th Ed. Philadelphia, Lea & Febiger, 1986, p. 322.)

when hemoglobin V or VII is present. Hemoglobin II, either alone or in combination with hemoglobins I, III, or IVb, is associated with the final development of a matchstick appearance after passing through the sickled stage (Fig. 3–8). Reindeer and montjac deer erythrocytes do not sickle when exposed to oxygen, unlike erythrocytes of many other species of Cervidae.

White-tailed deer have RBC, Hb, and PCV values that are considerably higher than those of normal domestic cattle, but WBC counts are lower than in cattle. Mule deer and black-tailed deer, including those from California, have lower RBC, Hb, and PCV values than the eastern white-tailed deer, but somewhat higher values than domestic cattle. Observations on several species of deer have revealed a direct relationship between red cell size and body size in members of the Cervidae (Hawkey and Hart, 1985). An indirect relationship between red cell size and number, as reported for other mammals, is also seen in deer.

The deer is one of the most excitable species. Hence, red cell values are significantly higher in excited deer than in resting deer, probably because of splenic contraction, which forces stored red cells into the circulation (Maede et al., 1990). A sex difference may be evident in some blood values of adult (>2 years)

sika deer (Cervus nippon yesoensis), but not in fawns (of about 10 months). For example, the WBC count with neutrophilia was markedly higher in excited wild females than in resting wild females, but this was not observed in excited and resting wild males. The RBC and PCV values were significantly higher and the MCH was lower in excited males than in excited females.

A study of clinically normal captive reindeers showed that the red cell values were lower in juveniles than in adults (Catley et al., 1990). Newborn animals were anemic compared with juveniles and adults and had high reticulocyte counts. It was shown that sick reindeers exhibit hematologic responses similar to those of other artiodactyla, with increases in erythrocyte sedimentation rate and fibrinogen level being of particular diagnostic significance. Eosinophilia occurred in animals with subclinical infections with intestinal parasites.

DONKEYS

The hematologic values of 217 donkeys (Equus asinus) are presented in Table 3–10 (Zinkl et al., 1990).

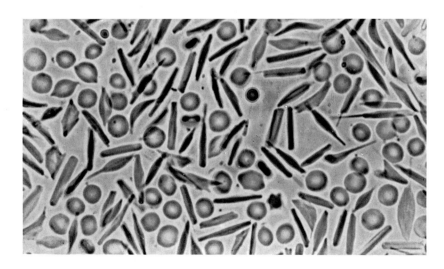

Fig. 3–8. Sickled erythrocytes of the deer, matchstick form, associated with hemoglobin II, either alone or in combination with hemoglobins I, III, or IVb. (From Jain, N.C.: Schalm's Veterinary Hematology. 4th Ed. Philadelphia, Lea & Febiger, 1986, p. 322.)

Donkeys had fewer but larger red cells and a lower icterus index and bilirubin concentration than horses. Erythrocyte, lymphocyte, and platelet counts and fibrinogen concentration decreased with age. Eosinophil counts, MCV and MCH values, and plasma protein and globulin concentrations increased with age. Females had significantly higher MCHC and MCH values and leukocyte and neutrophil counts than males.

ELEPHANTS

The Indian elephant, Elephas maximus, is of interest to the hematologist because of its large red blood cell and unusual differential leukocyte pattern. The erythrocyte is a biconcave disk that measures about 8.8 to 10.6 μm in diameter and forms rouleaux in drawn blood. The RBC count ranges from 1.98 to 4.0 million/μl, with a mean of 2.81 million. The low number of erythrocytes, as compared to other large animals, is compensated by large size and hemoglobin concentration in the red cells. Mean WBC counts range from 6,400 to 18,956/μl. Slight differences may be found in the hematologic values of Indian and African elephants.

The differential leukocyte count of the Indian elephant presents a problem in classification for a cell having a bilobed or, less commonly, a trilobed nucleus with clumped chromatin (Figs. 3–9 and 3–10; Plate VII–11); the cell has been misclassified as a lymphocyte. The nuclear lobes are connected by a thin filament. The cytoplasm of this cell is similar in staining quality to that of a typical monocyte, and both cell types may have small, cytoplasmic vacuoles. Furthermore, both the typical monocyte and the cell in question are peroxidase-positive. The bilobed cell is distinctly different from the peroxidase-positive neutrophil (heterophil or pseudoeosinophil) (Plate VII–12). The bilobed cell is nonspecific esterase-positive,

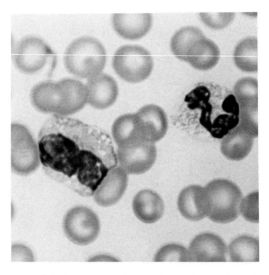

Fig. 3–10.   Bilobed monocyte (large cell) and heterophil leukocyte in the blood of Elephas maximus (× 2700). (From Jain, N.C.: Schalm's Veterinary Hematology. 4th Ed. Philadelphia, Lea & Febiger, 1986, p. 339.)

and this property is sensitive to sodium fluoride (typical of a monocyte reaction). On the basis of these morphologic and staining characteristics, the bilobed leukocyte can be classified as a monocyte. The heterophil has small pinkish granules. The eosinophil is characterized by numerous round granules that fill the cytoplasm.

FERRETS

Sex- and age-related changes in hematologic data have been reported for domestic ferrets (Mustela putorius) (Hoover and Baldwin, 1988). Male ferrets younger than 18 weeks of age had lower RBC, Hb, and PCV values than females and higher values as adults. Male ferrets showed an age-related increase in RBC, Hb, and PCV values and in segmented neutrophils and an age-related decrease in lymphocytes from 12 to 47 weeks of age. In comparison, female ferrets revealed an age-related increase in neutrophils and a decrease in PCV and lymphocytes.

GUINEA PIGS

A unique feature of guinea pig blood is the occurrence of a variable number of lymphocytes that contain a single, large, cytoplasmic inclusion or, rarely, several masses. These are called Kurloff bodies (Fig. 3–11). They stain diffusely red and appear homogeneous, finely granular, or slightly vacuolated. A relationship between the number of lymphocytes containing Kurloff bodies and sex hormones has been observed, particularly during the first 3 months of life. Kurloff bodies are lowest in number in males during the first 3 months of life. They are composed of a sulfated proteoglycan rich in neutral mucopolysaccharides. Thus, they stain with toluidine blue and are PAS-positive. The significance of the occurrence of Kurloff bodies remains to be determined. The tissue distri-

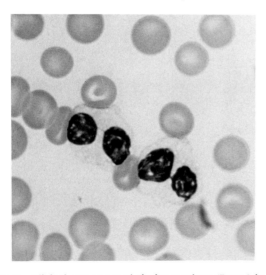

Fig. 3–9.   Bilobed monocytes of Elephas maximus (From Jain, N.C.: Schalm's Veterinary Hematology. 4th Ed. Philadelphia, Lea & Febiger, 1986, p. 338.)

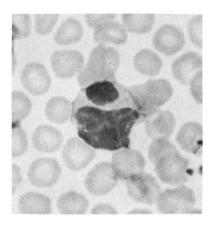

Fig. 3–11.   Guinea pig lymphocyte with Kurloff body (× 1400). (From Jain, N.C.: Schalm's Veterinary Hematology. 4th Ed. Philadelphia, Lea & Febiger, 1986, p. 288.)

bution of cells containing these inclusions in the guinea pig, however, appears to parallel that of lymphocytes with natural killer activity. Kurloff bodies have been found in four related South American rodents: the paca, capybara, cavy, and agouti (Messick and Willet, 1987). They are not found in the blood of the cuis (Galea musteloides), a relative of the domestic guinea pig.

The guinea pig has the largest erythrocytes of the more common laboratory animals. Animals with anemia in remission show polychromasia and macrocytosis because of reticulocytosis.

HAMSTERS

In the newborn golden hamster, 10 to 30% of circulating erythrocytes may be nucleated, whereas in the adult hamster, nucleated red cells are either absent or less than 2%.

The influence of hibernation on blood values has been studied in hamsters kept at 23°C (active) and at 5°C (hibernating). Blood volume, as well as RBC, Hb and PCV values, increase during hibernation. Hematopoiesis is suppressed, as indicated by a reduction in circulating reticulocytes and by a failure of a reticulocyte response to massive blood withdrawal. When hibernation was terminated, the long-delayed reticulocyte response took place. A retardation of RBC senescence and a virtual absence of random erythrocyte destruction occurs in the hibernating hamster. This is associated with an increased potential erythrocyte life span to 160 days, as compared to the normal erythrocyte life span of 60 to 70 days. During hibernation WBC counts are low, averaging about 2500/μl, with a neutrophil:lymphocyte ratio of 1.0:1.0. Platelet counts are also reduced.

MINKS

In Aleutian mink disease, hypergammaglobulinemia is a constant feature. Affected minks show functional and biochemical abnormalities of platelets and pro-

longed bleeding times with normal platelet counts. Large lysosomal granules are seen in leukocytes, as reported for Chédiak-Higashi syndrome of humans, cats, and cattle (Plates IX-10, IX-11, and IX-12).

The number of eosinophils in the blood of juvenile and adult minks increases markedly after repeated exposure to immobility stress and remains significantly elevated for 3 days after termination of the stress (Jeppesen and Heller, 1986). A single episode of an acute stress in juvenile mink, however, causes a pronounced decrease in circulating eosinophils. Thus, the eosinophil response of minks to stress depends on the duration and perhaps the severity of experimental stress.

RABBITS

The rabbit is unique among common laboratory animals in that the basophils are regularly present in blood in small to modest numbers. It is not unusual to find rabbits with 8 to 10% basophils and, rarely, counts up to 30% have been found. Pelger-Huët anomaly may be encountered in certain rabbits. Animals homozygous for the condition usually die.

Total plasma protein (3.73 ± 0.57 g/dl) and IgG concentrations (0.50 ± 0.18 g/dl) are low at birth and increase with age. Normal adult values are attained by the age of 12 weeks, 5.5 ± 0.37 and 0.94 ± 0.24 g/dl, respectively (Oppel et al., 1988).

RATS AND MICE

Hematopoiesis in rats and mice occurs in the bone marrow and spleen. Lymphocytes are present in considerable numbers in normal rat bone marrow; lymphocyte numbers as high as 45% have been found in rats at 3 weeks of age, with a rapid decline thereafter to attain a mean of about 5% in adult rats. Granulocytic maturation is peculiar in that some cells of this series develop a hole in the nucleus that gradually enlarges, giving the nucleus a "ring" or "doughnut" appearance. Ring forms occur as an intermediate stage between the myelocyte and metamyelocyte, but may appear as early as the promyelocyte stage. The ring may break and separate at the ends, or, instead of breaking in one place, the ring may begin to form constrictions at several points, leading to nuclear segmentation. The spleen of the adult mouse is actively engaged in hematopoiesis. Erythrocytic maturation is more pronounced and the granulocytic maturation series is less prominent in the spleen than in bone marrow. Numerous megakaryocytes are also found in the spleen.

In rats, leukocyte counts are markedly higher (about fourfold) in tail blood compared to heart blood, particularly at times of lowest muscular activity. Similarly, Hb and PCV values are lower in cardiac blood compared to blood from the tail vein or periorbital sinus. Regardless of the technique used, arterial blood has lower WBC counts and serum protein levels than venous blood. The tail vein technique is recommended for routine blood sampling in rats (Schwabenbauer, 1991).

Reticulocytes comprise almost all erythrocytes in the newborn and decrease with age. Age and sex related changes have been reported in blood values of rats and mice. In Sprague-Dawley rats, higher WBC counts were found in both young (<5 months) and old (>2 years) rats, particularly females (Wolford et al., 1987). The decrease in WBC counts in mid-life was mostly due to a decrease in lymphocytes, whereas the increase in WBC counts in old age was related to increases in neutrophils and eosinophils. RBC counts increased from 2 to 3 months of age and then decreased with age; females had lower counts than males throughout the lifespan. Platelet counts decreased sharply during the first year, then leveled off or increased gradually.

In rats and mice, the neutrophil:lymphocyte (N:L) ratio increases with age and leukocyte counts exhibit considerable diurnal variations, with lower counts occurring during periods of relative inactivity. The increase in N:L ratio results from an age-related decrease in lymphocyte numbers and an increase in neutrophil numbers (Wolford et al., 1987; Edwards and Fuller, 1992). Strain differences in rats may be reflected in hematologic values. For example, BB Wistar rats have significantly lower WBC and platelet counts, marked lymphopenia, and slight neutrophilia compared to outbred Wistar rats (Wright et al., 1983).

RHINOCEROSES

Acute hemolytic anemia is a major cause of death among captive black rhinoceroses (Diceros bicornis). Affected animals rarely show reticulocytes in blood despite a marked bone marrow erythroid hyperplasia. The mechanism of intravascular hemolysis remains undetermined, although erythrocytes of a rhinoceros with fatal hemolytic anemia had increased membrane coating by the third component of complement (Chaplin et al., 1986). Black rhinoceroses show a striking hemoglobin polymorphism, comprised of a major electrophoretically fast hemoglobin band and a slow (more cathodic) minor band. This hemoglobin polymorphism does not appear to be involved in acute hemolytic anemia and involvement of an unstable hemoglobin remains questionable (Fairbanks and Miller, 1990).

TORTOISES

Seasonal variations occur in the hematologic values of Mediterranean tortoises (Testudo gracea and T. hermanni) in captivity (Lawrence and Hawkey, 1986). A marked reduction in RBC count, Hb, and PCV occurs during hibernation. The WBC count also decreases, and heterophils and lymphocytes decrease in similar proportion during hibernation. Some desert tortoises may have basophil counts as high as 30%.

WATER BUFFALOES

Prominent features in the normal hemogram of water buffaloes (Bubalus bubalus) include an average red cell size (MCV) similar to that of cattle, low icterus index, conspicuous ESR, absence of reticulocytes, and predominance of lymphocytes over neutrophils. Morphologic features of erythrocytes, leukocytes, and platelets are similar to those of cells in cattle. Erythrocytes generally exhibit slight to marked rouleau formation. Polychromasia is absent and Howell-Jolly bodies are rare. Water buffaloes, like horses, do not show significant reticulocytosis in blood during recovery from acute blood loss anemia. Their leukocyte responses to corticosteroid and endotoxin administration are generally similar to those of cattle (Jain et al., 1989). Stress-related changes in differential leukocyte counts, similar to those in cattle, occur at parturition.

Important age-related changes in the hemogram include a slight decline in PCV by 3 months of age, followed by a gradual increase to adult levels after 24 months. The ESR increases gradually and is highest in adults; similarly, whole blood viscosity increases with age. The neutrophil:lymphocyte ratio decreases gradually from birth to 2 to 4 years of age because of a reduction in neutrophil numbers and a corresponding increase in lymphocytes (Sharma et al., 1985).

The American bison (Bison bison), or buffalo, shows some age-related variations in blood values (Sikarskie et al., 1990). Calves have higher red cell values and a leukogram typical of cattle in that lymphocytes exceed neutrophils, whereas adults have higher numbers of neutrophils and eosinophils and lower lymphocyte numbers.

YAKS

Yaks at high altitude have higher Hb (13.45 ± 1.25 g/dl) and PCV (38.5 ± 0.36%) values than yaks at lower altitudes (respective mean values, 10.9 g/dl and 31%) (Winter et al., 1989). The yak at high altitudes has hemoglobin with higher oxygen affinity than its lowland relatives. Its hemoglobin has two types of α and two types of β chains. One is a unique β chain in which valine is substituted for alanine, and this may be responsible for the high intrinsic oxygen affinity.

REFERENCES

Andreasen, C.B. and Latimer, K.S.: Cytochemical staining characteristics of chicken heterophils and eosinophils. Vet. Clin. Pathol, 19:51, 1990.

Brandt, A.: Haematology and Clinical Chemistry of Fur Animals. Tjele Scientifur, 1989.

Campbell, T.W.: Avian Hematology and Cytology. Ames, Iowa, Iowa State University Press, 1988.

Chaplin, H., Jr., Malecek, A.C., Miller, E., et al.: Acute intravascular hemolytic anemia in the black rhinoceros: Hematologic and immunohematologic observations. Am. J. Vet. Res., 47:1313, 1986.

Catley, A., Kock, R.A., Hart, M.G., et al.: Haematology of clinically normal and sick captive reindeer (Rangifer tarandus). Vet. Rec., 126:239, 1990.

Davis, J.R. and Avram, M.J.: Developmental changes in delta-aminolevulinic acid dehydratase (ALAD) activity and blood reticulocyte percent in the developing rat. A brief note. Mech. Aging Dev., 7:123, 1978.

Drag, M.D.: Hematologic values of captive Mexican wolves. Am. J. Vet. Res., 52:1891, 1991.

Edwards, C.J. and Fuller, J.: Notes on age-related changes in differential leucocyte counts of the Charles River outbred albino SD rat and CD1 mouse. Comp. Haematol. Int., 2:58, 1992.

Fairbanks, V.F. and Miller, E.: Beta-globin chain hemoglobin polymorphism and hemoglobin stability in black rhinoceroses (Diceros bicornis). Am. J. Vet. Res., 51:803, 1990.

Ferrer, M., Garcia-Rodriguez, T., and Carrillo, J.C.: Haematocrit and blood chemistry values in captive raptors (Gyps fulvus, Buteo, Milvus migrans, Aquila heliaca). Comp. Biochem. Physiol. [A], 87: 1123, 1987.

Fowler, M.E.: Zoo and Wild Animal Medicine. 2nd Ed. Philadelphia, W.B. Saunders Co., 1986.

Fowler, M.E. and Zinkl, J.G.: References ranges for hematologic and serum biochemical values in llamas (Lama glama). Am. J. Vet. Res., 50:2049, 1989.

Fredlin, P.J.: Destructive effect of heparin on avian erythrocytes. Avian Pathol., 14:531, 1985.

Frye, F.L.: Biomedical and Surgical Aspects of Captive Reptile Husbandry. 2nd ed. Malabar, Fla., Krieger Publishing Co., 1991.

George, E., Andrews, M., and Westmoreland, C.: Effects of azobenzene and aniline in the rodent bone marrow micronucleus test. Carcinogenesis, 11:1551, 1990.

Hawkey, C.M.: Comparative Haematology. London, William Heinemann Medical Books, 1975.

Hawkey, C.M.: The value of comparative haematological studies. Comp. Haematol. Int., 1:1, 1991.

Hawkey, C.M. and Dennett, T.B.: Colour atlas of comparative veterinary haematology. London, Wolfe, 1989.

Hawkey, C.M. and Gulland, F.M.D.: Haematology of clinically normal and abnormal captive llamas and guanacoes. Vet. Rec., 122:232, 1988.

Hawkey, C.M. and Hart, M.G.: Normal haematological values of axis deer (Axis), Pere David's deer (Elaphus davidianus) and barasingha (Cervus duvauceli). Res. Vet. Sci., 39:247, 1985.

Hawkey, C.M. and Hart, M.G.: Haematologic reference values for adult pumas, lions, tigers, leopards, jaguars and cheetahs. Res. Vet. Sci., 41:268, 1986.

Hawkey, C.M. and Hart, M.G.: An analysis of the incidence of hyperfibrinogenemia in birds with bacterial infections. Avian Pathol., 17:427, 1988.

Herbert, R., Nanney, J., Spano, J.S., et al.: Erythrocyte distribution in ducks. Am. J. Vet. Res., 50:958, 1989.

Hoover, J.P. and Baldwin, C.A.: Changes in physiologic and clinicopathologic values in domestic ferrets from 12 to 47 weeks of age. Companion Anim. Prac., 2:40, 1988.

Jain, N.C.: Schalm's Veterinary Hematology. 4th ed. Philadelphia, Lea & Febiger, 1986.

Jain, N.C., Vegad, J.L., Shrivastawa, A.B., et al.: Haematological changes in buffalo calves inoculated with Escherichia coli endotoxin and corticosteroids. Res. Vet. Sci., 47:305, 1989.

Jeppesen, L.L. and Heller, K.E.: Stress effects on circulating eosinophil leukocytes, breeding performance, and reproductive success of ranch mink. Scientifur, 10:15, 1986.

Jones, T.C., Ward, J.M., Mohr, U. and Hunt, R.D.: Hemopoietic System. Berlin, Springer-Verlag, 1990.

Latimer, K.S., Tang, K.N., Goodwin, M.A., et al.: Leukocyte changes associated with acute inflammation in chickens. Avian Dis., 32: 760, 1988.

Lawrence, K. and Hawkey, C.M.: Seasonal variations in haematological data from Mediterranean tortoises (Testudo gracea and Testudo hermanni) in captivity. Res. Vet. Sci., 40:225, 1986.

Leonard, R. and Ruben, Z.: Hematology reference values for peripheral blood of laboratory rats. Lab. Anim. Sci., 36:277, 1986.

Levi, A., Perelman, B., Waner, T., et al.: Haematological parameters of the ostrich (Struthio camelus). Avian Pathol., 18:321, 1989.

Long, R.E., Knutsen, G. and Robinson, M.: Myeloid hyperplasia in the SENCAR mouse: Differentiation from granulocytic leukemia. Environ. Health Perspect., 68:117, 1986.

Maede, Y., Yamanaka, Y., Sasaki, A., et al.: Hematology in sika deer (Cervus nippon yesoensis Heude, 1884). Jpn. J. Vet. Sci., 52:35, 1990.

Maxwell, M.H.: Fine structure and cytochemical studies of eosinophils from fowls and ducks and eosinophilia. Res. Vet. Sci., 41: 135, 1986a.

Maxwell, M.H.: Ultrastructural and cytochemical studies in normal Japanese quail (Coturnix japonica) eosinophils and in those from birds with experimentally induced eosinophilia. Res. Vet. Sci., 41:149, 1986b.

McLaughlin, B.G., Evans, N., McLaughlin, P., et al.: An Epierythrozoon-like parasite of llamas. J. Am. Vet. Med. Assoc., 197:1170, 1990.

Messick, J.B. and Willet, E.: Kurloff-like bodies in peripheral blood mononuclear cells from a capybara. Vet. Clin. Pathol., 16:88, 1987.

Omorphos, S.C., Rice-Evans, C. and Hawkey, C.: Heinz bodies do not modify the membrane characteristics of common marmoset (Callithrix jacchus) erythrocytes. Lab. Anim., 23:66, 1989a.

Omorphos, S.A., Hawkey, C.M. and Rice-Evans, C.: The elliptocyte: A study of the relationship between cell shape and membrane structure using the camelid erythrocyte as a model. Comp. Biochem. Physiol. [B], 94:789, 1989b.

Oppel, K., Bardos, L. and Puszatai, A.: Quantitative determination of serum total protein, albumin and IgG concentration in rabbit. Bulletin of the University of Agriculture Sciences, Godollo, No. 1:43, 1991.

Oyewale, J.O. and Durotoye, L.A.: Osmotic fragility of erythrocytes of two breeds of domestic fowl in the warm humid tropics. Lab. Anim., 22:250, 1988.

Peinado, V.I., Viscor, G. and Palomeque, J.: Erythrocyte osmotic fragility in some artidactylid mammals: Relationship with plasma osmolality and red cell dimensions. Comp. Haematol. Int., 2: 44, 1992.

Russo, E.A., McEntee, L., Applegate, L., et al.: Comparison of two methods for determination of white blood cell counts in macaws. J. Am. Vet. Med. Assoc., 189:1013, 1986.

Schindler, S.L., Gildersleeve, R.P., Thaxton, J.P., et al.: Hematological response of hemorrhaged Japanese quail after blood volume replacement with saline. Comp. Biochem. Physiol. [A], 87:933, 1987.

Schwabenbauer, C.: Influence of the blood sampling site on some haematological and clinical-chemical parameters in Sprague-Dawley rats. Comp. Haematol. Int., 1:112, 1991.

Sharma, M.C., Pathak, N.N., Verma, R.P., et al.: Normal haematology of Murrah buffaloes of various ages in the agroclimatic condition in Viet Nam. Indian Vet. J., 62:383, 1985.

Sikarskie, J.G., van Veen, T.W. S., van Selm, G., et al.: Comparative blood characteristics of ranched and free-ranging American bison (Bison). Am. J. Vet. Res., 51:955, 1990.

Smith, B.B., Reed, P.J., Pearson, E.G., et al.: Erythrocyte dyscrasia, anemia, and hypothyroidism in chronically underweight llamas. J. Am. Vet. Med. Assoc., 198:81, 1991.

Snow, D.H., Billah, A. and Ridha, A.: Effects of maximal exercise on the blood composition of the racing camel. Vet. Rec., 123: 311, 1988.

Swayne, D.E., Stockham, S.L. and Johnson, G.S.: Cytochemical properties of chicken blood cells resembling both thrombocytes and lymphocytes. Vet. Clin. Pathol., 15:17, 1986.

Tamburlin, J.H. and Glomski, C.A.: Leucocyte alkaline phosphatase in the Mongolian gerbil and other species: A comparative view. Lab. Anim., 22:202, 1988.

Winter, H., Tshewang, U., Gurung, B.J., et al.: Haemoglobin and packed cell volume of yaks at high altitude. Aust. Vet. J., 66: 299, 1989.

Wolford, S.T., Schroer, R.A., Gallo, P.P., et al.: Age-related changes in serum chemistry and hematology values in normal Sprague-Dawley rats. Fundamen. Appl. Toxicol., 8:80, 1987.

Wright, J.R., Jr., Yates, A.J., Shah, N.T. et al.: Hematologic characteristics of the BB Wistar rat. Vet. Clin. Pathol., 12:9, 1983.

Zinkl, J.G., Mae, D., Merid, G.P., et al.: Reference ranges and the influence of age and sex on hematologic and serum biochemical values in donkeys (Equus asinus). Am. J. Vet. Res., 51:408, 1990.

Chapter *4*

Hematopoiesis

Hematopoiesis (Gr., *haima*, blood, and *poiesis*, creation) means making blood, particularly the blood cells. The hematopoietic system is widely distributed and includes organs that have functions in addition to the formation of blood cells (Table 4–1).

HEMATOPOIESIS IN PRENATAL AND POSTNATAL LIFE

Hematopoiesis occurs extravascularly in mammalian marrow, whereas in the avian species granulopoiesis occurs at extravascular sites and erythropoiesis occurs intravascularly. No megakaryocytes are present in avian bone marrow and thrombocytes are believed to be produced intravascularly from a special cell line analogous to that for erythrocytes.

Hematopoiesis during intrauterine life begins in the yolk sac. Liver, spleen, and bone marrow successively become hematopoietically active, so that at birth the bone marrow is the principal site for hematopoiesis (Fig. 4–1). In general, hematopoietic activity in the dog and cat can be detected by the third week of prenatal life, and in the cow by the fourth week. During postnatal life, hematopoiesis in most mammals is restricted to the bone marrow, whereas the liver and spleen are usually inactive but retain hematopoietic potential. This potential (extramedullary hematopoiesis) is expanded at times of increased need, which is generally associated with bone marrow hypoplasia or aplasia. In mice, the spleen characteristically continues to be hematopoietically active during postnatal life. A feature common to prenatal hematopoiesis in all mammalian species is that erythrocytes are usually nucleated and large (Fig. 4–2). With advancing gestation, the erythrocytes gradually become non-nucleated and small and continue to follow this pattern for a few months after birth, until adult values have been attained (Fig. 4–3). The leukocyte count is low during early fetal life. It gradually becomes higher, mainly from increases in lymphocyte and neutrophil numbers, and near-normal values are attained by birth.

The marrow of all bones is hematopoietically active at birth and during early postnatal life. This activity involves the vigorous production of erythrocytes and other myeloid cells. The phase of rapid growth of the young and the associated expansion of blood volume places a heavy demand on the marrow for erythrocytes. As the demand for erythrocytes decreases with approaching maturity, hematopoiesis recedes from the shafts of the long bones. Red, hematopoietically active marrow is replaced by resting yellow marrow. Active hematopoiesis continues throughout life in all flat bones, such as the sternum, ribs, pelvis, vertebrae, and skull, and in the epiphyses of the long bones. The bone marrow, although widely distributed, constitutes an organ about two-thirds the size of the liver.

Bone marrow consists of various blood cells and their precursors, reticular cells and reticulin fibers, endothelium-lined sinusoids, and fat cells or adipocytes. Fat cells occupy space as hematopoiesis recedes and give up space as demand for the expansion of red marrow occurs—for example, in response to acute blood loss or hemolytic anemia. Blood is supplied to the marrow through a nutrient artery that ramifies within the marrow to form vascular sinuses, which carry the blood back to a central vein (Fig. 4–4). The hematopoietic islands in mammalian marrow lie between these broad venous sinuses (Fig. 4–5).

HEMATOPOETIC STEM CELLS

In the normal animal, the numbers of erythrocytes, various leukocyte types, and platelets remain relatively constant. Production and utilization or destruction of

Table 4–1.   Hematopoietic Organs and Tissues and Their Related Functions

Organ or Tissue	*Functions*
Bone marrow	1. Hematopoiesis—production of erythrocytes, granulocytes, monocytes, platelets, and B lymphocytes; supplies stem cells for lymphocyte production elsewhere 2. Stores iron
Thymus	1. Central lymphoid organ concerned with differentiation of bone marrow-derived precursor cells into immunologically competent T lymphocytes involved in cellular immunity, and production of lymphokines
Lymph nodes and follicles	1. Produce lymphocytes and plasma cells 2. Actively engage in antibody synthesis
Spleen	1. Produces lymphocytes and plasma cells 2. Antibody synthesis 3. Reservoir of erythrocytes and platelets 4. Destroys senescent and abnormal erythrocytes and degrades hemoglobin 5. Stores iron 6. Pitting function—removes Howell-Jolly bodies, Heinz bodies, nuclei, and parasites from erythrocytes and possibly returns purged cells to circulation 7. Retains its embryonic potential for hematopoiesis
Mononuclear phagocyte system (reticuloendothelial system)	1. Major phagocytic system of the body concerned with cellular defense in microbial infection 2. Destroys various blood cells 3. Degrades hemoglobin into iron, globin, and free bilirubin 4. Stores iron 5. Secretes macromolecules of biologic importance (e.g., colony-stimulating factors, complement)
Liver	1. Stores vitamin B_{12}, folate, and iron 2. Produces most of the coagulation factors, albumin, and some globulins 3. Converts free bilirubin to bilirubin glucuronide for excretion into bile, and participates in enterohepatic circulation of urobilinogen 4. Produces a precursor (an α-globulin) of erythropoietin or some actual erythropoietin 5. Retains its embryonic potential for hematopoiesis
Stomach and intestine	1. Stomach produces (*a*) HCl for release of iron from complex organic molecules and (*b*) intrinsic factor to facilitate absorption of vitamin B_{12} 2. Intestinal mucosa involved in absorption of vitamin B_{12} and folates and controls the rate of iron absorption in relation to body needs
Kidney	1. Produces erythropoietin and also thrombopoietin 2. Degrades excessively filtered hemoglobin to iron and bilirubin for excretion into urine

various cells remain in delicate balance. When this steady state is disturbed by reduced erythrocyte numbers, as in acute hemorrhage or hemolytic anemia, by increased utilization of neutrophil leukocytes, as in inflammatory diseases, or by increased destruction of platelets, as in immune-mediated thrombocytopenia, the hematopoietic centers are stimulated to increase production of the cells needed. This means that, for each cell type, a stimulatory feedback mechanism exists that responds to the decreased cell population. Bone marrow contains a small number of primitive stem cells that respond to these demands. They differentiate into progenitor cells, which multiply and mature into cells of the specific cell line that requires expansion.

In vitro and in vivo studies have revealed a structured hierarchy of multipotential, oligopotential, and unipotential stem cells in the bone marrow. The most primitive hematopoietic pluripotential stem cells are capable of self-renewal and of differentiating into oligopotential stem cells (cells able to produce progenitors of two or more cell lines), which in turn differentiate into unipotential stem cells committed to a single lineage. The morphologic identity of these stem cells remains uncertain, but they appear to be mononuclear, with some characteristics of a transitional lymphocyte. The unipotential progenitor cells develop into morphologically recognizable precursor cells (e.g., rubriblast, myeloblast, monoblast, and megakaryoblast), which ultimately give rise to mature cells of the series. Some studies have indicated the existence of subsets of the pluripotential stem cell and of committed lymphoid, erythroid, granulocyte-monocyte, and megakaryocytic progenitor cells.

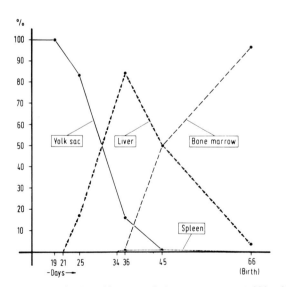

Fig. 4–1.   Contribution of hematopoietic organs to prenatal blood formation in the cat. (From Tiedemann, K., and Van Ooyen, B.: Prenatal hematopoiesis and blood characteristics of the cat. Anat. Embryol., 153:243, 1978.)

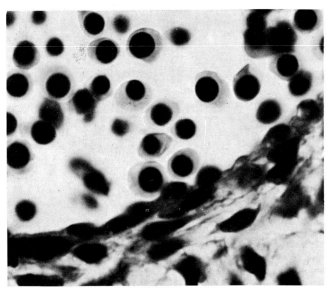

Fig. 4–2. Histologic section of the heart of a 1.0-cm bovine embryo. All erythrocytes are nucleated (× 3600). (From Jain, N.C: Schalm's Veterinary Hematology. 4th Ed. Philadelphia, Lea & Febiger, 1986, p. 355.)

Pluripotential Stem Cell

The current concept of hematopoiesis, based on the monophylactic or unitarian theory of blood cell formation, envisions the production of erythrocytes, all leukocyte types, macrophages, mast cells, and megakaryocytes from a pluripotential stem cell (Fig. 4–6).

This progenitor cell is known as the hematopoietic stem cell. Its existence was demonstrated in experiments in which normal mouse bone marrow cells were injected intravenously into heavily irradiated syngeneic mice. Macroscopic nodules (colonies), comprised of pure or mixed populations of erythroid, neutrophilic, megakaryocytic, and undifferentiated cells, were found to develop after 8 to 10 days on the surface of the spleen. Reinjection of cell suspensions from individual splenic colonies into irradiated mice produced similar colonies. By clonal and chromosomal analyses, these colonies were found to originate from a single progenitor cell, designated the colony-forming unit–spleen (CFU-S). The CFU-S is a heterogeneous population of cells capable of self-renewal and of differentiation into various types of progenitor cells. The presence of a small number of cells more primitive than CFU-S has been demonstrated in studies on marrow cells marked with retrovirus vectors and radiation-induced chromosomal abnormalities. These cells can differentiate into CFU-S and myeloid and lymphoid progenitor cells.

Studies on human leukemias have provided additional evidence for the existence of various stem cells. A chromosomal abnormality, designated Ph[1] for Philadelphia chromosome, has been demonstrated in erythrocytic, granulocytic, and possibly megakaryocytic cells of patients with chronic myelogenous leukemia (CML). This implicates a common progenitor cell for each of the three cell lines. The basic cytogenetic defect in CML is a translocation involving chromosomes 9 and 22. The Ph[1] was not found in lymphoid cells. Glucose-6-phosphate dehydrogenase (G-6-PD)

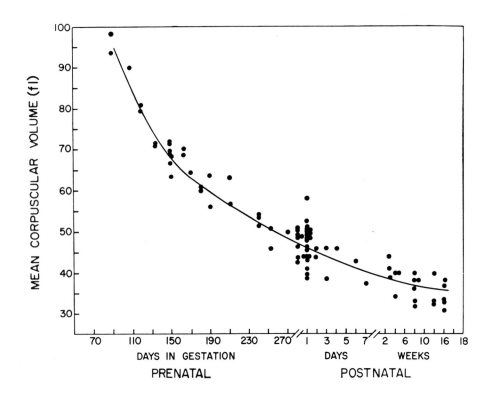

Fig. 4–3. Influence of advancing gestation and early postnatal life on the mean corpuscular volume of bovine erythrocytes. (From Jain, N.C.: Schalm's Veterinary Hematology. 4th Ed. Philadelphia, Lea & Febiger, 1985, p. 356.)

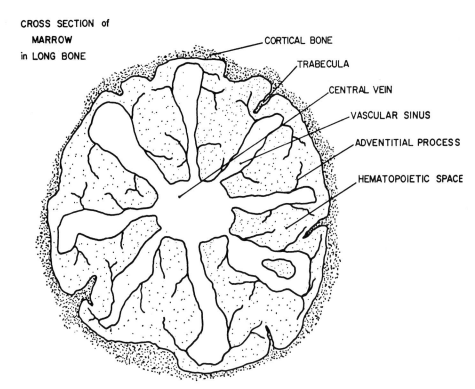

CROSS SECTION of MARROW in LONG BONE

CORTICAL BONE
TRABECULA
CENTRAL VEIN
VASCULAR SINUS
ADVENTITIAL PROCESS
HEMATOPOIETIC SPACE

Fig. 4–4. Organization of the venous vasculature of the marrow of a long bone. Thin-walled vascular sinuses originate at the periphery from the termination of transverse branches of the nutrient artery (not shown). The vascular sinuses run transversely toward the center to join the central vein. Hematopoiesis takes place in the space between the vascular sinuses. Adventitial processes project into the hematopoietic space, producing partial compartmentalization. (From Weiss, L.: The histophysiology of bone marrow. Clin Orthop., 52:13, 1967.)

has also been a useful marker. G-6-PD occurs in two isoenzyme forms, A and B. Females heterozygous for G-6-PD contain both isoenzymes in their somatic cells, including fibroblasts and bone marrow cells, although only one isoenzyme is found in an individual cell line

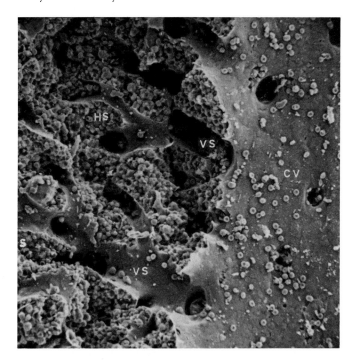

Fig. 4–5. Scanning electron micrograph of rat bone marrow showing developing cells in hematopoietic spaces (HS), anastomosing venous sinusoids (VS), and central vein (CV; × 290). (From Jain, N.C.: Schalm's Veterinary Hematology. 4th Ed. Philadelphia, Lea & Febiger, 1986, p. 362.)

because of random inactivation of the other isoenzyme during embryonic life. In such females, clonal proliferation of marrow cells, such as during CML, could be detected by the presence of one or the other isoenzyme in various myeloid cells. In CML patients heterozygous for G-6-PD, the same isoenzyme is found in erythrocytes, neutrophils, monocytes, eosinophils, and platelets.

The hematopoietic stem cell is considered to be a primitive cell of mesenchymal origin. During intrauterine life, these stem cells are first supplied by the embryonic yolk sac and then by the fetal liver, spleen, and bone marrow. In adult life, bone marrow is the principal source in most species. A small number of stem cells can be found in the peripheral blood (1/100,000 leukocytes). Normal beagles were found to have 40 to 400 committed stem cells/ml of blood and a 10-fold greater number was found after repeated injection of dextran sulfate, a stem cell mobilizing agent. The migration of granulocytic progenitor cells into blood can be induced by various stimuli (e.g., exercise, ACTH, dexamethasone, epinephrine, endotoxin, antigenic exposure, hypoxia, and localized irradiation). Experimental evidence has suggested that myeloid metaplasia involves the colonization of migrating bone marrow stem cells at suitable extramedullary sites.

A number of hematologic diseases originate from neoplastic and non-neoplastic disorders of stem cells. Hematopoietic neoplasms are clonal stem cell disorders and include acute and chronic myelogenous leukemias, essential thrombocythemia, and polycythemia vera. Non-neoplastic disorders result from stem cell dysfunction and include cyclic hematopoiesis in gray collie

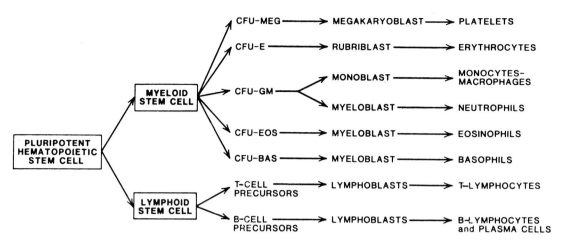

Fig. 4–6. Schematic representation of hematopoietic differentiation and production of various blood cells (CFU, colony-forming unit). (From Jain, N.C.: Schalm's Veterinary Hematology. 4th Ed. Philadelphia, Lea & Febiger, 1986, p. 366.)

dogs and pure red cell aplasia and aplastic anemia (pancytopenia) in humans. Some success has been achieved in correcting non-neoplastic disorders by the use of marrow transplantation.

Committed Stem Cells

Provision for a committed progenitor cell between the primitive stem cell and the differentiated blast cell of a series serves to explain the selective depression of a specific cell series under experimental and certain natural conditions. Both the multipotential and unipotential stem cell compartments are self-perpetuating and can supply large numbers of specific progenitor cells on demand, without exhaustion of the compartment. The stem cells are generally resting and require a serious insult to the hematopoietic tissue to increase their mitotic activity and furnish additional progenitor cells. The latter, under appropriate growth conditions, are diverted to differentiate into progenies of a particular cell line. For example, bone marrow cultures of endotoxin-treated and anemic calves exhibited a preferential increase of granulocyte-macrophage and erythroid progenitors, respectively, thereby indicating a directional proliferation of stem cells in response to the need for a particular cell type.

Information on committed stem cells and their regulators has become available primarily from in vitro studies of bone marrow culture in various semisolid media, including soft agar clot and methyl cellulose. Committed stem cells of granulocytes and monocytes (CFU-GM, CFU-Eos, CFU-Bas), erythrocytes (BFU-E and CFU-E), and megakaryocytes (CFU-Meg) have been cultured from human and murine bone marrows. Limited culture studies have also been conducted on hematopoietic, lymphopoietic, and stromal stem or progenitor cells of the dog, cow, cat, and sheep.

Factors Regulating Hematopoiesis

Various endogenous and exogenous factors influence hematopoiesis in vivo and in vitro (Tables 4–2 and 4–3). These also include the marrow microenvironment and locally produced humoral factors. Many hematopoietic growth factors act synergistically and affect the differentiation of multiple cell lines. Important growth factors include many interleukins, a family of glycoproteins known as colony-stimulating factors, and several specific poietins (Golde, 1990; Golde and Glaspy, 1990; Quesenberry, 1990; Shaw, 1991; Weisbart et al., 1989; Whetton and Dexter, 1989; Woodman, 1992). Specific poietins have been described for some cell lines (e.g., erythropoietin, eosinophilopoietin, thrombopoietin, granulocytopoietin, and monocytopoietin). Certain lymphokines such as lymphocyte mitogenic factor and T-cell growth factor have been found to have similar regulatory effects on lymphopoiesis. Abnormal hematopoiesis may involve pathologic disturbances of one or more humoral regulators, and immune suppression may occur in certain cases.

The concept that the hematopoietic inductive microenvironment (HIM) influences the differentiation of the hematopoietic stem cell was borne of experimental studies in mice. In normal mice, bone marrow is primarily engaged in granulopoiesis, whereas, the spleen is concerned with lymphopoiesis and erythropoiesis. Splenic colony assays in mice with irradiated bone marrow stroma implanted into the spleen have shown that granulocytic colonies still develop in marrow stroma localized within the spleen, but erythroid colonies develop in the adjacent splenic tissue. This hypothesis has been supported by several other observations. A genetically transmitted (recessive) macrocytic anemia is found in certain mutant (Sl/Sl[d]) mice as a result of defective HIM. Cells from these mice grow well in unaffected but not in mutant litter mates. Also, splenic transplantation corrects anemia in the

Table 4–2. Factors Influencing Hematopoiesis

Hematopoietic Process	Stimulators*	Inhibitors
Stem cell differentiation	HIM; IL-3; "short-range" hormonal factors	
Erythropoiesis	Burst-promoting activity (IL-3), erythropoietin, certain lymphokines such as IL-9, macrophages, PGE_1 and PGE_2, PGI_2, erythroblast-enhancing factor, erythropoietic stimulating cofactor, androgens, corticosteroids, growth hormone, thyroxine, cobalt, GM-CSF	Estrogen, a factor in urine, a factor in plasma, lithium, feline leukemia virus, suppressor T lymphocytes
Granulopoiesis	GM-CSF, G-CSF, (Syn. granulocytopoietin ?) antichalone, certain lymphokines such as IL-3, eosinophilopoietin, basophilopoietin, lithium, PGI_2, corticosteroids	Colony-inhibiting factor, chalone, lactoferrin, transferrin, acidic isoferritins, certain lymphokines, PGE_1 and PGE_2, macrophage products, unidentified plasma factors
Monocytopoiesis	M-CSF, monocytopoietin, GM-CSF, IL-3, IL-11	A serum inhibitor, PGE_1 and PGE_2, corticosteroids
Megakaryocytopoiesis and thrombopoiesis	Meg-CSF, thrombopoietin, iron, lithium, a factor in bovine bile, IL-3, IL-11	A splenic factor, iron in different amounts
Lymphopoiesis	Specific microenvironment, thymic hormones, antigens, interleukins (IL-1 to IL-7, IL-11, IL-12), tumor necrosis factor α, T-cell growth factor β, interferon α	Corticosteroids

* GM, granulocyte-macrophage; HIM, hematopoietic inductive microenvironment; IL, interleukin; M, monocyte; Meg, megakaryocyte; PG, prostaglandin; CSF, colony-stimulating factor.

mutant mice, whereas reconstitution with the hematopoietic stem cells has no effect. Similarly, W/Wᵛ mice develop a macrocytic anemia from a defect in the CFU-S compartment as a result of an abnormal regulatory mechanism. Chloramphenicol was found to have a suppressive effect on HIM in mice, thereby providing an explanation for the development of the aplastic anemia seen in certain human patients receiving this drug. Cyclic hematopoiesis in gray collie dogs can be transferred or corrected by bone marrow transplantation, suggesting the possibility of a defect in the stem cells (see below). The influence of microenvironment on lymphopoiesis is well known—the thymus influences the commitment of marrow-derived lymphoid progenitor cells into subsets of T lymphocytes. The bursa of Fabricius in birds and probably bone marrow in mammals similarly direct the development of lymphoid progenitor cells into B lymphocytes.

Cyclic Hematopoiesis in Silver-Gray Collie Dogs

Canine cyclic hematopoiesis, previously known as canine cyclic neutropenia, is an autosomal recessive,

Table 4–3. Properties and Functions of Colony-Stimulating Factors*

Factor	MW of Glycoprotein	Stimulates Production of	Source	Other Functional Role(s)
IL-3 or Multi-CSF	20,000	Neutrophils, monocytes, eosinophils, basophils, platelets, erythrocytes, mast cells	Activated T lymphocytes	Affects functions of mature eosinophils and monocytes, but not of neutrophils; acts synergistically with erythropoietin and other growth factors
GM-CSF	22,300	Neutrophils, monocytes, eosinophils, basophils, platelets, erythrocytes	Activated T lymphocytes, macrophages, endothelial cells, and fibroblasts	Enhances many neutrophil and some eosinophil and monocyte functions; also priming effects on neutrophils; acts, synergistically with other growth factors
G-CSF	19,600	Neutrophils	Macrophages, endothelial cells, and fibroblasts	Activates and primes neutrophils; acts synergistically with other growth factors
M-CSF	80,000–100,000	Monocytes	Macrophages, endothelial cells, and fibroblasts	Increases several functional activities and survival of macrophages; acts synergistically with other growth factors
Erythropoietin	34,000–39,000	Erythrocytes	Renal interstitial cells	Synergistic action with IL-3 to stimulate formation of BFU-E and promotes formation of CFU-E in vitro; in vivo, stimulates erythropoiesis and release of reticulocytes to blood

semilethal condition of silver-gray collies. It was originally characterized by neutropenic cycles, occurring in both sexes and resulting in premature deaths, most often from sudden overwhelming infection during a period of neutropenia. The affected pups are stunted or weak and less active at birth than their normal litter mates. Beginning within 12 days after birth, the pups show a marked cyclic neutropenia at 11- to 14-day intervals. The syndrome is remarkably similar to that of human cyclic neutropenia, which cycles at approximately 21 days.

The peripheral blood neutropenia results from a cyclic maturation arrest of the pluripotential hematopoietic stem cell, presumably the result of an intrinsic marrow defect. Neutrophil peroxidase is significantly reduced and platelets show decreased dense granule serotonin pools and diminished aggregation to agonists like collagen, platelet-activating factor, and thrombin (Pratt et al., 1990). Because cyclic activity of other blood cells, including reticulocytes, platelets, monocytes, and lymphocytes, also appears to occur, the defect is more aptly called canine cyclic hematopoiesis. Colony-stimulating activity, erythropoietin, and thrombopoietin concentrations also show cyclic patterns in relation to changes in blood neutrophil, reticulocyte, and platelet numbers, respectively. A cyclic effect on RBC count, hemoglobin concentration, and PCV is not seen, probably because of the longer red cell life span. An abnormality of the lymphoid system has been demonstrated and a periodic variation in lymphokine production has been observed.

Blood cell cycling can be induced in a normal dog by the irradiation and infusion of marrow cells from an affected gray collie. Conversely, the disorder in an affected dog can be corrected by total body irradiation followed by bone marrow transplantation from a normal dog. Cyclic changes in blood neutrophil, platelet, and reticulocyte numbers can also be eliminated by the administration of endotoxin or lithium carbonate. Treatment with human recombinant G-CSF (rhG-CSF) abrogated cyclic neutropenic episodes, but did not correct the cellular defects such as reduced myeloperoxidase activity in neutrophils and platelet defects (Pratt et al., 1990).

GRANULOPOIESIS

Granulopoiesis, or granulocytopoiesis, involves the production of neutrophils, eosinophils, and basophils. Under the proper stimulus, the pluripotential stem cell in the bone marrow gives rise to progenitor cells committed to produce granulocytes. Under the influence of interleukin-3 (Il-3) and granulocyte-macrophage colony-stimulating factor (GM-CSF), colony-forming units committed to producing neutrophils and monocytes (CFU-GM), eosinophils (CFU-Eos), and basophils (CFU-Bas) are produced (Fig. 4–6). The CFU-GM has a dual commitment; it subsequently differentiates to unipotential cells committed to produce either neutrophils or monocytes. Under appro-

priate stimuli, the granulocytic unipotential cells give rise to morphologically identifiable precursors known as myeloblasts, which divide, differentiate, and mature to yield blood granulocytes (Table 4–4). Similarly, the unipotential monocytic cell gives rise to monocytes, which later serve as a source of tissue macrophages.

The regulation of granulopoiesis has been studied most extensively for neutrophils (Golde, 1990; Whetton and Dexter, 1989). Various factors influence the differentiation and maturation of committed granulocytic progenitor cells. The main regulatory factors include IL-3 (multi-CSF) and various colony-stimulating factors (CSFs). Three CSFs have been characterized: GM-CSF, granulocyte colony-stimulating factor (G-CSF), and macrophage colony-stimulating factor (M-CSF). IL-3 is considered a multispecific growth factor (multi-CSF), whereas GM-CSF has broad specificity and G-CSF and M-CSF primarily stimulate granulocyte and monocyte production, respectively. G-CSF and M-CSF, however, may also influence the differentiation of other cell line (Table 4–3). Various hematopoietic growth factors have been found to act synergistically.

CSFs are produced by various cells, including activated T lymphocytes, macrophages, endothelial cells, fibroblasts, and marrow stromal cells. They are found in low concentration in serum and urine. Their production increases following antigenic exposure, bacterial infection, endotoxemia, cytotoxic chemotherapy, and whole body irradiation. CSFs are low-molecular-weight glycoproteins, but glycosylation is not necessary for the expression of functional activity.

Most studies have focused on human and murine CSFs, which have been genetically cloned to produce recombinant products, but some work has been done on bovine and canine CSFs. Restricted species specificity has been reported for some CSFs—for example, human GM-CSF has no effect on murine hematopoiesis, but it stimulates neutrophil production in the bovine. Injection of GM-CSF in animals and humans induces a dose-dependent increase in circulating neutrophils without any serious side effects (Fig. 4–7). In some species, increases in eosinophil and monocytes are also seen. Administration of rhG-CSF can stimulate myelopoiesis and induce neutrophilia in humans, dogs (Lothrop et al., 1988; Mishu et al., 1992; Pratt et al., 1990), and cats (Fulton et al., 1991). Some cats may also develop lymphocytosis and dogs in some studies have developed increases in monocytes and lymphocyte numbers and an accelerated production of platelets and granulocytes. Prolonged administration of rhG-CSF in dogs, however, may result in a chronic neutropenia because of immune-mediated neutralization of endogenous canine G-CSF (Hammond et al., 1991). Administration of recombinant canine G-CSF (rcG-CSF) induces a dose-dependent leukocytosis associated with neutrophilia and monocytosis in normal dogs. It prevents neutropenia and associated clinical signs in dogs with cyclic hematopoiesis, but may or may not completely eliminate the cycling of neutrophils.

Table 4–4. Developmental Stages of Myeloid and Lymphoid Cells*

CFU-E	CFU-GM	CFU-GM	CFU-Meg	Lymphoid Progenitor
Rubriblast	Myeloblast	Monoblast	Megakaryoblast	Prothymocyte Pre-B cells (cIgM; sIgM, sIgD)
Prorubricyte	Promyelocyte	Promonocyte	Promegakaryocyte	Thymocytes (CD4−, CD8−; CD4+, CD8+) Mature B cells (sIgA, sIgG, sIgE)
Basophilic rubricyte	Myelocyte: neutrophilic, eosinophilic, basophilic	Monocyte	Megakaryocyte	T lymphocytes (CD4+, CD8−; CD4−, CD8+) B lymphocytes, plasma cells
Polychromatic rubricyte	Metamyelocyte: neutrophilic, eosinophilic, basophilic	Macrophage	Platelets	
Metarubricyte	Band cell: neutrophilic, eosinophilic, basophilic			
Reticulocyte	Mature neutrophil, eosinophil, basophil			
Erythrocyte				

* Myeloid cells at various stages, from blast cells to definitive cells, can be identified morphologically, whereas various lymphocytic cells are recognized by differences in surface markers rather than cell morphology.

Neutrophil functions, such as chemotaxis, phagocytosis, oxidative metabolism, arachidonic acid metabolism, and cytotoxic effects, may be stimulated directly by GM-CSF and G-CSF or the cells become primed for enhanced functional responses to other agents. The precise mechanism of action of CSFs on hematopoietic cells or mature leukocytes is unknown, but specific cell surface receptors for various cytokines have been found on responsive cells.

The GM-CSF is believed to be a physiologic regulator of granulopoiesis and is also termed "granulocytopoietin," analogous to erythropoietin. The action of CSFs is regulated by a "colony-inhibiting factor," which is also produced by various cells. Granulocyte production is also thought to be controlled by a humoral feedback mechanism involving low-molecular-weight (MW) polypeptides: a specific inhibitor, chalone (MW, 2,000 to 4,000), and a specific stimulator, antichalone (MW, 30,000 to 35,000). Some additional simulators (prostaglandin I_2, or PGI_2, endotoxin, and lithium) and inhibitors (PGE_1, PGE_2, lactoferrin, and acidic isoferritins) of granulopoiesis have been recognized. Tumor necrosis factor, endotoxin, and interferons may induce macrophages, T lymphocytes, endothelial cells, or fibroblasts to produce CSFs, thus providing a mechanism for the neutrophil granulocytosis seen during infections and inflammatory conditions. Previous studies had shown that the number of neutrophils in blood is regulated by a humoral factor that influences cell release from bone marrow. This factor has been referred to as the neutrophil-releasing factor or leukocytosis-promoting factor, and it might represent an activity shared by the GM-CSF and G-CSF.

Eosinophil production and release is regulated by lymphokines produced by T lymphocytes—Eos-CSF (Eosinophil–colony-stimulating factor), eosinophilopoietin, and "eosinophil-releasing factor." The Eos-CSF (MW, 50,000) stimulates the development of CFU-Eos into myeloblasts committed to produce eosinophils, whereas the major activity of eosinophilopoietin (MW, 5,000) is to stimulate the proliferation of myeloblasts and their progenies in the mitotic compartment. Eosinophil-releasing factor promotes the release of eosinophils from bone marrow to blood. This is also helped by the chemotactic action of histamine in blood. Interleukin-5 acts in concert with IL-3 and GM-CSF to stimulate eosinophil production. Basophil production is said to be antigen-specific and is regulated by IL-3 and by an uncharacterized basophil-specific lymphokine ("basophilopoietin") produced by T lymphocytes.

The availability of recombinant CSFs has opened a new avenue of therapy for diseases of the hematopoietic system involving stem cell disorders. They could be used to improve general host defense in individuals with congenital and acquired neutropenias, defective or suboptimal neutrophil and macrophage functions, immunodeficiency diseases, and indolent infections (Weisbart et al., 1989). Their use in leukemic patients allows for the use of more intensive chemotherapy and irradiation to destroy all neoplastic clones of cells and subsequent stimulation of transplanted autologous marrow cells (Golde and Glaspy, 1990).

ERYTHROPOIESIS

In vitro clonal cultural assays have delineated two distinct types of erythroid progenitor cells, namely the burst-forming unit–erythroid (BFU-E) and colony-forming unit–erythroid (CFU-E). The differentiation of BFU-E from the pluripotential stem cell, of CFU-E from BFU-E, and of erythroid precursors from CFU-E is regulated by IL-3 and GM-CSF. In addition, the differentiation of BFU-E requires high concentrations of erythropoietin, but that of CFU-E requires relatively small amounts. Erythropoietin is a glycoprotein produced primarily by the kidney in response to

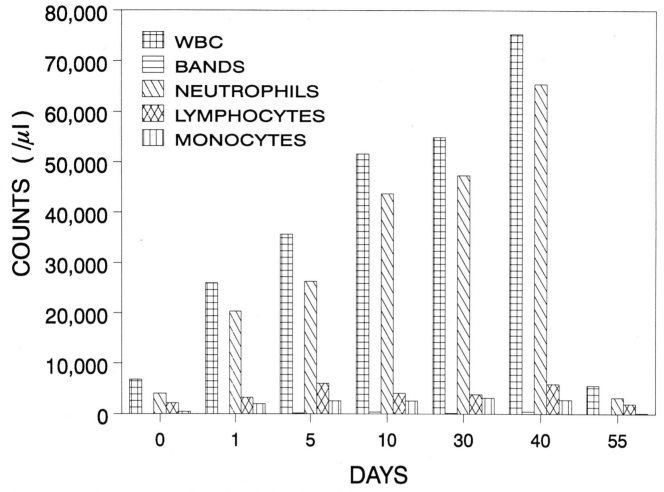

Fig. 4–7. Effect of granulocyte-macrophage colony-stimulating factor administration (5 µg/kg body weight/day subcutaneously for 6 weeks) on total and differential leukocyte counts in a dog. (Data collected in collaboration with Dr. J.G. Zinkl and Dr. G.R. Cain.)

renal tissue hypoxia. Some erythropoietin is also synthesized by the liver. Erythropoietin is needed for erythrocyte production involving progenitor cell differentiation, multiplication, and maturation through various morphologically recognizable stages (Table 4–4). High concentrations of erythropoietin increase protein synthesis in megakaryocytes in mice and platelet counts in rats, thereby suggesting a role in megakaryocytopoiesis and platelet production (Woodman, 1992).

Human recombinant erythropoietin (rHuEPO) has been produced and found to stimulate erythropoiesis in normal humans and to correct anemia in human, canine, and feline patients with renal failure. Preliminary investigations with rHuEPO have shown that profound refractory anemia in dogs and cats can be corrected by 3 to 4 weeks of therapy followed by maintenance follow-up dosage (Cowgill, 1991). In most patients, an increase of approximately one hematocrit point per week could be achieved, which resolved the anemia within 3 to 4 weeks. A few dogs and cats receiving rHuEPO for variable duration may develop antibodies to human erythropoietin and fail to respond. Such animals may develop a progressive un-

responsive anemia which reverses upon discontinuation of rHuEPO administration.

MEGAKARYOCYTOPOIESIS

Megakaryocyte production from pluripotential stem cells is regulated by IL-3, GM-CSF, the local microenvironment, and a specific poietin known as thrombopoietin (Jackson, 1989; Jain, 1986). Analogous to erythroid differentiation, intermediate stages of BFU-Meg and CFU-Meg have been recognized (Table 4–4). Megakaryocytopoiesis and platelet production are influenced by the platelet mass; thrombocytopenia has a stimulatory effect, whereas thrombocytosis is inhibitory. Platelet production is specifically controlled by thrombopoietin. The source of thrombopoietin is unknown, but a thrombocytopoiesis-stimulating factor has been isolated from human embryo kidney cells. Other growth factors, such as IL-1, IL-4, IL-6, erythropoietin, and G-CSF may have a synergistic stimulatory effect on megakaryocyte production. The production of IL-6 is increased during inflammatory responses and may result in increased platelet numbers and account, at least in part, for the secondary thrombocytosis seen in patients with an ongoing inflammatory process (Straneva et al., 1992).

A unique aspect of megakaryocytopoiesis is that megakaryoblasts undergo repeated endomitosis (nuclear division without cell division) so that cell size increases, unlike that associated with erythropoiesis or granulopoiesis. Furthermore, polyploid megakaryoblasts may begin to mature early, leading to the production of megakaryocytes with 8N to 32N (and sometimes 64N) nuclear chromatin. Obviously, small megakaryocytes produce fewer platelets than large megakaryocytes.

LYMPHOPOIESIS

Lymphopoiesis occurs in different tissues (bone marrow, thymus, spleen, and lymph nodes) and involves several cellular stages, unlike those in myelopoiesis. Lymphoid progenitor cells and their descendants are identified primarily by cell surface properties rather than on a morphologic basis (Table 4–4). Factors regulating the production, differentiation, and multiplication of lymphoid progenitor cells are complex and remain largely ill-defined. The local microenvironment, interleukins, and antigen are believed to play important roles. Several lymphocytic growth factors, most of which are interleukins, have been recognized (Quesenberry, 1990). T-cell production and maturation into different subsets are influenced by a complex interaction of IL-1, IL-2, IL-4, IL-5, IL-7, IL-12, tumor necrosis factor-α, T-cell growth factor-β, and interferon-α. Similarly a number of B-cell growth factors have been identified; these include IL-1, IL-2, IL-4, IL-5, IL-6, IL-7, IL-11, tumor necrosis factor-α, T-cell growth factor-β, and interferon-α. Current immunology texts should be consulted for a more detailed discussion of ongoing research in this fascinating area of hematology.

TRANSIT OF CELLS FROM BONE MARROW TO BLOOD

The process by which the extramedullary-produced mammalian blood cells enter the circulation is intriguing and still debated. Cell entry is selective and is regulated by various factors, including anatomic location of cells in the bone marrow, sinusoidal properties (e.g., blood flow, permissiveness of its wall, and surface characteristics of endothelial cells), maturity, deformability and surface properties of migrating cells, and hormonal factors. For example, inappropriate numbers of immature bone marrow cells may be delivered into the circulation following a breakage in the sinusoidal wall, as from tumor infiltration or myeloid malignancies, or increased permissiveness of the sinusoidal wall, as in shock and endotoxemia. Immature myeloid cells are less deformable and have a higher negative surface charge compared to mature cells, which retard their release from the bone marrow. Such cells are released into the blood in excessive numbers, generally in response to specific hormonal stimuli (e.g., reticulocytosis occurs from heightened erythropoietin production during responsive blood loss or hemolytic anemias).

Cell entry into the vascular spaces of bone marrow has been studied by electron microscopy. The entry of leukocytes and erythrocytes is believed to be transcellular. In addition, a variable but selective population of these cells may also enter through natural gaps or apertures that form in the sinusoidal wall during its constant remodeling in vivo. Studies in dogs have shown that the number of apertures in unilaminar sinuses is greater than that in multilamilar sinuses covered with adventitial layer, and that most of the apertures are occupied by cells in transit (Deldar et al., 1989). Megakaryocytes, being in apposition to the sinusoidal wall, usually extend long cytoplasmic processes (proplatelets) into the sinusoidal lumen, where they subsequently fragment into platelets. Megakaryocytes may also shed platelets directly into the sinusoidal lumen by surface budding (see Chap. 6).

REFERENCES

Cowgill, L.D.: Clinical experience and use of recombinant human erythropoietin in uremic dogs and cats. Proceedings of the 9th ACVIM Forum, 147, 1991.

Deldar, A., Lewis, H. and Bloom, J.: Electron microscopic study of the unique features and structural-morphologic relationship of canine bone marrow. Am. J. Vet. Res., 50:136, 1989.

Fulton, R., Gasper, P.W., Ogilvie, G.K., et al.: Effect of recombinant human granulocyte colony-stimulating factor on hematopoiesis in normal cats. Exp. Hematol., 19:759, 1991.

Golde, D.W.: Overview of myeloid growth factors. Semin. Hematol., 27:1, 1990.

Golde, D.W. and Glaspy, J.: Therapeutic use of granulocyte and monocyte colony-stimulating factors. In: Hematology, 4th Ed. Edited by W.J. Williams, E. Beutler, A.J. Erslev, et al. New York, McGraw-Hill, 1990, pp. 273–278.

Hammond, W.P., Csiba, E., Canin, A., et al.: Chronic neutropenia. A new canine model induced by human granulocyte colony-stimulating factor. J. Clin. Invest., 87:704, 1991.

Jackson, C.W.: Animal models with inherited hematopoietic abnormalities as tools to study thrombopoiesis. Blood Cells, 15:237, 1989.

Jain, N.C.: Schalm's Veterinary Hematology. 4th Ed. Philadelphia, Lea & Febiger, 1985, pp. 350–387.

Lothrop, C.D., Jr., Warren, C.D., Souza, L.M., et al.: Correction of canine cyclic hematopoiesis with recombinant human granulocyte colony-stimulating factor. Blood, 72:1324, 1988.

Mishu, L., Callahan, G., Allebban, Z., et al.: Effects of recombinant canine granulocyte colony-stimulating factor on white blood cell production in clinically normal and neutropenic dogs. J. Am. Vet. Med. Assoc., 200:1957, 1992.

Pratt, H.L., Carroll, R.C., McClendon, S., et al.: Effects of recombinant granulocyte colony-stimulating factor treatment on hematopoietic cycles and cellular defects associated with canine cyclic hematopoiesis. Exp. Hematol., 18:1199, 1990.

Quesenberry, P.J.: Hematopoietic stem cells, progenitor cells, and growth factors. In: Hematology, 4th Ed. Edited by W.J. Williams, E. Beutler, A.J. Erslev, et al. New York, McGraw-Hill, 1990, pp. 129–147.

Shaw, A.R.: Molecular biology of cytokines: An introduction. In: The Cytokine Handbook. Edited by A. Thomson, San Diego, Academic Press, 1991.

Straneva, J.E., ven Besien, K.W., Derigs, G., et al.: Is interleukin 6 the physiological regulator of thrombopoiesis? Exp. Hematol., 20:47, 1992.

Weisbart, R.H., Gasson, J.C. and Golde, D.W.: Colony-stimulating factors and hose defense. Ann. Intern. Med., 110:297, 1989.

Whetton, A.D. and Dexter, T.M.: Myeloid haemopoietic growth factors. Biochem. Biophys. Acta, 989:111, 1989.

Woodman, D.D.: Erythropoietin. Comp. Haematol. Int., 2:1, 1992.

Chapter 5

Coagulation and its Disorders

Blood clots when it is removed from normal, endothelium-lined blood vessels. Clotting is much more rapid in glass containers than in containers coated with silicone or similar materials, which suggests that, when blood comes into contact with glass, the clotting mechanism is activated. This phenomenon is called contact activation and indicates that all components necessary for clotting are present in normal blood. This type of clotting is brought about by the so-called intrinsic or endogenous system. Conversely, clotting is greatly accelerated if thromboplastins, which arise from damaged tissues, are added to the plasma. The clotting system involving tissue factors is called the extrinsic or exogenous system. Both systems are necessary to maintain normal hemostasis—that is, prevention of blood loss from damaged vessels.

PRIMARY HEMOSTASIS

Hemostasis entails a complex series of physiologic and biochemical events involving both promoters and inhibitors of blood coagulation. The hemostatic process is designed to maintain blood within the confines of blood vessels. Primary hemostasis is initiated when vascular injury disrupts endothelium, exposing subendothelial connective tissue to blood. Essentially, three functional components of hemostasis act in concert to arrest bleeding—blood vessels, platelets, and coagulation proteins or factors. Acquired or hereditary disorders of any of these three components can lead to defective hemostasis (Tables 5–1 and 5–2).

The mechanisms of arrest of bleeding differ, depending on the size of the blood vessels involved. During the first minutes after a small cut is made in the skin, the axon reflex leads to transient vasoconstriction, which contributes to hemostasis. Vasoconstriction alone, however, is insufficient to stop blood loss. The interaction of platelets and vascular endothelium may be sufficient to arrest bleeding. Severance of a larger vessel involves a more complex mechanism of platelet plug formation and activation of the blood coagulation system at the site of injury.

Table 5–1. Pathogenesis of Defective Hemostasis

Vascular defects
   Structural
   Immune-mediated
   Inflammation
Quantitative platelet abnormalities
   Failure of production
   Reduced survival
   Increased sequestration
Qualitative platelet abnormalities
   Failure to adhere or release adenosine diphosphate (ADP)
   Failure to aggregate
   Failure to make phospholipid available
Coagulation factor defects
   Absolute failure of synthesis
   Production of abnormal molecule
   Excessive destruction of coagulation factors
   Circulatory inhibitors

Table 5–2. Clinical Signs in Vascular, Platelet, or Coagulation Defects

Vascular or Platelet Defect	Coagulation Defect
Petechiae, superficial bruising	Deep-spreading hematoma
Bleeding in skin and mucous membranes	Hemarthroses or retroperitoneal bleeding
Immediate bleeding	Recurrent and late bleeding

Platelets do not adhere to normal intact endothelium and intact endothelium does not activate hemostasis. This property of endothelium is attributed both to active and passive processes.

Active Mechanisms.   Active mechanisms are associated with the direct or indirect participation of endothelial cells; these include the following (1) synthesis of prostacyclin (PGI$_2$), endothelium-derived relaxing factor (EDRF), plasminogen activators, thrombomodulin, protease nexin, and protein S; (2) uptake and/or degradation of adenosine diphosphate (ADP) and proaggregating vasoactive amines; and (3) inactivation of thrombin. PGI$_2$ is a potent vasodilator and stimulates membrane adenyl cyclase and increases platelet cyclic adenosine monophosphate (cAMP) concentrations. Increased cAMP concentration inhibits platelet adhesion to endothelium and impairs platelet-to-platelet cohesion (aggregation) and release of ADP and other platelet contents. A cAMP-stimulated, protein kinase-mediated phosphorylation of platelet membrane or cytoplasmic protein may cause these inhibitory effects. EDRF is a potent vasodilator and inhibitor of platelet aggregation and inhibition. Both PGI$_2$ and EDRF may act synergistically. Inactivation of thrombin may occur through the endocytosis of thrombin-thrombomodulin and thrombin-protease nexin complexes by endothelial cells and through localized production of plasmin by plasminogen activators.

Passive Mechanisms.   Passive mechanisms involve endothelial proteoglycans, heparan sulfate with anticoagulant properties, and a net negative surface charge that repels similarly charged blood cells. Heparan sulfate complexes with antithrombin III and inactivates thrombin.

Injury to endothelial cells and exposure of subendothelial collagen and microfibrils promote platelet adherence as well as coagulation (Fig. 5–1). Platelets adhere to the subendothelial collagen through the interaction of their surface receptors with von Willebrand factor (vWF), vitronectin, and fibronectin. Thrombospondin released from platelet α granules and platelet-activating factor (PAF) produced by endothelial cells may also be involved in platelet adhesion.

The adhered platelets undergo a shape change from disks to irregular spheres, exhibit centripetal movement of a circumferential band of microtubules that herds platelet storage granules toward the center, and begin to release their granule contents through the

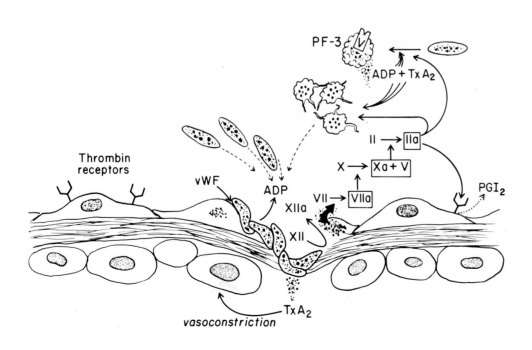

Fig. 5–1. Hemostatic events associated with vessel wall injury. These involve collagen-induced activation of platelets aided by adenosine diphosphate (ADP) and thromboxane (TxA$_2$) and the initiation of clotting through the activation of the intrinsic system (beginning at factor XII) and the extrinsic system (beginning at factor VII). See text for details. (From Jain, N.C.: Schalm's Veterinary Hematology. 4th Ed. Philadelphia, Lea & Febiger, 1986, p. 390.)

open canalicular system. Consequently, other platelets are recruited and platelet aggregation occurs, which eventually forms a large mass over the injured area. Within a short time, the opening in the vessel is filled and blood ceases to escape. Platelet aggregation, up to a certain point, may be reversible. The irreversible phase of platelet aggregation is called viscous metamorphosis. It occurs when prothrombin in the plasma is converted to thrombin.

During the process of platelet activation and release reaction, many factors are released into the microenvironment. These factors are stored preformed in various platelet organelles or are newly synthesized as a result of metabolic stimulation (see Table 6–1) and include ADP, adenosine triphosphate (ATP), serotonin, platelet factors 3 and 4 (PF-3 and PF-4), platelet fibrinogen, thromboxane A_2 (TxA_2), platelet-derived growth factor, β-thromboglobulin, and acid hydrolases. The release of ADP and the generation of TxA_2 recruit more platelets to the area to enlarge the hemostatic plug. ADP interacts with platelet membranes to expose a specific fibrinogen-binding receptor site associated with the glycoprotein IIb-IIIa complex on the platelet membrane. Bound fibrinogen serves as a primary recognition site for platelet aggregation.

Platelet adherence and aggregation create favorable conditions for localized activation of the clotting system. Platelets can activate the intrinsic clotting system through interactions with a factor XII receptor and high-molecular-weight (HMW) kininogen, through the release of PF-3, and through trapping of coagulation factors on their surfaces (Fig. 5–2). The release of tissue thromboplastin from injured endothelium and subendothelial connective tissue presumably activates the extrinsic clotting system as well. Thrombin gen-

erated by the activation of coagulation pathways amplifies platelet aggregation and release responses and induces platelet metamorphosis. Secretion, binding, and activation of coagulation factors by endothelial cells also promote the coagulation process.

The next stage involves fibrin formation, which enmeshes platelets and produces a compact mass (Fig. 5–2). An actinomycin-like contractile protein, thrombosthenin, present within platelet microfilaments, produces contraction of platelets; this tends to tense the fibrin strands and thereby reinforces and seals the hemostatic plug.

Thrombin activity is limited to the area of hemostasis by the action of plasma protease inhibitors, thrombin-antithrombin III complex formation, and endothelial activation of protein C, which destroys coagulation factors V and VIII. After it has served its purpose, the hemostatic plug dissolves through localized activation of the fibrinolytic system. Repair of the vessel wall is accomplished by the migration and proliferation of adjacent endothelial cells to cover the denuded surface. Similarly, the proliferation of fibroblasts and smooth muscle cells, stimulated by platelet-derived growth factors, aids the repair process.

COAGULATION

Blood coagulation occurs in a series of step-wise reactions that lead to the activation of coagulation factors (Table 5–3) and the formation of a stable fibrin clot (Fig. 5–3). The factors are numbered (in Roman numerals) according to the order of their discovery, not in order of their action. The coagulation factors

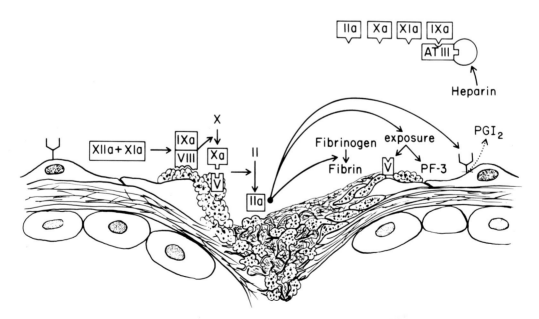

Fig. 5–2. Hemostatic events associated with vessel wall injury. These involve the organization of platelet plugs, fibrin deposition, and the regulatory actions of prostacyclin (PGI₂) and the heparin-antithrombin III (ATIII) complex. See text for details. (From Jain, N.C.: Schalm's Veterinary Hematology. 4th Ed. Philadelphia, Lea & Febiger, 1986, p. 391.)

Table 5–3. Nomenclature and Some Properties of Coagulation Factors

Factor	Common Name	Molecular Weight	Plasma Level (μg/ml)	Half-life (hr)	Turnover Rate (μg/ml/day)	Biosynthesis
I	Fibrinogen	340,000	2500	123	500	Liver, megakaryocytes
II	Prothrombin	70,000	100	100	40	Liver; vitamin K-dependent
III	Tissue thromboplastin	45,000	0	—	—	Virtually all tissues
IV	Calcium ions	—	—	—	—	
V	Proaccelerin	330,000	5–12	25	10	Liver, macrophages
VII	Proconvertin	63,000	1	5	2	Liver, vitamin K-dependent
VIII	Antihemophilic factor	1–2 million	7	10	25	VIII:C, probably liver vWF, endothelial cells, and megakaryocytes
IX	Christmas factor	62,000	4	20	2	Liver; vitamin K-dependent
X	Stuart-Prower factor	59,000	5	65	6	Liver; vitamin K-dependent
XI	Plasma thromboplastin antecedent	200,000	4	65	<2	Liver
XII	Hageman factor	80,000	29	60	<2	Liver
XIII	Fibrin-stabilizing factor	320,000	10	150	3	Liver; megakaryocytes
—	Prekallikrein	85,000	—	35	—	Liver
—	High-molecular-weight kininogen	120,000	—	156	—	Liver (?)

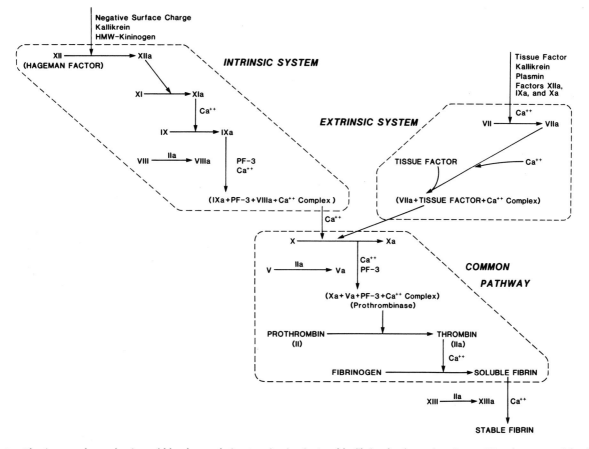

Fig. 5–3. Classic cascade mechanism of blood coagulation terminating in a stable fibrin clot formation. Factor XIIa plays a crucial role in the initiation of the intrinsic system, whereas factor VII and tissue factor complex initiate the extrinsic system. The two systems merge at the stage at which factor X is activated to Xa, the first step of the common pathway (HMW-kininogen, high-molecular-weight kininogen; PF-3, platelet phospholipid). See Figure 5–4 for interactions of the activated Hageman factor with other biologic systems and Figure 5–5 for fibrin(ogen)olysis. See text for details. (From Jain, N.C.: Schalm's Veterinary Hematology. 4th Ed. Philadelphia, Lea & Febiger, 1986, p. 392.)

are glycoproteins present in an inactive or precursor form. The activated forms of zymosans and cofactors are indicated by a lower case "a" following the Roman numeral, or given a special name. No factor VI is present, and some factors involved in the coagulation process have not been assigned a number. The only nonprotein factor is Ca^{2+} (factor IV), which is needed for most of the reactions. Factors V, VII, and VIII and tissue factor act as catalysts for the coagulation process, thereby increasing the efficiency of the enzymes with which they interact. The phospholipid membrane surface (tissue factor and PF-3) localizes the coagulation process at the site of vascular injury and protects membrane-bound coagulation proteins from the inhibitory action of antithrombin III. Laboratory tests have been developed to detect abnormalities of the steps involved in the coagulation process (Table 5–4).

With the exception of tissue thromboplastin (factor III), each factor is present in normal plasma. Serum is deficient in factors I, II, V, and VIII and has a reduced concentration of factor XIII and an increased concentration of factor IX compared to plasma. Activated factors XII, XI, X, IX, VII, and II and kallikrein, an active product of prekallikrein, possess serine at their active enzymatic sites, so are classified as serine proteases. Some of the coagulation proteins (e.g., factors II, VIII, IX, and X), have a sizable extravascular pool, which can be mobilized into the circulation by physiologic and pathologic stimuli. Highly purified coagulation factors have been obtained from human and bovine plasma and their amino acid sequences determined. Genes coding for most of the coagulation factors in humans have been cloned and sequenced.

Coagulation Factors and Their Interactions

FACTOR XII

The first step in the clotting sequence is the conversion of factor XII (Hageman factor) to its active state, XIIa, by contact activation or by proteolytic enzymes, such as kallikrein, plasmin, or trypsin. Ca^{2+} is not used during the activation of factor XII, but is required in all subsequent steps. Factor XIIa successively converts factors XI and IX to their activated forms, XIa and IXa. In vivo activation of factor XII occurs when collagen is exposed after tissue injury. Prekallikrein (also known as Fletcher factor) and HMW kininogen (also known as Fitzgerald factor, Williams factor, or Flaujeac factor) also participate in contact activation of factor XII. Kinin participation is needed for optimal activation of the intrinsic pathway; kallikrein can activate factors XII and XI. HMW kininogen mainly enhances the action of factor XIIa during the activation of factor XI. HMW kininogen is present in plasma complexed to prekallikrein and factor XI. Although activities of each of these contact factors may be reduced by acquired or hereditary disorders, only low concentrations of factor XI are associated with abnormal bleeding.

In addition to the coagulation system, the kinin, complement, and plasminogen systems also merge at this initial step of the coagulation cascade (Fig. 5–4). The Hageman factor also plays an important role in disseminated intravascular coagulation (DIC) and inflammation. Factor XIIa, in reacting with exposed collagen, activates the plasma kinin system by converting inactive prekallikrein to active kallikrein, which in turn converts kininogen to active kinins. Kinins are important in inflammation because they cause edema, vasodilation, and increased capillary permeability and induce chemotaxis of leukocytes. Factor XIIa leads to plasmin formation through the activation of plasminogen proactivators. Plasmin interaction with complement produces factors that participate in inflammatory response analogous to kinins.

FACTOR VIII

In the next sequence of the coagulation process, factor IXa forms a complex with PF-3 and factor VIIIa in the presence of Ca^{2+}. This complex then activates factor X to Xa. The action of thrombin on factor VIII greatly accelerates the generation of factor Xa.

Factor VIII, or antihemophilic factor (MW 25,000 to 340,000), normally circulates as a noncovalent complex of vWF (MW about 1 million), which serves as a carrier molecule. The procoagulant property of factor VIII is measured in clotting assays and designated VIII:C, factor VIII antigen determined by immunologic tests is designated VIII:Ag, and, similarly, vWF antigen is designated vWF:Ag. The term "factor VIII-related antigen" (VIIIR:Ag) is not recommended as another term for vWF. The term "factor VIII:C," however, is sometimes used interchangeably with factor VIII. The vWF does not participate in the intrinsic pathway of coagulation, but functions in hemostasis by promoting platelet adhesion and aggregation. The site of biosynthesis of factor VIII is not definitely known, but it is probably synthesized by macrophages in the liver. The half-life of factor VIII is estimated as 8 to 12 hours and that of vWF as 22 to 44 hours. Factor VIII is synthesized normally in patients with von Willebrand disease, but the half-life of factor VIII

Table 5–4. Common Laboratory Tests for Bleeding Disorders

Prothrombin time (PT)
    Assays extrinsic (factor VII) and common (factors X, V, II, and I) pathways
Activated partial thromboplastin time (APTT)
    Assays intrinsic (factors XII, XI, IX, and VIII) and common (factors X, V, II, and I) pathways
Thrombin time (TT)
    Assays fibrinogen (factor I)
Platelet count
    Examination of stained blood film for adequacy of platelet numbers
    Total platelet count is determined if smear indicates a decreased or markedly increased platelet number

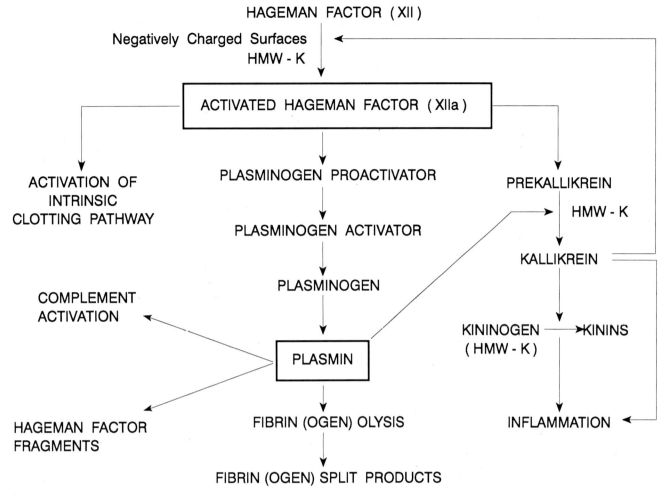

Fig. 5–4. Interactions among the coagulation, kinin, fibrinolytic, and complement systems (HMW-kininogen, high-molecular-weight kininogen). (Modified from Ruddy, S., Gigli, I., Austen, K. F. et al.: The complement system of man (first of four parts). N. Engl. J. Med., 287:489, 1972.)

is decreased because the vWF carrier molecule is decreased or absent.

A significant extravascular pool of factor VIII exists, principally in the spleen. Thus, plasma concentrations of factor VIII can increase under various conditions, such as vigorous exercise, pregnancy, chronic thrombocytopenia, and infusion of epinephrine and 2,3-diphosphoglycerate. Factor VIII also behaves as an acute phase protein, so its concentrations are increased during acute and chronic active inflammatory processes.

FACTOR X

The intrinsic and extrinsic systems converge at factor X (Stuart-Prower factor; Fig. 5–3) and, from this level onward, the two systems share a common pathway. In the intrinsic system, factor IXa, PF-3, factor VIIIa, and Ca^{2+} form a complex to activate factor X. In the extrinsic system, thromboplastin (tissue factor) released by tissue damage reacts with factor VIIa in the presence of Ca^{2+} to form a complex for the activation of factor X. Factor X can be activated in vitro by incubation with dilute trypsin or Russell's viper venom.

Activated factor Xa is the prime activator of prothrombin. Tissue factor and platelet phospholipids accelerate the coagulation process by participating in reactions involving factors VIII, VII, and V.

PROTHROMBIN AND THROMBIN

Prothrombin is converted to thrombin in the presence of factor Xa, PF-3, Ca^{2+}, and an accelerator (factor Va). Factors Xa and Va react with PF-3 in the presence of Ca^{2+} to form a particulate complex known as prothrombinase. Prothrombin is converted to thrombin by the enzymatic action of prothrombinase. During activation of the coagulation cascade by the extrinsic system, tissue thromboplastin substitutes for the phospholipid from platelets (PF-3).

Thrombin has both esterase and peptidase activities. It modifies or activates a number of reactions. Thrombin functions in the coagulation system at several stages—conversion of fibrinogen to fibrin, promotion of platelet aggregation and release reaction, and activation of factors XIII, XII, VIII, and V. Thrombin can activate its own production from prothrombin, but the reaction is slow. Thrombin also promotes conversion of plasminogen to plasmin and activation of the complement system. The enzymatic activity of thrombin is inhibited by heparin, fibrinopeptide A released from fibrinogen by thrombin action (see below), and natural antithrombins present in plasma.

FIBRINOGEN AND FIBRIN

Fibrinogen is a dimeric glycoprotein (MW, 340,000) having several Ca^{2+} binding sites. Each half of the fibrinogen molecule contains three pairs of polypeptide chains, α or A, β or B, and γ chains, having an MW of 73,000, 60,000, and 50,000 daltons, respectively. The chains are interconnected by disulfide bonds to form a symmetric dimer. Platelets contain plasma fibrinogen adsorbed to their surface and also intracellularly in α-granules. Rat and mouse megakaryocytes endocytose circulating proteins, including fibrinogen, albumin, and IgG, and incorporate them into α-granules (Handagama et al., 1990).

The proteolytic action of thrombin, in the presence of Ca^{2+}, results in the conversion of fibrinogen to fibrin monomers and four fibrinopeptides. Two of the fibrinopeptides are derived from the α chain (fibrinopeptides A) and two from the β chain (fibrinopeptides B). The rapid, spontaneous polymerization of the fibrin monomers results in formation of the clot, a gelatinous mass of fibrin strands. Initially, the clot is held together by weak, noncovalent forces between the fibrin monomers. Consequently, the clot is soluble in dilute acid and in concentrated urea solution. Within minutes, however, a stable clot is produced when the strands are joined covalently through the action of a cross-linking enzyme, factor XIIIa, in the presence of Ca^{2+} (Fig. 5–3). Factor XIIIa enables the clot to reach maturity and achieve its maximum strength. Factor XIII (fibrin-stabilizing factor) exists in plasma as a proenzyme and is also supplied by platelets. It is activated by thrombin in the absence of Ca^{2+}

TISSUE THROMBOPLASTIN

Tissue thromboplastin (factor III), or tissue phospholipid, provides a suitably charged surface for binding both Ca^{2+} and factor VIIa to form an enzymatic complex that activates factor X to Xa. Factor VII activity can be enhanced by the action of kallikrein, plasmin, factor XIIa, and factor IXa, and also by factor Xa. Factor VII has the shortest half-life of all the coagulation proteins (Table 5–3). The complex of tissue factor, factor VIIa, and Ca^{2+} may also activate factor IX to IXa in the normal coagulation process.

Tissue thromboplastin is not usually present in blood but is released when tissue is damaged. It is present in large amounts in the brain, lungs, and placenta, is secreted by activated leukocytes, and has been found in the intima of large vessels. Tissue thromboplastin is a protein-phospholipid complex associated with a microsomal fraction of cells. Lipid comprises one-third of the molecular weight of this factor and is essential for its activity. The action of tissue thromboplastin is species-specific, attributable to its protein moiety.

Endotoxin-activated monocytes express thromboplastin-like procoagulant activity on the cell surface; this may serve as a nidus for the formation of microvascular thrombi. Monocyte procoagulant activity is high in horses with acute gastrointestinal disease and may possibly play a role in the pathogenesis of equine endotoxemia and coagulopathy (Henry and Moore, 1991). Because neutropenia is an early event in endotoxemia, procoagulant substances may also be released from endotoxin-stimulated neurophils and activate the coagulation process resulting in DIC. PT and PTT are shortened and FDPs are increased in endotoxic horses (Duncan et al., 1985).

Summary of Coagulation and Platelet Interactions During Hemostasis

The hemostatic response is mediated by the cell surfaces and collagen exposed at the wound site (Fig. 5–1). Exposure of collagen initiates the activation of the intrinsic coagulation system locally, beginning with the conversion of factor XII to XIIa. Ruptured endothelial cells, smooth muscle cells, and other damaged cells exude tissue thromboplastin, which initiates the extrinsic pathway beginning with factor VII. Simultaneously, platelets become activated after coming into contact with exposed collagen or thrombin. Activated platelets then undergo the release reaction. Platelets release various substances, including ADP and TxA_2, both of which amplify platelet adherence and aggregation, thus enlarging the platelet plug. The availability of PF-3 and of adsorbed coagulation factors on the surface of platelets further potentiates the clotting process.

Factor V molecules on the surface of platelets in the hemostatic plug serve as binding sites for factor Xa (Fig. 5–2). This step markedly accelerates the clotting process. The activation of factor X triggers the formation of cross-linked fibrin molecules. Finally, within the platelet plug, thrombosthenin, contracts, strengthening the hemostatic plug and converting it into a tidy patch to arrest bleeding.

Several regulatory mechanisms act concurrently to keep the clotting process localized. Thrombin bound to cell surface receptors triggers the release of PGI_2 from uninjured endothelial cells to limit the spread of platelet aggregation. The heparin-antithrombin III complex stops further activation of the clotting process in the fluid phase. Plasmin activated early in the process begin to lyse the clot. Platelet-derived growth factors stimulate the multiplication of fibroblasts and smooth muscle cells to colonize the wound, enabling repair to occur. Simultaneously, endothelial cells migrate and proliferate to cover the denuded vessel wall.

BIOSYNTHESIS OF CLOTTING FACTORS AND THE ROLE OF VITAMIN K

The liver parenchyma synthesizes most of the clotting factors (Table 5–3). Factors II, VII, IX, and X are initially synthesized by hepatocytes as inactive precursors and require vitamin K for their activation—that is, γ carboxylation of glutamic acid residues on the N-terminal end of the molecules. This activation is necessary for Ca^{2+} binding and for binding to phospholipid membranes to express procoagulant activity. Most drugs with an anticoagulation action e.g., commonly used rodenticides and drugs used for long-term therapeutic anticoagulation, act by interfering with this activation. Their use results in the formation of abnormal coagulation factors that do not function in the clotting process. Most coagulation factors are in low concentrations in fetal blood, as shown by studies on ovine and bovine fetuses. The synthesis of vitamin K-dependent factors and protein C was found to be low in fetal lambs until the last 10 days, and then increased until birth (Moalic et al., 1989). Their fibrinolytic activity, however, was higher than in adults.

Vitamin K is also required for the production of the anticoagulant proteins known as protein C and protein M. Protein C is a single-chain glycoprotein (MW, about 62,000), but protein M remains to be characterized. Vitamin K is available in the diet (vitamin K_1, phylloquinone) or is synthesized in the gut (vitamin K_2, menaquinone). A deficiency of vitamin K can arise, hence, as the result of low dietary concentration, lack of synthesis in the bowel, lack of absorption, or lack of hepatic utilization.

Macrophages produce several coagulation factors, including factors II, V, VII, IX, and X and tissue factor. Factor V is also synthesized by megakaryocytes, and possibly by endothelial cells. The site of synthesis of factor VIII is not definitely known, but the liver may be the major site and other organs, such as the spleen, lungs, and lymph nodes, may be involved. The vWF is synthesized by the endothelial cells and megakaryocytes and is present in platelet α granules. Factor XIII synthesis involves the liver, megakaryocytes, and monocytes, and it is also synthesized by the placenta. Megakaryocytes also produce fibrinogen, which serves as an important source of intraplatelet fibrinogen. Fibrinogen is an acute phase reactant and its plasma concentration may be increased several fold in acute and chronic active inflammatory conditions. Hepatic synthesis of fibrinogen is triggered by interleukin-1, interleukin-6, and tumor necrosis factors produced from activated macrophages at the inflammation site (see Fig. 21–5).

REGULATION OF THE CLOTTING PROCESS

The clotting process is regulated by two general mechanisms—the elimination of activated clotting factors and the destruction of the fibrin clot. The elimination of activated clotting factors from the circulation involves cellular and humoral processes.

Cellular Processes

The cellular removal of activated coagulation factors involves the mononuclear phagocyte system (MPS),

liver, lungs, and neutrophils. The removal of activated coagulation factors by the liver involves both hepatocytes and the MPS. Soluble forms of activated coagulation proteins are cleared by hepatocytes. The MPS mainly removes particulate coagulation products (e.g., prothrombinase, tissue thromboplastin, and certain fibrin(ogen) degradation products). The coagulation factors are glycoproteins with a central protein core and carbohydrate side chains with terminal sialic acid residues. Removal of the sialic acid residues is associated with clearance of the coagulation factors by hepatocytes and macrophages through endocytosis by way of coated pits. A constant flow of blood also tends to diminish the local concentration of activated coagulation factors, thereby regulating the extent of clot formation.

Humoral Processes

The humoral process involves several natural inhibitors of coagulation that are found in blood and function by inhibiting protease activity. Five of these factors—antithrombin III, C_1 inactivator, α_2-macroglobulin, α_1-antitrypsin, and α_2-antiplasmin—act on one or more of the coagulation factors. Some clotting factors may also be directly inactivated by protein C and other humoral inactivators.

Antithrombin III is the principal physiologic inhibitor of coagulation found in plasma, as well as in extravascular sites. It is an α_2-glycoprotein (MW, 67,000) produced by the liver, with a half-life of less than 2 days. Antithrombin III works by combining with a clotting factor to form a stable, inactive complex. In this manner it acts against activated factors XII, XI, IX, X, and II. Antithrombin III is also active against plasmin and kallikrein. The action of antithrombin III is greatly potentiated by heparin. Heparin similarly accelerates the inactivation of thrombin by heparin cofactor II, which is present in plasma. Heparan sulfate, a compound closely related to heparin that is present in the vascular endothelium, also enhances antithrombin III action. Thus, patients with antithrombin III deficiency are at great risk for thrombosis.

Antithrombin III activity varies in different species. Normal canine, human, and bovine plasmas were found to have 65, 62, and 79% of antithrombin activity, respectively, compared to that of equine plasma (Johnstone et al., 1987). Cats have antithrombin III activity similar to that of dogs (Sugiyama and Furukawa, 1985). Antithrombin III activity in horses may vary with breed and age; for example, thoroughbreds have higher activity than standardbred horses, and younger horses (less than 16 months of age) have lower activity than mature (3-year-old) horses (Johnstone et al. 1989). Horses with acute diarrhea or colitis have reduced antithrombin III activity (74% of the reference plasma), and horses with liver disease have increased activity (127 to 177%) (Johnstone et al., 1987). Most dogs with DIC have decreased antithrombin III concentration in plasma. Antithrombin III activity is decreased in dogs naturally infected with heart worms probably from consumption in associated pulmonary thromboembolic phenomenon as a result of increased platelet reactivity (Baudreaux and Dillon, 1991).

C_1 inactivator is a plasma glycoprotein (MW, 135,000) with inhibitory activity against the first component of complement, factors XIIa and XIa, kallikrein, and plasmin. It is also present in platelet α granules and is secreted on activation.

α_2-Macroglobulin is a glycoprotein (MW, 725,000) that inhibits the activities of thrombin, kallikrein, plasmin, and other proteolytic enzymes by forming irreversible complexes. It has been identified in cell membranes. Its site of production is unknown, but cultured fibroblasts have been found to produce it. Its concentration in plasma decreases in severe liver disease.

α_1-Antitrypsin is an α-globulin (MW, 40,000 to 50,000) present in plasma and on platelets. It is the major trypsin inhibitor of plasma and also has inhibitory activity against chymotrypsin, urokinase, plasmin, and factors Xa and XIa.

α_2-Antiplasmin is an α_2-glycoprotein (MW, 65,000 to 70,000) that inactivates plasmin and urokinase, but not other coagulation proteins. It is the major inactivator of plasmin, and is also present in platelets.

Protein C is a vitamin K-dependent protein. When activated, it has potent anticoagulant and profibrinolytic properties. It is produced by the liver and has a half-life of about 16 hours. It cleaves the thrombin-activated forms of factors V and VIII and neutralizes the effects of plasminogen activator inhibitor, thus allowing the enhanced activation of plasminogen by tissue-plasminogen activator. Protein C therefore limits the size and expansion of thrombi by limiting fibrin deposition and promoting fibrin dissolution. Protein C can function only after it has been activated by thrombin, so its effect tends to be limited to regions in which active clotting is occurring. Its activation is enhanced by thrombomodulin present in the endothelial cell membrane. Protein C is complementary to antithrombin III, working on nonproteolytic clotting factors against which antithrombin III has no effect. Protein C also decreases the rate of thrombin formation. Protein S in plasma acts as a cofactor for the anticoagulation and antifibrinolytic activities of protein C. Protein S is present also in platelet α granules and megakaryocytes. Patients deficient in proteins C and S are at greatly increased risk of venous thrombosis. Similarly, decreased expression of thrombomodulin on endothelial cells during inflammatory conditions increases the risk of thrombosis. Horses with intestinal ischemia and endotoxemia have a low plasma protein C level and decreased plasminogen activity. Thus, it has been suggested that the determination of the plasma concentration of either one or both of these proteins may be useful as a predictor of hemostatic complications of equine colic (Wells et al., 1991). Coumarin administration in horses markedly reduces plasma protein C activity (Wells et al., 1989).

FIBRINOLYSIS

Fibrinolysis is the antithesis of blood coagulation. Fibrin is probably continuously laid down and removed along blood vessel walls. Removal of the clot formed at the site of injury is a necessary step in wound healing and in the restoration of circulation through thrombosed vessels. The clot is removed by the proteolytic action of plasmin bound to the clot, a process referred to as physiologic fibrinolysis, or simply fibrinolysis. Fibrinolysis is also involved in inflammation, the repair of connective tissue, and the promotion of healing.

Mechanisms of Action

Blood clots in vitro can lyse spontaneously, thereby indicating that the mechanisms for clot lysis reside within the clot itself. The clot is dissolved through a regulated system of proteolytic enzymes and their activators and inactivators; these include plasminogen proactivators, plasminogen activators, plasminogen, plasmin, inhibitors of plasminogen proactivators and activators, and antiplasmins (Fig. 5–5).

Plasminogen proactivator is a humoral precursor of plasminogen activator. It is converted to the activated form during contact activation of the clotting mechanism and by kallikrein, HMW kininogen, thrombin, and coagulation factors XIIa and XIa. Plasminogen proactivators and activators are also present in tissues.

Plasminogen activators can be found in the lysosomes of most cells (e.g., macrophages), in red cells, in endothelium (particularly of small vessels), and in body fluids, such as saliva, tears, urine, milk, and semen. Their plasma concentration is normally low because of constant clearance by the liver. Lysosomal and endothelial plasminogen activators are released by various stimuli, such as exercise, emotional stress, surgery, epinephrine, histamine, bacterial pyrogens, hypoxia, venous stasis, and thrombosis. These tissue plasminogen activators (TPAs) differ in immunologic and functional properties from urokinase-like plasminogen activators. A recombinant TPA is commercially available and has been found to be beneficial for dissolving intravascular clots in humans.

Plasminogen is a β-globulin (MW, 88,000) that is probably synthesized by the liver. It is present in plasma in low concentration (2.4 μM) and has a half-life of about 2.2 days. It is also found in extravascular locations. Plasminogen complexes with fibrinogen and fibrin and during clot formation is therefore incorporated within the clot. Plasminogen activators, which are released by endothelial damage and gain access to the clot by adsorption and diffusion, activate plasminogen. Plasminogen activators, by limited proteolysis, convert the plasminogen to an active serine protease, plasmin, which proteolyses fibrinogen and fibrin in an orderly manner into various fragments. Thus, fibrinolysis is a reflection of the activity of plasminogen activators located within the clot. Small amounts of

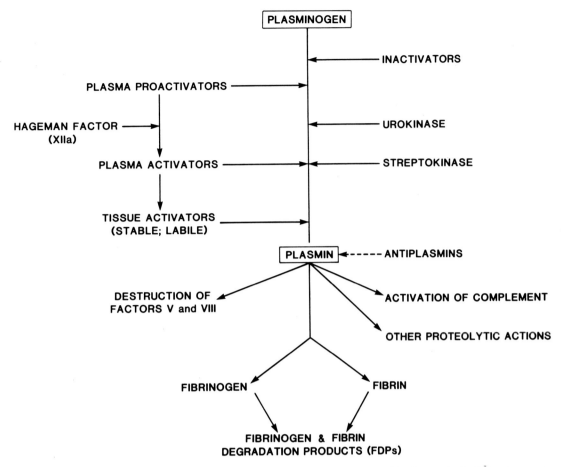

Fig. 5–5. The fibrinolytic system can be activated either intrinsically by factors present in the blood or extrinsically by tissue activators that are provided by damaged cells in the blood vessel wall. Both streptokinase and urokinase can convert plasminogen to plasmin to enhance fibrinolysis and can be used therapeutically as thrombolytic agents. Plasmin activity is normally regulated by antiplasmins in blood, but its excessive activity leads to increased fibrin(ogen)olysis with elevated concentrations of FDPs in blood. Other actions of plasmin are also shown. See text for details. (From Jain, N.C.: Schalm's Veterinary Hematology. 4th Ed. Philadelphia, Lea & Febiger, 1986, p. 400.)

plasminogen may be activated directly by factors XIIa and XIa and by kallikrein. Plasmin may also be produced by the action of other proteolytic enzymes, such as thrombin and trypsin, and by certain chemicals, such as fatty acids, benzene, and chloroform.

This mechanism of fibrinolysis is responsible for the formation of circulating fragments of fibrin(ogen) called fibrin(ogen) degradation products (FDPs) or fibrin(ogen) split products (FSPs) in patients with DIC and for the lower concentrations of factors V and VIII in such patients. FDPs impair hemostasis because they have antiplasmin activity, inhibit fibrin polymerization, and interfere with platelet function. FDPs are removed from the circulation by the liver, kidney, and MPS.

In addition, plasmin also hydrolyzes plasma coagulation factors V and VIII, complement components, and certain hormones such as ACTH, growth hormone, and glucagon. Plasmin can hydrolyze gelatin and casein, a feature that is useful in the assay of its activity.

Plasma inhibitors of fibrinolysis include antiplasmins, antiactivators (plasminogen activator inhibitors 1 and 2), and antiproactivators. At least five naturally occurring inhibitors of plasmin activity are present in plasma; of these, α_2-antiplasmin is the most potent and physiologic regulator of fibrinolysis, α_2-macroglobulin is of limited physiologic importance, and α_1-antitrypsin binds plasmin after the first two have become saturated. Antiplasmin activity has also been detected in platelets and endothelium.

Filtrates from β-hemolytic streptococci also cause the rapid liquefaction of fibrin clots. This streptococcal fibrinolysin is called streptokinase (MW, 48,000). Its mechanism of action remains to be elucidated, but one hypothesis is that streptokinase forms a complex with plasminogen (or plasmin) and this complex nonenzymatically activates plasminogen to plasmin, which then proteolyses the fibrin. Species variations have been noted with regard to the fibrinolytic system activated by streptokinase. Anititstreptokinase antibodies in plasma, formed as an immunologic response to streptokinase administration or infection with β-hemolytic streptococci, may limit the effect of streptokinase therapy. Urine and plasma also contain a powerful acti-

Table 5–5. Differences Between Primary Fibrin(ogen)olysis and Disseminated Intravascular Coagulation (DIC)

Parameter	Primary Fibrin(ogen)olysis	DIC
Platelet count	Normal	Low
Euglobulin lysis time	Shortened	Normal
Fibrin degradation products (FDPs)	Present	Present

vator of the fibrinolytic system, called urokinase or urokase (MW, 54,000), which has a trypsin-like protease action. It is synthesized by the kidney.

Measurement

The presence of plasmin in plasma indicates an advanced pathologic process, because its detection indicates that it is present in an amount sufficient to overcome the action of antiplasmins. Although fibrinolysis in the normal state is so low that it is often undetected, it is greatly enhanced in certain diseases. Accelerated fibrinolysis can be determined by demonstrating FDPs in serum or by finding increased plasminogen activation in plasma, as determined by the euglobulin lysis time test (Table 5–5). FDPs are potent inhibitors of coagulation and their presence may be suspected when abnormalities occur in the coagulation screening assays for prothrombin time (PT), activated partial prothrombin time (APTT), and especially thrombin time (TT). Lysis of extravascular fibrin(ogen), arising from internal hemorrhage, does not produce a clinically significant increase in circulating FDPs in dogs (McCaw et al., 1986).

Clinical Observations

Practical problems related to fibrinolysis in animals are rare, except perhaps as they relate to DIC and to the management of thrombosis and thromboembolism. Bleeding in patients with pathologic fibrinolysis is primarily a manifestation of the antihemostatic effects of FDPs, as in DIC. Consequently, treatment involves the use of antifibrinolytic agents, such as ε-aminocaproic acid, aprotinin (Trasylol), p-aminocyclohexane carbolic acid, and p-aminomethyl benzoic acid.

DISORDERS OF COAGULATION

This area of veterinary medicine is expanding rapidly. Both hereditary and acquired coagulopathies have been found.

Hereditary Coagulopathies

Hereditary coagulation abnormalities are less common than acquired coagulation disorders. They are generally a manifestation of a single factor deficiency resulting from inadequate or defective biosynthesis (Table 5–6). The hereditary disorders are characterized by appearance in early life and by the presence of a single abnormality that can account for the entire clinical picture. Multiple factor deficiencies are rare. Regardless of the type of coagulation abnormality, patients with hereditary coagulopathies show similar clinical signs. A prominent sign is either spontaneous hemorrhage or extensive hemorrhage after trauma or surgery.

INHERITANCE PATTERNS

With the exception of hemophilias A and B, all congenital coagulation defects have an autosomal inheritance pattern. Classic von Willebrand disease (vWD) in humans is transmitted as an autosomal dominant disorder—that is, a single autosomal gene (heterozygosity) causes the disease. The recessive form of vWD has been recognized in Poland-China swine, Scottish terriers, and Chesapeake Bay retrievers. The affected dogs are homozygous for vWD and almost

Table 5–6. Hereditary Coagulopathies in Animals

Disease	Species	Inheritance*
Congenital afibrinogenemia (hypofibrinogenemia)	Dogs, goats	Autosomal incomplete dominance
Factor II deficiency	Dogs	?
Factor VII deficiency	Dogs	Autosomal incomplete dominance
Hemophilia A (factor VIII deficiency)	Dogs, cats, horses, swine	X-linked recessive
von Willebrand disease	Dogs	Autosomal recessive; more commonly, incomplete dominance
	Poland-China swine	Autosomal recessive
	Cats	(?)
Hemophilia B (factor IX deficiency)	Dogs	X-linked
	Cats	(?)
Factor X deficiency	Dogs	Autosomal recessive or incomplete dominance
Factor XI deficiency	Dogs, cattle	Autosomal incomplete dominance
Factor XII (Hageman factor) deficiency†	Cats, dogs	Autosomal recessive
Prekallikrein deficiency	Dogs (one report), horses	Autosomal recessive (?)

* X-linked recessive—carried by females and manifested in their sons; affected males produce normal sons but all daughters are carriers; autosomal inheritance—seen in either sex.

† The Hageman factor is absent in marine mammals, fowl, and most reptiles.

deficient in vWF. The incompletely dominant form is much more common and has been recognized in many dog breeds, with some breeds having an incidence as high as 70% (Doberman pinschers). In this form, the affected dogs are heterozygous and have a variable decrease in plasma vWF. Doberman pinschers with severe vWF deficiency may develop a syndrome of osteochondrofibrosis that results in pelvic limb lameness, presumably because of an increased risk of microvascular bleeding (Dueland et al., 1990). A less severe form has been found in domestic cats and rabbits. Other defects, such as factor X or V deficiency, are autosomal recessive disorders (i.e., two abnormal genes—homozygosity—must be present for bleeding to occur). In contrast, hemophilias A and B are X-linked recessive disorders. Bleeding disorders occur in males who are hemizygous for the abnormal X chromosome, usually transmitted by a heterozygous, asymptomatic mother.

In hemophilia A, factor VIII is deficient, whereas factor IX is deficient in hemophilia B. Each disorder results from a different defect in the X chromosome. In most female carriers, the concentration of factor VIII or IX is about 40 to 60% of normal. Genetic probability indicates that a female carrier of hemophilia mated to a normal male transmits the defective X chromosome to half of her male offspring, who are hemophiliacs, and to half of her daughters, who are carriers. It is important to diagnose carriers, because they should be removed from breeding programs. If hemophilic males are bred to carrier females, hemophilic females (homozygous) can also be produced. In rare situations, both hemophilias A and B can be coinherited. A listing of various dog breeds in which inherited coagulopathies have been described has been prepared (Meyer et al., 1992).

HEMOPHILIA A

Hemophilia A is the classic form of hemophilia. As discussed above, hemophilia A has a sex-linked recessive mode of inheritance carried by females and manifested in males. Hemophilia A is one of the most common inherited bleeding disorders in humans as well as in animals, and appears in many dog and cat breeds and in horses. Being an X-chromosome linked recessive trait, hemophilia A is confined almost exclusively to males, but may rarely develop in a female (Murtaugh and Dodd, 1988). The synthesis or secretion of factor VIII is decreased in most patients with hemophilia A, and a defective form of factor VIII molecule is probably synthesized in others. Patients with hemophilia A have normal plasma and endothelial concentrations of vWF and may have normal or even slightly elevated vWF:Ag levels (Table 5–7).

The severity of the disease correlates directly with the concentration of factor VIII in the plasma. Bleeding can be severe if factor VIII activity is less than 5% of normal, or mild, with activity from 5 to 20% of normal. Spontaneous bleeding characteristically occurs in areas subject to mechanical stress, such as joints and

Table 5–7. Comparison of Hemophilia A and von Willebrand Disease

Parameter	Hemophilia A	von Willebrand Disease
Factor VIII:C	Decreased	Normal, decreased
vWF antigen	Normal, increased	Decreased, normal
vWF activity	Normal, increased	Decreased, absent
APTT	Prolonged	Normal, prolonged
Bleeding time	Normal	Prolonged
Platelet function	Normal	Abnormal

muscles. Hemarthroses, subcutaneous and intramuscular hematomas, and ecchymoses are frequent, and gastrointestinal and genitourinary bleeding may be present. Hematomas can cause neurologic or other tissue damage as a result of compression and diminished blood flow. Bleeding into any organ can follow trauma or surgery. In those with moderate and mild hemophilia, bleeding is usually a problem only during or after surgery, or in association with trauma.

In both hemophilias A and B the APTT is prolonged, whereas the PT, TT, bleeding time, fibrinogen concentration, and platelet count are normal or near-normal. An abnormal APTT is correctable by mixing the patient's plasma with normal plasma in a 1:1 ratio. Platelet function is normal in hemophilia A. For proper therapy, specific assays of factor VIII, vWF, and factor IX activity must be performed to distinguish hemophilia A from vWD and hemophilia B. Factor VIII activity in humans can increase nonspecifically from exercise, epinephrine response, pregnancy, or central nervous system stimulation. Submaximal treadmill exercise in dogs did not induce increase in plasma concentrations of Factor VIII or vWF (Turrentine et al., 1986a).

Bleeding episodes in patients with hemophilia A are treated by transfusing cryoprecipitate prepared from normal plasma. Cryoprecipitate contains both vWF and factor VIII, as well as fibrinogen and fibronectin. The half-life of cryoprecipitate in hemophilia A dogs is 7.7 to 32.3 hours and the therapeutic effect lasts for about a day or less. Cryoprecipitate infusion must be repeated to maintain normal hemostasis.

Lyophilized (human) factor VIII concentrates contain relatively large quantities of factor VIII:C and small quantities of factor vWF polymers, and are therefore ideal for treating hemophilia A in humans. The half-life of transfused factor VIII is 8 to 12 hours. Consequently, transfusions may have to be repeated two or three times daily. Because factor VIII is somehow closely bound to fibrinogen, the clotting defect is not correctable by the use of normal serum but can be corrected by the use of normal plasma.

The hepatic cells of patients with hemophilia A might produce a modest amount of functional factor VIII molecules. In these patients, 1-desamino-8-D-arginine vasopression (DDAVP, desmopressin), an analogue of vasopressin (antidiuretic hormone), has been used instead of cryoprecipitate or lyophilized factor VIII concentrate. DDAVP causes the endothelial release of stored factor VIII molecules. DDAVP produces a rise in factor VIII concentration in dogs in the same way as it does in humans, but the dose required is about twice that for humans, and repeated injections do not maintain the increase (Johnstone and Crane, 1986).

Some human patients with severe hemophilia A (approximately 20%) develop antibodies to factor VIII. A similar situation may occur in dogs. Treatment of these patients has been generally unsatisfactory because the antibodies rapidly inactivate the transfused factor VIII protein.

VON WILLEBRAND DISEASE

The deficiency of plasma vWF results in von Willebrand disease (vWD). This disease occurs in a number of dog breeds and in Poland-China swine (Table 5-6). It occurs in both sexes and is inherited as an autosomal incompletely dominant or autosomal recessive trait, as mentioned previously. Several variants (types I, II, and III) have been described in humans, dogs, and pigs. Type I vWD, the most common form in humans and dogs, is characterized by readily detectable but usually subnormal amounts of multimeric vWF in plasma. Type II vWF patients lack the larger vWF multimers, whereas plasma of type III vWD patients contain only traces or no vWF. A 3-day-old quarter horse filly was found to have a type II vWD (Brooks et al., 1991). Acquired forms of vWF deficiency have been observed in dogs in association with hypothyroidism (Avgeris et al., 1990). A case of vWD has been described in a Himalayan cat (French et al., 1987).

The vWF is produced by endothelial cells and megakaryocytes. Endothelial cells synthesize and store pre-vWF in secretory vesicles and cytoplasmic organelles known as Weible-Palade bodies. Injured endothelial cells release functionally active vWF (MW, 220,000 to 225,000) so that it become available in the subendothelium. Plasma contains dimers and multimers of vWF, ranging in molecular weight from 500,000 to at least 20 million daltons. In platelets, vWF is present in α granules and is released during platelet activation. Canine platelets contain much less vWF than do human, porcine, and feline platelets (Parker et al., 1991; Waters et al., 1989). Thrombin, histamine, and fibrin can cause the release of vWF from endothelial cells and induce the surface expression of platelet vWF. The plasma concentration of vWF increases in humans and dogs by stress, epinephrine, and vasopressin or its analogues. Its concentration also increases in pregnant women, mares, and bitches (Gentry et al., 1991).

The vWD clinically ranges from mild to severe in the same family or litter, and can be confused with hemophilia A. Although vWD is usually less severe than hemophilia A, the clinical signs are the same: bloody diarrhea, bleeding at estrus or postpartum, small surface hematomas as from vaccination procedures, excessive bleeding from trauma or nail clipping,

ear cropping, or tail docking, or other surgical procedures, and epistaxis and lameness. Although hemophilic newborns may die, most affected animals survive. Consequently, it is important to identify and remove carrier animals to halt the spread of the disease.

An epidemiologic study of vWD in three breeds of dogs, viz., Doberman pinschers, Scottish terriers, and Shetland sheepdogs, revealed significant differences between breeds with respect to age and plasma vWF:Ag concentrations of affected dogs (Brooks et al., 1992). The affected dobermans were older (mean age for respective breeds—4.6, 1.7, and 1.9 years) and had higher concentrations of plasma vWF:Ag (mean vWF:Ag concentrations for respective breeds—15%, 0%, and 8%). The prevalence of vWD in these dog breeds was higher in dobermans (73%) than in the other two dog breeds (28–30%).

In vWD, prolonged bleeding times are frequent, as opposed to hemophilia A (Table 5-7). Reduced platelet adhesiveness or retention in glass bead columns and abnormal platelet aggregation are seen. These properties of platelets are a function of platelet vWF surface receptors—GP (glycoprotein) Ib in normal platelets and also GPIIb-IIIa in activated platelets. Usually, the APTT is slightly to moderately prolonged and the PT and TT are normal. The definitive tests are the determinations of vWF and platelet function. In classic vWD, factor VIII:C is decreased or normal, whereas vWF activity is decreased to absent and vWF:Ag may be normal to decreased (Table 5-7). In comparison, vWF activity or vWF:Ag is not diminished in hemophilia A. Platelet vWF may decrease in some cases of vWD.

Cryoprecipitate fractions of normal plasma are transfused to arrest bleeding in a patient with vWD or to prepare a patient for surgery. In addition, because of the association of vWD with hypothyroidism in the Doberman pinschers and other breeds of dogs, thyroid extracts have been used to increase vWF antigen temporarily in canine patients prior to surgery (Avgeris et al., 1990). Lyophilized factor VIII concentrates contain relatively small quantities of factor vWF and are not effective in treating vWD in humans. Desmopressin causes a twofold or greater increase in plasma vWF levels in humans, but only an insignificant increase occurs in normal dogs and in Doberman Pinschers with mild to moderate type I vWD (Giger and Dodds, 1989).

HEMOPHILIA B

Hemophilia B (Christmas disease) is an X-linked recessive disorder characterized by decreased or defective synthesis or secretion of factor IX. Hemophilias A and B are indistinguishable clinically, and the diagnostic and screening tests used for hemophilia B are the same as those for hemophilia A. They are distinguished by performing specific coagulation factor assays on the patient's plasma. Hemophilia B has been reported in several breeds of dogs (Table 5-6) and the clinical signs are more severe in larger breeds.

The deficiency of factor IX is usually severe (frequently, about 1% of normal factor activity). Carrier females can be identified by having 40 to 60% of the normal concentration of factor IX. Bleeding episodes are treated with fresh plasma transfusions. Factor IX is stable in blood or plasma stored at 4°C. Transfused factor IX has a half-life of approximately 24 hours.

A family of Siamese-cross cats with combined factor IX and XII deficiencies has been identified, with factor levels of less than 5 and 20%, respectively (Boudreaux and Dillon, 1988). Clinical findings in affected male kittens included periodic lameness, gingival bleeding, conjunctival hemorrhage, and easy formation of subcutaneous hematomas. The dam and a female sibling did not exhibit abnormal bleeding, but the latter had reduced factor XII activity, which resulted in a prolonged APTT. Danazol, 5 mg/kg given orally once daily for 7 to 9 days, did not increase factor IX activity in the two male cats.

FACTOR VII DEFICIENCY

This rare autosomal recessive or incompletely dominant disease has been reported in dogs (Table 5–6). In dogs, it is a benign condition that usually does not manifest as a bleeding diathesis, as it does in people with factor VII deficiency. The affected animals also have a prolonged PT.

FACTORS X, XI, AND XII AND PREKALLIKREIN DEFICIENCIES

These deficiencies are rare (Table 5–6). Specific factors can be determined by immunologic and functional assays, and generally a moderate deficiency can be found. Deficiencies of these factors are associated with no clinical abnormalities of hemostasis or rarely cause minor bleeds.

In factor X deficiency, mild to moderate prolongation of the APTT, PT, Russell's viper venom time (RVVT), and whole blood clotting time have been noted.

Factor XI deficiency (sometimes called hemophilia C) in animals is similar to that in humans, generally manifesting as prolonged bleeding, particularly after surgery; spontaneous bleeding is rare. Whole blood clotting time and APTT are prolonged. Both sexes are affected, and carrier heterozygotes can be detected by suitable laboratory procedures. Cattle affected with factor XI deficiency seldom exhibit hemorrhagic problems.

Hageman factor (factor XII) deficiency in humans is manifested by a prolonged clotting time and a significantly prolonged APTT caused by the defective formation of thrombin by way of the intrinsic pathway. Patients lacking factor XII, HMW kininogen, and prekallikrein are usually asymptomatic, although minor bleeding may occur. Hereditary factor XII deficiency in cats is an autosomal recessive trait. Cats homozygous for Hageman factor have less than 10% of normal factor XII activity (Parker et al., 1988). Oral

mucosa bleeding times of these cats was normal, whereas cats homozygous for Chédiak-Higashi syndrome had a markedly prolonged time and cats heterozygous for Chédiak-Higashi syndrome had a slightly prolonged oral mucosa bleeding time. Factor XII deficiency is rare in the dog (Otto et al., 1991).

Prekallikrein deficiency has been described in a dog, in a family of miniature horses, and in a family of Belgian horses (Chinn et al., 1986; Geor et al., 1990; Turrentine et al., 1986b). The deficiency is characterized by a prolonged APTT in the presence of normal concentrations of all the other coagulation factors viz., factors VIII, IX, XI, and XII. Severe prekallikrein deficiency in the horse may be of clinical relevance during surgical procedures such as castration, although hemorrhagic manifestation is rare.

AFIBRINOGENEMIA AND DYSFIBRINOGENEMIA

Afibrinogenemia is rare in animals, but some cases have been noted in dogs and goats (Table 5–6). It is transmitted in humans as an autosomal recessive trait, often manifesting at birth as bleeding from the umbilical cord. The deficiency of fibrinogen prevents completion of the final step of coagulation, the conversion of fibrinogen to fibrin, and so the PT, APTT, TT, and clotting time are prolonged. Bleeding time may be prolonged in about half of patients.

Dysfibrinogenemia in humans is generally an autosomal dominant trait characterized by fibrinogen that is defective in its breakdown, polymerization, and stabilization. Heat precipitation and immunologic methods for quantitation of fibrinogen yield normal values, but the TT is prolonged and the PT may be variably prolonged. Patients are usually asymptomatic.

Acquired Coagulopathies

Acquired coagulation disorders are more common than inherited disorders. Unlike inherited disorders, acquired disorders are usually associated with multiple coagulation abnormalities, less severe bleeding that correlates poorly with laboratory test results, and less effective factor replacement therapy. The diagnosis of these disorders is often indicated by associated clinical features and by the results of screening tests such as the PT, APTT, and TT.

Some conditions associated with acquired coagulopathies are described briefly here. DIC and thrombosis, which are of major importance, are discussed separately. Qualitative and quantitative disorders of platelets, leading to abnormalities of hemostasis, are outlined in Table 5–1 and discussed in Chapter 6.

VITAMIN K DEFICIENCY AND ANTAGONISM

Vitamin K is essential in the formation of several vitamin K-dependent coagulation proteins—factors II, VII, IX, and X (Table 5–3). The role of the liver in the synthesis of these coagulation factors has been discussed earlier in this chapter.

A nutritional deficiency of vitamin K is rare in animals. Vitamin K deficiency develops with chronic gastrointestinal problems, such as malabsorption, and those brought about by long-term broad-spectrum antibiotic and sulfanilamide therapy. A lack of bile salts in the gut prevents absorption of the fat-soluble vitamin, obstructive jaundice thus leads to a deficiency and, finally, liver disease can result in a lack of utilization of the vitamin. Because of immaturity of the liver, human neonates exhibit a modest deficiency of vitamin K-dependent coagulation factors (20 to 50% of normal). Similar observations have been reported for sheep, cattle, and a foal.

Vitamin K antagonism is encountered in animals on ingestion of rodenticides, such as warfarin, indane-diones (diphacinone and pindone), bromadialone, and brodifacoum. The biochemical lesion of major importance is the inhibition of the enzyme epoxide reductase. Reductase activity is essential for the recycling of vitamin K (conversion of oxidized to reduced form) that is necessary for the activation of precursor forms of coagulation factors produced by the liver. The degree of enzyme inhibition contributes to species and rodenticide toxicity differences. The coccidiostat sulfaquinoxaline also produces coagulopathies caused by vitamin K antagonism. Dicumarol, a fungal metabolite in sweet clover hay, causes sweet clover poisoning (hypofibrinogenemia) in cattle feeding on such hay. The disease can be effectively treated by vitamin K_1 administration (Alstad et al., 1985).

The diagnosis of vitamin K deficiency is based on the history, clinical examination, laboratory evaluation of clotting abnormalities, and clinical and laboratory responses to vitamin K_1 therapy. Clinical signs of warfarin intoxication include anemia, weakness, pallor, hypovolemia, dyspnea, hematemesis, epistaxis, hematuria, melena (bloody stool), external hematomas, hemarthroses, and neurologic signs. Death may occur from acute intoxication. Detection of a factor VII deficiency confirms the diagnosis, as do prolonged PT, APTT, and activated clotting time (ACT) tests. Assays for coagulation factors II, VII, IX, and X reveal subnormal values. The PIVKA test, which detects *proteins induced by vitamin K absence* or antagonism, is considered the earliest indicator of vitamin K deficiency. Bleeding time and platelet counts are normal.

Vitamin K deficiency is treated with vitamin K_1 (phylloquinone series), K_2 (menaquinone derivatives) or the synthetic K_3 (menadione). Oral therapy is ineffective when an absorption problem exists. Menadione is converted to the vitamin K_2 series in vivo, but is poorly stored in the liver in comparison to K_1, so higher amounts are required to achieve the same physiologic effect. Adding menadione supplements to swine and poultry rations is a common practice to alleviate some forms of mycotoxin-induced bleeding syndrome.

Treatment in cases of vitamin K antagonism involves the administration of vitamin K preparations and fresh plasma transfusions. The mode of vitamin K therapy varies with the toxic compound incriminated. Poisoning with warfarin-related compounds may be successfully treated in dogs with vitamin K_1 given orally over a period of 4 to 6 days. In diphacinone poisoning, which causes vitamin K antagonism for a much longer period (about 3 to 4 weeks), a comparatively higher dose and longer therapy are indicated (Mount, 1988). Intravenous injection is not recommended because of the potential danger of an anaphylactic reaction. The half-life of vitamin K_1 is about 5 hours. At least a week is needed for most of the antagonist to be catabolized and removed from the body.

LIVER DISEASE

The liver is the site of synthesis of coagulation proteins of significance in hemostasis (Table 5–3), factors involved in fibrinolysis (plasminogen and plasminogen activator), and certain inhibitors of coagulation—antithrombin III, α_2-macroglobulin, and α_1-antitrypsin. Because the half-life of factor VII is the shortest (only 5 hours), determining factor VII activity seems to be the most useful measurement in both acute and chronic liver disease. The PT test also has a high prognostic value in acute liver disease.

In acute and chronic liver disease in humans, factor VII activity shows the greatest reduction, factor IX shows the least change, changes in factors II and X are intermediate, and factor VIII is often elevated. Factor VIII is, however, qualitatively abnormal. Factor deficiencies often correlate with hypoalbuminemia associated with liver disease in humans and dogs.

Bleeding in liver disease is usually mild to moderate, but severe bleeding may occur in patients with cirrhosis, fulminating hepatitis, and the terminal phase of chronic liver disease. Severe canine infectious hepatitis with bleeding problems has been reported. The routine screening tests of coagulation (e.g., PT, APTT) are unreliable guides of the risk of bleeding after liver biopsy.

A number of factors may contribute to the hemostatic defect in liver disease (Table 5–8). In addition, increased fibrinolytic activity may occur when patients with chronic liver disease are exposed to surgery or trauma. This is because of the impaired synthesis of antiplasmin by the diseased liver and of the inadequate clearance of plasminogen activator, which is released into the circulation following surgery or trauma.

Therapy of coagulopathies in liver disease varies with the cause and severity of the disease. It includes the administration of vitamin K, antifibrinolytic agents, and anticoagulants and the replacement of coagulation factors.

DYSPROTEINEMIAS

In multiple myeloma and other paraproteinemias (see Chap. 21), abnormal proteins may be adsorbed to fibrinogen and interfere with the fibrinogen-to-fibrin conversion and with fibrin polymerization. Vascular wall damage, thrombocytopenia, abnormal platelet

Table 5-8. Causes of Hemorrhagic Diathesis in Liver Disease

Deficiency in biosynthesis
  Various coagulation proteins (see Table 5-3)
  Prekallikrein
  HMW kininogen
  Plasminogen
  Antithrombin III
  Antiplasmins
Aberrant biosynthesis
  Fibrinogen
  Factor VIII
  Inhibitors of coagulation
Inadequate Clearance
  Activated clotting factors
  Plasminogen activators
  Hemostatic "debris," (e.g., fibrin monomers, fibrin degradation products—FDPs)
Accelerated destruction of coagulation factors
  Disseminated intravascular coagulation (DIC)
  Primary fibrin(ogen)olysis
Thrombocytopenia
  Splenic sequestration
  Other causes
Others
  Abnormal platelet function
  Poorly defined causes

function, hypercoagulability, and abnormal fibrinolysis may also be present. Bleeding time and the APTT may be prolonged.

PRIMARY PATHOLOGIC FIBRINOLYSIS

Primary pathologic fibrinolysis is a hemorrhagic state that can result from a marked increase in plasma fibrinolytic (plasmin) activity. It is an uncommon cause of bleeding, however, and may occur when large amounts of tissue plasminogen activators are released into the circulation as a result of extensive trauma, such as that associated with a major surgery or destruction of tumor tissue. Thus, bleeding caused by primary pathologic fibrin(ogen)olysis may occur in some of the same disorders that also produce DIC. The clinical picture in most of these cases is similar to that of DIC, but laboratory findings may differ remarkably (Table 5-5).

PATHOLOGIC INHIBITORS OF COAGULATION

Many abnormal anticoagulants that prevent normal coagulation have been found in the blood of human patients with acquired coagulopathies. These include antibodies to various coagulation proteins, such as those against factors V, VIII, IX, XI, and XIII, and "lupus inhibitors." Lupus inhibitors, originally found in patients with systemic lupus erythematosus, may be detected in various unrelated disorders, such as multiple myeloma, myelofibrosis, and rheumatoid arthritis, and following therapy with certain drugs (e.g., chlorpromazine and penicillin). They appear to be IgG and IgM antibodies, and probably act by interfering with the action of prothrombinase by complexing with the lipid moiety of the enzyme complex. Clinical

bleeding is rare. The APTT is prolonged and is not corrected by mixing equal volumes of normal plasma with the patient's plasma. Also, the PT and TT are often prolonged. Corticosteroids and other immunosuppressive drugs are effective, but therapy is seldom indicated.

Primary afibrinogenemia was found in a female Bichon Frise dog that had received multiple transfusions because of life-threatening hemorrhagic complications of ovariohysterectomy. The cause of the afibrinogenemia was the formation of alloantibodies to fibrinogen in the transfused blood (Wilkerson et al., 1989).

DISSEMINATED INTRAVASCULAR COAGULATION

DIC, or consumption coagulopathy, is a disorder in which diffuse intravascular thrombosis occurs in the microvasculature. It manifests as a hemostatic defect caused by the reduction of clotting factors and platelets resulting from their utilization in the thrombotic process. The anticoagulant properties of FDPs generated from the activation of the fibrinolytic system also contribute to the hemostatic defect.

Associated Conditions

DIC is rarely, if ever, a primary event. Most cases can be traced to platelet activation and/or the release of thromboplastins into the circulation from tissue damage in various conditions (Tables 5-9 and 5-10). DIC can be acute, subacute, or chronic, and can be localized or generalized. Its severity is related to the rate of release of thromboplastin, the duration of exposure to the causative agent, the ability of the liver to replace consumed coagulation factors, and the ability of the bone marrow to restore platelets.

Intravascular coagulation may be activated by relatively trivial stimuli, such as mild trauma. Fibrin is not being laid down continuously because of a composite action of several inherent protective mechanisms,

Table 5-9. Conditions Associated with Disseminated Intravascular Coagulation in Animals

Malignancies: metastasizing carcinomas, hemangiosarcomas, leukemias
Severe hemolysis
Infections: bacterial, viral, protozoal, mycotic, metazoal (heartworm)
Endotoxins
Massive trauma
Heat stroke
Liver disease
Pancreatitis
Obstetric complications
Incompatible blood transfusion
Snakebite
Purpura hemorrhagica
Acidosis

Table 5–10. Distribution of 41 Cases of DIC in Dogs by Major Disease Categories

Category	No.	%
Malignancy	16	39
Pancreatitis	12	30
Sepsis, hemolysis	1	2
Sepsis, shock	1	2
Chronic active hepatitis	6	15
Heat stroke	5	12
Total	41	100

From Feldman, B.F., Madewell, B.R., O'Neill, S., et al.: Disseminated intravascular coagulation: Antithrombin, plasminogen, and coagulation abnormalities in 41 dogs. J. Am. Vet. Med. Assoc. 179:151, 1981.

which include antagonism by circulating inhibitors of activated clotting factors, localized activation of the fibrinolytic system, and the rapid clearance of activated clotting factors by the MPS. Similarly, platelet aggregation is normally prevented by the action of plasma ADPase. Consequently, under normal circumstances, significant microthrombosis does not occur.

Tissue necrosis and inflammation are common inciting causes of DIC through the release of procoagulant or of thromboplastin-like substances and the

initiation of the coagulation sequence. Exposure of subendothelial collagen as a result of inflammation causes platelet activation, release of platelet factors, and subsequent initiation of coagulation. Red blood cells lysed at inflammatory sites release ADP, thus causing platelet activation. Intravascular hemolysis is a potential cause of DIC through contact activation of coagulation factors and platelets by red cell membranes. In sepsis, contact activation of coagulation may occur because of the presence of bacterial lipopolysaccharides. During viremia, antigen-antibody complexes may cause ADP release from platelets, contact activation of coagulation factors, or endothelial damage followed by a collagen-induced initiation of coagulation. Stagnant blood flow, acidosis, and hypoxia favor endothelial damage and DIC.

Pathophysiology

Tissue necrosis, inflammation, red cell or platelet damage, or endothelial damage induced by antigen-antibody or endotoxin initiates the coagulation process (see above) through thrombin generation (Fig. 5–6). Thrombin cleaves fibrinogen to fibrin monomers, which polymerize to form a firm clot. Simultaneously, the fibrinolytic and kinin systems are also activated.

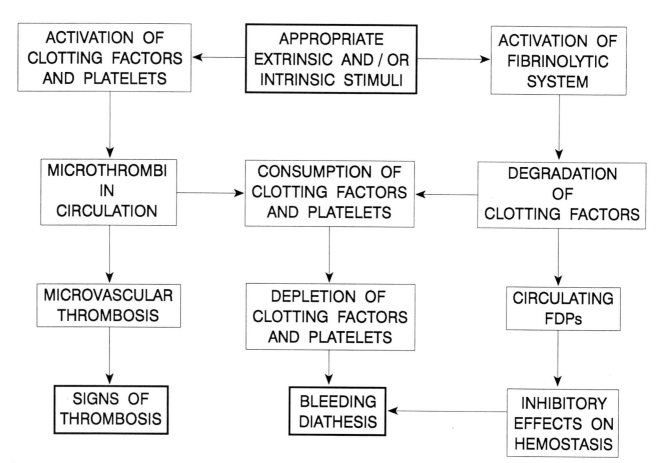

Fig. 5–6. Events associated with disseminated intravascular coagulation. (FDPs, fibrin(ogen) degradation products).

Plasmin, the active protease in fibrinolysis, degrades fibrinogen and fibrin, producing FDPs that have an affinity for soluble fibrin monomers preventing fibrin polymerization. Plasmin can also degrade coagulation factors. Thus, the bleeding tendency in DIC patients is a consequence of the depletion of coagulation factors and platelets and of the anticoagulant properties of FDPs. FDPs are cleared by the MPS, so MPS blockade augments DIC.

The resultant balance of coagulation and fibrinolysis is therefore affected by the two proteases, thrombin and plasmin. If thrombin is dominant, thrombosis occurs, whereas if plasmin is dominant, bleeding occurs. The production of kinins, mediators of vascular permeability and pain, is associated with vasodilation and vascular stasis and a vicious cycle ensues, with coagulation initiation, localized stasis, and organ ischemia.

Diagnosis

Clinically, DIC can be characterized by the widespread formation of fibrin thrombi, multiple coagulation defects, bleeding tendency, and impaired organ function. The syndrome has been reported principally in dogs, although it has also been described in other species. Presenting signs include shock of varying severity, generalized or localized bleeding, petechiae and ecchymoses of the skin and mucous membranes, evidence of intravascular hemolysis, and adrenocortical, pulmonary, renal, hepatic, pancreatic, and/or CNS involvement, with their accompanying signs and clinical effects.

The laboratory diagnosis of DIC (Tables 5–11 and 5–12) is usually based on the triad of prolonged PT, thrombocytopenia, and hypofibrinogenemia. The finding of FDPs, schistocytes (fragmented erythrocytes) in blood smears, and decreased concentrations of coagulation factors (usually factors V and VIII) and

antithrombin III add additional weight to the diagnosis. Also, the APTT and TT are prolonged. No single laboratory test is, however, pathognomic for the disease.

In chronic DIC, it is sometimes found that not all procoagulants are depleted, because the liver and bone marrow have varying capabilities for increasing the production of coagulation factors and platelets, respectively.

Therapy

The therapy of acute DIC should be approached in a logical and sequential fashion. The most important measure involves removal of the inciting cause. When this is not possible, specific treatment may be indicated. Specific therapeutic measures for DIC can be separated into several categories, including fluid therapy, administration of drugs to stop coagulation, and the replacement of depleted blood constituents.

FLUID THERAPY

Specific goals of fluid therapy are correction of hypovolemia, prevention or alleviation of vascular stasis, and dilution of thrombin, FDPs, and activators of fibrinolysis. The type of fluid administered is not critical and should be chosen on the basis of the primary disease and the acid-base, electrolyte, and hydration status of the patient.

INHIBITORS OF COAGULATION

Drugs for inhibiting coagulation are indicated if the patient manifests direct evidence of bleeding, thrombosis, or organ dysfunction. Heparin is the most common choice. Heparin potentiates the action of plasma antithrombin III; its primary action is the inactivation of thrombin and coagulation factors XIIa, XIa, Xa, and IXa. The most serious potential side effect of

Table 5–11. Coagulation Abnormalities in 41 Dogs with DIC

Parameter	Normal Range	Mean ± 1 SD in All Cases	Percentage Abnormal	Mean ± 1 SD in Abnormal Cases
Antithrombin III activity (%)	89–108	71 ± 14	85	62 ± 12
Prothrombin time (sec)	6.4–7.4	11.0 ± 5.4	80	12.3 ± 55
Activated partial thromboplastin time (sec)	9.5–10.5	16.7 ± 6.7	87	18.3 ± 61
Thrombin time (sec)	5.0–10.0	11.0 ± 6.6	55	16.4 ± 68
Platelet count (× 10^3/μl)	200–500	147 ± 98	80	111 ± 45
FDPs (μg/ml)	<10	—	61	>10–40
Protamine sulfate test (fibrin monomer*)	0	+	55	+ + +
Fibrinogen (g/dl)	0.20–0.40	0.24 ± 0.19	61	0.11 ± 0.05
Burr cells and red cell fragments†	Rare	+	71	+ +
Factor V activity (%)	80–120	81 ± 27	46	58 ± 18
Factor VIII:C activity (%)	75–125	88 ± 26	29	66 ± 13
Plasminogen activity (%)	88–120	82 ± 23	49	63 ± 17

Modified from Feldman, B.F., Madewell, B.R., O'Neill, S., et al.: Disseminated intravascular coagulation: Antithrombin, plasminogen, and coagulation abnormalities in 41 dogs. J. Am. Vet. Med. Assoc. 179:151, 1981.

* Presence of gel or fibrin strand was considered abnormal; graded trace to 4 +.

† Burr cells and fragmented red cells graded + = 5–10%; + + = 10–15%; + + + = >15%; greater than 5% was considered abnormal.

Table 5–12. Laboratory Findings in Disseminated Intravascular Coagulation

Parameter	Finding*	Parameter	Finding*
Platelets	↓	Antithrombin III	↓
Schistocytes	+	Plasmin	↑
Fibrinogen	↓	Plasminogen	↓
FDPs	↑	Complement	↓
APTT	↑	Fibrin monomers	↑
PT	↑	Fibronectin	↓
TT	↑	Factors V and VIII	↓
Clotting time	↑	Protamine sulfate test	+
Clot lysis time	↓	BUN	↑

* + = present; ↑ = increased; ↓ = decreased.

overzealous heparin therapy is bleeding from too much anticoagulation, which in some cases is aided by thrombocytopenia. The mechanism of heparin-induced thrombocytopenia is poorly understood, but it may partly involve an immune-mediated reaction. Heparinization in dogs and cats can be monitored using the ACT test. Heparin requirements may vary widely among individuals. When the plasma antithrombin III concentration is reduced from extensive DIC, even high-dose heparin therapy may be ineffective. In such patients, heparin therapy must be preceded or accompanied by fresh plasma administration to replenish the antithrombin III necessary for heparin action. Antithrombin III concentrates or fresh plasma incubated with heparin may also be given.

Inhibitors of platelet function such as aspirin may be used in DIC, but are contraindicated in severely thrombocytopenic patients.

BLOOD COMPONENT THERAPY

When patients with DIC bleed, replacement of some or all blood constituents is indicated to replenish depleted coagulation factors and platelets. Plasma infusion is preferred, but whole blood may be given if red cell infusion is necessary. The infusion of red cells, however, carries the risk of hemolysis and exacerbation of DIC.

The plasma fibronectin concentration and the MPS clearance of activated coagulation factors may be reduced in DIC. Fibronectin is a high-molecular-weight glycoprotein present on cell surfaces and in plasma. It is synthesized by hepatocytes and many other cells, including fibroblasts and endothelial cells. Fibronectin acts as an acute phase protein. Its synthesis increases after the administration of corticosteroids and at parturition (in mares). Fibronectin plays important roles in phagocytosis, embryonic differentiation, wound healing, cell-cell adhesion, oncogenic cell transformation, and attachment of fibrinogen or collagen to macrophages (Feldman et al., 1988; Gentry et al., 1991). It mediates the MPS clearance of bacteria and fibrin microaggregates. Fibronectin concentration is decreased in about 75% of dogs with metastatic neoplasias (Feldman et al., 1988). Fibronectin concentrations decrease after surgery, trauma, hemorrhage, and

DIC, and parallel the decrease in phagocytic activity of the MPS (Feldman et al., 1985). The administration of fibronectin in the form of cryoprecipitate of plasma restores MPS function and limits DIC.

MONITORS OF EFFECTIVE THERAPY

Various laboratory tests can be used to monitor anticoagulant therapy in DIC, including ACT, PT, APTT, and TT assays, quantitation of fibrinogen, assays for factors V and VIII, antithrombin III, and FDPs, and platelet count. Normalization of the screening coagulogram (PT, APTT, and FDPs) usually denotes successful therapy. The return of the normal fibrinogen concentration is a reliable long-term indicator of heparin therapy, but it may require 24 to 48 hours to normalize. Platelet counts may not normalize for 7 to 14 days after cessation of bleeding.

THROMBOSIS

A thrombus is an intravascular deposit composed of fibrin and formed elements of the blood. Thrombosis is the process of formation of this mass that partially or completely impedes the blood flow. Thrombi may form in the arteries, veins, heart, and microcirculation. A thromboembolism results when a thrombus formed locally or that dislodged from an upstream location occludes the vessel and shuts off the regional blood supply. DIC is a form of thrombosis in the microcirculation. Thromboembolic complications have been reported in both humans and dogs in nephrotic syndrome and hypercorticism. An increased thrombotic tendency is also noted in patients receiving long-term glucocorticoid therapy. A thromboembolism is of major importance in the pathogenesis of heart attack and stroke in humans. Calves with zinc toxicosis were found to develop a state of hypercoagulability in that their PT and APTT were significantly elevated compared to those of control calves, and lesions of thrombosis were common in affected calves (Graham et al., 1991).

Pathogenesis

The composition of arterial and venous thrombi differs because of differences in hemodynamics. Thrombi that form in a high-flow system (arteries) are mainly composed of platelet aggregates held together by a small amount of fibrin; these are known as platelet or white thrombi. Red cells and leukocytes form a small component of these thrombi. Thrombi that form in areas of slow to moderate blood flow are composed of a mixture of red cells, platelets, and fibrin; these are known as mixed platelet thrombi. Thrombi that form in areas of complete blood stasis are composed of red cells with a large amount of interspersed fibrin; these are known as coagulation or red thrombi. Platelets and leukocytes are randomly distributed in these

Table 5-13. Factors Implicated in the Pathogenesis of Thrombosis

Abnormalities of vessel wall
  Vascular injury—mechanical, chemical, immunologic, or infectious agents
  Diminished vascular tone
Abnormalities of blood flow
  Diminished or stagnant blood flow
  Turbulent or misdirected blood flow
  Hyperviscosity
Hypercoagulability of blood
  Elevated levels of coagulation proteins—increased synthesis or reduced catabolism
  In vivo activation of coagulation cascade—entrance of tissue thrombplastins in blood
  Platelet abnormalities—decreased survival; increased adhesion, aggregation and release reaction; marked thrombocytosis; thrombocythemia
  Abnormalities of inhibitory mechanisms—deficiency of antithrombin III and protein "C," reduced levels of α_2-antiplasmin, defective clearance of activated coagulation factors by the liver or MPS
Abnormalities of fibrinolysis
  Excessive α_1-antitrypsin inhibition of plasmin
  Deficiency of plasminogen activators
  Abnormal plasminogen

thrombi. Various thrombi may exhibit a lamellar arrangement of blood cells as they continue to grow gradually, and may become organized as a fibrous plaque.

Thrombosis results from an imbalance among stimuli that initiate clot formation and protective mechanisms that inhibit coagulation or control hemostasis. Basically, thrombus formation involves the same sequence of events that leads to the formation of a hemostatic plug, which is necessary to prevent the escape of blood from an injured vessel wall (Figs. 5–1 and 5–2). The only difference is that a thrombus results when these processes continue unabated by mechanisms that ordinarily cause dissolution of the hemostatic plug after it has served its purpose.

Factors promoting thrombosis include various circumstances that favor localized platelet adhesion and aggregation and the activation of the coagulation cascade (Table 5–13). Most probable thrombotic episodes recognized in animals are associated with infectious agents that cause inflammation and damage the vascular endothelium.

During inflammation, abnormalities of the endothelial mechanisms that normally regulate coagulation may promote in vivo clotting activity and predispose an animal to thrombotic complications. Three of these abnormalities are the following: (1) decreased thrombomodulin expression on the surface of endothelial cells, which reduces protein C activation necessary for controlling thrombin action; (2) increased release of tissue thromboplastin by the endothelial cells, which promotes coagulation by activating the extrinsic system; and (3) increased synthesis of C4b-binding protein by the endothelial cells that complexes protein S, thereby decreasing the availability of free protein S, which serves as a cofactor for protein C activation.

Diagnosis

The diagnosis of thrombosis is based on such procedures as angiography, impedance plethysmography, ^{125}I-fibrinogen scanning, and ultrasound. Generally, the diagnosis is difficult and, in veterinary medicine, thrombosis may often go unrecognized until it becomes a clinical emergency.

Laboratory findings associated with increased risk or the presence of thrombosis or thromboembolism include decreased antithrombin III concentration, deficient fibrinolysis, reduced platelet survival, increased platelet procoagulant activity (e.g., PF-4 and β-thromboglobulin), increased activity of clotting factors, and elevated levels of complexes of fibrin monomers, fibrinopeptide A, and FDPs.

A thrombus must be distinguished from a postmortem clot. A thrombus is an antemortem clot that is generally partly or completely attached to the vascular endothelium. It is irregular in shape, varies in color, and has a dull appearance and roughened surface. It is friable and usually appears lamellar on a cut surface. A postmortem clot, on the other hand, is entirely unattached to the vascular endothelium, dark red in color, molded to the vascular bed, and smooth and uniform in texture.

Therapy

Because of the important roles played by the coagulation system and the platelets in the pathogenesis of thrombosis, therapeutic measures for controlling thrombosis or thromboembolism must be directed toward inhibiting the abnormal activities of these blood constituents (Table 5–14). Anticoagulants, such as heparin, coumarin, and indanediones, and antiplatelet agents, such as aspirin, sulfinpyrazone, and dipyridamole, are commonly used to dampen the "hypercoagulable state" and to prevent the formation of new thrombi. In addition, fibrinolytic agents, such as streptokinase, human recombinant tissue plasminogen activator, and urokinase, have been used to dissolve preformed thrombi, particularly during early stages of the disease. Regardless of the therapeutic approach, if the patient is not selected and monitored carefully, serious bleeding complications can develop.

Antiplatelet drugs are used mainly to prevent thrombosis at the arterial side of the circulation, where clots are thought to originate as intravascular platelet aggregates (see above). These agents are less useful in combatting thrombosis on the venous side, because venous thrombosis appears to result mainly from inappropriate activation of the coagulation cascade. Thus, it should be obvious why heparin is beneficial in preventing venous thrombosis and is less effective in preventing arterial thrombosis. Prophylactic or long-term therapeutic management of the thrombotic patient, however, often involves the use of both anticoagulants and antiplatelet agents of choice.

Table 5-14. Mechanisms of Action of Selected Antithrombotic and Thrombolytic Agents

Agent	Effect	Mechanism of Action
Heparin	Inhibition of serine proteases involved in clot formation	Potentiates the anticoagulant effects of antithrombin III by complexing with it
Coumarin-type drugs	Decreased supply of vitamin K-dependent functional clotting factors II, VII, IX, and X	Inhibition of the enzyme system necessary to recycle vitamin K for γ carboxylation of the vitamin K-dependent clotting factors
Aspirin	Decreased thromboxane production—hence, inhibition of platelet aggregation and release reaction	Inactivation of platelet cyclo-oxygenase (irreversible)
Sulfinpyrazone	Decreased thromboxane production—hence, inhibition of platelet aggregation and release reaction	Inactivation of platelet cyclo-oxygenase (reversible)
Dipyridamole	Increased cAMP production—hence, inhibition of platelet aggregation and release reaction	Inactivation of platelet phosphodiesterase, inhibition of intracellular Ca^{2+}
Streptokinase	Conversion of plasminogen to plasmin → thrombolysis	Formation of a nonenzymatic complex with plasminogen or plasmin
Urokinase	Activation of plasminogen to plasmin → thrombolysis	Enzymatic cleavage of plasminogen

DIAGNOSTIC METHODS

A thorough medical history and clinical examination are essential for making a proper diagnosis of a bleeding problem. Screening tests (Table 5–4) for the clotting cascade are carried out in plasma separated from blood that has been anticoagulated with sodium citrate. These tests include the PT, APTT, and TT, which measure primarily components of the extrinsic system, intrinsic system, and fibrinogen in the common pathway, respectively (Fig. 5–3). Many tests are available for determining specific coagulation defects; these are useful in research on hemostasis, but are not routinely useful in clinical medicine. Also, some physiologic processes (e.g., exercise and pregnancy in horses) may introduce alterations in coagulation and fibrinolysis, as reflected by significant changes in test results, but these may not necessarily be associated with signs of bleeding (Feldman et al., 1990; Heuwieser et al., 1990; McKeever et al., 1990). Procedures for various clotting tests can be found in standard hematology texts (Brown, 1988; Jain, 1986; Williams et al., 1990).

Deficiencies of the extrinsic and intrinsic pathways are differentiated by the PT and APTT coagulation tests, respectively. Coagulopathies with a normal APTT but an abnormal PT suggest factor VII deficiency, whereas an abnormal APTT and a normal PT suggest factor VIII, IX, XI, or XII deficiency. To identify factor VIII deficiency, it is necessary to determine the concentrations of vWF and factor VIII:C. If factor VIII:C activity is low and vWF is normal or increased, hemophilia A is indicated. If factor VIII:C activity and vWF concentration are low, vWD is suspected (Table 5–7). A prolonged PT or APTT is usually corrected by mixing the deficient plasma with an equal volume of normal plasma or with a plasma lacking a different clotting factor. Failure of correction of an abnormal screening test using this technique indicates the presence of an inhibitor in the plasma.

Evaluation of Hemostasis

SCREENING TESTS

The bleeding time test, a crude but valuable screening test, is performed by measuring how long it takes for bleeding to stop from a fresh cut of determined size. A prolonged bleeding time usually indicates a platelet disorder (quantitative or qualitative) or probably an intrinsic blood vessel problem. In pure disorders of the clotting cascade, the bleeding time is almost invariably normal.

The clotting time is a measure of the overall functioning of the coagulation cascade. It is influenced by many factors, such as the manner of blood withdrawal, the size and surface of the test tube, and the temperature of incubation. Care must be taken not to traumatize the veins during bleeding, and it is essential that the needle be inserted immediately into the vein to avoid inclusion of tissue thromboplastin in the test sample.

The activated clotting time (ACT) is unique because immediate contact activation of freshly drawn blood occurs from mixing blood with diatomaceous earth in the collection tube, resulting in a shortened clotting time than that obtained with the Lee-White method. Thus, the ACT is a more sensitive method for detecting coagulation disorders of the intrinsic system. Substances interfering with the ACT include salicylates, anticoagulants, certain antibiotics, and barbiturates.

ROUTINE TESTS

The APTT involves incubating platelet-poor plasma with a platelet substitute ("partial" thromboplastin) and a factor XII activator, and then measuring the clotting time after recalcification. Plasma activated by kaolin, celite, or elagic acid gives shorter clotting times and more reliable results than nonactivated plasma. Animal phospholipids (cephalins) and vegetable phospholipids (purified soya phosphatides) available commercially can be used in the test with a manual or semiautomated format using a fibrometer.

The PT test is based on the fact that plasma obtained from blood to which an anticoagulant (that binds Ca^{2+}) has been added, clots in a few seconds when recalcified in the presence of tissue thromboplastin. The time recorded is the time elapsed between the addition of Ca^{2+} and the appearance of a visible clot. An abnormal PT can be found in patients, with DIC, liver disease, or deficiencies of factor VII and fibrinogen. It is a sensitive indicator of coagulation abnormality arising from vitamin K deficiency or antagonism. The PT can be used to monitor anticoagulant therapy and to screen patients with severe liver disease. Whole blood thrombotest clotting time requires a minute amount of blood (10 μl) and can be used as a more sensitive test than the PT to detect deficiency of vitamin K dependent coagulation factors in rats (Godsafe and Singleton, 1992).

The Russell's viper venom time (RVVT) test is performed when it is necessary to differentiate between a deficiency of factor VII and factor X. Russell's viper venom (Stypven) in high dilutions can activate factor X in recalcified normal plasma and in plasma from patients with deficiency of factors VII, VIII, and IX. A prolonged PT and normal RVVT are diagnostic of factor VII deficiency. The RVVT time is prolonged in factor X deficiency and in factor V deficiency.

The thrombin time measures the time required and rate at which fibrin is formed (i.e., conversion of fibrinogen to fibrin monomers to initial clot). Test results are abnormal in patients with quantitative and qualitative abnormalities of fibrinogen and in patients whose plasma contains inhibitors of the fibrinogen-to-fibrin conversion, such as heparin and FDPs. A prolonged TT with a normal quantity of fibrinogen suggests dysfibrinogenemia or the presence of inhibitors.

The PIVKA test (see above) is considered the earliest indicator of vitamin K deficiency (Mount, 1988). Healthy individuals do not have PIVKA in circulation. The reagent for this test contains standardized bovine brain thromboplastin and modified bovine plasma that is deficient in specific vitamin K-dependent coagulation factors II, VII, and X. The reagent is sensitive to both the deficiency of these coagulation proteins and to the presence of abnormal molecules of factors II, VII, and X that are produced as a result of coumarin toxicity. Therefore, an increase in assay time is attributable not only to a decrease in coagulation factors but also to an elevation in PIVKA. Normal PIVKA test values for the dog are 16.2 to 19 seconds (mean, 17.6 ± 0.87 seconds).

DIC AND FIBRINOLYSIS

A determination of inhibitors of blood clotting has diagnostic significance, as in DIC. Antithrombin III can be measured by the thrombin-agar gel diffusion method; it is decreased in DIC (Table 5–12). FDPs are commonly measured by a latex agglutination test; these are increased in DIC and fibrinolysis. Fibrinogen can be quantitated by various techniques, including a refractometer method. A clot lysis or euglobulin lysis time test is used to measure fibrinolysis to evaluate increased fibrinolytic activity, such as that seen during DIC or during treatment with streptokinase. The protamine sulfate test is used to detect fibrin monomers and early, clottable FDPs. The addition of protamine sulfate to citrated plasma causes a visible polymerization of monomer complexes, and the test is usually positive in those with DIC.

FIBRIN STABILIZATION

Factor XIII deficiency can be found by determining clot solubility. The initial clot, held together only by weak, noncovalent forces, is soluble in mild denaturing agents, whereas a clot cross-linked by factor XIIIa is insoluble. The solubility of a clot in a solution of mild denaturant (urea or monochromatic acid) is therefore used to measure factor XIII.

Detection of Platelet Abnormalities

See Chapter 6 for a discussion of the quantitative and qualitative evaluation of platelets.

REFERENCES

Alstad, A.D., Casper, H.H., and Johnson, L.J.: Vitamin K treatment of sweet clover poisoning in calves. J. Am. Vet. Med. Assoc., 187:729, 1985.

Avgeris, S., Lothrop, C.D., and McDonald, T.P.: Plasma von Willebrand factor concentration and thyroid function in dogs. J. Am. Vet. Med. Assoc., 196:921, 1990.

Boudreaux, M.K. and Dillon, A.R.: The effect of danazol treatment on factor IX deficiency in cats. Vet. Clin. Path., 17:84, 1988.

Boudreaux, M.K. and Dillon, A.R.: Platelet function, antithrombin-III activity, and fibrinogen concentration in heartworm-infected and heartworm-negative dogs treated with thiacetarsamide. Am. J. Vet. Res., 52:1986, 1991.

Brooks, M., Dodds, W.J., and Raymond, S.L.: Epidemiologic features of von Willebrand's disease in Doberman Pinschers, Scottish terriers, and Shetland sheepdogs: 260 cases (1984–1988). J. Am. Vet. Med. Assoc., 200:1123, 1992.

Brooks, M., Leith, G.S., Allen, A.K., et al.: Bleeding disorder (von Willebrandt disease) in a quarter horse. J. Am. Vet. Med. Assoc., 198:114, 1991.

Brown, B.A.: Hematology: Principles and Procedures. 5th Ed. Philadelphia, Lea & Febiger, 1988.

Chinn, D.R., Dodds, W.J. and Selcer, B.A.: Prekallikrein deficiency in a dog. J. Am. Vet. Med. Assoc., 188:69, 1986.

Dueland, R.T., Wagner, S.D., Parker, R.B., et al.: von Willebrandt heterotopic osteochondrofibrosis in Doberman Pinschers: Five cases (1980–1987). J. Am. Vet. Med. Assoc., 197:383, 1990.

Duncan, S.G., Meyers, K.M., Reed, S.M., et al.,: Alterations in coagulation and hemograms of horses given endotoxins for 24 hours via hepatic portal perfusions. Am. J. Vet. Res., 46:1287, 1985.

Feldman, B.F., Brummerstedt, E., Larsen, L.S., et al.: Plasma fibronectin concentration associated with various types of canine neoplasia. Am. J. Vet. Res., 49:1017, 1988.

Feldman, B.F., Gentry, P.A., O'Neill, S., et al.: Hemostatic analyte evaluation in the pre- and postparturient mare and in the neonate. Proceedings of the Annual Convention of the American Association of Equine Practitioners, 35:133, 1990.

Feldman, B.F., Thomson, D.B. and O'Neill, S.: Plasma fibronectin concentrations in dogs with disseminated intravascular coagulation. Am. J. Vet. Res., 46:1171, 1985.

French, T.W., Fox, L.E., Randolph, J.F., et al.: A bleeding disorder (von Willebrand's disease) in a Himalayan cat. J. Am. Vet. Med. Assoc., 190:437, 1987.

Gentry, P.A., Feldman, B.F. and Liptrap, R.M.: Hemostasis and parturition revisited: Comparative profiles in mammals. Comp. Haematol. Int., 1:150, 1991.

Geor, R.J., Jacson, M.L., Lewis, K.D., et al.: Prekallikrein deficiency in a family of Belgian horses. J. Am. Vet. Med. Assoc., 197:741, 1990.

Giger, R.J. and Dodds, W.J.: Effect of desmopressin in normal dogs and dogs with von Willebrandt's disease. Vet. Clin. Path., 18:39, 1989.

Godsafe, P.A. and Singleton, B.K.: The use of the whole blood thromboplast time (1/51) as a routine monitor of vitamin K-dependent blood coagulation factor levels in the rat. Comp. Haematol. Int., 2:51, 1992.

Graham, T.W., Feldman, B.F., Farver, T.B., et al.: Zinc toxicosis of Holstein veal calves and its relationship to haematological changes and an associated thrombotic state. Comp. Haematol. Int., 1:121, 1991.

Handagama, P., Rappolee, D.A., Werb, Z., et al.: Platelet alpha-granule fibrinogen, albumin, and immunoglobulin G are not synthesized by rat and mouse megakaryocytes. J. Clin. Invest., 86:1364, 1990.

Henry, M.M. and Moore, J.N.: Clinical relevance of monocyte procoagulant activity in horses with colic. J. Am. Vet. Med. Assoc., 198:843, 1991.

Heuwieser, W., Kauntni, J., Biesel, M., et al.: Coagulation profile of dairy cattle in the periparturient period. J. Vet. Med. (A), 37:8, 1990.

Jain, N.C.: Schalm's Veterinary Hematology. 4th Ed. Philadelphia, Lea & Febiger, 1986, pp. 388–430.

Johnstone, I.B. and Crane, S.: The effects of desmopressin hemostatic parameters in the normal dog. Can. J. Vet. Res., 50:265, 1986.

Johnstone, I.B., Petersen, D., and Crane, S.: Antithrombin III (ATIII) activity in plasmas from normal and diseased horses, and in normal canine, bovine and human plasmas. Vet. Clin. Pathol., 16:14, 1987.

Johnstone, I.B., Physick-Sheard, P., and Crane, S.: Breed, age, and gender differences in plasma antithrombin-III activity in clinically normal young horses. Am. J. Vet. Res., 50:1751, 1989.

McCaw, D.L., Jergens, A.E., Turrentine, M.A., et al.: Effect of internal hemorrhage on fibrin(ogen) degradation products in canine blood. Am. J. Vet. Res., 47:1620, 1986.

McKeever, K.H., Hinchcliff, K.W., Kociba, G.J., et al.: Changes in coagulation and fibrinolysis in horses during exercise. Am. J. Vet. Res., 51:1335, 1990.

Meyer, D.T., Coles, E.H. and Rich, L.J.: Veterinary Laboratory Medicine Interpretation and Diagnosis. Philadelphia, W.B. Saunders Co., 1992.

Moalic, P., Gruel, Y., Foloppe, P., et al.: Hemostasis development in the lamb fetus and neonate. Am. J. Vet. Res., 50:59, 1989.

Mount, M.E.: Diagnosis and therapy of anticoagulant rodenticide intoxications. Vet. Clin. North Am. Small Anim. Pract., 18:115, 1988.

Murtaugh, R.J. and Dodds, W.J.: Hemophilia A in a female dog. Am. J. Vet. Med. Assoc., 193:351, 1988.

Otto, C.M., Dodd, W.J. and Greene, C.E.: Factor XII and partial prekallikrein deficiencies in a dog with recurrent gastrointestinal hemorrhage. Am. J. Vet. Med. Assoc., 198:129, 1991.

Parker, M.T., Collier, L.L., Kier, A.B., et al.: Oral mucosa bleeding times of normal cats and cats with Chediak-Higashi syndrome or Hageman trait (Factor XII deficiency). Vet. Clin. Pathol., 17:9, 1988.

Parker, M.T., Turrentine, M.A. and Johnson, G.S.: von Willebrand factor in lysates of washed canine platelets. Am. J. Vet. Res., 52:119, 1991.

Sugiyama, F. and Furukawa, T.: Purification, electrophoretic characterization and plasma concentrations of feline or canine antithrombin III. Jpn. J. Vet. Sci., 47:987, 1985.

Turrentine, M.A., Hahn, A.W. and Johnson, G.S.: Factor VIII complex in canine plasma after submaximal treadmill exercise. Am. J. Vet Res., 47:39, 1986a.

Turrentine, M.A., Sculley, P.W., Green, E.M., et al.: Prekallikrein deficiency in a family of miniature horses. Am. J. Vet Res., 47:2464, 1986b.

Waters, D.C., Eaton, A.H., Steidley, K.R., et al.: Expression of von Willebrandt factor in plasma and platelets of cats. Am. J. Vet. Res., 50:201, 1989.

Wells, E.G., Prasse, K.W., Duncan, A., et al.: Equine protein C: An antigenic assay. Vet. Clin. Pathol., 18:15, 1989.

Wells, E.G., Prasse, K.W. and Moore, J.N.: Use of newly developed assays for protein C and plasminogen in horses with signs of colic. Am. J. Vet. Res., 52:345, 1991.

Wilkerson, M.J., Johnson, G.S., Riley, L.K., et al.: Afibrinogenemia and a circulating inhibitor to fibrinogen in a Bichon Frise. Vet. Clin. Pathol., 18:14, 1989.

Williams, W.J., Beutler, E., Erslev, A.J., et al.: Hematology. 4th Ed. New York, McGraw-Hill, 1990.

The terms "platelet" and "thrombocyte" can be used interchangeably, although originally thrombocyte was introduced to describe the nucleated cell of lower vertebrates, the counterpart of the non-nucleated mammalian platelet. Mammalian platelets are produced from the cytoplasmic fragmentation of megakaryocytes. In contrast, thrombocytes in lower vertebrates originate from a successive division of precursor cells (thromboblasts) within the marrow sinusoids. Platelets are crucial to the maintenance of hemostasis and vascular integrity. Therefore, knowledge of their mode of production, kinetics, structure, and function is essential for understanding the clinical conditions associated with the quantitative and qualitative abnormalities of platelets that lead to defective hemostasis (Jain, 1986; Williams et al., 1990)

MORPHOLOGIC FEATURES

Platelets of various mammalian species present a heterogeneous morphology in stained blood films (Figs. 6–1 and 6–2; Plate IX-1). Individual platelets appear as non-nucleated discoid, spheroid, or elongated flat objects, with fine, reddish-purple granules scattered throughout the cytoplasm or sometimes located centrally. The cytoplasm is clear and bounded by a delicate smooth membrane that sometimes bears a few fine, thread-like surface projections (Figs. 6–1A, B). Platelets may be distributed singly or found in small to large clumps. Platelet clumping can be minimized by careful venipuncture and by the use of EDTA as the anticoagulant. Infrequently, a platelet may lie over an erythrocyte. One or two platelets may sometimes be found attached to a neutrophil (Fig. 6–1C); this is known as platelet satellitism. It has been found in normal persons and in some patients with antiplatelet antibodies, lymphocytic leukemia, and myeloproliferative diseases. Its cause remains unknown.

The platelet volume varies in different species, with those of the dog, pig, and human being similar (7.6 to 8.3 fl), those of the ox, horse, sheep, rat, guinea pig, and mouse being smaller (3.2 to 5.4 fl), and those of the cat being larger (15.1 fl). Platelet counts in mammals vary inversely but nonlinearly with platelet volume within and among species. Larger platelets are considered to be metabolically and functionally more active than smaller platelets. Large platelets are often found in situations involving platelet destruction or consumption compared to platelet sequestration or failure of production, in which small platelets are a common finding.

Platelets of various mammalian species generally have a similar ultrastructure. Scanning electron microscopic studies have shown that "resting" platelets characteristically have a discoid or lentiform shape, with a

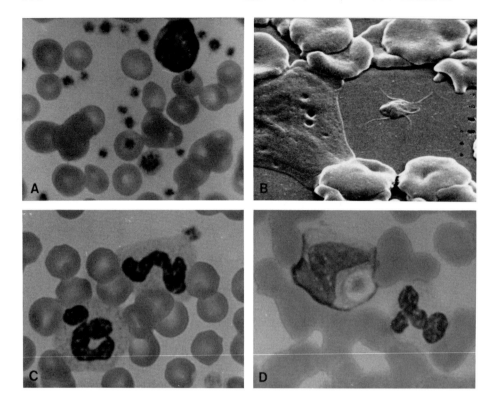

Fig. 6–1. *A*, Normal canine platelets exhibiting prominent granularity and some pleomorphism; an occasional platelet is as large as a red cell. *B*, Scanning electron photomicrograph of a blood film depicting a platelet with several distinctly visible fine dendritic processes; such processes are also seen in stained blood films examined with the light microscope, but they are difficult to depict photographically, as was the case with the platelets shown in *A*. *C*, An example of platelet satellitism in which a canine platelet has adhered to a neutrophil. *D*, A rare example of platelet phagocytosis by a monocyte in peripheral blood of a thrombocytopenic dog (platelet count, 18,000/µl of blood) (*A*, *C*, and *D* from Wright-stained blood films; *A*, *C*, and *D* × 1400; *B* × 2000.) (From Jain, N. C.: Schalm's Veterinary Hematology. 4th Ed. Philadelphia, Lea & Febiger, 1986, p. 447).

fairly smooth surface and slightly biconvex contour (Fig. 6–3). Some platelets may show shallow surface indentations and granularity (Figs. 6-3*A*, *B*, and *C*). The former presumably represent external openings of the open canalicular system (OCS) ramified within the body of the platelets, whereas the latter probably represent protracted platelet granules. A few dendritic or transformed platelets, with small to large pseudopods, may be found in the blood of normal animals (Fig. 6–3*F*), and these may represent activated platelets.

Transmission electron microscopic studies have revealed some unique ultrastructural features (Figs. 6–4 and 6–5). The unit membrane of normal platelets is covered with some amorphous material that forms a thin (150- to 200-nm) external coat. The external coat is rich in glycoproteins (GPs), and so is also known as the glycocalyx. Some microfilaments and a bundle of microtubules, consisting of one or several continuous coils, are found in the platelet matrix beneath the surface membrane. The internal structure is comprised of many α granules and glycogen particles, some dense bodies (granules), and a few mitochondria, lysosomes, and peroxisomes. A poorly developed Golgi apparatus may be seen in an occasional platelet, but cisternae of smooth or rough endoplasmic reticulum and free ribosomes are rarely found. Tubular channels of the OCS are randomly distributed and interconnected within the platelet matrix, and their openings (about 25 nm) may be seen on the platelet surface. Because the OCS is formed by the invagination of the platelet membrane, it is also covered with the exterior coat. Another series of channels, the dense tubular

system (DTS), is found just under the marginal band of microtubules. The DTS does not open on the platelet surface. It contains an isoenzyme of peroxidase that is considered to be specific for platelets. Bovine platelets characteristically have large α granules, are devoid of OCS, and secrete their contents directly to the exterior rather than by way of the OCS, as in humans (Smith et al., 1989).

The structural and functional relationships of various platelet components are listed in Table 6–1. Platelet α granules contain various proteins, all of which are secreted when platelets are stimulated with an agonist. Platelet factor 4, β-thromboglobulin, and basic protein are normally only present in platelets. Their presence in plasma indicates intravascular platelet activation.

BIOCHEMICAL CHARACTERISTICS

General Considerations

The chief source of energy in platelets is anaerobic glycolysis, although the pentose phosphate pathway and oxidative phosphorylation are also active. Resting discoid platelets contain a significant amount of cAMP that regulates platelet activity, probably through operation of the calcium pump. The ATP content of a platelet is about 150 times that of an erythrocyte, and both ATP and ADP are distributed in metabolic (one-third) and nonmetabolic or storage (two-thirds) pools, with an ATP:ADP ratio of 3 to 5:1 and 0.9:1 in respective pools. Inducers of shape change and release

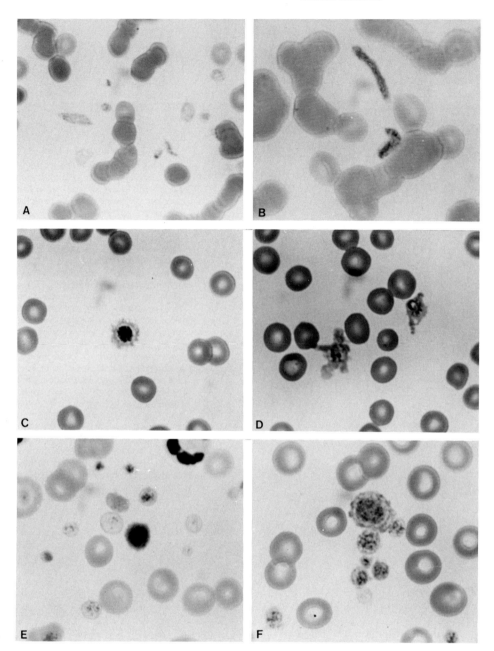

Fig. 6–2. *A,* Pleomorphic filamentous platelets in equine blood. *B,* Filamentous platelets in blood of a thrombocytopenic dog. *C,* Giant platelet with centripetal granularity. *D,* Abnormal giant platelets from a cat with lymphosarcoma. *E,* Excessively granular, several hypogranular, and a few small granular platelets in a canine patient with thrombocytosis (platelet count, 824,000/μl of blood). *F,* A megathrombocyte in a canine patient. (Wright-stained blood films; × 1200). (From Jain, N. C.: Schalm's Veterinary Hematology. 4th Ed. Philadelphia, Lea & Febiger, 1986, p. 448.)

reaction cause a profound increase in platelet metabolism and oxygen utilization. Activated platelets secrete not only substances stored in their cytoplasmic organelles, but also elaborate newly synthesized substances such as endoperoxides, prostaglandins, and thromboxanes. Platelets of various species differ in serotonin content; relatively low levels are found in platelets of humans, nonhuman primates, rats, and guinea pigs, medium levels are present in platelets of dogs and horses, and high levels are found in platelets of cats. Platelets are rich in glutathione, which provides important protection from oxidant damage.

Many GPs have been found in platelet plasma membrane. Seven of these GPs predominate in human platelets and have been isolated by solubilization with sodium dodecyl sulfate and subsequent electrophoresis in polyacrylamide gels. Species differences exist in the properties and relative abundance of various GPs. For example, bovine, canine, porcine, and rabbit platelets contain three to four major GPs, whereas feline platelets have only two such bands. Feline platelets lack the GPI band. Some of these GPs are important for platelet function, such as adherence, aggregation, and subsequent release reaction. GPIa mediates platelet interaction with collagen. GPIb is the receptor for von Willebrand factor (vWF) in unstimulated platelets, and the GPIIb-IIIa complex on stimulated platelets serves as a receptor for vWF, fibrinogen, fibronectin, and

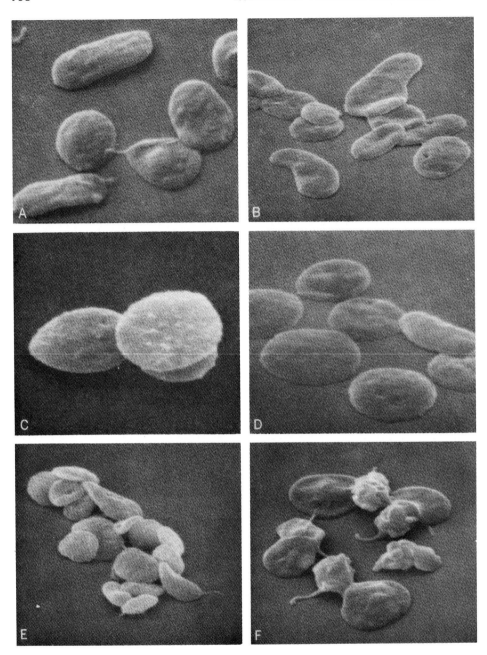

Fig. 6–3. Scanning electron photomicrographs of normal platelets from peripheral blood of various animal species. *A,* Canine platelets depicting discoid, oval, and elongated morphology, with or without surface projections. *B,* Equine platelets showing prominent pleomorphism, some with clearly visible surface pits. *C,* Uniformly discoid feline platelets with some surface roughness. *D,* Ovine platelets with relatively smooth surface, except for some surface depressions. *E,* Bovine platelets of variable shapes and sizes, one having a short thin filament. *F,* Normal canine discoid platelets and activated platelets with centripetal aggregation of internal organelles *(upper left)* comparable to those seen with the light microscope (Fig. 6–2*C*), many surface buds, and long pseudopods. (A × 8200; B × 5200; C × 13,200; D × 10,400; E × 6200; and F × 6200). (From Jain, N. C.: A scanning electron microscopic study of platelets of certain animal species. Thrombosis et Diathesis Haemorrhagica 33:501, 1975.)

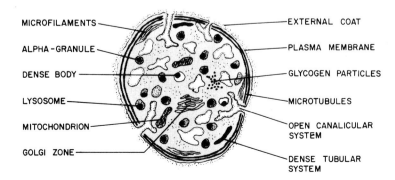

MICROFILAMENTS
ALPHA-GRANULE
DENSE BODY
LYSOSOME
MITOCHONDRION
GOLGI ZONE

EXTERNAL COAT
PLASMA MEMBRANE
GLYCOGEN PARTICLES
MICROTUBULES
OPEN CANALICULAR SYSTEM
DENSE TUBULAR SYSTEM

Fig. 6–4. Schematic representation of the ultrastructure of a platelet. (From Jain, N. C.: Schalm's Veterinary Hematology. 4th Ed. Philadelphia, Lea & Febiger, 1986, p. 450.)

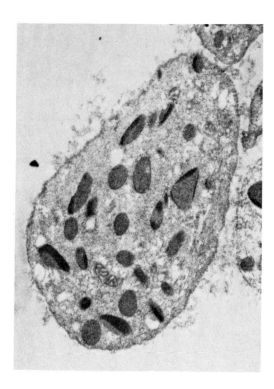

Fig. 6–5. Transmission electron photomicrograph of a bovine platelet showing prominent granularity, some vacuolar areas, a mitochondrion, and some profiles of microtubules near the surface membrane in the right area, (× 12000). (From Jain, N. C.: Schalm's Veterinary Hematology. 4th Ed. Philadelphia, Lea & Febiger, 1986, p. 450.)

Table 6–1.　Constituents and Possible Functions of Some Anatomic Units of Platelets

Anatomic Unit	Constituents	Possible Functions
Exterior coat	Fibrinogen	Platelet aggregation
	Glycoproteins	Platelet adhesion
Unit membrane	Arachidonic acid	Prostaglandin synthesis
	Platelet factor 3 (phospholipid)	Enhances coagulation
	cAMP	Inhibits release reaction
	Glycoproteins	Platelet adhesion and activation; GPIb is receptor for vWF
Microtubules	Tubulin	Provides cytoskeleton, forms contractile system
Microfilaments	Thrombosthenin	Shape change, clot retraction, release reaction
α Granules	β-Thromboglobulin	Impedes prostacyclin production by endothelial cells
	Catalase	Unknown
	Factor VIII-related antigen	Platelet adhesion to subendothelium
	Fibrinogen	Platelet aggregation and local coagulation
	Fibronectin	Adherence to extracellular matrix; promotes wound healing
	Growth factor(s)	Mitosis of endothelial and smooth muscle cells and fibroblasts
	High-molecular-weight kininogen	Blood coagulation
	Platelet factor 4	Binds glucosaminoglycans, antiheparin action
	Platelet factor 1	Acts as plasma coagulation factor V
	Thrombospondin	Platelet adhesion, bacterial adherence
	Platelet-specific basic protein	Source of Platelet factor 4 and β-thromboglobulin
	vWF	Platelet adhesion
	Cationic proteins	Vascular permeability, chemotactic and bactericidal factors
	Albumin	Humoral immunity
	IgG	Transport protein, colloidal osmotic pressure
	Osetonectin	?
Dense bodies	"Storage pool" of adenine nucleotides	Platelet metabolism and hemostasis
	Histamine	Increases vascular permeability
	Serotonin	Vasoconstriction, platelet aggregation
	Ca^{2+}	Platelet stimulation
Lysosomal granules	Acid hydrolases (e.g., acid phosphatase, β-glucuronidase, arylsulfatase, cathepsin)	Proteolysis
Dense tubular system	Ca^{2+}	Platelet stimulation
	Enzymes for prostaglandin synthesis	Prostaglandin synthesis
	Peroxidase	Platelet-specific peroxidase for identification
Open canicular system	Extensive surface area and canaliculi	Route for exocytosis, endocysois, phagocytosis
?	Antiplasmin	Inactivates plasmin
?	Epinephrine	Vasoconstriction

vitronectin. GPIc acts as a receptor for fibronectin and GPIV probably for thrombospondin. Abnormalities of platelet membrane GP have been found in humans and in dogs with thrombasthenic thrombopathia. Integrin receptors for collagen, laminin, fibronectin, and vitronectin have also been identified on human platelets.

Arachidonic Acid Metabolism

Arachidonic acid metabolites have diverse biologic functions, such as regulation of leukocyte functions, inflammation, hematopoiesis, platelet adhesion and aggregation, and allergic reactions. They are important in hemostasis and thrombosis involving platelet-vessel wall interactions. The following is a brief discussion of various aspects of arachidonic acid metabolism in animals and humans.

Prostaglandins (PGs) and thromboxanes (Txs) are synthesized and released from platelets, leukocytes, endothelial cells, and other body cells after appropriate stimulation (Fig. 6–6). They are not found as preformed substances in body cells. Arachidonic acid is liberated from membrane phospholipids of stimulated cells by phospholipase C or A. Platelet stimulation is achieved by thrombin, ADP, collagen, epinephrine, and calcium ionophores or stimulators. Free arachidonic acid is rapidly oxygenated by cyclo-oxygenase to its cyclic endoperoxides, PGG_2 and its reduction product PGH_2, or by lipoxygenase to 12-hydroperoxyeicosatetraenoic acid (HPETE) and 12-hydroxyeicosatetraenoic acid (HETE). Cyclo-oxygenase is also involved in the conversion of dihomolinoleic acid, a derivative of arachidonic acid, to PGG_1 and PGH_1, and the former is subsequently converted to PGE_1. The metabolism of arachidonic acid through another pathway in some leukocytes results in the production of leukotrienes and lipoxygenation products, which have important biologic functions in inflammation. PGG_2 and PGH_2 are nonenzymatically converted to hydroxyheptadecatrienoic acid (HHT) and malondialdehyde (MDA) or enzymatically to stable prostaglandins PGD_2, PGE_2, and $PGF_{2\alpha}$. PGD_2 is the main product formed in the platelets. The major pathway of PGG_2 and PGH_2 in platelets is conversion to TxA_2 by thromboxane synthetase. TxA_2 spontaneously hydrolyzes to TxB_2.

The arachidonic acid pathway is characteristic of platelets in general, but considerable differences have been found between and within species. It is most prominent in human platelets, intermediate in those of the horse, and poorly developed in platelets of cows, miniature pigs, and mink. In dogs and cats, individual differences are seen in the behavior of

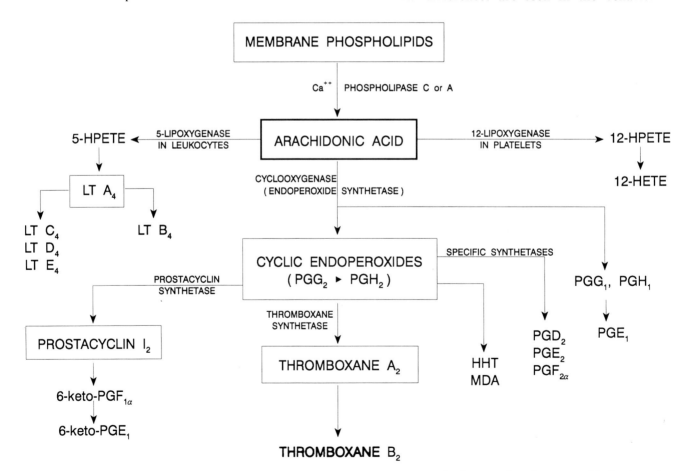

Fig. 6–6. Outline of arachidonic acid metabolism leading to the formation of various prostaglandins (PG), thromboxanes, and leukotrienes (LT). See text for details. (Modified from Jain, N. C.: Schalm's Veterinary Hematology. 4th Ed. Philadelphia, Lea & Febiger, 1986, p. 452.)

platelets in this regard with low to high activity. Similarly, species variation occurs in the generation of TxB₂ by platelets, with the dog producing the highest amounts (887.7 ± 123.7 ng/ml) and the sheep the lowest (2.7 ± 0.2 ng/ml) (McKeller et al., 1990).

Arachidonic acid metabolism in vascular endothelium differs from that in platelets in certain respects. The lipoxygenase pathway is absent, the nonenzymatic conversion of cyclic endoperoxides primarily produces PGE_2, and the thromboxane synthetase pathway is less active, producing small amounts of TxA_2. The major pathway is the conversion of cyclic endoperoxides to prostacyclin (PGI_2) by prostacyclin synthetase. PGI_2 is short-lived (half-life, 3 minutes) and is hydrolyzed to an inactive product, 6-keto-$PGF_{1\alpha}$.

Various functions have been ascribed to arachidonic acid metabolites. HPETE inhibits thromboxane synthetase, and both HPETE and HETE are chemotactic for neutrophils. MDA cross-links proteins and inhibits certain enzyme activities. TxA_2 lowers platelet cAMP levels, causes vasoconstriction, and is the most potent platelet-aggregating agent described. PGG_2 and PGH_2 also cause platelet aggregation. Platelet aggregation by ADP, epinephrine, and low concentrations of collagen and thrombin is induced through the production of TxA_2 and is, therefore, blocked by inhibitors of cyclo-oxygenase and thromboxane synthetase. Aggregation by high concentrations of collagen and thrombin or by calcium ionophores does not involve this mechanism. PGI_2 acts as a vasodilator and is the most potent platelet antiaggregating agent described. The relative concentration of PGI_2 needed to inhibit platelet aggregation varies among species—for example, sheep and horse platelets are much less sensitive than human platelets. PGI_2 acts primarily by increasing cellular levels of cAMP through the stimulation of adenylate cyclase. PGI_2 also inhibits platelet adhesion to exposed subendothelium in vitro.

Various drugs inhibit arachidonic acid metabolism and have proved to be effective or potentially important in controlling the pathologic manifestations of platelet functions. For example, glucocorticoids and anti-inflammatory steroids inhibit phospholipase activity, but are not potent enough to exert any antithrombotic action. Most of the clinically used inhibitors of prostaglandin or thromboxane synthesis inhibit cyclo-oxygenase activity. For example, aspirin irreversibly inactivates platelet cyclo-oxygenase within minutes. The defect persists for the life of platelets, but newly formed platelets exhibit cyclo-oxygenase activity. In contrast, indomethacin and sulfinpyrazone cause a transient and reversible inhibition of prostaglandin synthesis.

THROMBOPOIESIS

Megakaryocytes

DEVELOPMENTAL ASPECTS

Isotope labeling, electron microscopic, and in vitro bone marrow culture studies have provided informa-

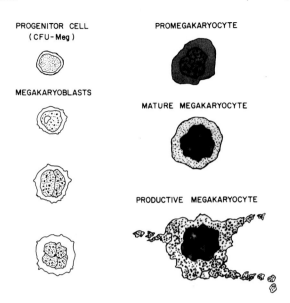

Fig. 6–7. Megakaryocyte development and maturation. The megakaryocytic progenitor cell is a descendant of the pluripotential hematopoietic stem cell and an immediate precursor of the earliest morphologically recognizable cell of the series, the megakaryoblast. The megakaryoblast is initially a diploid cell with a single nucleus but, because of endoreduplication (nuclear division without cytoplasmic division), it enlarges and becomes a polyploid cell with two to four nuclei. With progressive endoreduplication and maturation, a megakaryoblast develops into a promegakaryocyte and then into a megakaryocyte. The nuclei of the promegakaryocyte and megakaryocyte appear multilobed rather than individually separated, and the cytoplasm of the latter cell shows prominent azurophilic granulation. Platelets are produced by cytoplasmic fragmentation of a mature, productive megakaryocyte (also see Fig. 6–10). (From Jain, N. C.: Schalm's Veterinary Hematology. 4th Ed. Philadelphia, Lea & Febiger, 1986, p. 432.)

tion about the development and maturation of megakaryocytes and platelet production. The pluripotent stem cell (PPSC) in the bone marrow gives rise to two functionally recognizable megakaryocytic progenitor cells, the burst-forming unit-megakaryocyte (BFU-Meg) and the colony-forming unit–megakaryocyte (CFU-Meg) (Hoffman et al., 1990). The CFU-Meg then divides and differentiates into morphologically recognizable megakaryocytic precursors, which later mature to produce platelets (Fig. 6–7). Division and differentiation of the PPSC to the CFU-Meg are influenced by the hematopoietic microenvironment, cell-cell interactions, and/or short-range humoral factors, whereas division and differentiation of the CFU-Meg to megakaryoblast are regulated by a specific colony-stimulating factor (CSF-Meg) and other cytokines. The development of megakaryocytes and platelet production are influenced primarily by thrombopoietin. Megakaryocytopoiesis differs uniquely from erythropoiesis and granulocytopoiesis in that it involves polyploidization of the precursor cells as a result of endomitosis or endoreduplication (nuclear division without cytoplasmic division).

LIGHT MICROSCOPIC MORPHOLOGY

Megakaryocytes are the largest hematopoietic cells in the bone marrow, measuring over 20 to 160 μm in

Wright-stained smears. They are generally classified into three types, stages, or groups according to their cytoplasmic and nuclear characteristics. These are megakaryoblast, promegakaryocyte, and megakaryocyte or, respectively, stage I, II, and III cells, or group I, II, and III cells. The megakaryocyte engaged in platelet formation is considered a stage IV cell (Fig. 6–7).

The megakaryoblast is the most morphologically immature recognizable cell of the series. It has a highly basophilic, nongranular cytoplasm and a round nucleus, with finely stippled chromatin and one or more nucleoli. Small cells with two to four nuclei and basophilic agranular cytoplasm are also regarded as megakaryoblasts (Plates III-1 and III-3). The nucleus or nuclei occupy most of the cell, giving a high nucleus-to-cytoplasm ratio. Some megakaryoblasts have a few cytoplasmic vacuoles and small cytoplasmic twigs or blebs on the cell surface. Mitotic division of the nucleus without division of the cytoplasm (endoreduplication, endomitosis, or acytokinesis) leads to the production of a polyploid nucleus and an increase in cell size (Plates III-1, III-2, and III-3). Repeated nuclear division produces cells having a polyploid DNA content (4N, 8N, 16N, 32N, and sometimes 64N). The diploid cell committed to undergo polyploidy is known as the promegakaryoblast, whereas blast cells with higher ploidy are considered megakaryoblasts. Small mononuclear cells, with a ploidy of 2N or 4N, cannot be determined morphologically but are identified by special procedures, such as immunohistochemical staining with antibodies to GPIIb-IIIa and platelet factor 4, cytochemical staining for acetylcholinesterase in certain species (e.g., mouse, cat, dog, horse, but not humans), and staining for a platelet-specific peroxidase in the nuclear envelope, rough endoplasmic reticulum (RER), and demarcation membrane system (DMS).

Cells with more than four nuclei and moderately basophilic agranular cytoplasm are promegakaryocytes. Cells with separate nuclei are extremely rare in normal marrow, but can be found when megakaryocytopoiesis is markedly stimulated in response to thrombocytopenia. More commonly, promegakaryocytes have a mass of multilobed nuclei with indistinct separations. Their cytoplasm is less basophilic but copious, giving a lower nucleus:cytoplasm ratio than that of megakaryoblasts (Plate III-4). As promegakaryocytes begin to mature to megakaryocytes, patches of fine, reddish-purple (azurophilic) granules develop in the cytoplasm, particularly near the nucleus. With maturation, the nucleus becomes more lobulated, the nuclear chromatin condenses, and the cytoplasm increases in amount, becomes less basophilic, and acquires increasing granularity.

Thus, the megakaryocyte has a single, multilobed nuclear mass, abundant, pale staining cytoplasm, and numerous small azurophilic granules (Plates III-4 and III-5). Megakaryocytes are generally round, although an occasional cell may be distorted because of crowding or from smear making. An osteoclast, in contrast, has multiple separate nuclei, somewhat larger and fewer reddish-purple cytoplasmic granules, and an irregular shape (Plate III-6).

Endoreduplication in megakaryoblasts and promegakaryocytes requires the synthesis of DNA. Megakaryocytes and some promegakaryocytes do not synthesize DNA and may be at the 8N or higher ploidy level. Endoreduplication generally precedes cytoplasmic maturation, but both processes may occur simultaneously. Thus, it is possible to observe mature megakaryocytes with different cell sizes, nuclear masses, and cytoplasmic characteristics, depending on the degree of cytoplasmic maturation. Rarely, platelet-producing megakaryocytes may be found to have pseudopod-like extensions of the cytoplasm (proplatelets) or individual platelets breaking away from the cell surface (Plate III-5). The entire process of megakaryocyte differentiation and maturation takes about 6 days in humans, 3 days in dogs, and 2 to 3 days in rodents.

ULTRASTRUCTURE AND CYTOCHEMISTRY

Megakaryocytes appear spherical and reveal varied surface morphology with use of the scanning electron microscope. Principal surface features include numerous ruffles and ridges, microprocesses of variable sizes and shapes, and globular, bud-like protuberances and scaly structures resembling platelets (Fig. 6–8).

Principal features visible with the transmission electron microscope vary with the maturity of megakaryocytes and include the following: several distinct nucleoli only in the megakaryoblasts, a prominent Golgi apparatus, small and large mitochondria, polyribosomes and ribosomes, segments of RER, a convoluted DMS, an OCS, α granules, and some glycogen granules (Figs. 6–9 and 6–10). Formation of the DMS involves invagination of the megakaryocyte cell membrane and arborization throughout the cytoplasm, fusion of vesicles or vacuoles originating from the Golgi apparatus, or both mechanisms.

The Golgi apparatus is the site of production of the α granules and primary lysosomes. The α granules contain various proteins of biologic significance, including platelet factor 4, β-thromboglobulin, fibrinogen, vWf, factor V, and the platelet-derived growth factor. In addition, megakaryocytes contain thrombosthenin, an actomyosin-like protein, and some other cytoskeletal proteins, such as α-actinin and talin. The dense bodies, unique to the circulating platelets, are absent. Lysosomal granules stain positive for acid phosphatase and aryl sulfatase.

The internal organelles in megakaryocytes may be scattered in the cytoplasm or may be preferentially localized, so that the cell periphery is free of organelles, the intermediate cytoplasmic zone is rich in the DMS, and the perinuclear region chiefly contains the Golgi apparatus, RER, and developing granules. The external surface of the DMS in megakaryocytes becomes coated with GPs, which later constitute the exterior coat of the platelets. Pseudopod formation and clearly defined platelet zones, with groups of granules sepa-

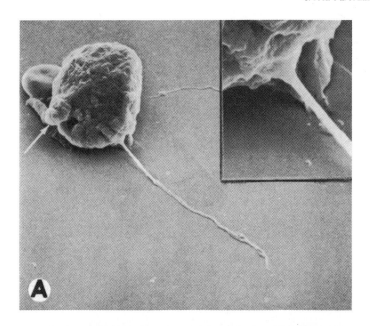

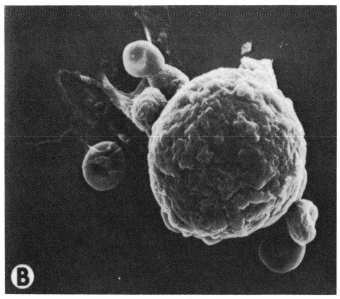

Fig. 6–8.   Scanning electron photomicrographs of canine mega-karyocytes in suspensions of bone marrow cells. *A,* megakaryocyte with a long, thin, proplatelet process, a short, thick, curled up process *(arrow),* and several surface protuberances (× 2000). The inset clearly shows the origin of the long process from the megakaryocyte (× 8000). *B,* Megakaryocyte with complex surface protuberances, some of which resemble budding platelets. Two processes having a thick stem and flat filamentous branches represent a broken proplatelet (× 2300). (From Handagama, P., Jain, N. C., Kono, C. S., et al.: Scanning electron microscopic studies of megakaryocytes and platelet formation in the dog and rat. Am. J. Vet. Res., 47:2454, 1986.)

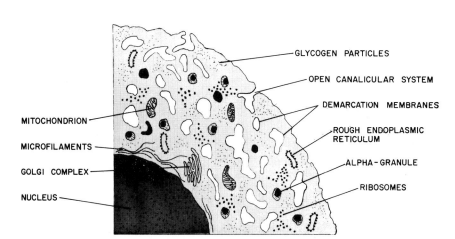

Fig. 6–9.   Schematic representation of the morphologic features of a megakaryocyte. Only a portion is drawn. (From Jain, N. C.: Schalm's Veterinary Hematology. 4th Ed. Philadelphia, Lea & Febiger, 1986, p. 435.)

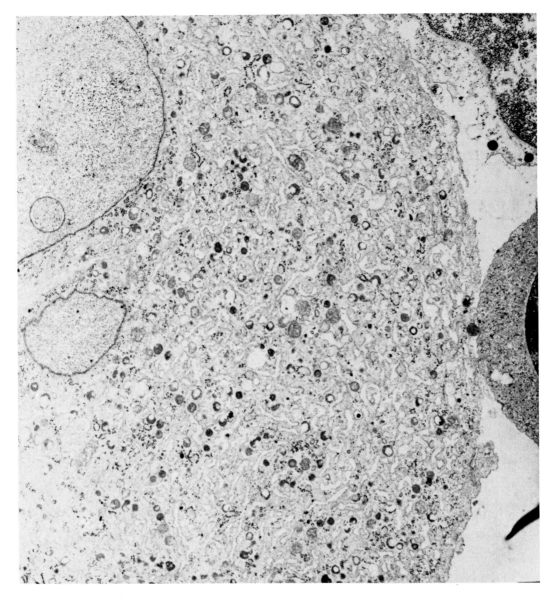

Fig. 6–10. Transmission electron photomicrograph of a portion of a canine megakaryocyte containing numerous granules, membranous tubules and vesicles, and ribosomes. Platelets are formed at the surface as a result of the separation of cytoplasmic fragments by membranous channels. Parts of the nucleus are also seen at the upper left corner (×8000). (From Jain, N. C.: Schalm's Veterinary Hematology. 4th Ed. Philadelphia, Lea & Febiger, 1986, p. 436.)

rated by the DMS, may be seen in some larger and more mature megakaryocytes.

Platelet Formation

In vivo and in vitro studies have revealed several modes of platelet formation. These include random fragmentation of megakaryocyte cytoplasm, extension of megakaryocyte cytoplasm into long, ribbon-like processes (proplatelets) and their segmentation in circulation, and possibly surface blebbing or budding. Megakaryocyte fragmentation may occur in the marrow or after translocation elsewhere in the body, primarily in the pulmonary circulation. In vitro studies

have shown that platelet release by megakaryocytes depends on an intact cytoskeleton (microtubules and microfilaments), active glycolysis, and cellular integrity (Handagama et al., 1987a, 1987b).

In 1910, Wright hypothesized that pseudopod-like projections arise from the surface of mature megakaryocytes and penetrate into the marrow sinusoids to shed platelets. This hypothesis has been confirmed. Megakaryocytes located in the hematopoietic islands extend long, ribbon-like cytoplasmic processes through the endothelial cells into the sinusoidal lumen (Fig. 6–11). These proplatelets ($\sim 2.5 \times 120$ μm) frequently present regional constrictions and beaded areas (a string of platelet fields) along their lengths. Fragmentation at these regions by a pinching-off process,

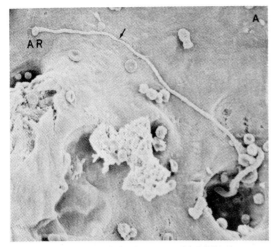

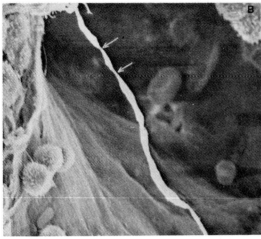

Fig. 6–11. Scanning electron photomicrographs of canine bone marrow depicting long, slender extensions of proplatelets within the sinusoidal lumen. Platelets may be shed by fragmentation of a proplatelet at the apical region (AR) or areas of intermittent constructions *(arrows; A,* × 721; *B,* × 2540). (From Jain, N. C.: Schalm's Veterinary Hematology. 4th Ed. Philadelphia, Lea & Febiger, 1986, p. 437.)

through the participation of microtubules and thrombosthenin, leads to the production of a heterogeneous population of platelets. Giant platelets, often seen during reactive thrombocytosis, may be composed of several platelet fields. Proplatelets have been found in the blood of several species (Handagama et al., 1987c). Proplatelets in healthy rats are more numerous in blood from right ventricles than in blood from left ventricles, and their number in heart blood was found to increase 24 hours after acute blood loss. These observations suggest platelet release through proplatelet formation in the lungs as well as in the circulation.

An additional mode of platelet formation through surface blebbing or budding has been described. In mouse and rat bone marrows, megakaryocytes were seen to lie near the sinusoidal wall and, at certain sites, the wall structure appeared to be completed by the megakaryocyte. In this position, platelets could be shed from cytoplasmic projections and surface blebs on the megakaryocyte, or the intact cell could enter the sinus

to shed its platelets in the sinusoid or elsewhere, particularly in the pulmonary circulation. Some megakaryocytes are found in extramedullary locations, such as the lungs and occasionally in the spleen, liver, kidneys, and heart, In the dog, seven megakaryocytes/ml of venous blood and two megakaryocytes/ml of arterial blood were found as elongated cells (20 to 50 µm).

It is estimated that a mature megakaryocyte normally produces about 2000 to 8000 platelets over a period of 3 to 12 hours. The number produced is proportional to the cytoplasmic volume and ploidy value of the megakaryocyte. A rough correlation between platelet size and platelet number has been observed in many species. Young platelets are larger, denser, and metabolically and functionally more active than old platelets. The heterogeneity of circulating platelets, with regard to size and density, stems from the origin of platelets from different populations of megakaryocytes. Small and young megakaryocytes produce large and dense platelets.

Regulatory Factors

The number of platelets in the circulation is remarkably constant in a healthy animal. The platelet number in blood is influenced both by positive and negative feedback mechanisms. Experimental studies in rats and humans have shown that platelet production can be increased up to sixfold.

Megakaryocytopoiesis is regulated by the number of circulating platelets. Thus, experimental thrombocytopenia stimulates megakaryocytopoiesis, leading to increases in megakaryocyte numbers, mitotic indices, nuclear ploidy, and cell size, and to a decrease in the megakaryocyte maturation time. In contrast, transfusion-induced thrombocytosis is associated with decreases in megakaryocyte number, cell size, and nuclear ploidy. The megakaryocyte maturation time remains normal or is prolonged. Furthermore, the number of megakaryocytes in bone marrow may influence the regulation of megakaryocytopoiesis even when there is thrombocytosis (Ebbe, 1991).

Megakaryocytopoiesis and thrombopoiesis are stimulated by various factors including, the hematopoietic microenvironment, a megakaryocyte colony-stimulating factor (Meg-CSF), a hormonal factor known as thrombocytosis-stimulating factor (TSF) or thrombopoietin, interleukin-3, (IL-3), GM-CSF, and G-CSF (Han et al., 1991; McDonald, 1992; Teramura et al., 1992). The Meg-CSF stimulates the proliferation and differentiation of specific progenitor cells to megakaryocytes, IL-3, GM-CSF, and G-CSF influence or potentiate the growth and maturation of megakaryocytes; and thrombopoietin influences the entire process. Meg-CSF is present in the urine of patients with aplastic anemia and idiopathic thrombocytopenia, and its plasma level is inversely related to the marrow megakaryocyte number. It is present in the plasma of dogs whose marrow has been depleted of megakaryocytes because of irradiation or chemotherapy. IL-1, IL-4, IL-6, and IL-11 may also have some stimulatory effects on megakaryocyte proliferation. Erythropoietin has been found to stimulate megakaryocytopoiesis in vitro.

Platelet production is specifically regulated by thrombopoietin (McDonald, 1992). Thrombopoietin has been isolated from the urine and plasma of normal humans and animals and from the plasma of thrombocytopenic individuals. Partially purified rat thrombopoietin is a glycoprotein (MW, 48,000). The site of thrombopoietin production remains to be determined, but the kidney is at least one such site. Thrombopoietin seems to influence megakaryocyte production in at least three ways: (1) by stimulating committed stem cells (i.e., increasing the rate of differentiation of unrecognizable megakaryocytic progenitors into megakaryocytic precursors); (2) by inducing additional endomitosis in immature megakaryocytes, resulting in increased ploidy and cell volume; and (3) by shortening the megakaryocyte maturation time. Thrombopoietin levels vary inversely with the circulating platelet mass. Thus, thrombocytopenia is associated with increased levels and thrombocytosis with decreased levels of thrombopoietin. The regulatory mechanisms of thrombocytoses seen in myeloproliferative disorders and in many other conditions, including iron deficiency anemia, remain unknown.

Inhibitors of thrombopoiesis have also been investigated. Normal human serum contains one or more factors that inhibit the formation of megakaryocytic colonies in vitro. For example, α- and β-interferons inhibit CFU-Meg as well as other hematopoietic progenitors. Other inhibitors of megakaryocytopoiesis include megakaryocyte-platelet products (transforming growth factor-β and platelet factor 4) and interferon-alpha and -gamma (Han et al., 1991). The spleen may produce an inhibitor of thrombopoiesis, as indicated by the occurrence of thrombocytosis in splenectomized animals. Suppressor T cells were found to inhibit megakaryocytopoiesis in human patients with acute myelogenous leukemia. Vincristine induces thrombocytosis in several species, and therefore is commonly used in the treatment of immune-mediated thrombocytopenia. It has been suggested that vincristine induces thrombocytosis by inhibition of a platelet regulatory function, probably the secretion of a substance that affects feedback inhibition of megakaryocytopoiesis.

SURVIVAL AND DISTRIBUTION

Intravascular Survival

The platelet has a finite life that is generally similar in humans and animals (Table 6–2). The use of labeling with ^{51}Cr and ^{111}In-oxime is satisfactory for estimating platelet survival and turnover. Platelet destruction occurs in the mononuclear phagocyte system and is essentially age-dependent (linear disappearance), but some random destruction (exponential removal) is also observed. Although damaged and senescent platelets are sequestered mainly in the spleen or liver, or at both sites, bone marrow is also important in platelet destruction.

Splenic and Nonsplenic Pools

Two rapidly mobilizable pools of platelets, one splenic and the other nonsplenic, are present in humans and animals. A transient increase in platelet numbers in blood occurs after epinephrine injection and after mild exercise. The increase caused by the former is attributed to the release of platelets from the spleen, whereas that resulting from exercise is associated with platelet release from the lungs. This is based on findings that epinephrine-induced platelet release is not seen in asplenic individuals, whereas exercise-induced change is not affected by splenectomy. Platelet counts in both cases return to normal levels within 30 minutes. Platelets from both pools could be released during vigorous muscular activity.

About 30 to 40% of the total platelet mass in humans, dogs, and rabbits is normally sequestered in the spleen and can be mobilized rapidly. In patients with splenomegaly, as much as 90% of the platelet mass may be sequestered in the spleen. The sequestered platelets include a disproportionately higher number of young platelets (megathrombocytes) in addition to senescent platelets. Normally, a dynamic exchange occurs between the splenic and circulating platelets. Splenectomy is followed by a protracted thrombocytosis that results largely from the removal of the splenic reservoir and circulation of the total intravascular platelet mass and partly from increased thrombopoiesis, probably because of the removal of an inhibitory splenic influence (see above).

The nonsplenic pool in the dog and rabbit represents approximately half of the total, rapidly mobilizable pool. Furthermore, in contrast to the splenic pool, the nonsplenic pool is not appreciably enriched with megathrombocytes. Possible sites of this nonsplenic pool include the lungs, liver, heart, and bone marrow. That such a nonsplenic pool of platelets may not be present in all species was revealed by a study of splenectomized ponies whose platelet counts and size were not significantly altered after exercise.

Table 6–2. Mean Platelet Survival In Different Species

Species	Days
Sheep	9–11
Bovine calves	5–10
Humans	6.9–9.9
Monkeys	8.0
Dogs	5–7
Horses	5.5 ± 0.49
Rats	5
Rabbits	3
Pigs	2.5

AGGREGATION AND RELEASE REACTION

A series of biochemical and morphologic events occurs in platelets after contact with damaged vascular surface in vivo or after exposure to various substances in vitro. Platelets have surface receptors for various agonist, and receptor-ligand interaction leads to various platelet responses through the activation of a signal transduction cascade. Four such separable events have been recognized—adhesion, aggregation, contraction, and release reaction or secretion—one or more of which may occur simultaneously or independently, depending on the stimulus and environmental conditions. Derangement of any one process can lead to a bleeding disorder.

Injury to the vascular endothelium initiates the adherence of platelets to the site of injury. This stickiness of platelets to a nonplatelet surface is known as adhesion. During this process, platelets first undergo a shape change; they become spherical and develop dendritic processes as a result of changes in the organization of microtubules and the release of intraplatelet calcium. The adherence of platelet to platelet is called aggregation. Primary aggregation from the initial activation of platelets by an agonist is reversible, whereas secondary aggregation induced after initiation of the release reaction is irreversible. The release reaction, or secretion, entails the fusion of platelet-dense bodies and α granules with membranes of the OCS, and exocytosis of the granular contents into the canaliculi and from there to the outside. This process is aided by internal contraction of the microtubules and by microfilaments inducing the central mobilization of platelet organelles. The release of material from dense bodies is called release reaction I, and release reaction II is characterized by the release of contents from the α granules and lysosomes.

The intracellular transmitter of aggregation and release reaction is calcium, and the basic reaction is cellular contraction requiring energy in the form of ATP. Many drugs inhibit platelet aggregation and the release reaction. For example, aspirin blocks the release reaction for the life of the platelet by blocking the generation of TxA_2 through the inhibition of cyclo-oxygenase. Dipyridamole interferes with platelet function by inhibiting the release of intracellular calcium needed for platelet aggregation. Sulfinpyrazone prevents the platelet release reaction by the reversible inactivation of cyclo-oxygenase. The latter two drugs are useful in the treatment of arterial thrombosis.

Various conditions and substances make the platelet membrane stickier, induce platelet adherence to endothelial surface, and promote platelet aggregation and secretion. Endothelial damage promoting platelet adhesion may occur as a result of numerous factors, both physiologic (e.g., epinephrine) and pathologic (e.g., endotoxin, viral and bacterial infections). Platelet adhesion in vivo is most often followed by platelet aggregation. Platelet aggregation in vitro can be induced by ADP, epinephrine, collagen, thrombin, serotonin, calcium ionophores, TxA_2, immune complexes, endotoxin, ristocetin, and viruses. These agents can also induce platelet aggregation in vivo. A reduction in the intracellular level of cAMP in the platelets is associated with increased platelet aggregation, whereas an increase in the cAMP level inhibits platelet responses. A similar influence of cGMP has also been observed.

Platelet aggregation can be measured in vitro and is a means of evaluating functional defects of platelets. Species variations occur, however, in the aggregation of platelets by various agents. Typically, human platelets undergo a biphasic aggregation, primary and secondary, in response to ADP and epinephrine. Such a response to ADP occurs irregularly in the dog and some monkeys, but most other animal species show a monophasic, primary response to ADP and no measurable response to epinephrine. Canine platelets do not aggregate with ristocetin, whereas human and baboon platelets do. Feline platelets exhibit biphasic aggregation with most aggregating agents. Equine platelets have a biphasic response to ADP and serotonin, but are nonresponsive to epinephrine. Platelets from all species respond to collagen. Responses to arachidonic acid vary within and among species; platelets of mink, miniature pigs, horses, and cows do not aggregate, those of dogs and cats show variable aggregation, and human, guinea pig, and rabbit platelets show irreversible aggregation. Bovine platelets are more sensitive to aggregation by platelet-activating factor than ADP or thrombin. Epinephrine, arachidonic acid, and serotonin do not aggregate bovine platelets, but do increase the aggregation response to other agonists (Bondy and Gentry, 1989). Bird and reptile thrombocytes respond only to thrombin.

Acquired functional defects of platelet aggregation have been found in various diseases in animals. Examples include the following: in horses, laminitis, exercise-induced pulmonary hemorrhage (bleeder horses), and platelet-associated hemorrhagic disorders (newborn foals); in cats, Chédiak-Higashi syndrome; in dogs, uremia, acute pancreatitis, Ehrlichia canis infection, and megakaryocytic leukemia. Platelets of dogs infected with Rickettsia rickettsii (Rocky Mountain spotted fever) have an increased tendency to aggregate. Platelets from basset hounds with a hereditary thrombocytopathia fail to aggregate with ADP.

FUNCTIONS

The primary function of platelets is the maintenance of hemostasis. By interacting with endothelial cells, platelets help maintain vascular integrity. Platelets are important in blood coagulation by providing platelet phospholipid (platelet factor 3) and by carrying several coagulation factors on their surfaces. Platelets are essential for clot retraction, which depends on their contractile protein system, including thrombosthenin. Other functions of platelets include roles in thrombosis and embolism, in the inflammatory response through the activation of chemotactic substances and the release of cationic proteins and vasoactive amines, in the phagocytosis of small particles and bacteria, in atherosclerosis, and in tumor metastasis. Thus, the platelet has become an intriguing component of blood, from a mere fragment of megakaryocyte cytoplasm essential for hemostasis to a biologically important secretory cell that releases a number of proteins with procoagulant, antiheparin, inflammatory, and growth-promoting activities. A brief description of various platelet functions is presented here.

Hemostasis

The main function of platelets is in hemostasis. An adequate number of functional platelets is essential for arresting hemorrhage after vascular injury and for preventing the diapedesis of red cells from seemingly uninjured vessels. Larger and younger platelets are more active in this respect. An abnormality of the hemostatic function of platelets characteristically results in increased bleeding time and purpura.

Platelets do not adhere to each other or to capillary endothelium under normal conditions. This lack of adherence is partly attributable to the thrombin-triggered production of PGI_2, a powerful inhibitor of platelet adherence and aggregation, by the normal endothelium. The denudation of capillary endothelium, with exposure of subendothelial collagen, immediately attracts platelets and triggers them to undergo a series of complex physical and biochemical changes that lead to the formation of a hemostatic plug (Fig. 6–12). Vasoconstriction, induced by neurohormonal mechanisms, is insufficient per se to prevent hemorrhage. The platelets at first undergo a shape change to spiny spheres and then begin to adhere to the site of injury.

Platelets also adhere to exposed basement membrane and elastic fibers. Adhesion to collagen in vitro requires the presence of calcium ions and vWF, but calcium is not required for adhesion to noncollagenous surfaces. Platelet adhesion to injured endothelium is effected through their surface receptors for collagen (GPIa) and vWF (GPIb and GPIIb-IIIa). Adhesion is followed by the release of platelet granule contents. The release reaction promotes the aggregation of assembled platelets and the accumulation of more platelets, and thus a chain reaction sets in to form a covering mass to arrest bleeding. Platelet aggregation is a basic response to the release of ADP in the presence of calcium. The ADP initially comes from the injured vessel wall and then from the platelets themselves through the degradation of ATP by ATPase. Activated platelets also synthesize and release several prostaglandins and thromboxanes from arachidonic acid. TxA_2 is the most potent platelet-aggregating agent and inducer of release reaction. Thus, a self-contained means of continuing platelet aggregation exists until an adequate mass has formed over the site of damage to the vessel wall.

Initially, the hemostatic plug is loosely constructed and cannot arrest bleeding. Fusion of the platelet mass follows, which forms a solid plug through the process of viscous metamorphosis brought about by the action of thrombin. Injury to the vessel wall and the availability of platelet factor 3 (PF-3) and other platelet coagulants activate the intrinsic system of coagulation at the site of injury. Thromboplastin (Tp) released from the injured vessel triggers activation of the extrinsic system of coagulation, leading to the conversion of prothrombin (factor II) to thrombin (factor IIa). In addition to causing viscous fusion of the platelets, thrombin acts on the fibrinogen present on the platelet surface and converts it to a lattice of fibrin

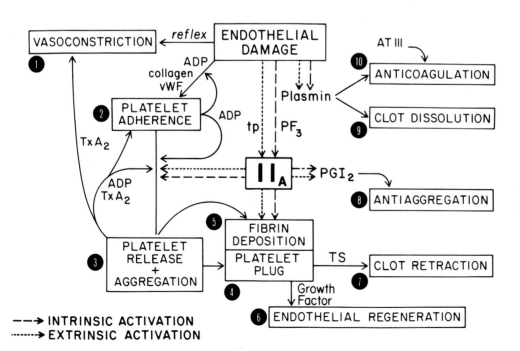

Fig. 6–12. Schematic representation of a series of complex reactions associated with hemostasis at the site of a vascular injury. See text for details. (From Jain, N. C.: Schalm's Veterinary Hematology. 4th Ed. Philadelphia, Lea & Febiger, 1986, p. 457.)

strands that extends throughout the plug. The fibrin strands interconnect the platelet pseudopods. Thrombosthenin (TS), a contractile protein released from the platelets, further strengthens the hemostatic plug by pulling the fibrin strands taut, thereby producing clot retraction. This same action occurs in blood removed from the body, leading to shrinkage of the clot and separation of serum. Clot retraction requires viable platelets with an intact energy metabolism and depends on the reaction between ATP and TS. In the absence of platelets, separation of serum from the clot does not occur in shed blood. Thus, a simple test for thrombocytopenia is the clot retraction test. Clot retraction also depends on the fibrinogen concentration. In thrombocytopenia, the blood clot that forms at the site of injury remains soft or gel-like, and is less effective in sealing a damaged vessel. Bleeding time may therefore be prolonged in severe thrombocytopenia. Blood vessel wall abnormalities and functional defects of platelets are also associated with similar abnormalities in hemostasis.

Vascular Integrity

The integrity of capillary endothelium depends on an adequate supply of circulating platelets. Petechiae, ecchymoses, and bleeding from body orifices may accompany severe thrombocytopenia. Erythrocytes escape from intact vessels in thrombocytopenic individuals by squeezing through the weakened endothelial cells. An almost straight-line relationship exists between platelet count and bleeding time. The transfusion of fresh platelets prevents bleeding by strengthening the endothelium of blood vessels. The incorporation of platelet material into capillary endothelium has been demonstrated in ultrastructural and autoradiographic studies.

Blood Coagulation

Platelets arrest bleeding from an injured vessel, not only by formation of a primary hemostatic (platelet) plug but also by promoting the production of the secondary hemostatic (fibrin) plug through the generation of thrombin. Almost all plasma coagulation factors are found in association with platelets. More important, various platelet proteins and lipoproteins, designated as platelet factors 1 through 4, play a significant role in blood coagulation (Table 6–1). The best known is PF-3, which acts as an accelerator of the coagulation process. It participates during the interaction of coagulation factors IXa and VIIIa and of Xa and Va to generate thrombin from prothrombin (see Fig. 5–3). The platelet surface membrane probably provides the reaction site for such an in vivo interaction. Platelets can promote the proteolytic activation of factors XI, XII, and XIII by kallikrein and of factor XI by factor XII-dependent and/or factor XII-independent mechanisms. Stimulated platelets may also secrete a factor that inhibits the activation of factor IX by factor XIa.

Clotted blood in vitro separates into serum and a compact clot. This phenomenon of clot retraction requires the presence of platelets. The force necessary for the fibrin meshwork to retract is provided by platelet thrombosthenin through the transmembrane GPIIb-IIIa complex, which binds to the ends of fibrin strands in the clot. The tensile strength of fibrin is increased by factor XIIIa, which enzymatically cross-links fibrin within the clot.

See Chapter 5 for additional information on the role of platelets in blood coagulation.

Inflammation and Tissue Damage

Platelets probably play a dual role in the inflammatory response. The release of platelet vasoactive substances and other substances (e.g., prostaglandins, cationic proteins, collagenase, elastase, histamine, serotonin, and a chemotactinogen) may initiate or contribute to persistence of an inflammatory response and influence tissue repair (de Gaetano et al., 1989). Some of these factors are also tissue-damaging. For example, prostaglandins have been implicated as mediators of tissue damage in many forms of renal disease.

Neutrophils and macrophages at the inflammatory site may promote the platelet release reaction. The myeloperoxidase-hydrogen peroxide-halide system of activated neutrophils can induce the release of platelet constituents at the site of inflammation. A platelet-activating factor, elaborated by neutrophils and macrophages, has been found to induce platelet aggregation and the release reaction. Thrombospondin released from activated platelets mediates bacterial adherence to tissues during inflammation and infection (Herrman et al., 1991).

Platelets were also found to exert some anti-inflammatory effects in studies of acute inflammation in rats. Platelets accumulated at the site of experimental inflammation and the inflammatory response was significantly enhanced in thrombocytopenic rats.

Phagocytic and Bactericidal Properties

Chicken thrombocytes were found to phagocytize bacteria and particulate matter. Human platelets have been found to phagocytize bacteria and latex particles. These materials were internalized through the OCS and not by pseudopod formation. Phagocytosis by leukocytes involves pseudopod formation, which is *not* the case with platelets. The process appears to be energy-dependent, but is not accompanied by degranulation. Platelets also bind endotoxin, possibly to detoxify and clear it from plasma.

β-Lysin, a thermostable bactericidal component of serum, has been localized in platelets and is secreted during blood coagulation, inflammation, antigen-antibody reactions, and bacteremia. It has been conjectured that platelet β-lysin plays a major role in maintaining sterile conditions in the body. β-Lysin is bactericidal to certain bacteria (Bacillus subtilis) and damaging to others (Escherichia coli). It can amplify the antibody and complement-mediated killing and lysis of gram-negative bacteria. A platelet-derived cationic protein (MW, 8,500) was found to have a potent bactericidal activity against Staphylococcus aureus (Yeaman et al., 1992).

In view of these platelet functions in host defense, it has been suggested that thrombocytopenic patients could be given a prophylactic transfusion therapy to enhance their resistance to bacterial infection.

Thrombosis

Arterial or white thrombi are composed primarily of platelets because of the high shear forces of circulating blood. Platelets are selectively consumed, but the fibrinogen level remains normal. Such thrombi may be seen in cerebral vascular disease, diabetes mellitus, and renal vascular disease. The selective consumption of platelets can be prevented by inhibitors of platelet function such as dipyridamole and sulfinpyrazone, but not by heparin. Venous or red thrombi involve the combined and equivalent consumption of both platelets and fibrinogen. These thrombi are composed of platelets, fibrin, and red cells because of low shear flow. Such thrombi are found in pulmonary embolisms and malignancy-induced deep venous thrombosis. Venous thrombosis may be prevented by heparin or warfarin, but not by drugs that inhibit platelet functions (see Chap. 5 for further details).

Atherosclerosis

Platelets contribute to the development of atherosclerosis by inflicting damage to the vascular endothelium through chemical mediators released after platelet activation and by initiating the proliferation of smooth muscle cells in the arterial wall (Seiss, 1990). A platelet-derived growth factor (PDGF) has been incriminated in the development of atherosclerotic lesions because of its mitogenic activity for smooth muscles and fibroblasts (Tennant and McGeachie, 1991). In addition, PDGF is chemotactic for monocytes and neutrophils. Macrophages also secrete potent stimulators of mitogenesis for cells such as fibroblasts and smooth muscles. Myelofibrosis in acute megakaryocytic leukemia has been associated with the local release of α-granule components from megakaryocytes in the bone marrow.

Role in Tumor Metastasis

Based on in vitro and in vivo experimental studies, it has been suggested that platelets play a role in the sequestration, adherence, and penetration of tumor cells through the vascular endothelium. Aggregated platelets prevent rapid clearance of tumor cells from the circulation, promote adherence to endothelial surface, and allow extravascular formation of nests of cells. Tumor cells can cause platelet aggregation and antiplatelet agents have been found to decrease tumor metastasis in laboratory animals (Tzanakakis et al., 1991).

PATHOLOGIC ASPECTS

Abnormalities of Megakaryocytes

Pathologic abnormalities of megakaryocytes can usually be attributed to myeloproliferative syndromes, toxic or infectious agents, and immune mechanisms. Various abnormalities include changes in the proportion of different maturative stages, altered cell size, and nuclear and cytoplasmic abnormalities. For example, degenerative changes such as cytoplasmic vacuolation and karyorrhexis may be seen in megakaryocytes in patients with immune-mediated thrombocytopenia (Fig. 6–13), and reduced ploidy and micromegakaryocytes may be seen in those with hematopoietic neoplasias or dysplasias (Plates XXI-3 and XXI-4). Antigenic cross-reactivity between platelets and megakaryocytes, although it may be incomplete, causes the antibody-mediated cytopathologic changes seen in megakaryocytes in dogs with immune-mediated thrombocytopenia.

A rare form of acute megakaryoblastic leukemia, classified as M7 by FAB (French-American-British) criteria (see Chap. 19), with circulating micromegakaryocytes has been reported in humans and dogs. These micromegakaryocytes may be confused with lymphoblasts and myeloblasts because of their ambiguous morphologic features in Wright-stained blood and bone marrow films. They are usually identified by positivity for specific platelet antigens (GPIIb-IIIa), acetylcholinesterase, and platelet peroxidase. Micromegakaryocytes and megakaryoblasts have been found in the blood and bone marrow of dogs with radiation-induced acute megakaryocytic leukemias (Plates XXI-3 and XXI-4).

Megakaryocytes may exhibit emperipolesis (transmigration) of neutrophils or other leukocytes (Fig. 6–14) as a rare, nonspecific phenomenon. It involves active penetration by the migrating cell. The frequency is less than 0.3% in young rats, 2 to 5% in 18- to 24-month old rats, and markedly increased in rats with hyperplastic bone marrow secondary to chronic suppurative or neoplastic lesions (Lee, 1989).

Qualitative and Quantitative Platelet Disorders

Platelet disorders are broadly categorized as quantitative or qualitative. Quantitative disorders include

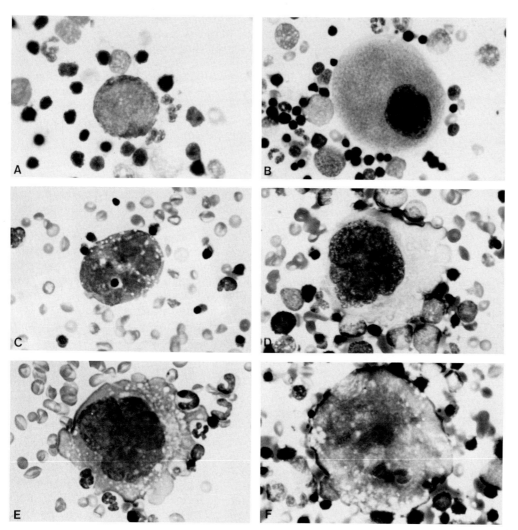

Fig. 6–13. Normal canine promegakaryocyte *(A)* and megakaryocyte *(B)* are compared with promegakaryocyte *(C)* and megakaryocytes *(D,E,F)* from dogs with autoimmune thrombocytopenia. Note morphologic abnormalities such as karyolysis *(F)*, cytoplasmic vacuolation *(C,E,F)*, and deficiency in *(F)* or lack of *(D,E)* cytoplasmic granularity, (Wright's stain; × 700). (From Jain, N. C.: Schalm's Veterinary Hematology. 4th Ed. Philadelphia, Lea & Febiger, 1986, p. 434.)

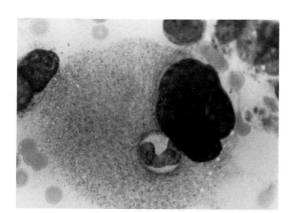

Fig. 6–14. Canine bone marrow showing emperipolesis (transmigration) of a neutrophil metamyelocyte through the cytoplasm of a mature megakaryocyte, (Wright's stain; × 900). (From Jain, N. C.: Schalm's Veterinary Hematology. 4th Ed. Philadelphia, Lea & Febiger, 1986, p. 435.)

thrombocytopenia (subnormal number of platelets) and thrombocytosis (above-normal number of platelets). Thrombocytopenia is the most common platelet abnormality encountered, and is probably the most common cause of hemorrhagic diathesis, both in humans and animals. Thrombocytosis, whether physiologic or reactive, occurs less frequently. A primary proliferative disorder of megakaryocytes in the bone marrow, associated with tremendous thrombocytosis, is known as essential thrombocythemia; it has been reported in humans but rarely in animals. Qualitative or functional disorders include rare hereditary abnormalities and more common acquired defects, thrombasthenia and thrombopathia. Thrombasthenia is a specific defect of platelet aggregation by ATP and thrombopathia is a general term describing functional defects of platelets. Abnormalities of both platelet number and function may occur simultaneously, as in cases of kidney disease with uremia, liver disease, and myeloproliferative disorders, such as chronic myelogenous leukemia and essential thrombocythemia.

Both qualitative and quantitative platelet disorders may arise because of primary abnormalities in megakaryocytes or platelets (primary platelet disorders) or as a consequence of other diseases (secondary platelet disorders). These platelet disorders may also be accompanied by abnormal platelet morphology.

The finding of abnormal platelets in Wright-stained blood films may be the first clue of a disturbance of thrombopoiesis or platelet function. For example, megathrombocytes (large platelets) usually occur in reactive or compensatory thrombocytoses and myeloproliferative disorders, particularly in cats, whereas microthrombocytes (small platelets) are found in iron deficiency anemia and in idiopathic or immune-mediated thrombocytopenia. Megathrombocytes may occasionally be found in normal animals. Platelet volume determination using an electronic particle counter is a reliable means of detecting megathrombocytes and microthrombocytes in the blood. Platelet volume measurements for dogs should be carried out on citrated blood samples kept at 37° C, because blood collected in EDTA and kept at 4° C may show a spurious increase in platelet volume as a result of changes in platelet morphology, from a smooth disk to an irregular sphere with filopodia (Handagama et al, 1986).

FUNCTIONAL AND/OR MORPHOLOGIC DEFECTS

Defects of platelet function may be hereditary or acquired. These disorders vary in severity, often involve multiple functional abnormalities, and may stem from extrinsic abnormalities or defects of the morphologic and biochemical components of the platelets or megakaryocytes. Clinical manifestations referable to platelet dysfunction, however, are generally similar.

Morphologic alterations, such as sphering, budding, and pseudopod formation, occur in platelets coming in contact with nonphysiologic surfaces or after storage at low temperatures (Fig. 6–3F). These changes can be attributed to the disintegration and disappearance of microtubules. The exposure of platelets to aggregating agents causes extensive surface and ultrastructural changes, which lead to the secretion of internal contents into the external milieu.

A functional platelet disorder may be suspected when an increased tendency to bleed (petechia, ecchymosis, and purpura) and/or prolonged bleeding times are observed in the presence of a normal or increased platelet count. Early onset in life and familial occurrence indicate a hereditary disorder. The initial evaluation of a patient with a bleeding diathesis includes platelet count, examination of blood film for platelet distribution and morphology, bleeding time, and screening tests to rule out coagulation abnormalities. Further evaluation includes tests for platelet adherence, aggregation, secretion, and availability of platelet phospholipid.

Von Willebrand disease (vWD) is not actually a platelet disorder. The increased bleeding tendency in this disorder is ascribed to the absence of vWF:Ag; because of this, platelets do not adhere adequately to injured blood vessels and to glass beads.

Hereditary Disorders. Several hereditary disorders of platelet morphology and/or specific functional abnormalities have been found in humans (Williams et al., 1990). Some of the more common disorders are summarized here, but similar information about such disorders in animals is limited.

Microthrombocytes are seen in Wiskott-Aldrich syndrome, a hereditary disorder of male children characterized by thrombocytopenia and increased susceptibility to infection. These platelets are deficient in α granules, dense bodies, mitochondria, adenine nucleotides, and serotonin.

Platelets of patients with Glanzmann's thrombasthenia show defective adhesiveness or aggregation resulting from a lack of GPIIIa and a markedly reduced amount of GPIIb. These platelets are also deficient in fibrinogen and α-actinin. Glanzmann's thrombasthenia is an autosomal recessive disorder. A hereditary disorder resembling Glanzmann's thrombasthenia has been described in dogs, and a hereditary thrombopathia with an autosomal inheritance pattern and markedly abnormal platelet function has been described in basset hounds. The rate and extent of ADP-induced and collagen-induced aggregation of platelets were significantly depressed. Bleeding time was slightly prolonged, clot retraction was normal, and no platelet glycoprotein abnormality was detectable.

Bernard-Soulier syndrome is an autosomal recessive bleeding disorder characterized by a mild thrombocytopenia, a prolonged bleeding time, and giant platelets that are not aggregated by ristocetin, human or bovine factor VIII, or bovine fibrinogen. The platelets of these patients lack GPIb, a receptor for vWF, resulting in a defective adhesion of platelets to subendothelial surfaces. GPIb is normal in the platelets of patients with von Willebrand disease (vWD) and Glanzmann's thrombasthenia. The platelets also lack α granules and contain disorganized microtubules.

Platelets of patients with "gray platelet syndrome" are devoid of morphologically recognizable α granules and contain numerous vacuoles, so they acquire peculiar gray staining in Wright-stained blood films. Similarly, megakaryocytes lack α granules. Some studies have indicated that gray platelets contain a 140,000-dalton protein, normally present in α-granule membranes, in the membranes of the cytoplasmic vacuoles, and that this protein is expressed on the surface of thrombin-stimulated platelets. Thus, the basic defect seems to be the inability of megakaryocytes to transfer endogenously synthesized secretory proteins into the membrane-bound α granules so that they can acquire normal tinctorial properties.

Hermansky-Pudlak syndrome is an autosomal recessive disorder characterized by bleeding diathesis and impaired in vitro platelet functions. A marked reduction in or absence of dense bodies occurs, and low levels of serotonin and of the nonmetabolic pool of adenine nucleotides are present.

Chédiak Higashi syndrome occurs as an autosomal recessive disorder in cattle, mink, and cats. Platelets of these animals are almost devoid of dense bodies and show a marked deficiency of the storage pool of adenine nucleotides and of serotonin. Granulocytes characteristically contain giant lysosomal granules that are considered diagnostic of the syndrome. Platelets generally lack such giant granules. The platelets of cats with the Chédiak-Higashi syndrome have a storage pool deficiency and almost no dense granules as a result of similar defects in their megakaryocytes (Menard et al., 1990). These cats show abnormal hemostasis, with a prolonged bleeding time but a normal coagulation time. Their platelets show abnormal in vitro aggregation, as do platelets of affected mink and cattle.

A storage pool deficiency involving a large decrease in the dense bodies of platelets was found in a breeding colony of pigs homozygous and heterozygous for vWD. Pigs homozygous for vWD were characterized by extremely low levels of vWD:Ag and ristocetin cofactor (RCof), low levels of factor VIII, bleeding times longer than 15 minutes, and a severe bleeding tendency. Pigs heterozygous for vWD (vWD carriers) had low mean values of vWF:Ag and RCof, normal levels of factor VIII, normal bleeding times, and no bleeding tendency. Pigs with storage pool deficiency had factor VIII, vWF:Ag, and RCof levels similar to those of vWD carriers, but in contrast, had bleeding times of greater than or equal to 15 minutes and a severe bleeding tendency. The mode of inheritance was autosomal recessive (Daniels et al., 1986).

Acquired Disorders. Acquired functional disorders of platelets, with or without hemorrhagic manifestations, have been described in humans with various diseases, including systemic disorders such as kidney disease with uremia, liver disease, immune-mediated disorders such as systemic lupus erythematosus, or disseminated intravascular coagulation (DIC), myeloproliferative and lymphoproliferative disorders, dysproteinemias such as Waldenström's macroglobulinemia and plasma cell myeloma, and therapy with certain drugs, particularly nonsteroidal anti-inflammatory drugs (NSAIDs) that affect platelet functions (Williams et al., 1990). Similar abnormalities seem to occur in animals, but they have not been as well documented (Jain, 1986). Platelet activity is enhanced in heartworm-infected dogs (Boudreaux et al., 1989).

Acquired platelet functional disorders are multifactorial, but essentially involve defects of platelet activation, adherence, aggregation, and release reaction because of abnormal substances in the plasma or an acquired structural abnormality. Platelet abnormalities in patients with kidney disease include reduced in vivo adhesiveness to endothelium and in vitro defects of adherence, aggregation, platelet phospholipid availability, and clot retraction. These platelet abnormalities are ascribed not to urea but to its metabolites, guanidinosuccinic and phenolic acids. Decreased production of prostaglandin endoperoxides by platelets and increased production of PGI_2, an inhibitor of platelet adhesion and aggregation, by the blood vessels of uremic patients are thought to act synergistically and contribute to bleeding tendencies in such patients. Intensive dialysis, the administration of desmopressin, a vasopressin analogue that causes the release of vWF from tissue stores such as endothelial cells, and infusion of cryoprecipitate have been used to correct the bleeding diathesis in uremic patients.

Patients with liver disease may show similar functional abnormalities of platelets and, in some cases, thrombocytopenia may also be present. Bleeding diathesis associated with severe liver disease may also involve the decreased production of coagulation factors, dysfibrinogenemia, fibrinolysis, and DIC.

Both hemostatic and in vitro abnormalities of platelets in dysproteinemias are generally proportional to the amount of paraprotein in the circulation, and are largely correctable by plasmapheresis. It is believed that myeloma proteins and macroglobulins coat platelet surfaces and nonspecifically result in decreased platelet adhesiveness, aggregation, and secretion. Platelet abnormalities in myeloproliferative disorders include defective adhesiveness, aggregation, and availability of platelet phospholipid, as well as abnormal morphology. Abnormalities of the coagulation system are also present in some cases. It has been reported that some human patients may paradoxically develop both thrombotic and bleeding complications because of qualitative defects in platelets.

Drug-induced platelet functional defects are mainly related to a derangement of arachidonic acid metabolism. Patients receiving such drugs in large doses may show prolonged bleeding times with or without a bleeding diathesis. NSAIDs, such as aspirin, indomethacin, and phenylbutazone, inhibit cyclo-oxygenase activity, thereby curtailing the production of TxA_2, a potent agonist of platelet aggregation. The defect caused by aspirin is irreversible, persisting for the life of the platelet, but that caused by indomethacin and phenylbutazone is transient. Sulfinpyrazone probably acts as a competitive inhibitor of cyclo-oxygenase, but its mechanism of action is largely unknown. Dipyridamole inhibits phosphodiesterase, thus increasing the intracellular level of cAMP, which inhibits TxA_2. Because these drugs interfere with platelet function, they are often used in the treatment of arterial thrombosis and for other conditions ascribed to hyperaggregability of platelets.

QUANTITATIVE DISORDERS

Platelet counts vary among species (Table 6–3). Platelet counts in small laboratory animals exceed 1 million/μl and those in domestic animals are generally below 1 million/μl. Age and sex have little influence on platelet counts. Platelet counts are lower in the newborn, but normal adult values are reached at about 3 months of age.

Thrombocytosis. Thrombocytosis may occur because of a physiologic response, may be secondary to a disease process, or may be autonomous because of a neoplastic process. The increase in platelet count in

124   ESSENTIALS OF VETERINARY HEMATOLOGY

Table 6–3. Normal Platelet Numbers in Various Animals

Animal Species	Platelet Count/μl of Blood Range	Mean
Dog	200,000–500,000	300,000
Cat	300,000–800,000	450,000
Cow	100,000–800,000	500,000
Sheep	250,000–750,000	400,000
Goat	300,000–600,000	450,000
Horse	100,000–350,000	225,000
Pig	100,000–900,000	520,000

patients with thrombocytosis is usually modest, of short duration, and asymptomatic. Sometimes substantially high platelet counts, particularly greater than 1 million/μl, may be encountered, which could endanger life by thromboembolism. Generally, a mild thrombocytosis is more prevalent than marked increases in platelet numbers, as shown in Figure 6–15 for the dog. Fictitious hyperkalemia occurs in dogs with thrombocytosis and thrombocythemia as a result of the release of intracellular potassium from platelets during the clotting process (Mandell et al., 1988; Reimann et al., 1989). In such cases, plasma rather than serum should be used to measure potassium concentration.

Physiologic thrombocytosis is usually transient and results from the increased mobilization of platelets from splenic and nonsplenic body pools. The nonsplenic (largely pulmonary) pool is mobilized during mild muscular activity, whereas epinephrine injection mobilizes the splenic pool. Platelets from both pools are mobilized during vigorous physical activity. Species variation, however, may be found in this regard. Transient thrombocytosis also occurs during pregnancy and during the growth period of many species of mammals.

Reactive or secondary thrombocytosis is seen in association with various conditions, including acute or chronic inflammatory conditions, acute hemorrhage, iron deficiency anemia, hemolytic anemia, malignancies, severe trauma and fractures, postsurgery, splenectomy, asplenic or hyposplenic state, Cushing's disease, and therapy with glucocorticoids and Vinca alkaloids (Tables 6–4 and 6–5). In dogs and cats, the most common disease categories associated with thrombocytosis were neoplasia (25%), gastrointestinal disorders (19%), and endocrine disorders (10%), and the most common drug classes were corticosteroids and antineoplastic agents (Hammer, 1991).

Platelet production in reactive thrombocytosis increases because of increases in plasma levels of thrombopoietin. The megakaryocyte number increases in the bone marrow and the platelet count is directly proportional to the megakaryocytic mass. Reactive thrombocytosis is prolonged, lasting from days to weeks, whereas physiologic thrombocytosis is transient, peaking in about 15 minutes and returning to baseline level in about 30 minutes. Platelet survival time is normal or decreases and platelet function tests are

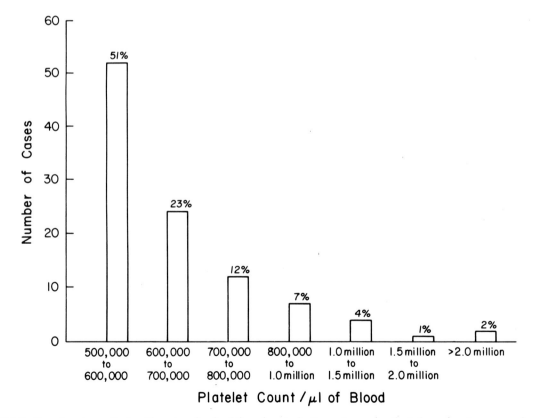

Fig. 6–15. Distribution of canine patients with various levels of thrombocytosis. Percentages of patients in each category are shown above the bar graphs. (From Jain, N. C.: Schalm's Veterinary Hematology. 4th Ed. Philadelphia, Lea & Febiger, 1986, p. 471.)

Table 6–4. Selected Examples of Thrombocytosis in the Dog, Cat, and Horse

Animal	Platelet Count/μl of Blood	Clinical Diagnosis or Finding
Dog	200,000–500,000	Normal range
	2,073,000	Vincristine and immunosuppressive therapy for autoimmune thrombocytopenia
	1,988,000	Suppurative bronchitis and enteritis
	1,148,000	Iron deficiency anemia
	828,000	Iron deficiency anemia
	755,000	Cushing's disease
	738,000	Squamous cell carcinoma
	737,000	Adenocarcinoma
	713,000	Prednisolone and immunosuppressive therapy for autoimmune hemolytic anemia
	673,000	Mastocytoma
	618,000	Nasal trauma
	613,000	Chronic inflammation or infection
Cat	300,000–800,000	Normal range
	2,046,000	Lymphocytic leukemia
	1,470,000	Anemia and bleeding disorder
	1,432,000	Mast cell sarcoma
	1,378,000	Myelogenous leukemia
	1,256,000	Myeloproliferative disorder
	1,163,000	Six days posttherapy for thrombocytopenia
	876,000	Erythremic myelosis
	872,000	Lymphocytic leukemia
Horse	100,000–350,000	Normal range
	632,000	Pleuritis
	611,000	Foal pneumonia
	510,000	Fluctuating temperature
	474,000	Combined immune deficiency
	472,000	CNS ataxia, abscess
	450,000	Strangles
	405,000	Pleuritis; heparin therapy for DIC

usually normal. Therapy is directed at the primary disease causing the thrombocytosis.

An extensive study of the diagnostic value of platelet counts on 6294 blood samples from 3172 adult mammals of more than 200 different species revealed that reactive thrombocytosis associated with bacterial infection often parallels neutrophilia in those species of mammals whose neutrophils respond well to bacterial infection (Hawkey et al., 1990). In some cases, particularly in the bovine and other species whose neutrophil response to bacterial infection is minimal, the platelet count may be more useful than the neutrophil count for identifying and following the course of a bacterial infection.

Table 6–5. Postsplenectomy Thrombocytosis in a Dog with an Idiopathic Anemia

Status	Platelet Count/μl of Blood
Presplenectomy	377,000
Postsplenectomy	
1 days	1,197,000
5 days	1,395,000
12 days	1,305,000
26 days	1,061,000
40 days	617,000

Autonomous thrombocytosis is a myeloproliferative disorder. It occurs as a primary disease of the bone marrow, (e.g., essential thrombocythemia; see below) or in association with other hematopoietic neoplastic diseases (e.g., polycythemia vera, chronic myelogenous leukemia).

Essential Thrombocythemia. Essential thrombocythemia, autonomous or primary thrombocythemia, or megakaryocytic leukemia is a hemorrhagic syndrome associated with marked increases in circulating platelets (>1 million/μl of blood) resulting from the neoplastic proliferation of megakaryocytes. The disease is characterized by recurrent spontaneous hemorrhages, purpura, epistaxis, gastrointestinal bleeding, splenomegaly, abnormalities of platelet morphology and function, thromboembolic episodes, and pseudohyperkalemia (Degen et al., 1989; Hopper et al., 1989). Morphologic abnormalities of megakaryocytes may also occur (Tablin et al., 1989). Therapy is directed toward reducing the platelet count by plateletpheresis, irradiation, and the use of alkylating and antimitotic agents (Smith and Turrel, 1989).

Thrombocytopenia. Pathophysiologic mechanisms of thrombocytopenia include decreased production, accelerated destruction or utilization, abnormal distribution, and excessive loss of platelets from the body (Tables 6–6 and 6–7). The first two are more common and occasionally more than one mechanism may be involved. Selected examples are given for platelet counts in thrombocytopenic dogs, cats, and horses (Table 6–8) and for the distribution of platelet counts in thrombocytopenic dogs (Fig. 6–16).

An epidemiologic survey of thrombocytopenia in 987 dogs revealed immune-mediated thrombocytopenia in 5%, neoplasia-associated thrombocytopenia in

Table 6–6. Pathophysiologic Classification of Thrombocytopenia

Decreased platelet production
  Hereditary: Wiskott-Aldrich syndrome, May-Hegglin anomaly
  Congenital: pancytopenia resulting from marrow aplasia (Fanconi's syndrome), amegakaryocytic thrombocytopenia with congenital malformations
  Acquired: drug toxicity; x-irradiation, mycotoxins, viral, rickettsial, or protozoan infection, renal disease, pregnancy, cyclic thrombocytopenia, selective aplasia of megakaryocytes
  Dysthrombopoiesis: vitamin B_{12} or folate deficiency, uremia, myeloproliferative disorders, myelophthisis, aplastic anemia, severe iron deficiency, protozoan parasites
  Defective thrombopoietin production
  Miscellaneous
Accelerated platelet destruction or utilization
  Immune mediated: autoimmune, isoimmune, or neonatal, in association with other immune-mediated disorders, bacterial, viral, rickettsial, or protozoan infection, drug-induced and other causes such as neoplasia
  Nonimmune: anaphylaxis, DIC, microangiopathies, acute bacterial or viral infection, uremia, transfusion of stored blood, cirrhosis
  Structural defects of platelets: Glanzmann's thrombasthenia, other hereditary or acquired defects
Abnormal distribution
  Splenomegaly, hypothermia, neoplasia
Excessive loss from blood
  Massive blood loss, exchange blood transfusion

Table 6–7.   Causes of Thrombocytopenia in Different Species

Species	Causes
Cats	Lymphoma, myeloproliferative disorders, ribavirin, DIC, immune-mediated thrombocytopenia, immune-mediated hemolytic anemia, feline leukemia virus infection, septicemia, squamous cell carcinoma
Cattle	DIC, bracken fern poisoning, trichloroethylene poisoning, furazolidone, food additives, toxic fungi, East Coast fever, bovine viral diarrhea virus, and Trypanosoma congolense, T. vivax, and T. lawrencei
Dogs	Lymphoma, ehrlichiosis (Ehrlichia canis, E. platys), experimental Rocky mountain spotted fever, infectious canine hepatitis virus, distemper vaccination, endotoxin, peritonitis, dapsone therapy, myasthenia gravis, immune-mediated thrombocytopenia, immune-mediated hemolytic anemia, levamisole, antibiotics and sulfonamide, splenomegaly, estrogen, DIC, chronic hepatopathy, myelogenous leukemia, hemangiosarcoma and other neoplasias, Addison's disease
Horses	Marrow hypoplasia, equine infectious anemia, septicemia, epistaxis, ehrlichiosis, idiopathic immune-mediated thrombocytopenia, immune-mediated hemolytic anemia, myelogenous leukemia, DIC
Pigs	Neonatal thrombocytopenia, swine fever, hog cholera, DIC, endotoxic shock, anaphylaxis with ovalbumin
Sheep	Radiation, tick infection with Amblyomma variegatum and Hyalomma rufipes, amprolium poisoning, Stachybotrys alternans-contaminated hay
Water buffaloes	T. lawrencei

13%, inflammatory or infectious thrombocytopenia in 23%, and miscellaneous thrombocytopenia in 59% of cases (Grindem et al., 1991). Dogs with immune-mediated thrombocytopenia had significantly lower platelet counts (mean, 36,760 ± 50,288/µl) than dogs in the other three groups, and Doberman pinschers were overrepresented in all groups except the former.

Idiopathic thrombocytopenic purpura is defined as thrombocytopenia associated with purpuric lesions in the absence of a defined cause, and with normal or increased numbers of megakaryocytes in the bone marrow. A compensated thrombocytopenic state exists when an increase in platelet destruction is present but platelet counts are within the normal range. This may be seen in conditions such as cirrhosis, systemic lupus erythematosus, and chronic DIC. Platelet life span is shortened and the platelet turnover rate is increased in such cases.

Diagnostic evaluation of a thrombocytopenic patient involves clinical evaluation for bleeding, determination of platelet count, examination of Wright-stained blood films for platelet distribution and morphology, and examination of the bone marrow for megakaryocyte number and morphology. Platelet function tests and survival studies may be performed, if necessary.

A crude estimate of platelet count may be made from the stained blood film; when platelets are uniformly distributed, one platelet/oil immersion field (100×) generally equals 20,000 platelets/µl of blood. It should be realized that platelet counts performed by hemocytometer techniques may be in error by as

much as 25%. Platelet counts determined with an electronic counter are much more accurate. Low platelet counts may be artifactual, resulting from antibody-mediated clumping of platelets in vitro and from platelet satellitism (platelet adherence to neutrophils) or rosette formation (platelet adherence to lymphocytes and monocytes), particularly in EDTA-anticoagulated blood. Pseudothrombocytopenia may also occur from macrothrombocytosis, particularly if an inadequate threshold is used for the electronic enumeration of platelets. Such spurious thrombocytopenias can be confirmed by the examination of a well-prepared blood film, and are not associated with systemic signs of thrombocytopenia.

Platelet distribution width, obtained by the use of an electronic counter, provides useful information about mean platelet volume (MPV). The MPV in humans is increased in thrombocytopenias resulting from increased platelet destruction, dysthrombocytopoiesis associated with acute or chronic myelogenous leukemias, and abnormalities of megakaryocyte fragmentation. Microthrombocytosis has been observed in dogs suspected of having immune-mediated thrombocytopenia (IMT) (Northern and Tvedten, 1992).

Table 6–8.   Selected Examples of Thrombocytopenia in the Dog, Cat, and Horse

Animal	Platelet Count/µl of Blood	Clinical Diagnosis, Finding, or Suspected Cause
Dog	200,000–500,000	Normal range
	0	Sulfonamides, antibiotics
	5,000	Estrogen toxicity
	6,000	Ehrlichiosis
	7,000	Autoimmune thrombocytopenia
	10,000	Consumption coagulopathy
	21,000	Myelogenous leukemia
	34,000	Autoimmune thrombocytopenia
	40,000	Splenomegaly
	47,000	Hemangiosarcoma
	64,000	Acute exacerbation of chronic hepatopathy
	102,000	Lymphosarcoma
	131,000	Addison's disease
	170,000	Autoimmune hemolytic anemia and thrombocytopenia
Cat	300,000–800,000	Normal range
	26,000	Feline leukemia virus infection
	51,000	Myelomonocytic leukemia
	101,000	Lymphosarcoma
	131,000	Autoimmune hemolytic anemia
	139,000	Squamous cell carcinoma
	160,000	Septicemia
	174,000	Erythremic myelosis
	188,000	DIC
Horse	100,000–350,000	Normal range
	11,000	Autoimmune hemolytic anemia
	12,000	Myelogenous leukemia
	19,000	Anemia associated with marrow hypoplasia
	31,000	DIC
	69,000	Salmonellosis with DIC
	53,000	Equine infectious anemia
	56,000	Ehrlichiosis
	61,000	Epistaxis
	88,000	Septicemia

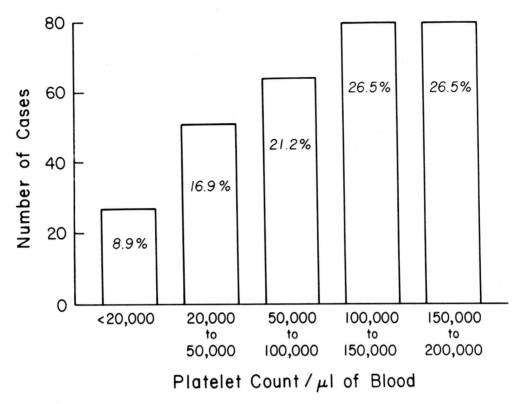

Fig. 6–16.   Distribution of canine patients with various levels of thrombocytopenia. Percentages of patients in each category are shown in the bar graphs. (From Jain, N. C.: Schalm's Veterinary Hematology. 4th Ed. Philadelphia, Lea & Febiger, 1986, p. 475.)

Platelet volume measurements may be influenced by anticoagulation and technical factors, and thus require standardization for accurate clinical application (Waner et al., 1989).

Certain substances released into the plasma from intravascular platelet destruction (e.g., platelet factor 4, β-thromboglobulin) can be measured by sensitive radioimmunoassays. An inverse relationship between β-thromboglobulin and platelet life span has been found in humans.

Bone marrow examination is essential for distinguishing hypoproliferative and hyperdestructive causes of thrombocytopenia. In thrombocytopenia resulting from increased platelet destruction, megakaryocytes are usually abundant, with a normal to left-shifted maturation sequence, and with or without morphologic abnormalities, (see above, Abnormalities of Megakaryocytes, for additional comments).

Decreased platelet production may involve marrow hypoplasia, ineffective thrombopoiesis and, rarely, thrombopoietin deficiency. The platelet life span is usually normal or modestly decreased. The bone marrow megakaryocyte population diminishes in thrombocytopenia from marrow hypoplasia, whereas it increases in thrombocytopenia because of dysthrombopoiesis or ineffective thrombopoiesis. Common causes of marrow hypoplasia are marrow damage by various drugs, chemicals, or x-irradiation. Estrogen toxicity is a classic example in the dog. Myelosuppressive drugs used in cancer chemotherapy can cause thrombocytopenia, depending on the dose and duration of therapy. In humans, marrow hypoplasia or megakaryocytic aplasia may occur rarely as a congenital abnormality. Platelet counts may progressively decrease by 20% during pregnancy, but a thrombocytopenia may not necessarily be evident.

Increased platelet destruction or utilization as a mechanism of thrombocytopenia may involve an immunologic or nonimmunologic process. Platelet survival is markedly reduced, whereas megakaryocytopoiesis increases in some cases but decreases in others. In IMT, antibody-coated platelets are largely removed by cells of the mononuclear phagocyte system, although some destruction may occur intravascularly through complement activation. The formation of autoantibody to platelets may occur for unknown reasons (idiopathic) or may be secondary to a disease or drug therapy. The transfer of maternal antiplatelet antibodies to the fetus or newborn results in isoimmune thrombocytopenia, a situation analogous to neonatal isoerythrolysis. Nonimmunologic thrombocytopenia may occur as a complication of various bacterial, viral, rickettsial, or fungal infections. Thrombocytopenia is an early manifestation of most septicemic bacterial infections. It results from the induction of DIC, direct interaction of micro-organisms with platelets, and/or platelet binding to vascular endothelium damaged by bacterial action. Virus-induced thrombocytopenia may result from decreased megakaryocytopoiesis from the viral invasion of precursor cells in the bone marrow, increased destruction of platelets by the virus or antigen-antibody complexes, or, rarely, may be secondary to DIC (Axthelm and Krakowska, 1987; Edwards et al., 1985).

Abnormal distribution of platelets within the vasculature is a rare cause of thrombocytopenia. Normally, about one-third of the circulating platelet mass is preferentially sequestered in the spleen. During splenomegaly and hypersplenism, abnormal platelet pooling (up to 90%) occurs in the spleen and, in most cases, some shortening of the platelet life span occurs. The degree of thrombocytopenia in such cases is related to the size of the spleen. The thrombocytopenia is caused either by a humoral factor suppressing the marrow or by the accelerated destruction of platelets in the spleen. Splenomegaly is rare in animals, but a few cases have been described in the dog. Splenectomy in these patients corrected the thrombocytopenia and accompanying bleeding problem. Normally, the liver is an important site of platelet pooling, and abnormal portal sequestration may also cause thrombocytopenia. Hypothermia (body temperature, <25° C) causes morphologic changes in platelets and usually results in a transient thrombocytopenia because of abnormal pooling in the spleen, liver, and possibly other sites. Platelets may clump and become trapped in the lungs of dogs or pigs experiencing soft tissue trauma.

Excessive loss of platelets to the level of thrombocytopenia may occur under unusual circumstances of extensive external hemorrhage. Patients undergoing massive transfusion therapy may develop severe thrombocytopenia from inadequate replacement of platelets and reduced production. Extracorporeal perfusion of blood and hemodialysis may cause platelet damage and formation of platelet aggregates, and may lead to a slight to marked thrombocytopenia.

Bleeding Tendency During Thrombocytopenic State. As the circulating platelet number decreases, blood vessel integrity diminishes proportionately and the possibility of the escape of erythrocytes through the capillary walls increases. Bleeding may occur in the form of petechiae and ecchymoses in the tissues, and/or frank blood may appear in the body cavities. Bleeding occurs almost invariably at platelet counts below 10,000/µl of blood, commonly at counts below 20,000, and infrequently at counts below 100,000. In some cases, however, an obvious relation between the platelet count and clinical bleeding is lacking. This dissociation may be the result of variations in accompanied stress, platelet function, and endothelial receptors for platelets.

In addition to a lack of platelets, stress on blood vessels plays a significant role in enhancing bleeding in the thrombocytopenic state (Jain, 1986). This is evidenced by the tissue distribution and location of hemorrhage associated with thrombocytopenia compared to bleeding associated with a coagulation factor abnormality. Purpura and petechiae are observed most commonly in the dog on the skin of the ventral portion of the chest, abdomen, and inner thighs and in the oral mucous membranes (Figs. 6–17, 6–18, and 6–19). These areas of the body are most susceptible to pressure stresses on surface capillaries. Bleeding into the gut also occurs

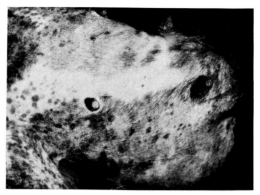

Fig. 6–17. Severe purpura on the ventral thorax and abdomen resulting from an overdose of estradiol cyclo-pentylpropionate for the prevention of pregnancy because of mismating. (From Jain, N. C.: Schalm's Veterinary Hematology. 4th Ed. Philadelphia, Lea & Febiger, 1986, p. 477.)

rather frequently in thrombocytopenic dogs. Vessels close to the surface, with little intervening tissue, are at a disadvantage from comparatively light traumatic influences. Thus, the small vessels running parallel to the surface of the upper respiratory, gastrointestinal, and urogenital tracts are commonly involved in hemorrhagic episodes associated with disorders of hemostasis.

Disorders or Diseases Associated with Thrombocytopenia. Thrombocytopenia has been found in various diseases or disorders in animals (Tables 6–7 and 6–8). A few situations are summarized here.

Estrogen toxicity in the dog may be associated with hemorrhagic purpura (Figs. 6–17 and 6–18), thrombocytopenia, profound leukocytosis followed by leukopenia, and progressive anemia. Bone marrow changes include depressed megakaryocytopoiesis and erythropoiesis and increased neutrophilic granulopoiesis followed by suppressed granulopoiesis. Dogs vary with regard to their sensitivity to changes in platelet and leukocyte numbers. Experimental studies have suggested that platelet counts show an initial increase, with a peak between 5 and 7 days, followed by a precipitous decrease to a level of 50,000/µl on

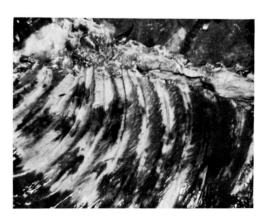

Fig. 6–18. Ecchymotic hemorrhage in the costal pleura of the same dog as presented in Figure 6–17. (From Jain, N. C.: Schalm's Veterinary Hematology. 4th Ed. Philadelphia, Lea & Febiger, 1986, p. 477.)

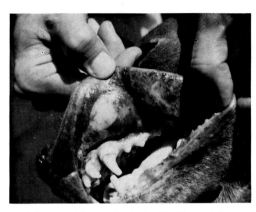

Fig. 6–19. Edema and hemorrhagic foci in the oral tissue of a dog with thrombotic thrombocytopenic purpura. (From Jain, N. C.: Schalm's Veterinary Hematology. 4th Ed. Philadelphia, Lea & Febiger, 1986, p. 480.)

day 13 and persistent thrombocytopenia thereafter. Leukocytosis resulting from neutrophilia and monocytosis develops, with a peak between 17 and 23 days, followed by a rapid decline. The severity and duration of thrombocytopenia and leukopenia seem to be age- and dose-dependent.

Drug sensitivity leading to thrombocytopenia may develop within a few days of initiation of drug therapy. A number of drugs have been implicated in humans, but limited observations have been reported in animals. Discontinuance of the offending drug is rapidly accompanied with return of thrombocyte counts to the normal range. Mechanisms of drug-induced thrombocytopenia include direct bone marrow suppression of megakaryocytopoiesis and the destruction of platelets by immune and nonimmune mechanisms.

Immune-mediated or autoimmune thrombocytopenia has been seen in the dog, cat, and horse. Females and small breeds of dogs, such as poodles and cocker spaniels, appear predisposed to immune-mediated thrombocytopenia (Williams and Maggio-Price, 1984). The pathogenesis of autoantibody formation remains unknown. Presenting clinical complaints and signs of IMT are those of bleeding related to thrombocytopenia. A definitive diagnosis requires the demonstration of antiplatelet antibody, either in serum or associated with circulating platelets or marrow megakaryocytes. In cases in which antiplatelet antibody is not demonstrated, a presumptive diagnosis is made following successful management of thrombocytopenia with corticosteroids or other immunosuppressive drugs. For further details see Chapter 22.

Isoimmune or neonatal thrombocytopenia is a consequence of transfer of maternal antibodies to the newborn either in utero or through the colostrum. A hemorrhagic syndrome of piglets resulting from thrombocytopenia caused by maternal isoimmunization has been described. It was attributed to the transfer of isoantibodies against the platelets through colostrum consumption. Thrombocytopenia developed within a few days or weeks after birth, but

generally a spontaneous recovery occurred. The affected animals developed prominent, generalized petechial and ecchymotic hemorrhages and death occurred in some cases, usually as a result of intracranial hemorrhage.

Thrombocytopenia associated with DIC is common in animals. Extensive intravascular clotting with disseminated thrombi is associated with the significant consumption of blood clotting factors and thrombocytopenia. Clotting factors and platelets may be used up to such a degree that hemostasis is no longer possible, and hemorrhagic diathesis results. Various conditions may trigger the complex phenomenon of DIC—septicemia, hemolytic transfusion reactions, surgery, snakebite (venoms), heat stroke, hypersensitivity reactions, certain viral infections, neoplasias, and leukemias. DIC is commonly an acute disorder, but may be subacute or chronic.

Tropical canine pancytopenia is a tick-borne disease caused by Ehrlichia canis. Rhipicephalus sanguineus is the tick that transmits the disease. Typically, the organism is found as cytoplasmic inclusions, primarily in monocytes and lymphocytes. In Wright-stained blood or bone marrow films, it appears as single or multiple aggregates of fine bluish to slightly azurophilic coccoid or rod-shaped structures (elementary bodies) that form inclusions (morulae) in the leukocytes (Plates XIII-5, XIII-6, and XIV-4). The disease is best diagnosed serologically, because the organisms are not always found in blood cells. The characteristic mild to severe pancytopenia of acute and chronic ehrlichiosis is attributed to marrow hypoplasia, but its pathogenesis appears multifactorial. Thrombocytopenia appears to be the result of megakaryocyte hypoplasia and reduced platelet survival, which may be partly immune-mediated and partly consumptive. Platelet function may also be defective, because platelet adhesiveness is reduced. The anemia may result from several mechanisms, including blood loss from thrombocytopenia, bone marrow suppression, and immune-mediated red cell destruction. The depletion of granulocytic precursors contributes to leukopenia, but some other factors may also be involved. Mortality is high in dogs with WBC counts of less than 2,000/μl. Some infected dogs may also show hypergammaglobulinemia and hyperviscocity syndrome. High antibody titers to E. canis and hyperglobulinemia are usually present and proteinuria is common in dogs with subclinical infections (Codner and Farris-Smith, 1986). Subclinical infections in naturally infected dogs may persist up to 5 years compared to a 1 to 4 month duration in experimentally infected dogs.

The organism found primarily in canine neutrophils and eosinophils and causing an acute polyarthritis produces what is known as canine granulocytic ehrlichiosis (Stockham et al., 1990, 1992). The organism may be a variant of Ehrlichia canis or an antigenically related Ehrlichia species. It produces a subclinical infection and causes fever and most of the hematologic abnormalities (e.g., neutropenia, lymphocytosis, and thrombocytopenia) between 18 and 24 days of infection. Infected dogs may recover spontaneously or can be treated with tetracycline.

Infection of dogs by Ehrlichia platys causes cyclic parasitemia and thrombocytopenia at approximately 7- to 14-day intervals and decreased platelet aggregation in vitro (Gaunt et al., 1990; Kontos et al., 1991; Simpson et al., 1991) Acute infection also produces anemia, leukopenia, hypergammaglobulinemia, generalized lymphadenopathy, and lymphoid hyperplasia. Anemia is mild and is accompanied by normocytic normochromic red cell morphology and decreased serum iron and iron binding capacity as seen in anemia of inflammatory disease (Baker et al., 1988). The organism is found in platelets, but is difficult to visualize by light microscopy, although electron microscopy clearly reveals the elementary bodies (Fig. 6–20). The diagnosis is best made by an immunofluorescent antibody assay on serum. Serum antibodies to E. canis and E. platys do not cross-react, but concurrent infection is frequent.

Ehrlichia equi causes a peracute disease of horses characterized by high fever, anorexia, depression, limb edema, ataxia, icterus, leukopenia, and thrombocytopenia (Madigan and Gribble, 1987). The organism

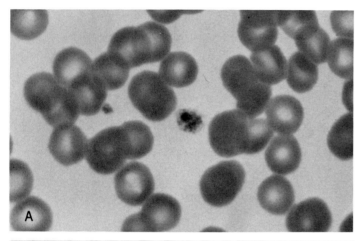
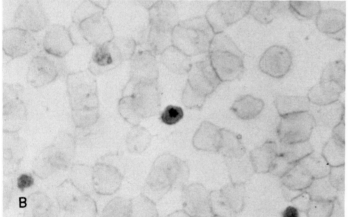
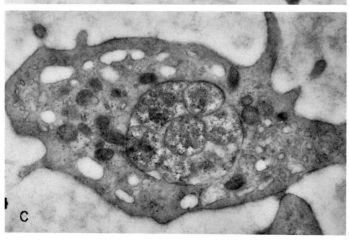

Fig. 6–20. *Ehrlichia platys* in blood of a dog. *A*, Wright's stain; *B*, New methylene blue stain; *C*, Electron photomicrograph of a platelet containing a microorganism with seven subunits. (Courtesy of Dr. John Harvey). (From Jain, N. C.: Schalm's Veterinary Hematology. 4th Ed. Philadelphia, Lea & Febiger, 1986, p. 482.)

presents elementary bodies and morulae in the cytoplasm of neutrophils (Plates XIV-1, XIV-2, and XIV-3) and, occasionally, in eosinophils during the period of pyrexia. E. equi has a broad host specificity in that it can infect dogs, cats, sheep, goats, and nonhuman primates, whereas E. canis infects only domestic and wild canines. Dogs infected with E. equi may develop mild or no clinical signs.

Potomac horse fever, caused by Ehrlichia risticii, is usually characterized by fever, depression, anorexia, leukopenia, and frequently mild to severe diarrhea. Leukopenia results from neutropenia with a left shift, lymphopenia, and monocytopenia; leukocytosis may follow leukopenia in many cases (Ziemer et al., 1987). Severely affected animals develop hemostatic abnormalities, viz., increased fibrinogen, factor VIII:coagulant, and APTT values and decreased factor V concentrations (Morris et al., 1988). The disease is diagnosed by an indirect immunofluorescence test (Ristic et al., 1986). The causative organisms are not found in leukocytes in stained blood films, but can be found in cultured blood monocytes, hence the disease is also referred to as equine monocytic ehrlichiosis. Thus, E. equi is a neutrophil parasite, whereas E. risticii infection is restricted to monocytes.

E. phagocytophilia causes the tick-borne fever of sheep and cattle. The organism in sheep is found as an intracytoplasmic inclusion in neutrophils and monocytes and causes a marked transient thrombocytopenia and neutropenia.

Bovine viral diarrhea virus causes thrombocytopenia in cattle and, with increasing frequency, among veal calves (Corapi et al., 1990). In experimentally infected calves, clinical signs of the disease, fever and diarrhea, were mild and often preceded the development of hemorrhage by several days. A severe thrombocytopenia ($\leq$5,000 platelets/μl) and hemorrhage developed by 3 to 11 days after inoculation. After 11 days postinoculation, the virus was detected on platelets by immunofluorescence, but evidence of surface-bound immunoglobulin was not found. The mechanism of thrombocytopenia remains unknown. Surviving animals recovered from thrombocytopenia at 3 to 7 weeks with the development of viral neutralizing antibody.

Therapy. The treatment of thrombocytopenia from varied causes is generally similar, except for correction of the inciting cause (if possible). In rare cases, spontaneous recovery may occur. If drug-induced thrombocytopenia is suspected, administration of the putative drug should be stopped. In IMT, therapy consists primarily of corticosteroids alone or in conjunction with immunosuppressive drugs such as cyclophosphamide, azathioprine, and/or Vinca alkaloids. Whole blood or platelet transfusions are given as supportive therapy in life-threatening situations. Splenectomy has been performed in cases refractory to corticosteroid therapy, but with variable success. Treatment with danazol, a synthetic analog of androgen steroids and progesterone, and prednisone was used to induce remission in a corticosteroid-resistant IMT in a dog (Bloom et al., 1989). IMT patients generally require continuous maintenance therapy with corticosteroids and careful management and follow-up. (For further details see Chapter 22).

Abnormalities of Survival and Distribution

Abnormalities of platelet life span and distribution may occur in pathologic conditions. The sequestration of platelets in idiopathic thrombocytopenia may be mainly splenic or hepatic, or may be diffuse, with bone marrow as the major site. The platelet life span is markedly reduced in various conditions in humans and animals (e.g., IMT, acute myelogenous leukemia, and heparin therapy in humans, IMT and localized and metastatic tumors in dogs, and viral infection in rabbits).

REFERENCES

Axthelm, M.K. and Krakowka, S.: Canine distemper virus-induced thrombocytopenia. Am J. Vet. Res., 48:1269, 1987.

Baker, D.C., Guant, S.D. and Babin, S.S.: Anemia of inflammation in dogs infected with *Ehrlichia platys.* Am. J. Vet. Res., 49:1014, 1988.

Bloom, J.C., Meunier, L., Thiem, P.A., et al.: Use of danazol for treatment of corticosteroid-resistant immune-mediated thrombocytopenia in a dog. J. Am. Vet. Med. Assoc., 194:76, 1989.

Bondy, G.S. and Gentry, P.A.: Characterization of the normal bovine platelet aggregation response. Comp. Biochem. Physiol. [C], 92:67, 1989.

Boudreaux, M.K., Dillon, A.R. and Spano, J.S.: Enhanced platelet reactivity in heartworm-infected dogs. Am J. Vet. Res., 50:1544, 1989.

Codner, E.C. and Farris-Smith, L.L.: Characterization of the subclinical phase of ehrlichiosis in dogs. J. Am. Vet. Med. Assoc., 189:47, 1986.

Corapi, W.V., Elliot, D., French, T.W., et al.: Thrombocytopenia and hemorrhage in veal calves infected with bovine viral diarrhea virus. J. Am. Vet. Med. Assoc., 196:590, 1990.

Daniels, T.M., Fass, D.N., White J.G., et al.: Platelet storage pool deficiency in pigs. Blood, 67:1043, 1986.

de Gaetano, G., Cerletti, C., Nanni-Costa, M.P., et al.: The blood platelet as an inflammatory cell. Eur. Respir. J. Suppl., 6:441s, 1989.

Degen, M.A.. Feldman, B.F., Turrel, J.M., et al.: Thrombocytosis associated with a myeloproliferative disorder in a dog. J. Am. Vet. Med. Assoc., 194:1456, 1989.

Ebbe, S.: Regulation of murine megakaryocyte size and ploidy by non-platelet-dependent mechanisms in radiation-induced megakaryocytopenia. Radiat. Res., 127:278, 1991.

Edwards, J.F., Dodds, J. and Slauson, D.O.: Mechanism of thrombocytopenia in African swine fever. Am. J. Vet. Res., 46:2058, 1985.

Gaunt, S.D., Baker, D.C. and Babin, S.S.: Platelet aggregation studies in dogs with acute *Equine platys* infection. Am. J. Vet. Res., 51:290, 1990.

Grindem, C.G., Breitschwerdt, E.B., Corbett, W.T., et al.: Epidemiologic survey of thrombocytopenia in dogs: A report on 987 cases. Vet. Clin. Pathol., 20:38, 1991.

Hammer, A.S.: Thrombocytosis in dogs and cats: A retrospective study. Comp. Haematol. Int., 1:181, 1991.

Han, Z.C., Bellucci, S., and Caen, J.P.: Megakaryocytopoiesis: characterization and regulation in normal and pathologic states. Int. J. Hematol., 54:3, 1991.

Handagama, P., Feldman, B., Kono, C., et al.: Mean platelet volume artifacts: The effect of anticoagulants and temperature on canine platelets. Vet. Clin. Pathol., 15:13, 1986.

Handagama, P.J., Feldman, B.F., Jain, N.C., et al.: Circulating proplatelets: isolation and quantitation in healthy rats and in rats with induced acute blood loss. Am. J. Vet. Res., 48:962, 1987a.

Handagama, P.J., Feldman, B.F., Jain, N.C., et al.: In vitro platelet release by rat megakaryocytes: effect of inhibitors and cytoskeletal disrupting agents. Am. J. Vet. Res., 48:1142, 1987b.

Handagama, P.J., Jain, N.C., Feldman, B.F., et al.: In vitro platelet release by rat megakaryocytes: effect of heterologous antiplatelet serum. Am. J. Vet. Res., 48:1147, 1987c.

Hawkey, C.M., Hart, M.G., Bennett, P.M., et al.: Diagnostic value of platelet counts in mammals. Vet. Rec., 127:18, 1990.

Herrmann, M. Suchard, S.J., Boxer, L.A., et al.: Thrombospondin binds to Staphylococcus aureus and promotes staphylococcal adherence to surfaces. Infect. Immun., 59:279, 1991.

Hoffman, R., Briddell, R. and Bruno, E.: Numerous growth factors can influence in vitro megakaryocytopoiesis. Yale J. Biol. Med., 63:411, 1990.

Hopper, P.E., Mandell, C.P., Turrel, J.M., et al.: Probable essential thrombocythemia in a dog. J. Vet. Intern. Med., 3:79, 1989.

Jain, N.C.: Schalm's Veterinary Hematology. 4th Ed. Philadelphia, Lea & Febiger, pp. 431–486, 1986.

Kontos, V.I., Papadopoulos, O., and French, T.W.: Natural and experimental canine infections with a Greek strain of Ehrlichia platys. Vet. Clin. Pathol., 20:101, 1991.

Lee, K.P.: Emperipolesis of hematopoietic cells within megakaryocytes in bone marrow of the rat. Vet. Pathol., 26:473, 1989.

Madigan, J.E. and Gribble, D.: Equine ehrlichiosis in northern California: 49 cases (1968–1981). J. Am. Vet. Med. Assoc., 190:445, 1987.

Mandell, C.P., Goding, B., Degen, M.A., et al.: Spurious elevation of serum potassium in two cases of thrombocytopenia. Vet. Clin. Pathol., 17:32, 1988.

McDonald, T.P.: Thrombopoietin. Its biology, clinical aspects, and possibilities. Am. J. Pediatr. Hematol. Oncol., 14:8, 1992.

McKellar, Q.A., Nolan, A.M. and Galbraith, E.A.: Serum thromboxane generation by platelets in several domestic animal species. Br. Vet. J., 146:398, 1990.

Menard, M., Meyers, K.M. and Prieur, D.J.: Absence of dense granule precursors in megakaryocytes from cats with the Chediak-Higashi syndrome. Vet. Clin. Pathol., 19:6, 1990.

Morris, D.D., Messick, J. and Whitlock, R.H.: Effect of equine ehrlichial colitis on the hemostatic system in ponies. Am. J. Vet. Res., 49:1030, 1988.

Northern, J., Jr. and Tvedten, H.W.: Diagnosis of microthrombocytosis and immune-mediated thrombocytopenia in dogs with thrombocytopenia: 68 cases (1987–1989). J. Am. Vet. Med. Assoc., 200:368, 1992.

Reimann, K.A., Knowlen, G.G. and Tvedten, H.W.: Factitious hyperkalemia in dogs with thrombocytosis. J. Vet. Intern. Med., 3:47, 1989.

Ristic, M., Holland, C.J., Dawson, J.E., et al.: Diagnosis of equine monocytic ehrlichiosis (Potomac horse fever) by indirect immunofluorescence. J. Am. Vet. Med. Assoc., 189:39, 1986.

Siess, W.: Platelets in the pathogenesis of atherosclerosis. Adv. Exp. Med. Biol., 273:119, 1990.

Simpson, R.M., Gaunt, S.D., Hair, J.A., et al.: Evaluation of Rhipicephalus sanguineus as a potential biologic vector of Ehrlichia platys. Am. J. Vet. Res., 52:1537, 1991.

Smith, C.M., Burris, S.M., Weiss, D.J., et al.: Comparison of bovine and human platelet deformability, using micropipette elastimetry. Am. J. Vet. Res., 50:34, 1989.

Smith, M. and Turrel, J.M.: Radiophosphorus (^{32}P) treatment of bone marrow disorders in dogs: 11 cases (1970–1987). J. Am. Vet. Med. Assoc., 194:98, 1989.

Stockham, S.L., Schmidt, D.A., Curtis, K.S., et al.: Evaluation of granulocytic ehrlichiosis in dogs of Missouri, including serologic status to Ehrlichia canis, Ehrlichia equi, and Borrelia burgdorferi. Am. J. Vet. Res., 53:63, 1992.

Stockham, S.L., Tyler, J.W., Schmidt, D.A., et al.: Experimental transmission of granulocytic ehrlichial organism in dogs. Vet. Clin. Pathol., 19:99, 1990.

Tablin, F., Jain, N.C., Mandell, C.P., et al.: Ultrastructural analysis of platelets and megakaryocytes from a dog with probable essential thrombocythemia. Vet. Pathol., 26:289, 1989.

Tennant, M. and McGeachie, J.K.: Platelet-derived growth factor and its role in atherogenesis: A brief review. Aust. N. Z. J. Surg., 61:482, 1991.

Teramura, M., Kobayashi, S., Hoshino, S., et al.: Interleukin-11 enhances human megakaryocytopoiesis in vitro. Blood, 79:327, 1992.

Tzanakakis, G.N., Agarwal, K.C., Veronikis, D.K. et al.: Effects of antiplatelet agents alone or in combinations on platelet aggregation and on liver metastases from a human pancreatic adenocarcinoma in the nude mouse. J. Surg. Oncol., 48:45, 1991.

Waner, T., Yuval, D. and Nyska, A.: Electronic measurement of canine mean platelet volume. Vet. Clin. Pathol., 18:84, 1989.

Williams, D.A. and Maggio-Price, L.: Canine idiopathic thrombocytopenia: Clinical observations and long-term follow up in 54 cases. J. Am. Vet. Med. Assoc., 185:660, 1984.

Williams, W.J., Beutler, E., Erslev, A.J., et al.: Hematology. 4th Ed. New York, McGraw-Hill, 1990.

Yeaman, M.R., Puentes, S.M., Norman, D.C., et al.: Partial characterization and staphylocidal activity of thrombin-induced platelet microbicidal protein. Infect. Immun., 60:1202, 1992.

Ziemer, E.L., Whitlock, R.H., Palmer, J.E., et al.: Clinical and hematologic variables in ponies with experimentally induced ehrlichial colitis (Potomac horse fever). Am. J. Vet. Res., 48:63, 1987.

Chapter **7**

Erythrocyte Physiology and Changes in Disease

Hematopoietic organs in vertebrates include the bone marrow, spleen, and liver. The bone marrow is the principal organ of erythropoiesis during postnatal life, whereas the spleen and liver are active during fetal life and resume this activity in times of need after birth. Active erythropoiesis, however, continues to occur in mice during postnatal life. The current concept of hematopoiesis is shown in Figure 4–6. Erythrocyte production and survival and hemoglobin synthesis and degradation are discussed in this chapter.

ERYTHROPOIESIS AND ITS REGULATION

Experimental studies have shown that the primitive pluripotential stem cell (PPSC) in the bone marrow differentiates and gives rise to unipotential cells, each committed to the erythrocytic, granulocytic, monocytic, or megakaryocytic series. Such differentiation occurs under the influence of the local microenvironment and cytokines produced by macrophages and activated T lymphocytes. Erythropoiesis begins with the differentiation of the PPSC to an early erythroid progenitor cell, burst-forming unit–erythrocyte (BFU-E), which gives rise to a late progenitor cell, the colony-forming unit–erythrocyte (CFU-E). The CFU-E then gives rise to morphologically identifiable erythroid precursors, rubriblasts, which further differentiate, divide and mature, ultimately producing red cells (Figs. 7–1 and 7–2). The formation of erythroid progenitors is regulated by interleukin-3 and colony-stimulating factor–granulocyte-monocyte (GM-CSF). The BFU-E is also stimulated by a burst-promoting activity produced by various cells, including macrophages and T lymphocytes, whereas the CFU-E and its progeny are sensitive to erythropoietin. The erythroid progenitors remain morphologically unidentifiable. The nomenclature system for morphologically identifiable cells of the erythroid series is presented in Table 7–1.

Erythropoietic Islands and the Nurse Cell

The process of erythropoiesis occurs in clusters of cells, erythroblastic islands, comprised of a central macrophage known as the "nurse cell" and a surrounding ring of developing erythroid cells (Fig. 7–3). The erythroblastic islands are fragile and are therefore extremely rare in bone marrow aspirates. The macrophage-erythroid cell contact is mediated by fibronectin and possibly by thrombospondin, a thrombin-sensitive glycoprotein present in platelet α granules, endothelial cells, and fibroblasts. Maturing erythroid cells move away from the nurse cell and then make contact with the abluminal side of the sinusoidal endothelial cells to gain entry into the circulation. The nurse cell is believed to provide nutrients for cell growth and iron for hemoglobin synthesis. Iron is taken up by the erythroid cells, largely through the endocytosis of ferritin by a process known as ropheocytosis and to some extent through transferrin, an iron transport sialoprotein. Ferritin and transferrin receptors are present in clathrin-coated pits on the outer membrane of developing erythroid cells (Fig. 7–4). Receptor-bound transferrin and ferritin are internalized by endocytosis, iron is released in the cytosol, and the apotransferrin-transferrin receptors are recycled to the cell membrane where apotransferrin is released into the milieu for transport of more iron. Apoferritin is also recycled. The synthesis of transferrin receptors is stimulated in iron deficiency.

133

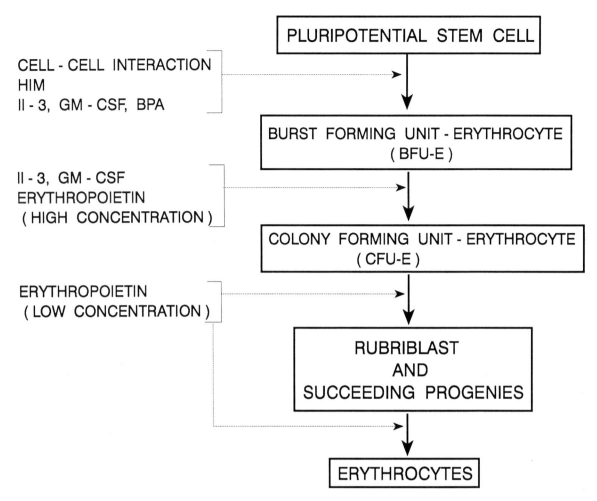

Fig. 7–1. Development of morphologically recognizable rubriblasts from morphologically unidentifiable but functionally recognizable progenitor cells. Also depicted are possible sites of interaction of various factors found to stimulate erythropoiesis in vitro and in vivo (also see Fig. 7–8). (From Jain, N. C.: Schalm's Veterinary Hematology. 4th Ed. Philadelphia, Lea & Febiger, 1986, p. 488.)

Ferritin and Hemosiderin

Ferritin molecules (MW, 441,000 to 800,000) consist of thousands of iron atoms embedded in a protein shell (apoferritin). Ferritin can be visualized as tiny, electron-dense particles localized on the cell membrane or (Figs. 7–4B and E) in the cytosol of erythroid cells

Table 7–1. Nomenclature for Morphologically Identifiable Cells of the Erythrocytic Series

Recommended Term	Other Terms
Rubriblast	Pronormoblast, proerythroblast
Prorubricyte	Basophilic (or early) normoblast or erythroblast
Basophilic rubricyte	(included in the above category)
Polychromatic rubricyte	Early polychromatic normoblast or erythroblast
Metarubricyte	Late polychromatic normoblast or erythroblast, orthochromatic normoblast, or erythroblast
Reticulocyte	Polychromatic erythrocyte
Erythrocyte	Red blood cell, red cell

and macrophages. The degradation of the protein shell by intracellular lysosomal enzymes in macrophages converts ferritin to hemosiderin, a golden, iron-containing protein visible on light microscopy of iron-loaded tissues. Thus, hemosiderin is found primarily in cells of the mononuclear phagocyte system (macrophages in the bone marrow and spleen and Kupffer cells of the liver). Ferritin is water-soluble, and hemosiderin is not, but both serve as stores of iron that can be mobilized for heme synthesis. In anemias of chronic disease, the storage of iron in macrophages increases because of a reduction in the rate of iron release.

A minute amount of ferritin is normally found in plasma and can be quantitated to evaluate total body iron stores. A significant correlation was found between serum ferritin concentration and nonheme iron stores in humans, dogs, horses, pigs, and rats (Adams et al., 1988; Andrews et al., 1992; Harvey et al., 1987; Weeks et al., 1989). The serum ferritin concentration increased with increasing body iron stores in iron-loaded pigs. Serum ferritin levels increase in foals at 1 day of age because of colostrum consumption and

Patterns of Erythropoiesis

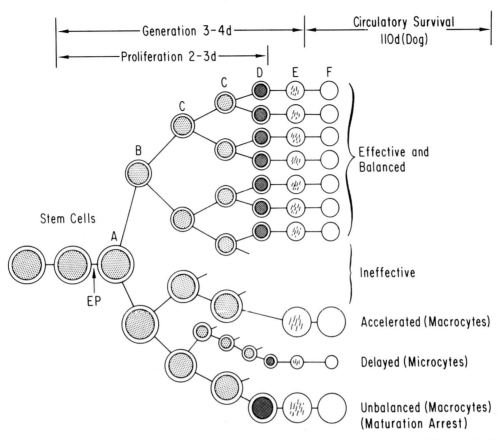

Fig. 7–2. Patterns of development and maturation of erythroid cells in health and disease. Erythropoiesis in health is mostly effective and balanced, although some ineffective erythropoiesis may occur. Examples of altered erythropoiesis shown are accelerated erythropoiesis seen in responsive anemia, delayed erythropoiesis of iron deficiency, and unbalanced erythropoiesis of vitamin B_{12}-folate deficiency (A, rubriblast; B, prorubricyte; C, rubricyte; D, metarubricyte; E, reticulocyte; F, erythrocyte). The average marrow proliferation and generation times of erythroid cells in days are given at the top, along with the life span of circulating red cells of the dog. (From Kaneko, J. J.: Clinical Biochemistry of Domestic Animals. 3rd Ed. New York, Academic Press, 1980.)

then diminish gradually by 3 weeks of age and increase again to reach normal adult levels by 6 months of age.

The nucleated erythroid cells that contain cytoplasmic aggregates of ferritin, siderosomes, are called sideroblasts. Siderosomes are demonstrated as small, cytoplasmic iron particles by Prussian blue stain. Normally, a few particles are seen scattered in the cytoplasm. In contrast, ringed sideroblasts contain excessive iron deposited in mitochondria and arranged as a ring around the nucleus. The mitochondrial iron is antigenically distinct from ferritin and is known as ferruginous micelles. Reticulocytes and mature erythrocytes containing siderosomes are called siderocytes (Plate XII-10). Pappenheimer bodies are siderosomes that stain with Wright stain. The iron in these cells is present in the form of ferritin aggregates (normal siderocytes) or ferruginous micelles in mitochondria (pathologic siderocytes).

Effective and Ineffective Erythropoiesis

Normal erythropoiesis entails a minimum of four mitoses—one each at the rubriblast and prorubricyte

stages and two at the basophilic rubricyte stage (Fig. 7–2). The basophilic rubricyte then matures into a polychromatic rubricyte, which in turn matures to become a metarubricyte. Occasionally, the polychromatic rubricyte may also divide. Denucleation of the metarubricyte leads to the formation of a reticulocyte, which finally matures into a red cell. The entire process of erythrogenesis that results in the formation of mature red cells in known as effective erythropoiesis, and takes about 7 to 8 days. The extruded nuclei are phagocytosed and disposed of by local macrophages.

A small number of developing erythroid cells in the bone marrow may not reach the final stage because of premature death. This process is called ineffective erythropoiesis (Fig. 7–2). An increase in ineffective erythropoiesis would lead to anemia, as in lead toxicity in dogs and erythropoietic porphyria in cattle. Ineffective erythropoiesis is suspected when the reticulocyte count in blood is normal or disproportionately low compared to erythroid hyperplasia in marrow. The extent of effective erythropoiesis can be estimated from the myeloid:erythroid ratio interpreted in conjunction with the reticulocyte count in blood and bone

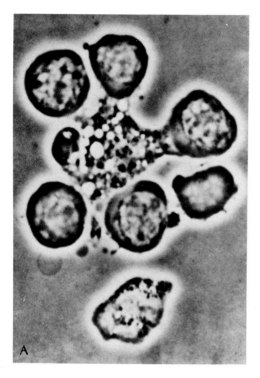

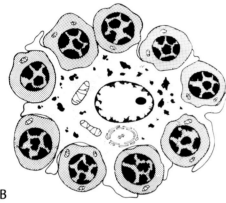

Fig. 7–3. *A,* Erythroblastic island examined in the living state by phase contrast microscopy; the cytoplasm of the macrophage can be identified by its many refractile inclusions. *B,* Schematic representation of an erythroblastic island; a corona of erythroid cells encircles the macrophage, in which masses of hemosiderin can be seen. (From Bessis, M.: Living Blood Cells and Their Ultrastructure. New York, Springer-Verlag, 1973.)

marrow. A better estimate of effective erythropoiesis can be obtained, however, by measuring the rate of erythropoiesis (ferrokinetics) or red cell turnover using radioisotopes. Usually, ^{59}Fe is used to study ferrokinetics and ^{51}Cr to estimate red cell survival.

Morphologic Features of Developing Erythroid Cells

Developing erythroid cells in the bone marrow can readily be identified because of their deeper nuclear and cytoplasmic staining compared to that of cells of the leukocytic series. These features are attributable to their high DNA and RNA contents. The cytoplasm of erythroid cells is nongranular, whereas the myeloid series shows azurophilic and specific cytoplasmic granules in more developed cells. The rubriblast is recognized by its relatively large size, round nucleus with stippled chromatin and a nucleolus, and deep blue cytoplasm. The prorubricyte has identical features, but lacks a nucleolus. Rubricytes are identified by their coarsely clumped chromatin and cytoplasmic color; the one with blue cytoplasm is called a basophilic rubricyte, and that with gray cytoplasm is designated as a polychromatic rubricyte. The gray color of the cytoplasm is attributed to increasing hemoglobin synthesis and decreasing basophilia from a reduction in the rough endoplasmic reticulum and ribosomes. Hemoglobin synthesis in the erythroid cells begins early, but is not appreciated until the polychromatic rubricyte stage. The smallest nucleated erythroid cell with a highly condensed, almost solid nucleus and an usually gray cytoplasm is called a metarubricyte. Rarely, a metarubricyte may have an orthochromic (normal red cell color) cytoplasm. A reticulocyte is a non-nucleated, polychromatic (grayish) red cell (See Chap. 1 for details).

Reticulocytes

Reticulocytes display a variable degree of membranous folds and minute surface invaginations, or pits (Fig. 7–5). They contain ribosomes, polyribosomes, and mitochondria, which enable them to synthesize up to 20% of the final hemoglobin content (Figs. 7–6*A,* *B,* and *C*). Rarely, remnants of other cytoplasmic organelles such as the centriole and Golgi apparatus may be found, but not endoplasmic reticulum. The ribosomes and polyribosomes contribute to their polychromasia, as seen in Wright-stained blood and marrow films. A bluish reticular meshwork of aggregated ribosomes, mitochondria, and other cytoplasmic organelles appears in reticulocytes after staining with a supravital stain, such as new methylene blue (Fig. 7–6*D*)—thus, the name of the cell. Reticulocytes in canine blood can be enumerated more accurately by flow cytometry after staining them with the nucleic acid staining dye thiazole orange (Abbot and McGrath, 1991).

Reticulocytes may stay in the bone marrow for 2 to 3 days before entering the blood by diapedesis through the endothelial cells that line the marrow sinusoids. Their release into the blood is controlled by a number of factors acting in concert, including erythropoietin concentration and their cellular deformability and surface charge. Species variation may occur in regard to the number of reticulocytes released into the blood under physiologic and pathologic conditions. For example, the horse does not normally release reticulocytes into the peripheral blood, and only rarely is a reticulocyte found in blood, even in marked anemia. Dogs and cats respond vigorously with reticulocytosis

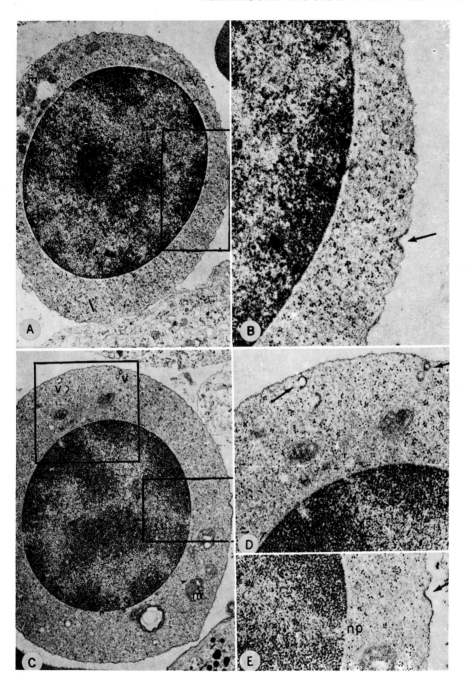

Fig. 7–4.   Early (A, ×10,560) and late (C, ×9,860) rubricytes. The nuclei in these cells are typically round and present areas of chromatin condensations having fuzzy demarcation zones that become distinct with maturation. The cytoplasm contains some ribosomes and polyribosomes, mitochondria (m), and endocytotic vesicles (v). Insets show areas enlarged. B (×31,680) and E (×19,710) depict areas of surface membrane with fuzzy coating of ferritin granules and beginning's of endocytotic invaginations (arrows); a nuclear pore (np) can be seen clearly in E. Endocytotic vesicles (arrows) in the cytoplasm of the late rubricyte (D, ×19,710) are clearly visible at higher magnification. (From Jain, N. C.: Schalm's Veterinary Hematology. 4th Ed. Philadelphia, Lea & Febiger, 1986, p. 493.)

in blood during responsive anemia, but ruminants usually have a slight response.

Reticulocytes mature to erythrocytes in 24 to 48 hours in the circulation or in the spleen, where they may sequester temporarily. The maturation process involves the loss of some surface membrane, transferrin and fibronectin receptors, ribosomes, and other organelles, attainment of the normal hemoglobin content, final assembly of the submembrane skeleton, reduction in cell size, and shape change to the biconcave form (Fig. 7–7).

Reticulocytes and young red cells may occasionally display additional morphologic features. Nuclear fragmentation or incomplete extrusion of the metarubricyte nucleus results in the retention of a small nuclear remnant, a Howell-Jolly body. The Howell-Jolly body is pitted from the reticulocyte when it passes through the spleen, and is often encountered in splenectomized individuals or when splenic function is compromised. Reticulocytes in humans with megaloblastic anemia may display Cabot rings. These are ring-like filamentous structures, sometimes twisted into the form of a figure eight. They probably originate from mitotic spindles. Cabot rings have been observed in red cells

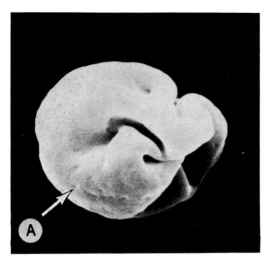

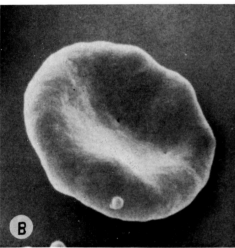

Fig. 7–5. Scanning electron photomicrographs of a reticulocyte and an erythrocyte from a dog. *A,* Reticulocyte shows characteristic irregular shape, membrane folding, invaginations of the surface, and many small, shallow pits on the surface (*arrow*). The pits probably represent areas of endocytotic activity (×7700). *B,* Discoid erythrocyte with concave shape of maturity. The presence of a few surface pits indicates its young age (×8900). (*A* from Jain, N. C.: Schalm's Veterinary Hematology. 4th Ed. Philadelphia, Lea & Febiger, 1986, p. 498; *B* from Keeton, K. W., and Jain, N. C.: Erythrocyte morphology during response to blood loss. Cal. Vet., 27:13, 1973.)

Erythropoietin

The fundamental stimulus for erythropoiesis is tissue oxygen tension (Po_2). Tissue hypoxia triggers the production of erythropoietin, a humoral factor specifically concerned with red cell production. The erythropoietin is produced by the kidney (cortical endothelial, glomerular, and interstitial cells) and to a smaller extent by the liver (Kupffer cells, hepatocytes, and endothelial cells). The kidney is believed to be the sole source in the dog and the liver is the predominant site in the fetus. Erythropoietin is generated by the activation of erythropoietinogen, an α_2-globulin, by the renal erythropoietic factor or erythrogenin, or by the activation of proerythropoietin produced in the kidney by a plasma factor (Fig. 7–8). Erythropoietin is found in plasma, urine, milk, and other body fluids, including amniotic fluid. It is a glycoprotein (MW, 38,000) with a blood half-life of about 7 to 10 hours in the dog and 3 to 6 hours in humans. Because it is a large molecule, it cannot cross the placental barrier. Increases in the renal concentrations of prostaglandin E (PGE), prostacyclin I (PGI), and cyclic AMP are associated with the increased production of erythropoietin. The human gene for erythropoietin has been cloned, and recombinant erythropoietin is now commercially available for the treatment of erythropoietin-responsive anemias. Erythropoietins from different species show weak antigenic cross-reactivity, but have similar biologic activity. Erythropoietin stimulates erythropoiesis at several steps by inducing the differentiation of erythroid progenitors cells to rubriblasts, stimulating the mitosis of erythroid cells and reducing their maturation time, and increasing the delivery of reticulocytes and young red cells to the peripheral blood. It acts through erythropoietin receptors present on the surface of various responsive cells. The role of erythropoietin and some of the recent advances relating to its production, regulation, action, and clinical use have been reviewed (Giger, 1992; Woodman, 1992).

The erythropoietin concentration is elevated during blood loss and hemolytic anemia, but is diminished in anemias associated with end-stage kidney disease. Erythropoiesis is more vigorous in hemolytic anemias than in blood loss anemias, but the precise cause of this difference is not known. The erythropoietin concentration is usually elevated in secondary polycythemia, but primary polycythemia is erythropoietin-independent. Primary polycythemia has been reported in cattle, dogs, and cats. Various endocrine organs have been found to influence erythropoiesis, largely through their effects on erythropoietin synthesis. The pituitary mediates its effect through the production of prolactin, TSH, ACTH, and growth hormone, the adrenals through corticosteroid production, the thyroid glands through the secretion of thyroxin, and the gonads through the production of androgens and estrogen. The only negative influence is that of estrogen.

Mean normal serum erythropoietin levels, assayed

of the camel, but not in those of other animal species. In certain diseases, such as lead toxicity, ribosomes may aggregate into large clumps and appear as bluish granules scattered in the reticulocytes and young red cells in Wright-stained films. This feature is referred to as basophilic stippling or punctate basophilia. The enzyme pyrimidine 5'-nucleotidase that is present in reticulocytes normally catabolizes ribosomes and polyribosomes. The activity of this enzyme is reduced in lead toxicosis. Basophilic stippling may also occur during an intense response to anemia in dogs and cats. Basophilic stippling is a species-specific characteristic of the reticulocytes of ruminants (Plate XVII-10).

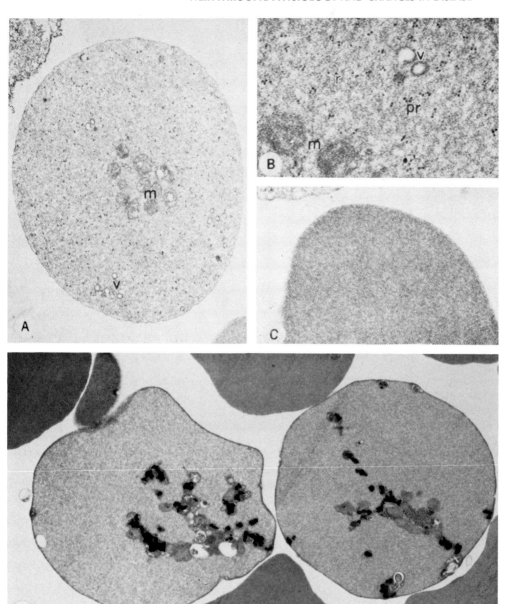

Fig. 7–6. A reticulocyte (A, ×12,740) and its enlarged portion (B, ×35,280) contain many ribosomes (r) and polyribosomes (pr). These form the characteristic reticulum when blood films are stained with new methylene blue vital stain. Mitochondria (m) and endocytotic vesicles (v) are also present. The fuzzy, finely granular material in B is the hemoglobin. A portion of the mature erythrocyte shown in C exhibits homogeneous cytoplasm (×15,680). Two reticulocytes in D are from canine blood stained with new methylene blue to demonstrate their reticulum by electron microscopy. Cytoplasmic aggregates contain dense, stringy ribosomal material with entangled electron-light mitochondria (×11,500). (From Jain, N. C.: Schalm's Veterinary Hematology. 4th Ed. Philadelphia, Lea & Febiger, 1986, p. 497.)

by the mouse spleen cell culture method, are higher in dogs (88.2 ± 30.7 mU/ml) than in horses (55.2 ± 8.9 mU/ml), cows (41.7 ± 10.3 mU/ml), and cats (39.4 ± 5.4 mU/ml). Puppies have higher levels of serum erythropoietin than 1- to 7-year-old dogs, but dogs aged 8 to 13 years have comparatively lower levels (Ikeda et al., 1990).

Essential Nutrients

Adequate erythropoiesis requires a continual supply of necessary nutrients, vitamins, and minerals. A deficiency of such factors from any cause would lead to anemia. A common cause, indeed, is iron deficiency.

Nutritional anemias in humans and animals have included those caused by deficiencies of protein, vitamin B_{12}, folate, niacin, vitamin E, selenium, copper, and cobalt. Dietary vitamin E supplementation does not alter the antioxidant status in equine red cells (Ji et al., 1990).

ERYTHROCYTES

The primary function of the red cell is carrying hemoglobin for the transport of oxygen. The biconcave shape of the mammalian erythrocyte is functionally the most suited morphologic form. Typical biconcave red cells are seen in the dog, cow, and sheep,

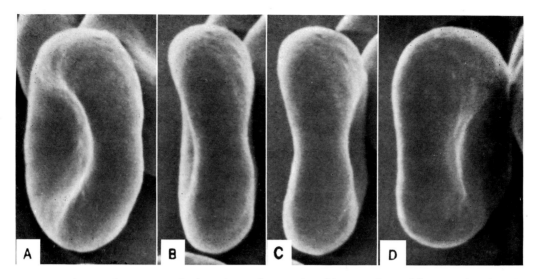

Fig. 7–7. *A–D,* Scanning electron photomicrograph of a canine erythrocyte viewed in succession at different angles of rotation to demonstrate its distinctive biconcave morphology (×500). (From Jain, N. C.: Schalm's Veterinary Hematology. 4th Ed. Philadelphia, Lea & Febiger, 1986, p. 499.)

cells with shallow concavity occur in the cat and horse, and slightly concave to rather flat cells are found in the goat (Figs. 7–9 and 7–10). Some uniconcave red cells may occur in cattle and sheep. A few wart-like protuberances representing cell fragmentation may be found on some red cells. The cell surface is smooth, except in reticulocytes, which have a relatively rough surface and many small pits corresponding to the sites of iron intake (see Fig. 7–5). Species differences in erythrocyte morphology include ovalocytes in the family Camelidae, sickle cells in deer, poikilocytes in goats, fusiform cells in Angora goats, and nucleated oval cells in nonmammalian vertebrates (Fig. 7–10; Plate XXVII).

Red Cell Membrane

The erythrocyte membrane is the most studied cell membrane. It is composed of two electron-dense layers, each about 25 Å thick, separated by a 20 to 30 Å thick electronlucent area. Biochemically, the membrane is composed of proteins (48%), lipids (44%), and carbohydrates (8%). The fluid mosaic model of the cell membrane most satisfactorily represents the biochemical structure (Fig. 7–11). It envisions a lipid bilayer composed of phospholipid molecules arranged so that their hydrophobic nonpolar groups are directed inward, toward each other, and their hydrophilic polar groups are directed outward, into the hydrophilic

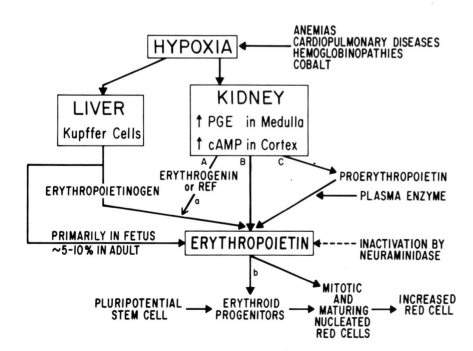

Fig. 7–8. Various views (A, B, C) on the synthesis of erythropoietin in response to various stimuli. Primary sites of stimulation of erythroid precursors by erythropoietin and sites of estrogen inhibition (a, large dose; b, small dose) of erythropoietin production or erythropoiesis are also shown (REF, renal erythropoietic factor). (From Jain, N. C.: Schalm's Veterinary Hematology. 4th Ed. Philadelphia, Lea & Febiger, 1986, p. 504.)

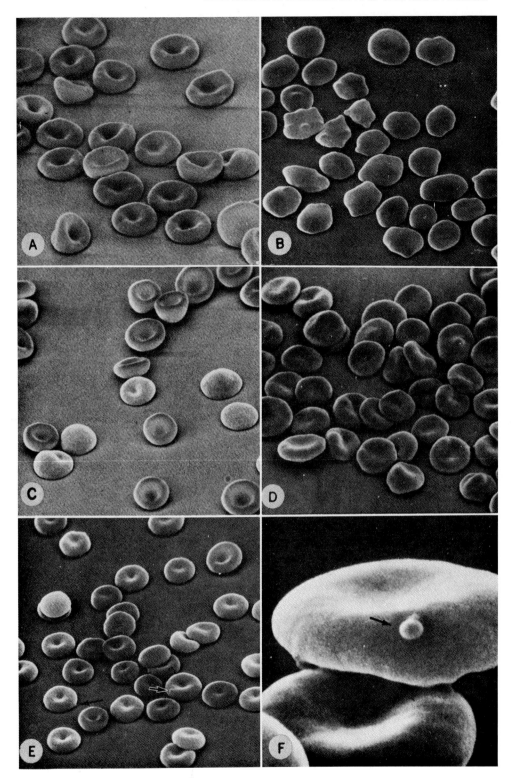

Fig. 7–9. Scanning electron photomicrographs of erythrocytes from a clinically normal dog (*A*, × 2600), cat (*B*, ×2500), cow (*C*, ×2500), horse (*D*, ×2550), and sheep (*E*, ×2430; *F*, ×12,000). The arrows in *E* and *F* point to small protuberances on the cell surface; such structures are often seen on sheep and goat erythrocytes, but rarely on dog red cells. (*A, B, D, F* from Jain, N. C., and Kono, C. S.: Scanning electromicroscopy of erythrocytes of dog, cat, cow, horse, sheep, and goat. Res. Vet. Sci., 13:489, 1972; *C* from Jain, N. C.: Morphology of blood cells in three dimensions. Cal. Vet., 26:16, 1972.)

cytoplasm on one side and the plasma on the other side. The lipids are distributed asymmetrically between the inner and outer leaflets of the membrane. Cholesterol molecules are interspersed between the phospholipid molecules and remain in equilibrium with unesterified plasma cholesterol. The normal cholesterol-to-phospholipid ratio in the human red cell membrane is 1:1.1. Any significant change in this ratio results in altered cell morphology and reduced red cell survival. In horses, the phospholipids of the erythrocyte membrane are greatly reduced after endurance exercise, leading to an increase in the choles-

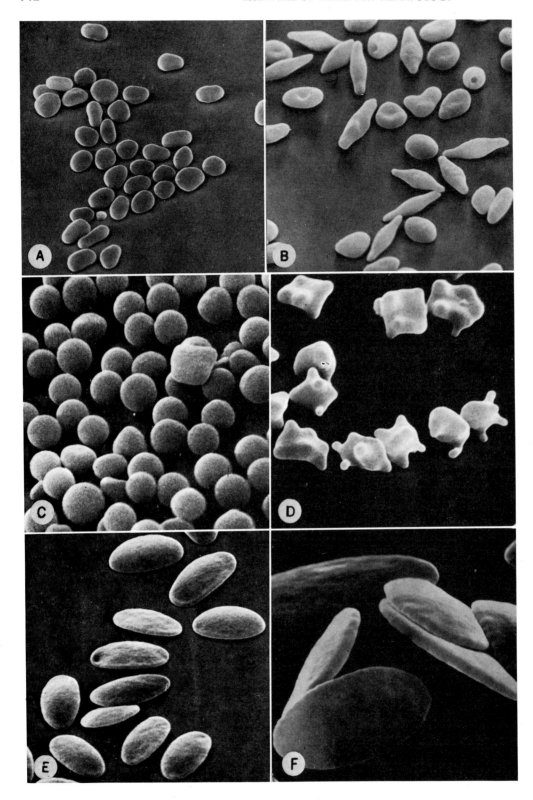

Fig. 7–10. Scanning electron photomicrographs of erythrocytes. *A* (×2500), *B* (×3150), and *C* (×3275) are from clinically healthy goats, *D* (×3000) shows acanthocytes from a normal cow, and *E* (×2400) and *F* (×6500) are erythrocytes from a camel; the side view in *F* shows their wafer-like thinness. (*A* from Jain, N. C., and Kono, C. S.: Scanning electromicroscopy of erythrocytes of dog, cat, cow, horse, sheep, and goat. Res. Vet. Sci., 13:489, 1972; *F* from Jain, N. C., and Keeton, K. S.: Morphology of camel and llama erythrocytes as viewed with the scanning electron microscope. Br. Vet. J., 130:288, 1974.)

terol:phospholipid ratio (Hambitzer, 1987), but the influence of such a change in membrane lipid composition on red cell morphology remains to be determined. Erythrocytes from sheep inoculated with Corynebacterium pseudotuberculosis, which produces a sphingomyelin-specific phospholipase D endotoxin, developed alterations in phospholipid composition and morphologic changes, such as spherostomatocytosis and surface pits (Brogden and Engen, 1990).

A number of red cell proteins have been characterized (Smith, 1987; Williams et al., 1990), including spectrin (bands 1 and 2), ankyrin or syndein (band

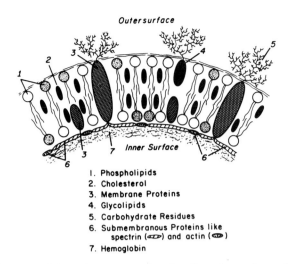

Fig. 7–11. Schematic representation of erythrocyte membrane showing different structural components. (Modified from Zucker-Franklin, D., et al: Atlas of Blood Cells. Philadelphia, Lea & Febiger, 1981.)

2.1), bands 3 and 4.1, glycophorins A, B, and C, and actin (band 5). These proteins constitute the integral part of the erythrocyte membrane and submembrane skeleton (Fig. 7–12). Spectrin is the predominant protein of the red cell membrane. It occurs as heterodimers linked together into a fibrous network by direct contact between the "heads" of the complimentary strands of the heterodimer and by linkage of the "tail" ends by actin and band 4.1. The lipid bilayer is anchored to the spectrin network by one or two integral membrane proteins; band 2 of spectrin is attached to protein band 3 of the membrane by band 2.1 and glycophorin C or A in the membrane binds to band 4.1. Most of these erythrocyte membrane proteins have been found in the dog and sheep (Barker, 1991).

Many morphologic abnormalities of red cells and hemolytic conditions in humans have been associated with changes in membrane lipid and protein compositions and their interactions, depletion of ATP, and accumulation of calcium. These include a quantitative deficiency of spectrin, protein band 4.1, and ankyrin, as well as qualitative abnormalities of spectrin. Similar abnormalities of red cells in animals are rare.

Red Cell Metabolism

The mature red cell derives energy solely from glucose metabolism, predominantly (95%) through anaerobic glycolysis (Embden-Meyerhof, or EM, pathway) and to a minor extent (5%) through the oxidative pentose phosphate pathway (Fig. 7–13). Reticulocytes are metabolically more active than mature red cells because of their high glycolytic enzyme activity and more "machinery" to produce energy. No tricarboxylic acid (TCA) cycle and oxidative phosphorylation occur in mature erythrocytes because they lack mitochondria. Senescent red cells have decreased activity of several key enzymes necessary for survival—hexokinase, glucose-6-phosphate dehydrogenase (G-6-PD), phosphofructokinase (PFK), and pyruvate kinase (PK). The metabolic activity of the red cell varies with individuals, species, breed, and age. For example, erythrocytes of the neonatal pig use glucose as a source of energy, but those of the adult pig use inositol instead. Glucose is transported across the red cell membrane through a carrier protein present in the cell membrane.

Metabolic activities of the red cell are directed toward its enhanced survival and functional performance. Metabolic energy is not needed for binding, transport, or delivery of oxygen. Energy from adenosine tri-

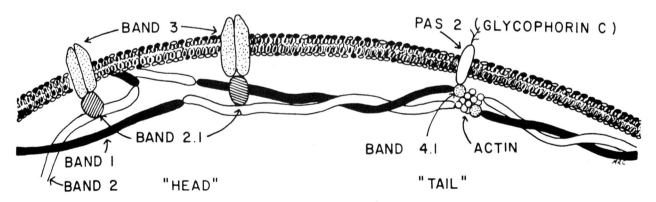

Fig. 7–12. Diagrammatic cross section of red cell membrane bilayer and supporting "skeleton." The outer leaflet of the bilayer is composed predominantly of choline-containing phospholipids (*black head groups*), and the inner leaflet is predominantly composed of acidic phospholipids, such as phosphatidylethanolamine and phosphatidylserine (*white head groups*). Cholesterol (*black ovals*) is shown embedded symmetrically in each leaflet among the fatty acid side groups of the phospholipids. The predominant protein of the membrane, spectrin, occurs as a heterodimer (bands 1 and 2) linked together into a fibrous network. The linkage between the "tail" of the dimers appears to be mediated by actin (band 5) and band 4.1. Linkage between the "head" ends of the dimers occurs by direct contact between complimentary strands of the heterodimer (the carboxy terminus of the beta chain and the amino terminus of the alpha chains). Attachment of the skeleton to the membrane is produced by a specific association between band 2 of spectrin and band 3 in the lipid bilayer through the spectrin-binding protein, band 2.1 (ankyrin), near the head end of the spectrin dimer. An additional association of the skeletal complex with the lipid bilayer may be provided by a connection between spectrin and another bilayer protein, glycophorin C or A, through band 4.1. (From Williams, J. W., Beutler, E., Erslev, A. J., et al.: Hematology. 4th Ed. New York, McGraw-Hill, 1990, p. 373.)

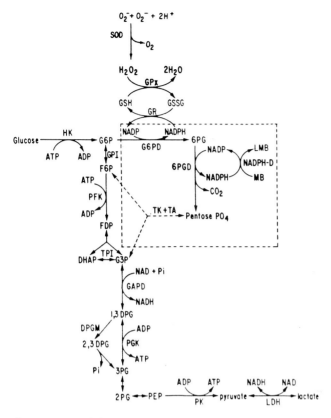

Fig. 7–13. Metabolic pathways of the mature RBC. Pentose phosphate pathway-related reactions are shown in dashed box. (From Kaneko, J. J.: Clinical Biochemistry of Domestic Animals. 4th Ed. San Diego, Academic Press, 1989, p. 207.) (For abbreviations, see footnote, p. 158.)

phosphate (ATP), generated from the anaerobic glycolysis, is used for the maintenance of the following: (1) adequate cellular deformability; (2) cell shape, by controlling the active ionic movement of sodium out of and potassium into the cell; and (3) membrane fluidity. Species differences exist in the ionic gradients of sodium and potassium in the red cells and plasma; for example, compared to the plasma, red cells of the dog and cat have high sodium and low potassium concentrations, and the reverse occurs in humans. Breed differences may also occur in this regard— some Japanese Shiba dogs were found to have high K^+ and low Na^+ concentrations together with high Na^+, K^+-ATPase activity, whereas other Shibas and other breeds examined showed low K^+ and high Na^+ concentrations and no Na^+, K^+-ATPase activity (Maede et al., 1991). The high K^+ Shiba dogs also had high reduced glutathione concentration and these characteristics followed an autosomal recessive mode of inheritance (Yamoto and Maede, 1992). Some Akitas also have high red cell K^+, and spontaneous in vitro hemolysis in such cases produces pseudohyperkalemia (Degen, 1987). The intraerythrocytic concentration of Na^+ is also increased in some Siberian huskies (Wilson and Dixon, 1991).

Reduced nicotinamide-adenine dinucleotide

(NADH) generated from the anaerobic glycolysis is used for the enzymatic reduction of methemoglobin (ferric iron) to functional hemoglobin (ferrous iron) for the transport of oxygen. The enzyme involved in this process is NADH-methemoglobin reductase, also known as NADH-diaphorase or cytochrome b_5 reductase. Erythrocytes also contain another enzyme, NADPH-methemoglobin reductase (NADPH-diaphorase or dehydrogenase) that can reduce methemoglobin. This enzyme contributes little physiologically to this process, but it can be activated by various flavins or redox dyes, such as methylene blue used to treat methemoglobinemia (Fig. 7–13).

Reduced nicotinamide-adenine dinucleotide phosphate (NADPH) generated in the pentose phosphate pathway is used for the conversion of oxidized glutathione (GSSG) to reduced glutathione (GSH), which is important for maintaining the structural integrity of the hemoglobin molecule (Fig. 7–13). Glutathione reductase and glutathione peroxidase are involved in glutathione metabolism.

Reduced glutathione prevents the oxidative denaturation of hemoglobin by oxidant drugs that cause Heinz body formation and hemolytic anemia. Heinz bodies are large amorphous precipitates of denatured hemoglobin within the red cells. They appear as small, pale areas near the periphery or as slightly protruding objects. They are best seen in blood films stained with supravital stains such as new methylene blue or crystal violet. GSH is also important for the conversion of methemoglobin to functional hemoglobin, thereby preventing the accumulation of small amounts of methemoglobin normally produced in circulating erythrocytes. The red cell GSH content may vary in health and disease; a bimodal physiologic distribution is seen in sheep and goats. The red cell glutathione peroxidase is a selenium-containing enzyme and has been used as an indicator of selenium deficiency in humans and animals.

Only a few metabolic defects of red cells have been reported in animals, as compared to many in humans. It is important to recognize that enzyme deficiencies in the EM pathway cause hemolytic anemias without Heinz body formation. In contrast, enzymatic defects of the pentose phosphate pathway and oxidative damage to the hemoglobin result in anemias associated with Heinz body formation. Examples of metabolic defects of red cells in animals include the following: (1) PFK deficiency associated with persistent, compensated hemolytic anemia in English springer spaniels; (2) PK deficiency associated with hereditary hemolytic anemia in the basenji and beagle; (3) NADH-methemoglobin reductase deficiency leading to methemoglobinemia in several breeds of dogs; and (4) decreased glutathione reductase and GSH levels leading to hemolytic anemia reported in a horse (Kaneko, 1989). Erythrocytes of stress-susceptible pigs have an increased glutathione concentration and an antioxidant abnormality that leads to increased lipid peroxidation of the cell membrane (Duthie et al., 1989).

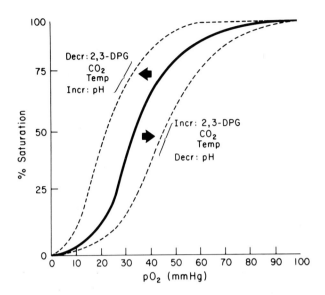

Fig. 7–14. Oxygen dissociation curve of hemoglobin and factors influencing the position of the curve. (From Kaneko, J. J.: Clinical Biochemistry of Domestic Animals. 4th Ed. San Diego, Academic Press, 1989, p. 210.)

2,3-Diphosphoglycerate and Oxygen Affinity of Hemoglobin

The erythrocytes of many mammalian species contain 2,3-diphosphoglycerate (2,3-DPG) in high concentration. It is generated in the diphosphoglycerate or Rapoport-Luebering pathway of anaerobic glycolysis (Fig. 7–13). This compound acts as a potential regulator of energy through the EM pathway, but it also is important in regulating the release of oxygen from hemoglobin. The oxygen affinity of hemoglobin is primarily influenced by temperature, pH, and red cell 2,3-DPG concentration (Fig. 7–14). The oxygen affinity of hemoglobin is usually expressed as the P_{50}, the oxygen tension at which hemoglobin is half saturated. Higher values of P_{50} indicate a lower oxygen affinity of the hemoglobin or red cells. A left shift in the oxygen dissociation curve indicates increasing oxygen affinity and a right shift suggests efficient oxygen delivery to the tissues. The oxygen affinity increases with a decrease in temperature, decreased red cell 2,3-DPG concentration, and increased pH. An increase in 2,3-DPG concentration produces a corresponding decrease in the intracellular pH, which then decreases the oxygen affinity of human hemoglobin by the Bohr effect (the binding of more protons by deoxyhemoglobin than by oxyhemoglobin), Thus, more oxygen is delivered to tissues, as in hypoxia, anemia, and exercise. The concentration of 2,3-DPG in human erythrocytes negatively correlates with blood hemoglobin concentration—for example, it increases during anemia and decreases during polycythemia. The higher oxygen affinity of fetal hemoglobin compared to that of adult hemoglobin is little influenced by 2,3-DPG concentration.

The effect of 2,3-DPG on animal hemoglobins is variable because of species differences in the relative reactivity of the hemoglobin to this compound. Hemoglobins of the horse, dog, pig, rabbit, guinea pig, mouse, and rat react strongly and red cells of these species have high concentrations of 2,3-DPG. In contrast, hemoglobins of the sheep, goat, cattle, and cat react weakly and have low concentrations of red cell 2,3-DPG. The 2,3-DPG concentration of equine erythrocytes is influenced by the physical activity of the horse. It increases after a short bout of exercise, but an increase (Stull and Lawrence, 1986) or decrease (Debski, 1985) is observed after conditioning horses for 6 to 16 weeks. Equine hemoglobin has a higher oxygen affinity compared to that of human hemoglobin (Clerbaux et al., 1986). Changes in pH have an effect similar to that in humans, but changes in temperature have comparatively less effect. Hemoglobin types A and B of sheep differ in their oxygen affinity (Maginniss et al., 1986).

Red Cell Survival and Destruction

The erythrocyte of each species has a finite, characteristic intravascular life span (Table 7–2). The loss of erythrocytes is continually balanced by the release of reticulocytes or young red cells from the bone marrow. Red cell destruction may occur intravascularly or extravascularly. Intravascular destruction can involve changes in erythrocyte membrane permeability and cell fragmentation. Extravascular destruction involves phagocytosis by macrophages in the mononuclear phagocyte system (MPS). Erythrocyte deformability is important for normal cell survival. Deformability depends on at least three factors: (1) maintenance

Table 7–2. Erythrocyte Life Span in Various Animals

Species	Life Span, Mean or Range (Days)
Birds	<50
Cat	68
Cattle	
Calf (3 months)	48–63
Adults	160
Dog	110
Guinea pig	83
Goat	125
Guanaco	225
Hamster	60–70
Horse	140–150
Human	120
Nonhuman primate	98
Mouse	20–30
Pig	63
Pigeon	17–25
Rabbit	68
Rat	45–50
Sheep	
Lamb (3 months)	46
Adult	70–153
Tortoise	330 (half-life)

of cell shape; (2) normal internal fluidity of hemoglobin; and (3) intrinsic membrane viscoelastic properties. Red cells can be destroyed when they lose metabolic components essential for generating energy to maintain cell shape and ionic balance and to protect hemoglobin and the lipid bilayer from oxidative damage. The mature red cell cannot synthese depleted enzymes because it lacks the necessary organelles (see above).

A gradual reduction of surface charge from the loss of sialic acid residues during red cell aging may contribute to the normal destruction of red cells. The accelerated reduction of erythrocyte sialic acids by sialidase cleavage is associated with reduced red cell life span in several species. The development of a severe hemolytic anemia in Zebu cattle infected with Trypanosoma vivax is associated with a reduction in erythrocyte sialic acid concentration by trypanosome sialidase, with increased susceptibility of desialated erythrocytes to phagocytosis by the MPS. Ndama cattle, the West African dwarf breed, are more tolerant to the pathogenic effects of African trypanosomes, probably because their erythrocyte surface sialic acid concentration is much higher (about sevenfold) than that of the susceptible Zebu cattle (Esievo et al., 1986, 1990).

Sheep		4.5
Goat		3.2

aFrom Perk et al., 1964a.
bMean RBC sizes taken from Chapters 4 through 10 and

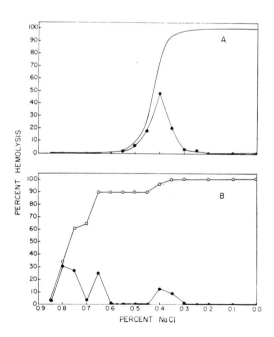

Fig. 7–15. *A,* Normal cumulative (—) and derivative (●—●) erythrocyte osmotic fragility curves drawn from mean values for 51 clinically healthy dogs. *B,* Cumulative (○—○) and derivative (●—●) curves for a dog with autoimmune hemolytic anemia. Three osmotically different populations of erythrocytes are apparent clearly from the derivative curve. (From Jain, N. C.: Osmotic fragility of erythrocytes of dogs and cats in health and in certain hematologic disorders. Cornell Vet., 63:411, 1973.)

Table 7–3. Osmotic Fragility of Erythrocytes of Normal Adult Animals*

Animal	RBC Diameter (μm)	Buffered NaCl Solution (%)	
		Maximum	Minimum
Camel	7.5 × 4.4	0.21	0.30
Dog	7.0	0.29	0.50
Pig	6.0	0.29	0.52
Rat	6.3	0.30	0.42
Rabbit	6.7	0.30	0.50
Mouse	6.1	0.30	0.50
Guinea pig	7.5	0.30	0.52
Hamster	6.5	0.30	0.51
Horse	5.8	0.34	0.54
Donkey	6.2	0.35	0.54
Cat	5.8	0.36	0.60
Cow	5.8	0.38	0.59
Sheep	4.5	0.43	0.56
Goat	3.2	0.44	0.66

*As indicated by maximum and minimum resistance to hypotonic saline solutions.

Changes in membrane permeability to electrolytes increase the osmotic fragility of erythrocytes and shorten red cell survival (Fig. 7–15). Various factors may influence osmotic fragility, the most important being a linear relationship between the red cell size (MCV) and the critical hemolytic volume that a cell can attain before lysing from the formation of holes or a large tear. In other words, the greater the MCV, the greater the osmotic resistance. Such differences are reflected in species differences in minimum and maximum resistance to hemolysis in hypotonic saline (Table 7–3). The small red cells of the goat can swell only 25% and soon lyse, whereas the large red cells of the horse can swell up to 42% and camel erythrocytes can swell remarkably, up to 200%. Breed differences may occur in red cell fragility; for example, the red cells of Pygmy goats seem to be more susceptible to osmotic and mechanical stress than those of Toggenburg goats, probably because of differences in red cell membrane composition and not in red cell size (Fairley et al., 1988). The osmotic resistance of red cells is high in pregnant ewes compared to dry ewes and rams, and is probably related to their red cell size (MCV, 39.4, 33.2, and 32.6 fl, respectively) (Durotoye, 1987). Fetal erythrocytes are osmotically more resistant than adult red cells. Spherocytes formed in autoimmune hemolytic anemia in dogs (Fig. 7–15) and cats (see Fig. 22–2) have increased osmotic fragility because their critical hemolytic volume is reached earlier than normal. This is because the maximum expansion of the spherocytes is compromised as a result of reduced cell volume from the loss of surface membrane through partial erythrophagocytosis by the mononuclear phagocytes.

Erythrocyte fragmentation into fine hemoglobin dust, because of membrane damage from the repeated trauma of microcirculation, is another mechanism of intravascular red cell destruction. The red cell membrane is intolerant to excessive stretching. Pathologic fragmentation of red cells has been observed in various diseases with a component of hemolytic anemia.

The phagocytic destruction of red cells by macrophages occurs primarily in the spleen and liver, but bone marrow may also be involved. It has been shown that an antierythrocyte IgG (100 to 600 molecules) selectively binds to an age-specific antigen on the senescent red cells and initiates phagocytosis. The senescent antigen is antigenically related to the red cell membrane protein band 3. The macrophages recognize the Fc portion of the IgG molecule through their Fc receptors. It has been shown that the spleen can sense minor changes in the red cell surface membrane, but the liver is adapted to recognize greater membrane damage.

Accelerated erythrocyte destruction may occur from various causes. Abnormalities in membrane lipid and skeletal proteins and in lipid-protein interactions can result in altered red cell shape and decreased survival from increased sensitivity to osmotic lysis. The association of hemoglobin and inner membrane proteins, particularly spectrin, progressively increases in aging red cells, and oxidative damage may enhance this association. Red cells coated with IgG antibody and complement component C3b are readily phagocytosed by macrophages or destroyed from increased osmotic fragility in the splenic sinusoids and in the circulation. Complement activation, leading to the formation of the membrane attack complex (C5 through C9), disrupts membrane integrity and creates membrane pores that result in leakage of hemoglobin. Activated neutrophils may alter the antigenic nature of the erythrocyte membrane through the generation of toxic oxygen radicals and promote immunoglobulin binding to the cell membrane. This mechanism may be a potential cause of erythrocyte destruction in anemias of inflammatory disease (Weiss and Klausner, 1988). Similarly, increased activity of the MPS, as in splenomegaly or hypersplenism, can cause excessive phagocytic destruction of red cells and result in anemia. Red cell fragmentation from thermal, physical, or enzymatic injuries is associated with decreased red cell survival. Phospholipase C from Clostridium welchii and phospholipase in cobra venom induce hemolysis by cleaving the glycerol phosphate bond of membrane lecithin.

Abnormalities of Red Cell Shape

The descriptive terminology of red cell morphology has been derived mostly from Greek and sometimes from Latin roots (Table 7–4; Bessis, 1977; Jain, 1986). It is based on the shape of red cells in stained blood films examined by light microscopy (Figs. 7–16 and 7–17) or on their three-dimensional appearance on scanning electron microscopy (Figs. 7–18, 7–19, and 7–20). A red cell may sometimes display features befitting the use of a compound term such as spheroechinocyte or spherostomatocyte. Abnormalities of red cell shape have been found in many human diseases,

Table 7–4. Terms Describing Erythrocyte Morphology and Their Greek or Latin Roots*

Term	Greek or Latin Root and Its Meaning
-cyte	Gr., *kytos* cell
Acanthocyte	Gr., *akantha*, thorn, spicule, spine
Acuminocyte	L. *acuminatus*, fusiform
Codocyte	Gr., *kodea*, helmet, hat, cup-shaped
Cryohydrocyte	Gr., *kryos* + *hydros*, frost
Dacryocyte	Gr., *dakryon*, tear
Desicyte	L., *de-siccus*, completely dry
Discocyte	Gr., *diskoeites, diskos*, disk, round plate
Drepanocyte	Gr., *drepano, drepanē*, sickle
Eccentrocyte	Gr., *ekkentros*, out of the center
Echinocyte	Gr., *echinos*, sea urchin
Elliptocyte	Gr., *elleipsis*, defect
Fusocyte	L., *fusus*, spindle
Hydrocyte	Gr., *hydōr*, water
Keratocyte	Gr., *keras, keratos*, horn
Knizocyte	Gr., *knizo*, dimple
Leptocyte	Gr., *leptos*, thin
Macrocyte	Gr., *makros*, long
Megalocyte	Gr., *megas*, large, great
Microcyte	Gr., *mikros*, small
Ovalocyte	L., *ovum*; N.L., *ovalis*, egg
Poikilocyte	Gr., *poikilos*, variegated
Pyknocyte	Gr., *pyknos*, compact
Pyropoikilocyte	Gr., *pyr, pyros* + *poikilos*, fire + variegated
Schistocyte	Gr., *schistos*, divided, divisible, split
Schizocyte	Gr., *schizein*, cut, cleave, split
Selenocyte	Gr., *selēnē*, moon
Siderocyte	Gr., *siderōs*, iron
Spherocyte	Gr., *sphaira*, sphere, ball
Stomatocyte	Gr., *stoma, stomatos*, mouth
Torocyte	L., *torus*, bulge, protuberance
Xerocyte	Gr., *xeros*, dry

* The Greek root is preferred. The Latin root is substituted for lack of an appropriate Greek root.

but such occurrences have been documented less in animal species (Table 7–5). The precise basis of the abnormal shape is usually unknown, but it may involve changes in the intrinsic properties of the cell—such as membrane composition, submembrane skeletal proteins, and hemoglobin—or in its milieu.

An acanthocyte or spur cell is an irregular, spiculated, red cell with less numerous, unevenly distributed surface projections of variable length and diameter (Figs. 7–10*D*, 7–17*C*, and 7–19*E*).

An acuminocyte or fusocyte is a spindle-shaped or fusiform red cell (Figs. 7–10*B* and 7–19*H*). Its shape results from the polymerization of hemoglobin in the form of longitudinal tubules, analogous to those in the sickle cells of humans with sickle cell anemia. Such red cells are found in certain normal goats, particularly of the Angora breed (Fig. 7–10*B*). These cells are less prone to shape changes induced in vitro by stomatocytic and echinocytic agents such as chlorpromazine and lysolecithin, respectively (Jain and Kono, 1989).

A codocyte or target cell is a bell-shaped red cell that may appear to have a dense central area of hemoglobin separated partially or completely by a clear area encircled by the peripheral hemoglobinized region (Figs. 7–16*H* and 7–18*L*). Both acanthocytes

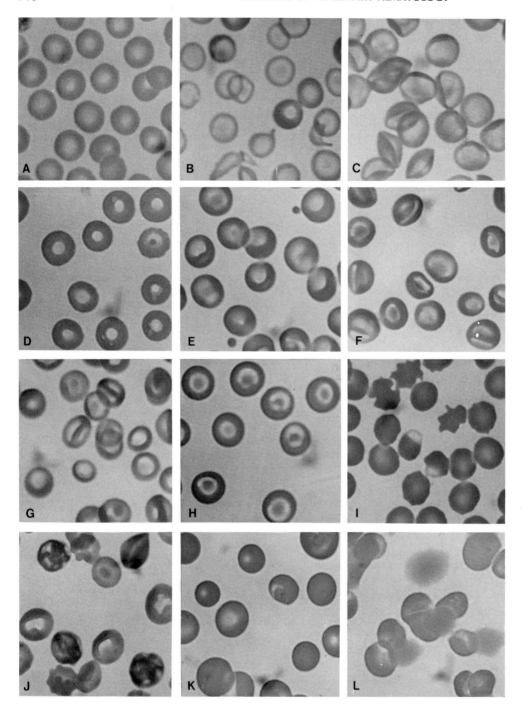

Fig. 7–16. Erythrocyte morphology in Wright-stained canine blood films examined with the light microscope. A, Normal discoid red cells with central pallor. B, Hypochromic erythrocytes with a thin rim of hemoglobin and extended central pallor. C, Thin leptocytes with variable foldings. D, Punched-out red cells (torocytes). E and F, Various forms of stomatocytes; a few small red cell fragments are also present in E. G, Microcytic hypochromic red cells and a few leptocytic red cells with a central membranous fold (knizocytes). H, Target cells (codocytes). I, Hemoglobin crystallization in an occasional red cell. J, Several polychromatic red cells with membranous folds typical of reticulocytes examined with the scanning electron microscope (see Fig. 7–5A). K, Spherocytic red cells; those with a slight clear area are called spherostomatocytes. L, Smudge cells, these are partically lysed, lightly stained red cells without membranes. (From Jain, N. C.: Schalm's Veterinary Hematology. 4th Ed. Philadelphia, Lea & Febiger, 1986, p. 535.)

and codocytes result from an increase in the cholesterol:phospholipid ratio of the cell membrane because of elevations in cholesterol or both cholesterol and phospholipid levels, respectively.

A dacryocyte (Figs. 7–17J and 7–20E) is a teardrop-shaped red cell. It is formed probably because of the inability of deformed red cells to resume a normal shape after passage through narrow splenic or marrow sinusoids. It is believed that a change in membrane skeletal proteins must occur as an associated event to make the normally highly deformable cell assume a distorted shape permanently. Dacryocytes may also occur as artifacts of smear making, particularly along

the feather edge of the blood film. Dacryocytes have been found in dogs and cats with myeloproliferative disorders. They were seen in a dog with hypersplenism (Kuehn and Gaunt, 1986).

A discocyte is a normal biconcave discoid erythrocyte seen in most mammals (Figs. 7–16A, 7–18A, B and C). The biconcave form provides increased surface area to facilitate the exchange of oxygen and carbon dioxide by the red cell.

A drepanocyte is a sickle-shaped red cell (Fig. 7–19G). It is found in humans with sickle cell anemia and is produced as the result of the polymerization of hemoglobin S (or other abnormal hemoglobins) on

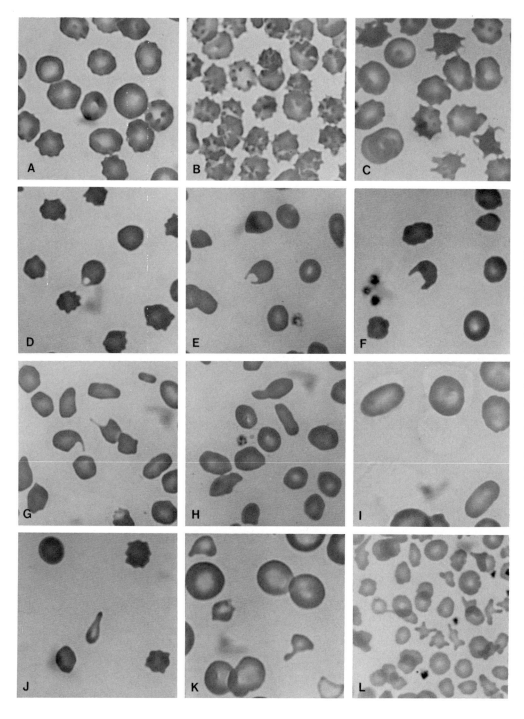

Fig. 7–17. Erythrocyte morphology in Wright-stained blood films examined with the light microscope. A, Discoid erythrocytes and slightly crenated (echinocytic) canine red cells. B, Highly crenated (echinocytic) red cells and a few burr cells in dog blood. C, Acanthocytes in a dog blood. D–G, Stages leading to formation of a keratocyte from a blister cell in cat blood. H, Ovalocytic and matchstick forms of red cells in cat blood. I, Ovalocytes in dog blood. J, Teardrop red cell (dacryocyte) in cat blood. K, Schistocytes in dog blood. L, Poikilocytes in a calf with congenital erythropoietic porphyria.

deoxygenation of blood. Deer red cells sickle in vitro when blood becomes oxygenated after withdrawal from the body (see Fig. 3–6). An occasional sickle-shaped red cell may be found in sheep and goats, but rarely in other species. Hemoglobin crystallization, seen in an occasional red cell in humans and animals with hemoglobin C disease, is a different phenomenon than hemoglobin polymerization that leads to the formation of drepanocytes. Hemoglobin crystals, unassociated with hemoglobin C disease, have been found in occasional red cells of dogs, cats (Figs. 7–16I and 7–19L), and llamas (Plate XVIII-6) (Tvedten, 1990).

An eccentrocyte or pyknocyte is a red cell with condensed hemoglobin in one area of the cell. It probably results from oxidative injury to the cell.

An echinocyte, commonly known as a *crenated* red cell, has numerous short, evenly spaced, blunt to sharp, surface projections of uniform dimension (Figs. 7–17A and B, 7–19B, C, and D). Echinocytes are usually artifactual and some are invariably found in blood films. Nonartifactual echinocytes may occur in some dogs with lymphoma and glomerulonephritis (Weiss et al., 1990) and chronic doxorubicin toxicosis (Badylak et al., 1985). Echinocytes are found in the blood of exercising horses, possibly because of a depletion in erythrocyte ATP, increased levels of ionic potassium,

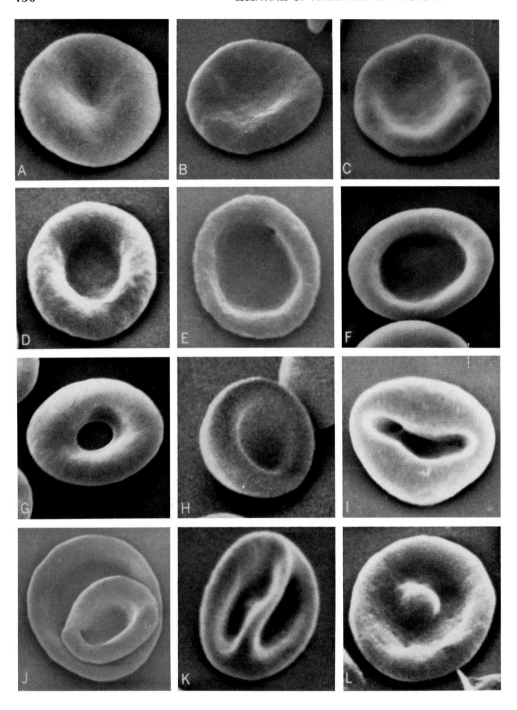

Fig. 7–18. Scanning electron photomicrographs of various morphologic forms of erythrocytes. *A–C,* Normal discoid forms with varying degrees of concavity. *D,* Red cell with extreme concavity—such cells appear as punched-out cells (torocytes) with light microscopy. *E* and *F,* Hypochromic red cells with a narrow rim of hemoglobin and extended central concavity. *G,* Torocyte. *H* and *I,* Stomatocytes. *J,* Microcyte and macrocyte. *K,* Knizocyte. *L,* Codocyte, ×4500. (From Jain, N. C.: Schalm's Veterinary Hematology. 4th Ed. Philadelphia, Lea & Febiger, 1986, p. 537.)

and reduced pH of plasma (Snow and Martin, 1990). Highly crenated red cells (burr cells) have been found in uremic humans.

An elliptocyte or ovalocyte is an ellipsoid or oval red cell; it includes other variants, such as matchstick or cigar-shaped forms (Figs. 7–17*H* and *I,* 7–20*A, B,* and *C*). Ovalocytes are characteristic of the family Camelidae (Fig. 7–10*E* and *F*). Nucleated ovalocytes are peculiar to birds, fish, and reptiles (Plate XXVII). Qualitative and quantitative abnormalities of spectrin and membrane protein band 4.1 have been associated with hereditary elliptocytosis in humans. A deficiency of protein band 4.1 was associated with hereditary

elliptocytosis in the dog, presumably as an autosomal recessive trait (Smith, 1987).

A keratocyte is a spiculated red cell with one or usually two or more pointed projections (Figs. 7–17*E, F,* and *G,* 7–19*I, J,* and *K*). It results from the rupture of a vacuole formed near the cell surface (Fig. 7–17*D* and *E*), probably because of physical or chemical injury.

A knizocyte is a triconcave red cell that in blood films appears to have a central bar of hemoglobin and somewhat clear spaces on either side (Figs. 7–16*G* and 7–18*K*).

A leptocyte is a thin red cell with excessive surface

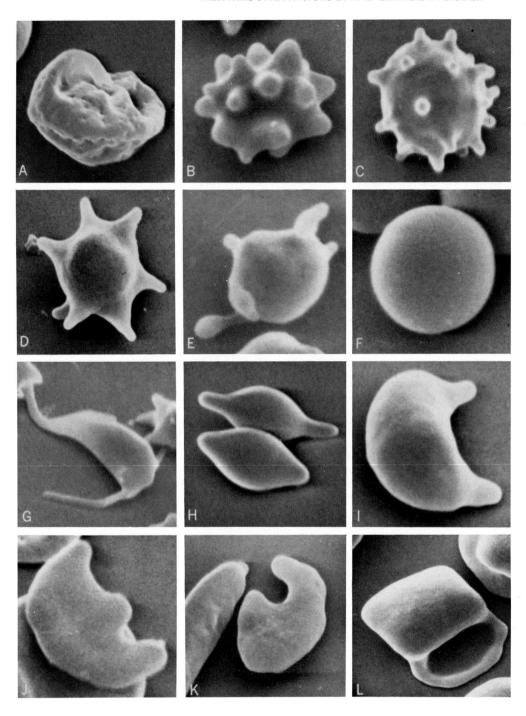

Fig. 7–19. Scanning electron photomicrographs of various morphologic forms of erythrocytes. *A*, Reticulocyte. *B–D*, various forms of echinocytes (the cell in *D* may be called a burr cell). *E*, Acanthocyte. *F*, Spherocyte. *G*, Drepanocyte. *H*, Acuminocyte and fusocyte; *I–K*, Keratocytes. *L*, Hemoglobin crystal in a feline red cell. (×4500). (From Jain, N. C.: Schalm's Veterinary Hematology. 4th Ed. Philadelphia, Lea & Febiger, 1986, p. 538.)

area compared to its contents. These cells tend to fold and may appear as target cells, folded bowl-shaped cells, knizocytes, or stomatocytes (Figs. 7–16*C*, *G*, and *J*, 7–18*E*, *K*, and *L*, 7–20*F*). In Wright-stained blood films, polychromatic leptocytes are generally reticulocytes, whereas orthochromatic leptocytes are usually mature red cells altered by chronic disease.

A macrocyte or megalocyte is a large red cell that has an MCV greater than normal for the species in question. In contrast, a microcyte is a small red cell with an MCV smaller than normal (Figs. 7–18*J* and 7–20*F*). Red cell size is characteristic of a species and varies within a narrow range. For unknown reasons,

however, certain dogs of the poodle breed exhibit macrocytosis, whereas dogs of the Japanese Akita breed normally have microcytic cells compared to dogs of other breeds. A gigantocyte is a large red cell (more than 1.5 to 2 times the normal diameter).

The term "poikilocyte" refers to a red cell of any morphology other than the normal and should be used to refer to shapes that cannot be properly categorized, or when a general description is desired (Figs. 7–17*L*, 7–20*D* and *E*).

A schistocyte or schizocyte is an irregular red cell fragment resulting from mechanical trauma to the circulating erythrocyte (Figs. 7–17*K* and 7–20D). It is

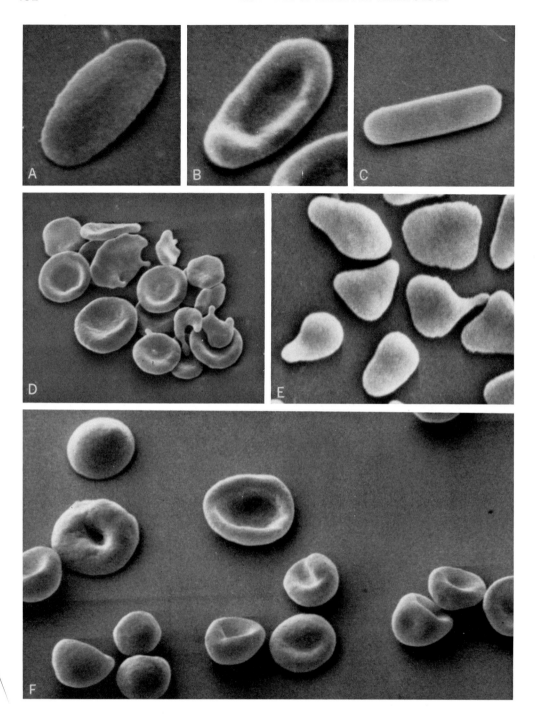

Fig. 7–20. Scanning electron photomicrographs of various morphologic forms of erythrocytes. *A* and *B*, Ovalocytes. *C*, Matchstick form. *D*, Schistocytes admixed with normal-appearing red cells of varying sizes. *E*, Dacryocytes and triangular cells. *F*, Leptocytes and stomatocytes in different profiles, (×4500). (From Jain, N. C.: Schalm's Veterinary Hematology. 4th Ed. Philadelphia, Lea & Febiger, 1986.)

the hallmark of red cell fragmentation associated with disseminated intravascular coagulation and microvascular angiopathic hemolytic anemias. Schistocytes have been found in dogs with chronic doxorubicin toxicosis (Badylak et al., 1985) and in a dog with hypersplenism (Kuehn and Gaunt, 1986).

A spiculated cell is a red cell with one or more surface spicules. It is a general term that encompasses several well-recognized forms such as echinocytes, acanthocytes, dacryocytes, drepanocytes, keratocytes, and schistocytes. It may be used for red cells with spicules that cannot be categorized exactly (Fig. 7–17G).

A stomatocyte is a cup-shaped red cell that, in Wright-stained blood films, appears to have a slit-like or mouth-like clear opening near the cell center (Figs. 7–16E and F, 7–18H and I, and 7–20F). Chemicals that preferentially expand the inner leaflet of the red cell bilayer are stomatocytogenic, and those that expand the outer leaflet are echinocytogenic.

A spherocyte is a small, densely stained spherical red cell with a reduced surface area-to-volume ratio (Figs. 7–16K and 7–19F). A spherocyte may have a small depression or dimple that becomes clearly visible on scanning electron microscopy (Fig. 22–1). Spherocytes are almost pathognomic of immune-mediated

Table 7–5. Diseases or Conditions Associated With Abnormalities of Erythrocyte Shape

Morphology	*Disease or Condition*
Acanthocyte	In humans with congenital abetalipoproteinemia, liver disease, postsplenectomy state, malabsorptive state, heparin therapy; in dogs with splenic hemangioma or hemangiosarcoma, diffuse liver disease, portocaval shunts, high-cholesterol diets
Acuminocyte (fusocyte)	Normal in certain goats, particularly of the Angora breed
Codocyte	In humans with iron deficiency anemias, liver disease with cholestasis, postsplenectomy state, thalassemia, lecithin-cholesterol acyltransferase deficiency, hemoglobinopathies (S,C); in dogs with first three conditions listed for humans
Dacryocyte	In humans with myelofibrosis with myeloid metaplasia, myelophthisic anemias, thalassemia; in dogs and cats with myeloproliferative disorders and in normal goat kids. Hypersplenism in a dog
Drepanocyte	In humans with sickle cell disorders, hemoglobin C disease, certain other hemoglobinopathies; normally in deer, infrequently in sheep and goats, rarely in other species
Eccentrocyte	In dogs with hemolytic anemia from acetylphenylhydrazine and onion toxicoses
Echinocyte	Usually artifactual and in old blood; in humans with kidney disease with uremia (burr cells), pyruvate kinase deficiency, carcinoma of the stomach and bleeding peptic ulcers, low-potassium red cells; in dogs with lymphoma, glomerulonephritis, and chronic doxorubicin toxicosis
Elliptocyte (ovalocyte)	In humans with hereditary elliptocytosis, megaloblastic anemia, thalassemia, iron deficiency, myelophthisic anemias; in dogs with hereditary deficiency of protein band 4.1; normal in Camelidae family
Knizocyte	During responsive anemias in humans and dogs
Leptocyte	Polychromatic leptocytes are seen in responsive anemias, whereas orthochromic leptocytes may be found in liver disease, obstructive jaundice, and iron deficiency in humans and animals; in humans with thalassemia
Macrocyte, megalocyte	In humans during response to anemia and in vitamin B_{12} and folate deficiency; normal in certain dogs of the poodle breed; in dogs and cats with myeloproliferative diseases; in dogs on antifolate therapy
Microcyte	Iron deficiency anemia and anemia of chronic disease; in dogs with portosystemic shunts; normal in dogs of the Japanese Akita breed
Poikilocyte	Iron deficiency anemias; normal in goats, particularly in kids
Schistocyte, schizocyte	In humans with disseminated intravascular coagulation (DIC), microangiopathic hemolytic anemia (MHA), severe burns, heart valve hemolysis, march hemoglobinuria; in dogs with DIC, MHA, congestive heart failure, glomerulonephritis, myelofibrosis, chronic doxorubicin toxicosis, hypersplenism, and neoplasms, particularly hemangiosarcoma; in other animal species with DIC
Spherocyte	Immune-mediated hemolytic anemias, Heinz body anemias, post-transfusion; in humans with hereditary spherocytosis, water dilution hemolysis, fragmentation hemolysis; hereditary spherocytosis in goats, anaplasmosis in cows.
Stomatocyte	In Alaskan malamutes with hereditary stomatocytosis; in humans with hereditary spherocytosis, stomatocytosis, hydrocytosis, cirrhosis, obstructive liver disease; in dogs with chronic anemias; occasional stomatocytes are found in normal cattle and sheep
Torocyte	Iron deficiency anemias and sometimes as artifacts

anemia and are seen occasionally in Heinz body anemia. They result from an excessive loss of surface membrane relative to the contents because of partial erythrophagocytosis of antibody and/or complement-coated red cells by macrophages in the MPS. Similarly, pitting of the Heinz body by macrophages may result in spherocyte formation. Spherocytes are readily detected in immune-mediated hemolytic anemia in the dog (Plate XVI-4), but are difficult to recognize in blood films of other species, although they have been found occasionally in the cat (see Fig. 22–1). Spherocytes have reduced deformability and consequently exhibit increased osmotic fragility (Figs. 7–15 and 22–2). A possible instance of hereditary spherocytosis was recorded in the goat (Fig. 7–10C). Spherocytes may rarely occur in cows with acute anaplasmosis.

A torocyte, commonly known as a punched-out cell, is a ring-shaped red cell with a sharply defined clear central area and a thickened peripheral rim of hemoglobin (Figs. 7–16D, 7–18D and G). It is believed to result from the peripheral redistribution of hemoglobin. Microcytic hypochromic red cells, seen in iron deficiency, have increased central pallor from reduced hemoglobin content and may resemble torocytes. In such cells, the clear area gradually merges with the peripheral hemoglobinized zone, as opposed to abrupt

separation in torocytes (compare Figs. 7–16B and D with Figs. 7–18F and G).

Rare abnormalities of ionic transport function and thermal reactivity of erythrocytes have been recognized in humans. The former has been associated with shape changes such as xerocytosis and hydrocytosis, and the latter with pyropoikilocytosis.

HEMOGLOBIN

Hemoglobin is essential to maintain life because it carries and delivers oxygen to tissues. About 400 million molecules of hemoglobin are present in the red cell and comprise 95% of its dry weight. Hemoglobin synthesis and destruction are balanced under physiologic conditions, and the disturbance of either one can lead to a significant hematologic disorder.

Synthesis

Hemoglobin is a conjugated protein composed of heme and globin (MW, 64,458). Each gram of hemoglobin contains 3.34 mg of iron and carries 1.34 ml of oxygen at complete saturation. At a Po$_2$ of 100 mm

Hg (approximate P_{O_2} of arterial blood), hemoglobin is about 97.5% saturated with oxygen. Each hemoglobin molecule consists of four heme units, and each is associated with a single globin chain that has amino acid residues arranged in an α helix. Each globin chain has eight helical areas, numbered A to H. Heme consists of a protoporphyrin IX ring (formerly called type III) with an atom of ferrous iron in the center. Heme occupies a precise location between the E and F helices of each chain, the heme pocket, through linkage of its two propionyl side chains with two lysyl residues of the globin chain. The ferrous atom of heme has six electron pairs; four are bound to the four nitrogens of the protoporphyrin ring, one is linked to a histidyl residue (α87, β92) of the globin chain, and one remains available to bind and transport oxygen. Oxyhemoglobin delivers oxygen to the tissues and then reverts to its native form. Methemoglobin (oxidized hemoglobin) cannot bind oxygen reversibly, because its ferric atom has only five pairs of electrons and lacks the electron pair necessary to bind the oxygen.

Various steps involved in the biogenesis of heme are outlined in Figure 7–21. Heme is synthesized in the mitochondria, so it is produced only in immature erythroid cells up to the reticulocyte stage. Mature mammalian erythrocytes cannot synthesize heme because they lack mitochondria. The rate-limiting step in the entire sequence of heme synthesis involves the enzyme δ-aminolevulinic acid (ALA) synthetase. Heme and globin concentrations in the developing red cell control their own synthesis by negative feedback mechanisms. Prolonged interference with heme synthesis at any stage manifests as microcytic hypochromic anemias, analogous to iron deficiency.

Heme synthesis is disturbed by lead poisoning, during which the intraerythrocytic concentration of free protoporphyrin builds up. Lead reduces heme synthesis by inhibiting ALA dehydrase and heme synthetase. Congenital erythropoietic porphyria in humans (Günther disease), cattle, pigs, and cats results from an autosomal recessive deficiency of uroporphyrinogen III cosynthetase. In comparison, erythropoietic protoporphyria in humans is caused by an autosomal dominant deficiency of heme synthetase (ferrochelatase). Affected animals accumulate porphyrins in the

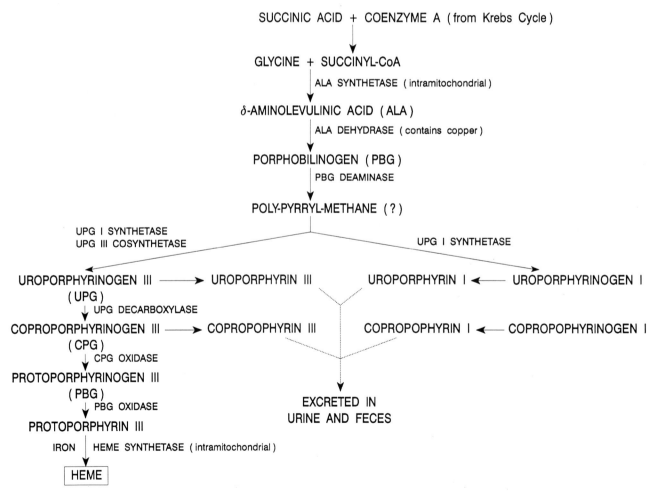

Fig. 7–21.   Schematic representation of the steps involved in the biogenesis of heme. (Modified from Jain, N. C.: Schalm's Veterinary Hematology. 4th Ed. Philadelphia, Lea & Febiger, 1986, p. 515.)

teeth, bones, and skin and excrete large amounts in the urine, which acquires a brown to wine color. The porphyrins are photosensitive; therefore, white areas of the skin (as in Holstein cattle), if unprotected, develop lesions typical of photosensitization.

Methemoglobin is a useless form of hemoglobin. Its ferric ions are continuously reduced to the native ferrous state by the NADH-cytochrome b_5 reductase-cytochrome b_5 system and by glutathione. Other forms of hemoglobin, such as sulfhemoglobin and carboxyhemoglobin, formed after exposure to some toxic agents and carbon monoxide, respectively, bind oxygen strongly and thus cannot deliver it to tissues. Hemin is an oxidized halide (chloride) of free heme and hematin contains hydroxyl ions in place of halides. Hemin and hematin are formed after the dissociation of heme from globin.

Globin synthesis occurs in the cytoplasmic ribosomes of nucleated red cells. Normal mammalian hemoglobin contains two α-like and two non-α (β, δ, or γ) chains. The human adult hemoglobin A molecule consists of two α- and two β-polypeptide chains ($\alpha_2\beta_2$), with 141 and 146 amino acid residues, respectively. Fetal hemoglobin has, instead of β chains, two γ chains ($\alpha_2\gamma_2$) and, similarly, hemoglobin A_2 has two δ chains ($\alpha_2\delta_2$). Embryonic hemoglobin is composed of two α or ζ chains and two γ or ε chains (Gower 1, $\zeta_2\epsilon_2$; Gower 2, $\alpha_2\epsilon_2$; and Portland, $\zeta_2\gamma_2$). Differences in the amino acid sequence of globin chains account for the differences in various hemoglobins within and among species. A greater heterogeneity exists in animal hemoglobins than in human hemoglobins.

Hemoglobinopathies result from abnormalities of globin synthesis. Both qualitative and quantitative abnormalities have been reported in humans, but none (so far) in animals. It is remarkable that the substitution of a single amino acid (valine for glutamic acid, at position 6 in the β chain) results in the formation of hemoglobin S and causes sickle cell anemia in humans.

A nonenzymatic irreversible linkage of glucose to hemoglobin in the erythrocytes produces a glycosylated hemoglobin. In humans, the major glycosylated hemoglobin is HbA_{1c} and is used as an index of long-term blood sugar concentration and to monitor therapy of patients with diabetes mellitus. Glycosylated hemoglobin (HbA_1) is found in normal dogs (mean normal value, 7.1% ± 1.1) and its concentration is increased (10.1 to 15.4%) in diabetic dogs (Easley, 1986).

Types

Embryonic, fetal, and adult hemoglobins have been found in various animal species, as in humans, but their number varies (Table 7–6). One type of embryonic hemoglobin (HbE) is found in the goat and rabbit, two are found in the sheep and humans, two to three in the cow, three in the cat and mouse, and two to four in the pig. One type of fetal hemoglobin (HbF) is found in the cow, sheep, goat, rabbit, pig, rat,

humans, and subhuman primates; and one to two in the white-tailed deer. HbE or HbF in the dog and horse are electrophoretically indistinguishable from adult hemoglobins.

The concentration of fetal hemoglobin is highest at birth and gradually diminishes with age as it is replaced by the adult hemoglobin, within a few weeks of life in most animals and in a few months in some. Different hemoglobins may be found in the same red cell. Fetal hemoglobin production is influenced by erythropoietin and it is produced by progenies of the BFU-E. Adult sheep and goats have three types of hemoglobins: HbA, HbB, and HbAB. The concentration of HbB in sheep varies with age, increasing between 0.5 to 4.5 years of age and then declining slightly. Sheep and goats with phenotypes A and AB but not B synthesize HbC and replace HbA during response to anemia. Such a switch does not occur in the cat and bovine. The factor responsible for the A to C switch is erythropoietin. Ovine red cells with fetal hemoglobin are osmotically more resistant then those with adult hemoglobin (Facello et al., 1985).

Degradation and Bilirubin Metabolism

Hemoglobin is released in the free form when hemolysis occurs and the bond between the hemoglobin and red cell stroma is broken by a hemolytic agent. Free hemoglobin in plasma is quickly disposed (half-life, 1 to 7 hours) by oxidation to useless forms, is lost through the kidney, or is destroyed by the MPS (Fig. 7–22). Hemoglobin imparts a pink to red color to the plasma and the condition is then called hemoglobinemia. Free hemoglobin in plasma is first bound to haptoglobin and the complex is rapidly removed and degraded by macrophages. Excess hemoglobin undergoes degradation to hemoglobin dimers or monomers for excretion by the kidney, resulting in hemoglobinuria or hemosiderinuria. Part of the free hemoglobin in the circulation is oxidized to methemoglobin, which in turn dissociates and liberates hematin. This hematin binds to hemopexin and albumin successively, and the hematin-hemopexin and methemalbumin complexes are removed by the hepatocytes. The formation of methemalbumin is a characteristic of human and simian albumin, whereas the albumin of most other mammalian species, including the dog, cow, horse, goat, and pig, does not bind hematin to form methemalbumin (George, 1988).

Hemoglobin released from senescent red cells destroyed by the macrophages in the MPS, is catabolized in a step-wise manner (Fig. 7–23). In the macrophages, the iron from heme and amino acids from globin are recycled for use. The protoporphyrin moiety is degraded to biliverdin by microsomal heme oxygenase in the presence of oxygen and NADPH. The biliverdin is then converted to bilirubin by bilirubin reductase in the presence of NADPH. Birds excrete only biliverdin because they lack biliverdin reductase. Bilirubin released into the plasma is bound to albumin for trans-

Table 7–6. Hemoglobin Types in Animal Species

Species	Hemoglobin Type			Comments
	Embryonic	Fetal	Adult	
Dog	0	*	1–2	No embryonic or fetal Hb distinguishable from adult Hb
Cat	3	0	1–2	Three types of embryonic Hb present at 21 days after conception, but disappear between 30 and 35 days; adult Hb present between 20 and 30 days after conception and varies considerably in proportion
Cow	2–3	1	1–5	Embryonic Hb clearly shown at 4 weeks after conception and disappears between 6 and 10 weeks; fetal Hb appears at 6–8 weeks after conception and persists to 3–10 weeks after birth; Hb types vary in different breeds, types A and B most common
Horse	0	*	1–2	No embryonic or fetal Hb component distinguishable from adult Hb; most horses have two types of Hb in a ratio of approximately 70:30, but certain breeds may have only one component
Sheep	2	1	1–4	Trace of embryonic Hb present only at early development; fetal Hb present at 40 days, begins to decrease at birth, and disappears between 40 and 50 days of age; HbC appears soon after birth, with a rise to about 15% followed by a gradual disappearance; HbC reappears in response to blood loss
Goat	1	1	1–6	Embryonic and fetal Hb patterns same as in sheep; HbC appears soon after birth, approaching 100% at about 60 days with gradual disappearance and replacement with final adult Hb types; HbC reappears in response to blood loss
Rabbit	1	1	1–4	At 12 days after conception, three types of Hb are present: two embryonic and one indistinguishable from the adult type, but major component is embryonic; at 20 days of gestation, two components present, major one is adult type; near term, only adult type is present
Mouse	3	0	2–6	Embryonic types of Hb are present at day 12 and disappear by day 15 after conception; disappearance of embryonic components is followed by appearance of adult types
Guinea pig	0	0	1–2	No embryonic or fetal Hb detected in blood studied approximately 20–25 days after conception
Pig	2–4	1	1	Fetal and embryonic Hb present at 30 days after conception; embryonic Hb disappears between 45 and 60 days and fetal Hb is present at birth; fetal Hb is electrophoretically indistinguishable from adult Hb, and can be identified only by peptide mapping
Rat	0	1	4	Four Hb components present at birth, one component disappears 8–12 days after birth; four types of Hb are present in adult
White-tailed deer	0	1–2	1–8	At birth, 95% of Hb present is of fetal type, completely replaced by adult Hb 8–12 weeks after birth; presence of high levels of fetal Hb precludes sickling in young deer

Modified from Kitchen, H.: Fetal hemoglobins. Am. Soc. Vet. Clin. Pathol., 1:25, 1972.
* Prenatal hemoglobins indistinguishable from adult types by electrophoresis or peptide mapping techniques.

port to hepatic cells, where it is conjugated to glucuronic acid by the enzyme UDP-glucuronyltransferase. The hepatic uptake of bilirubin is facilitated by two types of protein (ligandins and the Z protein). Conjugated bilirubin is normally secreted across the biliary canalicular membrane in the bile for excretion into the intestine. In the intestinal tract, bilirubin is degraded to urobilinogen for excretion in feces, but some enters the general circulation for re-excretion in the bile. This process is known as the enterohepatic circulation of bile. A small amount of conjugated bilirubin and urobilinogen normally escapes re-excretion by the liver and is eliminated into the urine, and increased amounts are often excreted in those with hepatic disease.

Hereditary defects in the conjugation of bilirubin have been reported in humans, rats, and sheep (Kaneko, 1989). Severe unconjugated hyperbilirubinemia occurs from the congenital absence of the UDP-glucuronyltransferase (Gunn rats and Crigler-Najjar syndrome in humans) and from the defective uptake of bilirubin (Gilbert's syndrome in humans and South-

down mutant sheep). Defective hepatic secretion of bilirubin is associated with conjugated hyperbilirubinemia (Dubin-Johnson syndrome in humans, mutant Wistar rats, and Corriedale mutant sheep).

The two major forms of bilirubin in plasma have various names—unconjugated, free, albumin-bound, or indirect bilirubin, and conjugated or direct bilirubin or bilirubin diglucuronide. Unconjugated bilirubin does not filter through the kidney, but conjugated bilirubin does. In the van den Bergh test, bilirubin glucuronide is the direct-reacting bilirubin, whereas albumin-bound bilirubin is the indirect-reacting bilirubin. The increased accumulation of bilirubin in blood leads to jaundice or icterus. In hemolytic anemias, most of the bilirubin in blood is unconjugated, but it is largely conjugated in extrahepatic obstruction of the bile duct and mixed in hepatocellular disease. Although the major source of plasma bilirubin is senescent red cells, some may be derived from ineffective erythropoiesis in the bone marrow, degradation of hemoglobin associated with extruded metarubricyte nuclei during the birth of the reticulocyte, or surface

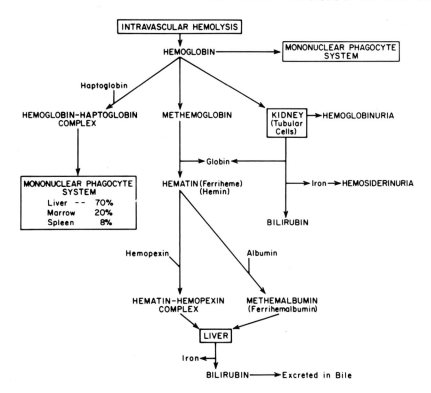

Fig. 7–22. Outline of steps involved in the catabolism of free hemoglobin in the plasma. (From Jain, N. C.: Schalm's Veterinary Hematology. 4th Ed. Philadelphia, Lea & Febiger, 1986, p. 521.)

remodeling of circulating reticulocytes in the spleen. Hypobilirubinemia may occur during decreased erythropoiesis.

The horse is unique in that its plasma bilirubin concentration is high compared to other species, and most of it is unconjugated. Its bilirubin concentration increases during anorexia and febrile conditions because of inappropriate hepatic uptake. Bilirubin concentration is high at birth, particularly in foals. Although the precise cause of neonatal hyperbilirubinemia in animals is unknown, similar observations in the human neonate indicate that it may involve several mechanisms. These include loss of the placental excretory mechanism for bilirubin, a low level of UDP-glucuronyltransferase activity in the neonatal liver, and a greater concentration of β-glucuronidase in the intestine, which degrades bilirubin glucuronide to free bilirubin that is reabsorbed.

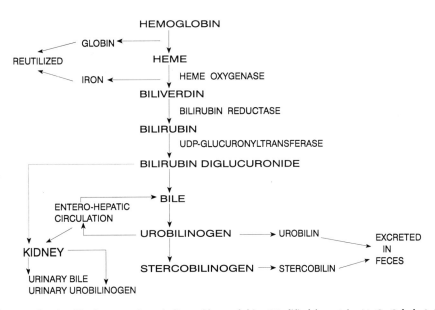

Fig. 7–23. Outline of the steps involved in the normal catabolism of hemoglobin. (Modified from Jain, N. C.: Schalm's Veterinary Hematology. 4th Ed. Philadelphia, Lea & Febiger, 1986, p. 523.)

REFERENCES

Abbot, D.L., and McGrath, J.P.: Evaluation of flow cytometric counting procedure for canine reticulocytes by use of thiazole orange. Am. J. Vet. Res., 52:723, 1991.

Adams, P.C., Powell, L.W., and Halliday, J.W.: Solid phase immunoradiometric assay for procine serum. Comp. Biochem. Physiol. [B], 89:355, 1988.

Andrews, G.A., Smith, J.E., Gray, M., et al.: An improved ferritin assay for canine sera. Vet. Clin. Path., 21:57, 1992.

Badylak, S.F., Van Vleet, J.F., Herman, E.H., et al.: Poikilocytosis in dogs with chronic doxorubicin toxicosis. Am. J. Vet. Res., 46:505, 1985.

Barker, R.N.: Electrophoretic analysis of erythrocyte membrane proteins and glycoproteins from different species. Comp. Haematol. Int., 1:155, 1991.

Bessis, M.: Blood smear reinterpreted. Berlin, Springer International, 1977.

Brogden, K.A., and Engen, R.L.: Alterations in the phospholipid composition and morphology of ovine erythrocytes after intravenous inoculation of *Corynebacterium pseudotuberculosis*. Am. J. Vet. Res., 51:874, 1990.

Clerbaux, T., Serteyn, D., Willems, E., et al.: Determination of the standard dissociation curve for equine oxyhemoglobin and the effect of temperature, pH and diphosphoglycerate. Can. J. Vet. Res., 50:188, 1986.

Debski, B.: The effect of training and physical exercise on the energetic metabolism of equine erythrocytes. Zentralbl. Veterinarmed. [A], 32:190, 1985.

Degen, M.: Pseudohyperkalemia in Akitas. J. Am. Vet. Med. Assoc., 190:541, 1987.

Durotoye, L.A.: The effect of sex, pregnancy and lactation on the osmotic fragility of erythrocytes of the West African dwarf sheep. Bull. Animal Hlth. Prod. Africa, 35:29, 1987.

Duthie, G.G., Arthur, J.R., Bremner, P., et al.: Increased peroxidation of erythrocytes of stress-susceptible pigs: An improved diagnostic test for porcine stress syndrome. Am. J. Vet. Res., 50:84, 1989.

Easley, J.R.: Glycosylated hemoglobin in dogs: Precision, stability, and diagnostic utility. Vet. Clin. Pathol., 15:12, 1986.

Esievo, K.A.N., Jaye, A.N., Andrews, J.J.N., et al.: Electrophoresis of bovine erythrocyte sialic acids: existence of additional band in trypanotolerant Ndama cattle. J. Comp. Pathol., 102:357, 1990.

Esievo, K.A.N., Saror, D.I., Kolo, M.N., et al.: Erythrocyte surface sialic acid in Ndama and Zebu cattle. J. Comp. Pathol., 96:95, 1986.

Facello, C., Guglielmino, R., Quaranta, G., et al.: Haemoglobin and erythrocyte osmotic fragility in sheep. Variations in relations to haemoglobin polymorphism. Summa, 2:247, 1985.

Fairley, N.M., Price, G.S. and Meuten, D.J.: Evaluation of red blood cell fragility in Pygmy goats. Am. J. Vet. Res., 49:1598, 1988.

George, J.W.: Methemalbumin: reality and myth. Vet. Clin. Pathol., 17:43, 1988.

Giger, U.R.S.: Erythropoietin and its clinical use. Compend. Contin. Educ. Pract. Vet., 14:25, 1992.

Hambitzer, R.: Changes in equine red blood cells during endurance exercise. Israel J. Vet. Med., 43:91, 1987.

Harvey, J.W., Asquith, R.L., Sussman, W.A., et al.: Serum ferritin, serum iron, and erythrocyte values in foals. Am. J. Vet. Res., 48:1348, 1987.

Ikeda, T., Inaba, M. and Maede, Y.: Serum erythropoietin level in normal dogs. Jap. J. Vet. Sci., 52:877, 1990.

Jain, N.C.: Schalm's Veterinary Hematology. 4th ed. Philadelphia, Lea & Febiger, pp. 487–562, 1986.

Jain, N.C. and Kono, C.S.: Shape changes in caprine erythrocytes exposed to chlorpromazine and lysolecithin. Vet. Clin. Path., 18:75, 1989.

Ji, L.L., Dillon, D.A., Bump, K.D., et al.: Antioxidant enzyme response to exercise in equine erythrocytes. J. Equine Vet. Sci., 10:380, 1990.

Kaneko, J.J.: Clinical Biochemistry of Domestic Animals. 4th ed. San Diego, Academic Press, 1989.

Kuehn, N.F. and Gaunt, S.D.: Hypocellular marrow and extramedullary hematopoiesis in a dog: hematologic recovery after splenectomy. J. Am. Vet. Med. Assoc., 188:1313, 1986.

Maede, Y., Amano, Y., Nishida, A., et al.: Hereditary high-potassium erythrocytes with high Na, K-ATPase activity in Japanese Shiba dogs. Res. Vet. Sci., 50:123, 1991.

Maginniss, L.A., Olszowka, A.J. and Reeves, R.B.: Oxygen equilibrium curve shape and allohemoglobin interaction in sheep whole blood. Am. J. Physiol., 250:R298, 1986.

Smith, J.E.: Erythrocyte membrane: structure, function, and pathophysiology. Vet. Pathol., 24:471, 1987.

Snow, D.H. and Martin, M.: Effects of exercise and adrenaline on equine erythrocyte ATP content. Res. Vet. Sci., 49:77, 1990.

Stull, C.L. and Lawrence, L.M.: The effect of exercise and conditioning on equine red blood cell characteristics. J. Equine Vet. Sci., 6:170, 1986.

Tvedten, H.W.: What is your diagnosis? Vet. Clin. Pathol., 19:77, 1990.

Weeks, B.R., Smith, J.E. and Northrop, J.K.: Relationship of serum ferritin and iron concentrations and serum total iron-binding capacity to nonheme iron stores in dogs. Am. J. Vet. Res., 50: 198, 1989.

Weiss, D.J. and Klausner, J.S.: Neutrophil-induced erythrocyte injury: A potential cause of erythrocyte destruction in anemia with inflammatory disease. Vet. Pathol., 25:450, 1988.

Weiss, D.J., Kristensen, A., Papenfuss, N., et al.: Quantitative evaluation of echinocytes in the dog. Vet. Clin. Pathol., 19:114, 1990.

Williams, W.J., Beutler, E., Erslev, A.J., et al.: Hematology. 4th ed. New York, McGraw-Hill, 1990.

Wilson, O. and Dixon, E.: Erythrocyte cation content and sodium transport in Siberian Huskies. Am. J. Vet. Res., 52:1427, 1991.

Woodman, D.D.: Erythropoietin. Comp. Haematol. Int., 2:1, 1992.

Yamoto, O. and Maede, Y.: Susceptibility to onion-induced hemolysis in dogs with hereditary high erythrocyte reduced glutathione and potassium concentrations. Am. J. Vet. Res., 53:134, 1992.

Abbreviations for Fig. 7–13.

ADP, adenosine diphosphate; ATP, adenosine triphosphate; DHAP, dihydroxyacetone phosphate; 1,3DPG, 1,3-diphosphoglycerate; 2,3DPG, 2,3-diphosphoglycerate; DPGM, diphosphoglycerate mutase; F6P, fructose 6-phosphate; FDP, fructose 1,6-diphosphate; G3P, glyceraldehyde 3-phosphate; G6P, glucose 6-phosphate; G6PD, glucose 6-phosphate dehydrogenase; GAPD, glyceraldehyde 3-phosphate dehydrogenase; GPI, glucose phosphate isomerase; GPx, glutathione peroxidase; GR, glutathione reductase; GSH, reduced glutathione; GSSG, oxidized glutathione; H_2O_2, hydrogen peroxide; HK, hexokinase; LDH, lactate dehydrogenase; LMB, leukomethylene blue; MB, methylene blue, NAD, nicotinamide adenine dinucleotide; NADH, reduced nicotinamide adenine dinucleotide; NADP, nicotinamide adenine dinucleotide phosphate; NADPH, reduced nicotinamide adenine dinucleotide phosphate; NADPH-D, NADPH dehydrogenase or diaphorase; PEP, phosphoenolpyruvate; PFK, phosphofructokinase; 2PG, 2-phosphoglycerate; 3PG, 3-phosphoglycerate; 6PGD, 6-phosphogluconate dehydrogenase; PGK, phosphoglycerate kinase; Pi, inorganic phosphate; PK, pyruvate kinase; SOD, superoxide dismutase; TA, transaldolase; TK, transketolase; TPI, triosephosphate isomerase.

Evaluation of Anemias and Polycythemias

Anemia is defined as the presence of a below-normal red cell count, hemoglobin concentration, and/or packed cell volume (PCV). The reverse indicates erythrocytosis or polycythemia. Anemia is rarely a primary disease—more commonly, it is one of the results of a generalized disease process. Anemia may be suspected from clinical signs and presenting history of a patient. Once anemia has been detected, its pathogenesis or cause should be thoroughly investigated to determine the proper therapeutic management of the patient. Treatment is not to be directed at the anemia per se except as an emergency measure; the cause must be found and corrected, if possible. The interpretation of erythrocyte parameters and other laboratory tests for the investigation of anemia and polycythemia are summarized in Figure 8–1.

CLINICAL SIGNS OF ANEMIA

The clinical signs referable to anemia result from the reduced oxygen-carrying capacity of the blood and from certain physiologic adjustments designed to increase the efficiency of the reduced circulating red cell mass and reduce the workload of the heart. The development of various clinical signs and their magnitude depend on rapidity of onset, degree, and cause of the anemia, as well as the physical activity of the animal. Signs common to anemias of diverse causes include exertional dyspnea, reduced exercise tolerance, pallor of the mucous membranes, increased heart rate, sometimes with murmurs (usually systolic), increased inappropriate respiratory rate, depression, and dementia.

In acute blood loss, when one-third of the blood volume has been lost in a short period, shock occurs and death may ensue. Tachycardia and dyspnea become prominent signs. In these cases, blood transfusion or the administration of plasma expanders is indicated to prevent death.

Clinical signs resulting from acute hemolytic anemia include icterus, hemoglobinemia, hemoglobinuria, and fever. Icterus without hemoglobinuria is observed when accelerated destruction of the erythrocytes occurs within the mononuclear phagocyte system (MPS), whereas massive hemolysis of red cells within the bloodstream is followed by hemoglobinemia and sometimes by hemoglobinuria. Nephrosis may develop from hemoglobinuria. The sudden release of hemoglobin and the end products of erythrocyte breakdown lead to pyrexia. Significant intravascular hemolysis may lead to disseminated intravascular coagulation.

In chronic blood loss or hemolytic anemias and in depression anemias, the hemoglobin level may drop to as low as 50% of the minimum normal without overt signs of hypoxemia, unless the patient is exerted. Compensatory adjustments occur in chronic anemia—increases occur in the heart rate and, later, in the heart size, to lessen the circulation time of the erythrocytes.

CLASSIFICATION OF ANEMIAS

Anemia may be relative or absolute in terms of the total red cell mass, which is normal in the former and reduced in the latter (Fig. 8–2). Relative anemia may develop from the expansion of plasma volume, as in pregnant females and neonates or after fluid therapy.

INTERPRETATION OF ERYTHROCYTE PARAMETERS

RBC\PCV\Hb
- ☐ Normal
- ☐ Increased
- ☐ Decreased

PLASMA PROTEINS
- ☐ Normal
- ☐ Increased
- ☐ Decreased

ICTERUS INDEX
- ☐ Normal
- ☐ Increased

NUCLEATED RBC
- ☐ Present
- ☐ Absent

RETICULOCYTES
- ☐ Normal
- ☐ Increased
- ☐ Decreased
- ☐ Aggregate
- ☐ Punctate
- ☐ RPI: N/↑/↓

PLATELET COUNT
- ☐ Normal
- ☐ Increased
- ☐ Decreased

RBC MORPHOLOGY
- ☐ Acanthocytes
- ☐ Accuminocytes
- ☐ Codocytes
- ☐ Dacrocytes
- ☐ Discocytes
- ☐ Drepanocytes
- ☐ Echinocytes
- ☐ Elliptocytes
- ☐ Keratocytes
- ☐ Knizocytes
- ☐ Leptocytes
- ☐ Macrocytes
- ☐ Microcytes
- ☐ Poikilocytes
- ☐ Schistocytes
- ☐ Siderocytes
- ☐ Spherocytes
- ☐ Stomatocytes
- ☐ Torocytes

- ☐ Agglutination
- ☐ Anisocytosis
- ☐ Basoph stippling
- ☐ Heinz bodies
- ☐ Hb crystals
- ☐ H-J bodies
- ☐ Pappenhmr bodies
- ☐ Polychromasia
- ☐ RBC inclusions
- ☐ RBC parasite
- ☐ Rouleau
- ☐ Other _____

RBC INDEXES
- ☐ MCV: N/↑/↓
- ☐ MCHC: N/↑/↓
- ☐ MCH: N/↑/↓

ADDITIONAL TESTS
- ☐ Coagulopathy
- ☐ Coombs test
- ☐ Cross match
- ☐ ESR: +/-/diphasic
- ☐ Fecal occult blood
- ☐ Hemoglobinemia
- ☐ Serum haptoglobin
- ☐ Serum methemoglobin
- ☐ RBC saline fragility
- ☐ RBC life span
- ☐ Serum bilirubin
- ☐ Serum iron/TIBC
- ☐ Transfusion: _____
- ☐ Parasitic exam
- ☐ Urinalysis
  - ☐ Bilirubinuria
  - ☐ Hematuria
  - ☐ Hemoglobinuria
  - ☐ Proteinuria

BONE MARROW ERYTHROPOIESIS
- ☐ DysEP
- ☐ Hypoplasia
- ☐ Hyperplasia
- ☐ Effect EP
- ☐ Ineffect EP
- ☐ Megaloblasts
- ☐ BM iron
- ☐ M:E -- N/↑/↓
- ☐ Reticulocytes

RBC METABOLISM
- ☐ ATP
- ☐ G6PD
- ☐ GSH
- ☐ PK
- ☐ PFK
- ☐ Porphyrins
- ☐ Other

INTERPRETATION
- ☐ Normal
- ☐ Age-related
- ☐ Breed specific
- ☐ Species specific
- ☐ Spurious
- ☐ Anemia
- ☐ Polycythemia
- ☐ MPD
- ☐ Erythroleukemia
- ☐ Erythremic myelosis
- ☐ Other _____

◼ TYPE OF ANEMIA

ERYTHROPOIETIC RESPONSE
- ☐ Responsive
- ☐ Nonresponsive

MORPHOLOGIC
- ☐ Normocytic Normochromic
- ☐ Normocytic Hypochromic
- ☐ Microcytic Normochromic
- ☐ Microcytic Hypochromic
- ☐ Macrocytic Normochromic
- ☐ Macrocytic Hypochromic
- ☐ Other _____

PATHOPHYSIOLOGIC
- ☐ Blood loss
  - ☐ Acute
  - ☐ Chronic
  - Cause? _____
- ☐ Depression
  - Cause? _____
- ☐ Hemolytic
  - Cause? _____

◼ POLYCYTHEMIA

RELATIVE
- ☐ Dehydration
- ☐ Splenic contraction

ABSOLUTE
- ☐ Primary
- ☐ Secondary

Arterial oxygen
- ☐ Increased
- ☐ Normal

Serum Erythropoietin
- ☐ Increased
  - ☐ Autonomous
  - ☐ Hypoxic
- ☐ Normal

Fig. 8–1. An approach to the interpretation of erythrocyte parameters and other laboratory tests in the investigation of the type and cause of anemia and polycythemia.

RED CELL MASS   PLASMA VOLUME   PCV (%)

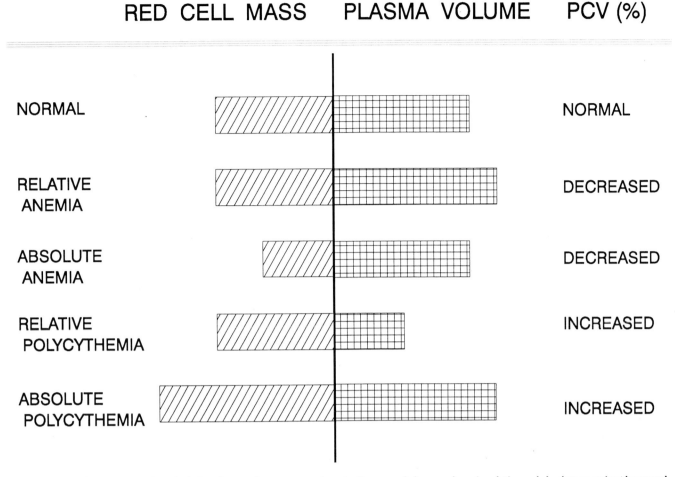

Fig. 8–2. Graphic representation of relative changes that may occur in red cell mass and plasma volume in relative and absolute anemias (decreased packed cell volume, PCV) and polycythemias (increased PCV). *Relative anemia* results from the expansion of plasma volume with normal red cell mass, as in pregnant females and neonates. *Absolute anemia* manifests when the red cell mass is reduced but the plasma volume remains normal, as in hemolytic or depression anemia. *Relative polycythemia* occurs when the plasma volume is reduced but the red cell mass remains normal, as in dehydration. *Primary polycythemia* is associated with a marked expansion in the red cell mass and some increase in the plasma volume.

Absolute anemia is clinically important and deserves thorough investigation. It is the most common form of anemia. Absolute anemias can be classified based on erythrocyte morphology, pathogenetic mechanisms, and bone marrow erythroid response. Although none of these is completely satisfactory by itself, they are complementary, and together provide a logical means of analyzing the anemia. The purpose of classifying anemias in various ways is to determine possible pathophysiologic mechanisms and probable causes. Anemia of a particular cause may involve more than one pathogenetic mechanism (e.g., a hemolytic component as well as suppression of erythropoiesis). A common practice is initial evaluation of a hemogram to classify the anemia morphologically on the basis of the MCV (mean corpuscular volume) and MCHC (mean corpuscular hemoglobin concentration). Evidence of the bone marrow response to anemia is then obtained by determining the degree of reticulocytosis or polychromasia in the blood.

Pathophysiologic Classification

Various causes of anemia include acute or chronic blood loss, intravascular or extravascular hemolysis, and selective or generalized hypoplasia or aplasia of the bone marrow, including deficiency or defective utilization of the nutrients essential for erythrocyte production (Table 8–1). Details of different types of anemias are given in Chapters 9 through 12. This classification scheme considers possible mechanisms of anemia and provides a rationale for appropriate therapy on that basis. Blood loss anemias generally result from the external loss of both red cells and plasma proteins, and hemolytic anemias are characterized by the destruction of circulating red cells. Hypoproliferative anemias result from reduced effective erythropoiesis from various causes. The red cell life span is usually normal in blood loss anemias and hypoproliferative anemias, but it is characteristically reduced in hemolytic anemias.

Table 8–1. Pathophysiologic Classification of Anemias

Blood loss or hemorrhagic anemias (see Table 9–3)
  Acute and chronic blood loss from various causes
Hemolytic anemias (see Tables 10–1 and 11–1)
  Blood parasites, bacterial, viral, and rickettsial agents
  Chemicals and drugs
  Poisonous plants
  Metabolic diseases
  Intraerythrocytic defects
  Immune-mediated disorders
  Miscellaneous causes
Depression or hypoproliferative anemias (see Table 12–1)
  Nutritional deficiency anemias
  Anemia of inflammatory disease
  Organic or tissue disorders
  Parasitic diseases
  Aplastic or hypoplastic anemias
  Myeloproliferative disorders

Morphologic Classification

Anemias may be classified on the basis of erythrocyte morphology using the two red cell indices, MCV and MCHC (Table 8–2). The morphologic categorization of anemia must be confirmed by the microscopic examination of erythrocyte populations. The morphologic classification of anemia is nonspecific as to cause, but is helpful in providing clues about pathophysiologic mechanisms. It also forms a basis for consideration and selection of treatment program.

Macrocytic normochromic anemia in humans is characteristic of vitamin B_{12} and folate deficiency. Such an anemia results from asynchrony of erythropoiesis whereby maturation arrest occurs at the prorubricyte-basophilic rubricyte stages, which produces megaloblastic erythroid cells in the bone marrow. Cattle on cobalt-deficient or molybdenum-rich pasture have developed macrocytic normochromic anemia, but this is rare. Macrocytic normochromic erythrocytes unaccompanied by anemia have been observed in some poodle dogs.

Macrocytic hypochromic anemia is typically observed during remission in acute blood loss or acute hemolytic anemia. The degree of macrocytosis and hypochromasia depends on the severity of anemia and on the associated intensified erythropoietic bone marrow response that leads to reticulocytosis in the blood. Reticulocytosis in response to the anemia increases the MCV and decreases the MCHC (Fig. 8–3). Several

days must elapse from the onset of anemia, however, before such a red cell morphology is apparent.

Normocytic normochromic anemia occurs from the selective depression of erythropoiesis in chronic diseases (e.g., infections, nephritis with uremia, malignancies, and certain endocrine disorders). In such cases, the reticulocyte response is absent or insignificant. Hematinics are not indicated, because the erythropoietic tissue cannot use these substances. Efforts should be directed toward diagnosis of the primary disease rather than treatment of the anemia.

Microcytic hypochromic anemia results from iron deficiency or failure to use iron for hemoglobin synthesis. Changes in erythrocyte morphology depend on the duration and severity of the anemia. Determination of the iron-binding capacity and serum iron, ferritin, and bone marrow iron levels is helpful in evaluating iron supply, utilization, and stores (see Chap. 9). Chronic blood loss or iron, copper, and pyridoxine deficiencies must be considered. Microcytic normochromic and normocytic hypochromic red cell morphology may be found during the development of the typical iron deficiency that would manifest later as microcytic hypochromic anemia. Microcytic normochromic red cells are a normal finding in some Akitas.

Classification Based on Bone Marrow Response to Anemia

Erythropoiesis is regulated by erythropoietin that is produced primarily by the kidneys in response to renal tissue hypoxia. Erythropoietin synthesis is inversely proportional to red cell mass and hemoglobin concentration. Erythropoiesis is stimulated by increased recruitment of progenitor cells, accelerated mitosis and maturation of erythroid cells, and speedy delivery of reticulocytes or young red cells to the circulation. The release of large ("stress" or "shift") reticulocytes into blood may be accompanied by the release of a small number of nucleated red cells (normoblastemia).

Based on the bone marrow erythropoietic response evident in the peripheral blood, anemias can be classified as responsive or regenerative and as nonresponsive or nonregenerative. This is helpful in differentiating blood loss and hemolytic anemias (generally responsive) from depression anemias (nonresponsive). Diminished erythropoietin production, inadequate re-

Table 8–2. Morphologic Classification of Erythrocyte Populations or Anemias

Based on MCV	Based on MCHC	Clinical Interpretation
Normocytic	Normochromic	Normal erythrocyte morphology; depression anemias (see Table 12–1), excluding certain nutritional deficiencies and some cases of myeloproliferative disorders in the cat (see below)
Normocytic	Hypochromic	Early iron deficiency
Macrocytic	Normochromic	Pernicious anemia in humans and primates; vitamin B_{12} and folate deficiencies; cobalt deficiency in ruminants; erythremic myelosis and erythroleukemia in cats; defective erythrogenesis, as in poodle macrocytosis
Macrocytic	Hypochromic	Anemia in remission, either blood loss (see Table 9–3) or hemolytic (see Table 10–1)
Microcytic	Normochromic	Characteristic of the Japanese Akita dogs; iron deficiency in progression
Microcytic	Hypochromic	Iron and copper deficiencies and chronic blood loss (see Table 9–3); pyridoxine deficiency

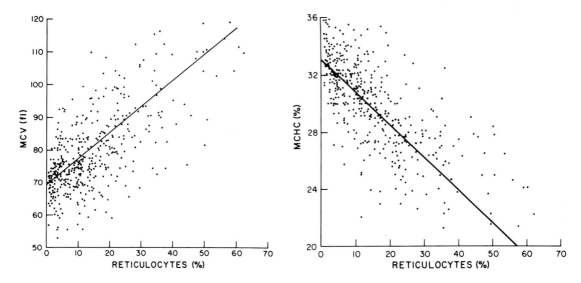

Fig. 8–3. Correlation of MCV *(left)* and MCHC *(right)* with reticulocyte count for anemic canine patients. (From Jain, N. C.: Hematologic characteristics of anemia. I. Pathophysiologic features of the erythrocyte. Cal. Vet., 33:9, 1979.)

sponse of the erythroid tissue to appropriate stimuli, or increased ineffective erythropoiesis manifests as nonresponsive anemia.

LABORATORY EVALUATION OF ANEMIAS

In this section, only brief comments of a general and comparative nature are made about various anemias. Details of specific types of anemias are found in Chapters 9 through 12 and in comprehensive hematology texts (Jain, 1986; Williams et al., 1990).

Red Cell Parameters

Anemia is indicated when one or more of the red cell parameters (PCV, hemoglobin, and RBC count) are below the normal level for the age, sex, and breed of the species concerned. Geographic location with regard to altitude and laboratory errors affecting red cell parameters should be considered. Of these three parameters, the PCV provides a simple, quick, and accurate means of detecting anemia, but should not be considered a reliable indicator if the animal is known to have an exceptionally high (poodles) or low (Akitas) MCV in health. In such cases, the hemoglobin concentration should be considered for establishing the presence (or absence) of anemia. During the latter half or last trimester of pregnancy, females may have lower red cell values ("spurious anemia") than nonpregnant females because of increased plasma volume and, occasionally, iron deficiency. Dehydration and splenic contraction may mask the anemia, whereas hemodilution may cause a temporary reduction in red cell parameters. Determination of both the PCV and total plasma protein concentration may help in differentiating these variables. Dehydration is associated with increases in plasma protein concentration and PCV, but splenic contraction elevates only the PCV.

Hemodilution following acute blood loss or fluid therapy is associated with decreases in both the plasma protein level and PCV, whereas hemolytic anemias are usually associated only with a reduction in the PCV. The degree of anemia varies with the nature, extent, and duration of the disease process. In general, a mild anemia is more common than a marked anemia.

Reticulocyte Count

The reticulocyte count is the best semiquantitative indicator of effective marrow erythropoietic activity, but reticulocyte counts should be interpreted in relation to species differences in erythropoiesis and to the release of young red cells into the circulation. Reticulocytes are normally found in the peripheral blood in small numbers in dogs and cats, rarely in cattle, sheep, and goats, and not in horses. Dogs respond to increased erythroid stimulation, as do humans. The varied morphology of reticulocytes in the cat (see Chap. 2) presents great difficulty in obtaining a valid reticulocyte count and interpreting it properly; "punctate" reticulocytes exceed "aggregate" reticulocytes and persist in blood much longer. In ruminants, the magnitude of reticulocytosis is lower and the presence of even some reticulocytes in blood is considered evidence of responsive anemia. Horses do not exhibit reticulocytosis, even when the anemia is extreme. Sometimes, a horse may respond with a marked anisocytosis as a result of macrocytosis from the erythropoietic response to anemia.

The reticulocyte count during responsive anemias generally varies with the degree of anemia (Table 8–3). *The greater the stimulation of marrow erythropoiesis, the greater the reticulocytosis.* Such is not the case in nonresponsive anemias. Therefore, the degree of reticulocytosis must be viewed in concert with the degree of anemia. This can be done by calculating a corrected reticulocyte count (%) or an absolute reticulocyte count

Table 8–3. Degree of Anemia and its Relationship to Reticulocyte Counts in Blood of Canine Patients

PCV (%)*	Patients		Number of Patients†	Reticulocyte Count (%)	
	Number	%		Range	Mean
>10	10	1.0	10	0–48.6	12.66
11–15	25	2.5	23	0–35.4	11.06
16–20	39	3.9	36	0–29.5	5.45
21–25	74	7.4	73	0–27.0	5.44
26–30	189	18.9	176	0–21.6	2.29
31–36	663	66.3	455	0–15.6	1.48

From Jain, N.C.: Hematologic characteristics of anemia. 33:15, 1979.

* Degree of anemia determined by packed cell volume (PCV) evaluation, normal range being 37–55%. A total of 1000 patients was evaluated.

† Reticulocyte counts were performed only for 773 patients.

(numbers/μl of blood). A reticulocyte production index (RPI) is calculated to eliminate errors arising from both the degree of anemia and the premature release of large ("shift") reticulocytes from the bone marrow into the circulation.

The absolute reticulocyte count is calculated by multiplying the percentage of reticulocytes by the RBC count. Alternatively, the percentage of reticulocytes can be corrected for the degree of anemia by the formula: corrected reticulocyte % = (observed reticulocyte count) × (PCV of the patient / mean normal PCV for the species). Mean normal PCV is 45% for the dog and 37% for the cat. Hemoglobin concentration or RBC count may be substituted for PCV in the above formula for similar calculations. A correction for the premature release of reticulocytes and their prolonged maturation time in the peripheral blood is made to calculate the RPI by the formula: RPI = corrected % reticulocyte count divided by the reticulocyte maturation time for the degree of anemia. The maturation of reticulocytes in the peripheral blood for humans is estimated as 1 day for a PCV of 45, 1.5 days for a PCV of 35, 2.0 days for a PCV of 25, and 2.5 days for a PCV of 15.0. Data for the animal species are not available, but similar values have been used to calculate the RPI for the dog. For example, a reticulocyte count of 5.0%, RBC count of 3.0 million/μl, and PCV of 25% in an anemic dog would equal an absolute reticulocyte count of 0.05 × 3.0 million or 150,000/μl of blood, a corrected reticulocyte count of 5.0 × 25/45 or 2.77%, and an RPI of 2.77/2.0 or 1.39.

A corrected reticulocyte count above 1% in the dog and cat indicates active erythropoiesis (responsive anemia). An absolute reticulocyte count of greater than 60,000/μl of blood in the dog is evidence of a responsive anemia. Similarly, greater than 50,000 aggregated reticulocytes/μl of blood in the cat indicate a responsive anemia (Kociba, 1989). An RPI lower than 1 usually indicates nonresponsive anemia, an RPI between 1 and 2 indicates erythropoietically active marrow with some response to anemia, and an RPI of greater than 2 is suggestive of accelerated erythropoiesis.

The magnitude of reticulocytosis is generally greater

in hemolytic anemia and is evident earlier than in blood loss anemia. Usually, it takes about 3 to 4 days for a significant reticulocytosis to be found in blood after an acute hemolytic or hemorrhagic episode, and a maximum response may take 1 to 2 weeks or longer. In a severe hemolytic anemia of rapid onset, however, a "shift" reticulocytosis (accelerated release of reticulocytes from the bone marrow pool) may develop in 1 to 2 days and be followed by reticulocytosis from intensified erythropoiesis. In studies on phenylhydrazine-induced Heinz body anemia in dogs, the mean PCV and peak reticulocyte counts varied with the dosage given, as follows: 5 mg/kg—32.5%, 5.9%; 8 mg/kg—25%, 8.2%; 11 mg/kg—25%, 11%; and 15 mg/kg—17%, 55% (Brock et al., 1989). With the highest dosage given, marked reticulocytosis in blood was evident by the second day and enhanced erythropoiesis was reflected in a decreased myeloid:erythroid ratio as early as the third day after induction of the anemia. Infection with canine parvovirus did not induce an inhibitory effect on erythropoiesis in these dogs.

Thus, reticulocytosis in an anemic patient indicates increased red cell destruction or blood loss. Reticulocytosis in the absence of anemia may indicate reduced oxygenation of the blood or diminished tissue perfusion. Hypoxic situations lead to increased erythropoietin production, which in turn stimulates erythropoiesis and the release of reticulocytes from the bone marrow. Conversely, the absence of reticulocytosis in an anemic patient suggests reduced erythropoietin production, marrow depression or failure, defective iron utilization, and/or increased ineffective erythropoiesis. A bone marrow examination is necessary to evaluate erythrogenesis in such patients.

Red Cell Indices and Erythrocyte Morphology

Erythrocyte morphology, noted on careful examination of the blood film, must always be considered in conjunction with the MCV and MCHC values to interpret these red cell indices properly. Important clues about the specific cause(s) or pathophysiologic process(es) of anemia and marrow erythropoietic activity may be obtained by carefully examining the erythrocyte morphology in a good, Wright-stained film (see Tables 1–3 and 7–4).

Erythrogram and Red Cell Distribution Width

The erythropoietic response to different types of anemias in humans can be evaluated from the erythrocyte histogram (erythrogram) and the red cell distribution width (RDW) parameter obtained through the use of newly developed automated blood analyzers. The erythrogram depicts the distribution of red cells according to cell size. Normal erythrograms are typically gaussian curves with minimal right skew; therefore, the presence of increased numbers of smaller or larger erythrocytes distorts the histogram, enabling earlier detection of abnormalities in red cell size than indicated by use of the MCV. The RDW provides an index of anisocytosis and is more sensitive than the MCV or light microscopic evaluation of red cell size in stained blood films for detecting changes in erythrocyte subpopulations. Humans with hypoproliferative anemias generally have a normal RDW regardless of the MCV, whereas the RDW increases during response to acute and chronic blood loss anemias, immune-mediated hemolytic anemias, and anemias from maturational defects (Bessman et al., 1983).

Observations on healthy and anemic dogs, cats, horses, cows, and goats have shown the usefulness of these newer measures of red cell heterogeneity in the evaluation of the erythropoietic response to anemias in animals (Dorr et al., 1986; Easley, 1985; Radin et al., 1986; Weiser, 1982; Weiser and Kociba, 1982, 1983; Weiser and O'Grady, 1983). For example, the RDW was found to be more sensitive than the MCV in detecting changes in erythrocyte subpopulations during response to iron deficiency anemia in kittens. Acute blood loss and acute Heinz body hemolytic anemias in horses were found to cause mild to moderate increases in the RDW and MCV in 2 weeks, and such changes lasted for 4 to 6 weeks. Erythrograms showed an extension of the right slope or a shift to the right of the entire histogram by 2 to 3 weeks, and lasted for 4 to 6 weeks. Greater changes occurred during a response to hemolytic anemia as compared to a response to acute blood loss anemia. In chronic blood loss (partial iron deficiency) anemia, the RDW did not change significantly, the MCV progressively decreased from days 21 to 56, and the erythrogram shifted slightly to the left. These findings are important, because reticulocytes do not appear in the blood of horses, even under intense erythropoietic response to anemia. Observations on goats recovering from acute blood loss anemia indicated that erythrograms can be used for a retrospective diagnosis of severe hemorrhage, because a distinct subpopulation of macrocytes, producing a right skew in histograms, persisted for several weeks in the absence of a demonstrable reticulocytosis or increase in the MCV beyond the normal range.

Other Abnormalities in Blood

The icterus index may be increased in hemolytic anemias, but it is normal in depression anemias and in anemias from blood loss, except when hemorrhage occurs in body cavities. Hemoglobinemia is an early manifestation of a severe hemolytic anemia developing from intravascular lysis of red cells. The total plasma protein concentration is usually reduced in anemias from external blood loss and infestation with blood-sucking parasites, whereas depression or hemolytic anemias do not show such a change in plasma protein concentration. Total and differential leukocyte counts are variable, more so because of the primary disease responsible for anemia than because of the anemia itself. During an intense response to anemia, however, reticulocytosis may be accompanied by a neutrophilia

with a left shift. This is particularly common in hemolytic anemias in the dog. Monocytosis is often encountered in autoimmune hemolytic anemia in the dog. Erythrocyte osmotic fragility increases in hemolytic anemias from various causes.

Bone Marrow Examination

Bone marrow examination in anemias is performed primarily to evaluate the erythropoietic response. Generally, hemolytic and blood loss anemias, during the responsive phase, are accompanied by increased erythropoiesis and a reduced myeloid:erythroid ratio. This is often evident from reticulocytosis in the peripheral blood and a bone marrow examination is usually unnecessary in such cases. Erythropoiesis is reduced in depression anemias, yielding an elevated myeloid:erythroid ratio. Erythropoiesis is disturbed in anemias of nutritional deficiencies, such as those of iron (see Chap. 9) and vitamin B_{12} (see Chap. 12). Megaloblastic erythroid cells are a remarkable finding in the bone marrow of cats with erythremic myelosis and erythroleukemia (see Chap. 20).

The bone marrow of poodles with macrocytosis simulating vitamin B_{12}-folate deficiency exhibits hypersegmented neutrophils, giant metamyelocytes, erythrocytes with multiple Howell-Jolly bodies, megaloblasts, and aberrant nuclear mitosis and fragmentation in erythroid cells. The bone marrow iron level, estimated after Prussian blue staining, decreases in iron deficiency anemias but increases in anemias of inflammatory disease. Both situations are associated with decreased numbers of marrow sideroblasts, whereas sideroblasts are increased in iron overload situations and in "sideroblastic" anemia. Siderocytes (red cells with iron granules) in blood and sideroblasts in bone marrow were found in a dog on high-dose chloramphenicol therapy (Harvey et al., 1985) and in a dog with idiopathic dyserythropoiesis (Canfield et al., 1987). The latter dog also showed intraerythrocytic hemoglobin crystallization in an occasional red cell.

A bone marrow examination is essential for evaluating the response to anemia in the horse. In this species, reticulocytes normally mature in the bone marrow prior to their release as red cells into the circulation. This is true both in health and during response to anemia, whether from blood loss or a hemolytic process. In such instances, a marrow reticulocyte count greater than 5% suggests effective erythropoiesis.

Other Laboratory Test Abnormalities

Fecal examination for occult blood usually yields positive results during bleeding into the gastrointestinal tract. Omnivores often have a positive fecal blood test because of hemoglobin in their diet, which includes meat. The excretion of urobilinogen into the urine increases during hemolytic anemias. The urinary excretion of bile also increases in hemolytic anemia as long as the liver can conjugate the excessive hemoglobin released during the hemolytic process. Hemoglobinemia, methemoglobinemia, and hemoglobinuria may be evident in hemolytic anemias. The total serum bilirubin concentration is normal in depression anemias and in anemias from external blood loss. A van den Bergh test, for direct- and indirect-reacting bilirubin in plasma, may help differentiate the hyperbilirubinemia of hemolytic anemia and hepatic disease or cholestasis from posthepatic obstruction of the bile duct, particularly in the dog and cat. Haptoglobin, hemopexin, and methemalbumin determinations may also be helpful in defining hemolytic anemias. Radiologic examination and other diagnostic tests may need to be performed to determine the primary cause of the anemia.

THERAPEUTIC ASPECTS OF ANEMIA

It is important to determine the cause and duration of the anemia and their effects on the patient to initiate appropriate therapy. A mild anemia may be of little consequence to the patient but may have a serious cause, such as a bleeding tumor. A moderate anemia affects the patient's well-being, and marked anemia may undoubtedly be life-threatening, regardless of the cause. Similarly, an acute anemia is more serious than a chronic anemia in which physiologic adjustments have occurred. Massive blood loss within a short period requires immediate treatment for shock and the restoration of blood volume for adequate oxygenation. Subsequently, materials essential for erythrocyte production (nutritious diet and hematinics) must be provided to ensure a rapid and appropriate bone marrow response. Specific measures may vary from surgical intervention to treatment with antibiotics, specific drugs, and various immunosuppressive agents. Corticosteroids and androgens can be used to stimulate red cell production.

A blood transfusion is given for several reasons: (1) to prevent shock from the loss of blood volume in acute hemorrhage; (2) to improve the oxygen-carrying

Table 8–4. Classification of Polycythemias in Humans and Animals

Absolute polycythemias
  Primary polycythemia
    Polycythemia vera, a malignant hematopoietic stem cell disorder
  Secondary polycythemia
    Hypoxic increase in erythropoietin production
      Reduced atmospheric oxygen
      Pulmonary hypoxia
      Cardiovascular disease (right-to-left shunts), tetralogy of Fallot
      Reduced oxygen transport by hemoglobin
    Autonomous increase in erythropoietin production
      Non-neoplastic renal diseases, (e.g., cysts, hydronephrosis, and polycystic kidneys)
      Neoplastic diseases (e.g., renal tumors, hepatomas, uterine leiomyomas, cerebellar hemangioblastomas)
      Familial erythrocytosis in humans
Relative polycythemias
  Dehydration from various causes
  Splenic contraction

Table 8–5. Hematologic and Other Laboratory Findings in Primary and Secondary Polycythemias in the Dog

Parameter	Case 1; Primary Polycythemia Vera	Case 2; Secondary Polycythemia (Tetralogy of Fallot)
RBC ($\times 10^6/\mu l$)	13.78	13.06
Hemoglobin (g/dl)	29.6	28.2
PCV (%)	83.0	83.0
MCV (fl)	60.2	63.5
MCHC (%)	35.6	34.0
MCH (pg)	21.4	21.6
Reticulocytes (%)	—	—
nRBC/100 WBC	0.0	2.0
ESR (mm/hr)	0	
Anisocytosis	Slight	Slight
Polychromasia	Slight	Slight
Icterus Index (units)	Slight hemolysis	Hemolyzed
Plasma proteins (g/dl)	7.0	9.5
Fibrinogen (mg/dl)	200	500
WBC/μl	9,900	11,862
Bands	0	0
Neutrophils	5,940	10,319
Lymphocytes	2,673	1,186
Monocytes	693	0
Eosinophils	594	355
Platelets (/μl)	94,000	—
Total blood volume (ml/kg)*	160	163
Plasma volume (ml/kg)	54	62.5
RBC volume (ml/kg)	106	100.5
RBC ^{51}Cr half-life (days)‡	56	28
Arterial P$_{O_2}$ (mm Hg)	90 (normal)	65%

* Normal total blood volume, 80–90 ml/kg.
‡ Normal ^{51}Cr half-life, 20–29 days.

capacity of the blood, which permits the patient to function more normally; and (3) to attempt to restore normal maturation of erythrocytes in certain idiopathic anemias by temporarily giving the erythropoietic tissue (bone marrow) a rest. The mere existence of anemia does not justify a blood transfusion.

POLYCYTHEMIA

An increase in erythrocyte numbers above normal in the blood is generally referred to as polycythemia. Polycythemia may be relative or absolute (Fig. 8–2), and the latter may be primary or secondary (Table 8–4). A PCV greater than 60% should arouse suspicion of polycythemia, relative or absolute, and a PCV greater than 70% usually suggests primary polycythemia (Table 8–5). The clinical manifestations of absolute polycythemia result from a persistent increase in red cell mass and associated expansion of blood volume. The characteristic congestion and cyanosis of mucous membranes is caused by the sluggish flow of deoxygenated blood that is exorbitantly rich in red cells. An excessive red cell mass increases the blood viscosity and pulmonary vascular resistance and decreases cardiac output. These abnormalities lead to decreased blood flow, reduced tissue oxygenation, neurological disturbances, and increased risk of thrombosis. The

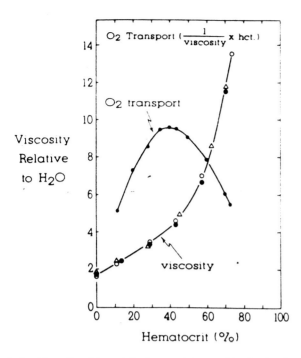

Fig. 8–4. Viscosity of heparinized normal human blood related to hematocrit (Hct). Viscosity is measured with an Ostwald viscosimeter at 37° C and expressed in relation to the viscosity of a saline solution. Oxygen transport is computed from Hct and O_2 flow (1/viscosity) and is recorded in arbitrary units. (From Williams, W. J., Beutler, E., Erslev, A. J., et al.: Hematology. 4th Ed. New York, McGraw-Hill, 1990, p. 428.)

blood viscosity and degree of oxygen transport change disproportionately with increases in the PCV above 50% (Fig. 8–4).

Relative Polycythemia

Relative polycythemia is commonly encountered in animals as a result of a reduction in the plasma volume caused by dehydration. Water intake by sick animals is generally inadequate to maintain the normal body water content. Diseases accompanied by excessive loss of water (e.g., diarrhea, vomiting, or polyuria from electrolyte imbalance) can quickly produce dehydration. Profuse sweating in horses, as during endurance rides, can cause hemoconcentration. Another form of relative polycythemia occurs as a result of the injection of a mass of concentrated erythrocytes into the circulation on contraction of the spleen. For example, the ovine spleen can sequester up to 25% of the red cell mass and can release the stored cells into the circulation within approximately 3 minutes, causing the circulating red cell mass to increase up to 38% (Torrington et al., 1989). This type of response is particularly prominent in more excitable animals and the females of some species. Splenic contraction may also occur under conditions of severe pain (e.g., in horses with colic). Relative polycythemia reverts to normal as the dehydration is relieved or when the circumstances leading to the splenic contraction are no longer present.

Primary Polycythemia

Primary polycythemia or polycythemia vera is a myeloproliferative disease. It is an acquired clonal disorder of the pluripotential stem cell that results in the expansion of committed stem cell pools, primarily of the erythrocytic line. Thus, polycythemia vera mainly involves overproduction of red cells, but slight leukocytosis and thrombocytosis often accompany the disorder. Erythropoiesis is erythropoietin-independent and the red cell life span is normal. Polycythemia vera may eventually terminate in myelofibrosis or acute myelogenous leukemia. Polycythemia vera is a rare disease in animals, although it has been described in the dog, cat, and cattle (Campbell, 1990; Jain, 1986). Therapy is directed at reducing the red cell count by phlebotomy and at reducing the erythropoiesis by chemotherapy and ^{32}P-irradiation. A balanced erythropoiesis with a normal PCV is, however, difficult to achieve in animals with primary polycythemia. Death occurs from vascular complications or other undetermined causes. Treatment involves repeated phlebotomies and therapy with hydroxyurea (in the dog, 30 mg/kg/day orally for 7 days, tapered to 15 mg/kg daily). Doxorubicin (20 mg/m², IV) at 3-week intervals has been used in conjunction with repeated phlebotomies (800 to 1000 ml every 3 weeks) to stabilize the PCV in a dog with primary polycythemia (Page et al., 1990) A series of 3 phlebotomies with fluid replacement was sufficient to decrease PCV from 74% to 45% in a dog with transient erythrocytosis (primary polycythemia) (Codner, 1992).

Secondary Polycythemia

Secondary polycythemia, sometimes called erythrocytosis, is unaccompanied by increases in the leukocyte and platelet counts. Secondary polycythemia has been observed in dogs, cats, and rabbits (Foster and Lothrop, 1988; Gorse 1988; Jain, 1986; Lipman et al., 1985). Secondary polycythemia is a result of increased erythropoiesis mediated usually by the overproduction of erythropoietin. Erythropoietin levels increase as a compensatory physiologic response by the kidney to tissue hypoxia (e.g., in animals at high altitudes and in tetralogy of Fallot in the dog, cat, cattle, and horse) or as a result of autonomous production independent of tissue oxygen supply (e.g., renal carcinoma in a dog, hepatocellular carcinoma in a horse). Measurement of the red cell mass using ^{51}Cr-labelled red cells and of the plasma volume using ^{131}I-labelled albumin or another suitable method is indicated in patients with suspected polycythemia. An increase in red cell mass without a significant decrease in the plasma volume suggests primary or secondary polycythemia (Table 8–5), whereas relative polycythemia (erythrocytosis) is characterized by a normal red cell mass and a decreased plasma volume. Therapy in secondary polycythemia is directed toward finding and eliminating the cause of the increased erythropoietin production.

The differentiation of primary and secondary polycythemias requires a detailed history, thorough physical examination, chest radiography, and laboratory tests necessary to establish the diagnosis. Determination of the arterial P_{O_2} is particularly essential, and measuring the serum or urine erythropoietin concentration may be necessary to confirm the type of polycythemia. The aterial P_{O_2} is low and the erythropoietin concentration is usually high in secondary polycythemia, the arterial P_{O_2} is normal and the erythropoietin concentration is usually below normal in primary polycythemia, and both parameters are normal in relative polycythemia (Table 8–5). Erythropoietin levels may be normal in some cases of primary or secondary polycythemia. In such cases intermittent secretion of erythropoietin (Giger, 1992) or increased sensitivity of the bone marrow may be involved in causation of polycythemia (Juvonen et al., 1991).

REFERENCES

Bessman, J.D., Gilmer, P.R., and Gardner, F.H.: Improved classification of anemias by MCV and RDW. Am. J. Clin. Pathol., 80: 332, 1983.
Brock, K.V., Jones, J.B., Shull, R.M., et al.: Effect of canine parvovirus on erythroid progenitors in phenylhydrazine-induced regenerative hemolytic anemia in dogs. Am. J. Vet. Res., 50:965, 1989.
Campbell, K.L.: Diagnosis and management of polycythemia in dogs. Compend. Contin. Educ. Pract. Vet., 12:543, 1990.
Canfield, P.J., Watson, A.D.J., and Ratcliffe, R.C.C.: Dyserythropoiesis, sideroblasts/siderocytes and hemoglobin crystallization in a dog. Vet. Clin. Pathol., 16:21, 1987.
Codner, E.C.: Transient erythrocytosis (primary polycythemia) in a dog. Comp. Haematol. Int. Vol 2, 1992 (In Press).
Dorr, L., Pearce, P.C., Shine, T., et al.: Changes in red cell volume distribution frequency after acute blood loss in goats (Capra hircus). Res. Vet. Sci., 40:322, 1986.
Easley, J.R.: Erythrogram and red cell distribution width of equidae

with experimentally induced anemia. Am. J. Vet. Res., 46:2378, 1985.
Foster, E.S. and Lothrop, C.D.: Polycythemia vera in a cat with cardiac hypertrophy. J. Am. Vet. Med. Assoc., 192:1736, 1988.
Giger, U.R. S.: Erythropoietin and its clinical use. Compend. Contin. Educ. Pract. Vet., 14:25, 1992.
Gorse, M.J.: Polycythemia associated with renal fibrosarcoma in a dog. J. Am. Vet. Med. Assoc., 192:793, 1988.
Harvey, J.W., Wolfsheimer, K.J., Simpson, C.F., et al.: Pathologic sideroblasts and siderocytes associated with chloramphenicol therapy in a dog. Vet. Clin. Pathol., 14:36, 1985.
Jain, N.C.: Schalm's Veterinary Hematology. 4th ed. Philadelphia, Lea & Febiger, 1986, pp. 563–576.
Juvonen, E., Ikkala, E., Fyhrquist, F., et al.: Autosomal dominant erythrocytosis caused by increased sensitivity to erythropoietin. Blood, 78:3066, 1991.
Kociba, G.J.: Feline anemia. In: Kirk, R.W. (eds), Current veterinary therapy X. Small animal practice. Philadelphia, W.B. Saunders Company, 1989, p. 425.
Lipman, N.S., Murphy, J.C. and Newcomer, C.E.: Polycythemia in a New Zealand White rabbit with an embryonal nephroma. J. Am. Vet. Med. Assoc., 187:1255, 1985.
Page, R.L., Stiff, M.E. and McEntee, M.C.: Transient glomerulonephropathy associated with primary erythrocytosis in a dog. J. Am. Vet. Med. Assoc., 196:620, 1990.
Radin, M.J., Eubank, M.C. and Weiser, M.G.: Electronic measurement of erythrocyte volume and volume heterogeneity in horses during erythrocyte regeneration associated with experimental anemias. Vet. Pathol., 23:656, 1986.
Torrington, K.G., McNeil, J.S., Phillips, Y.Y., et al.: Blood volume determinations in sheep before and after splenectomy. Lab. Anim. Sci., 39:598, 1989.
Weiser, M.G.: Erythrocyte volume distribution analysis in healthy dogs, cats, horses, and dairy cows. Am. J. Vet. Res., 43:163, 1982.
Weiser, M.G. and Kociba, G.J.: Persistent macrocytosis assessed by erythrocyte subpopulation analysis following erythrocyte regeneration in cats. Blood, 60:295, 1982.
Weiser, M.G. and Kociba, G.J.: Sequential change in erythrocyte volume distribution and microcytosis associated with iron deficiency anemia in kittens. Vet. Pathol., 20:1, 1983.
Weiser, M.J. and O'Grady, M.: Erythrocyte volume distribution analysis and hematologic changes in dogs with iron deficiency anemia. Vet. Pathol., 20:230, 1983.
Williams, W.J., Beutler, E., Erslev, A.J., et al.: Hematology. 4th ed. New York, McGraw-Hill, 1990, Chap. 42.

Blood Loss or Hemorrhagic Anemias

Acute and chronic blood losses are associated with hemodynamic effects, changes in total blood volume and plasma volume, and changes in composition of the blood and bone marrow. A reduction in blood volume below the normal level is known as hypovolemia or oligemia, whereas a reduction in the red cell volume is known as oligocythemia. The converse are, respectively, hypervolemia and polycythemia.

BLOOD VOLUME

The total blood volume is a function of lean body weight. It is influenced by various physiologic and environmental factors, such as climate, age, sex, breed, body size, pregnancy, lactation status, and physical activity. Blood volume is high at birth, decreases markedly during the neonatal period, and stabilizes to adult levels within a few weeks to a few months. Studies on the young of several animal species have shown that changes in blood volume during the neonatal period are related to increases in plasma volume caused by a shift in body water among various body compartments, colostrum consumption, a decrease in red cell number from the destruction of short-lived fetal erythrocytes, and a relative increase in body weight.

The total blood volume can be estimated by various techniques that measure its two components separately, the plasma volume and the red cell volume. A traditional method for determining the plasma volume has been the intravenous injection of Evans blue dye (T-1824). The dye concentration in blood samples collected at short intervals is measured spectrophotometrically and the total blood volume is calculated from the relative proportion of plasma to red cells as determined by a hematocrit test. Newer methods are based on the principle of isotope dilution using ^{131}I-labelled albumin to determine plasma volume and ^{51}Cr-labelling of autologous erythrocytes to determine the red cell mass. The use of indocyanine green provides a reliable estimate of plasma volume in ponies (Clarke et al., 1990). For practical purposes, the blood volume can be estimated on the basis of percentage of body weight or ml/kg body weight (Table 9-1). In common domestic animals it generally measures about 6 to 11%, or about 50 to 110 ml/kg of body weight. Studies in sheep have indicated that splenectomy produces a modest reduction in blood volume (Torrington et al., 1989).

Homeostasis of total blood volume is maintained by physiologic adjustments in the plasma volume and red cell mass. Following acute blood loss, the blood volume is mainly regulated by neurohormonal mechanisms triggered to prevent hypovolemic shock (shock from reduced blood volume) and death. Hypovolemic shock generally develops when the blood volume is reduced to 60 to 70% of normal and death follows when it is reduced below 60%. Events associated with the rapid replacement of lost plasma include a shift of body water from interstitial and intracellular compartments into the intravascular compartment and increased absorption of water from the gastrointestinal tract and from the urine into the kidneys. Immediate replacement of erythrocytes occurs from the ejection of red cells stored in the spleen. In contrast, replacement from increased erythropoiesis begins within a few days and may take several weeks to restore normal red cell mass. Studies in normal and splenectomized dogs and horses (Table 9-2) have shown that fluid and protein replacement can begin within hours and be complete within a few days. Protein replacement is from the extravascular compartment of body protein, aided by a decrease in protein catabolism and probably by increased synthesis.

Hemodilution from excessive replacement of fluid in relation to red cell number and plasma protein

Table 9–1. Blood Volume in Relation to Body Weight

	Body Weight	
Animals	ml/kg	%
Young dairy calves, hot-blooded horses	88–110	10–11
Dogs	77–78	8–9
Lactating cows, growing calves	66–77	7–8
Nonlactating cows, yearling calves, sheep, goats, cold-blooded horses, cats	62–66	6–7
Mature pigs	55	5–6
Laboratory animals	—	6–7

concentration results in anemia and hypoproteinemia, which become evident within hours of a significant episode of acute blood loss (Jain, 1986). This type of anemia is initially characterized by normal (normocytic-normochromic) red cell morphology. Subsequently (usually after 3 days), the erythropoietic response of bone marrow to anemia manifests in the blood of most species as polychromasia (Plate XVI-3) and reticulocytosis (Plate IV-6). The horse is an exception because reticulocytes are rarely found in its blood, even in a most severe case of anemia, although increased numbers of reticulocytes from intensified erythropoiesis might be observed in the bone marrow (Plate V-1).

ACUTE BLOOD LOSS ANEMIA

A significant loss of blood within a period of a few minutes to several hours constitutes acute blood loss.

Table 9–3. Causes of Blood Loss or Hemorrhagic Anemias

Acute blood loss
  Trauma and surgical procedures
  Bleeding lesions
  Coagulation disorders
    Bracken fern poisoning in cattle
    Sweet clover hay (dicumarol) poisoning in cattle
    Warfarin poisoning
    Disseminated intravascular coagulation from various causes
  Thrombocytopenia (see Table 6–6)
  Parasites: hemonchus; hookworms; coccidia
Chronic blood loss
  Gastrointestinal lesions: neoplasms, particularly leiomyomas; ulcers; parasitism, such as coccidiosis
  Neoplasms with bleeding into body cavities and tissues: hemangiosarcoma in the dog
  Coagulation disorders
    Vitamin K and prothrombin deficiencies
    Hemophilia A in dogs and foals
  Thrombocytopenia
  Parasites: ticks, bloodsucking lice, sticktight fleas; hookworms; hemonchus

Such losses have various causes (Table 9–3). Hemodynamic, blood volume, and hematologic changes vary with the degree of blood loss and its location. Blood may be lost externally or internally into the body cavities. A small amount of blood loss in relation to body weight is well tolerated, whereas a larger volume of blood loss may have significant immediate effects, and could be fatal.

Clinical manifestations differ with the magnitude of blood loss. Hemodynamic and circulatory adjustments

Table 9–2. Effect of Massive Hemorrhage in the Normal and Splenectomized Horse on Circulating Red Blood Cell Mass and on Plasma Volume as Measured by the T-1824 Dye Dilution Method

Horse Number	Status and Weight*	Amount of Blood Withdrawn and Time†	Sampling Time in Hours‡	PCV (%)	RBC ($\times 10^6/\mu l$)	Hb (g/dl)	Plasma Proteins (g/dl)§	Plasma Volume ml	Plasma Volume %
1	Normal; 364 kg	9.05 L withdrawn in 40 min	Prebleeding	35	6.8	12.8	—	15,788	100
			0	37	7.3	13.6	—	10,722	68
			1	37.5	—	—	—	13,424	85
			4	34	6.7	12.4	—	14,974	95
			24	27	5.16	9.8	—	18,202	115
1	Splenectomized; 334 kg	7.3 L withdrawn in 28 min	Prebleeding	35	7.05	12.1	6.95	12,230	100
			0	32	6.25	11.5	6.35	8,459	69
			1	30	—	—	5.9	9,275	76
			4	28	5.35	9.8	5.8	10,610	87
			24	25	4.47	9.1	6.35	15,541	127
2	Normal; 452 kg	11.2 L withdrawn in 53 min	Prebleeding	43	8.05	15.8	—	18,669	100
			0	47	8.1	16.8	—	14,954	80
			1	43	—	—	—	15,765	84
			4	41	7.5	14.7	—	20,410	109
			24	34	6.45	12.2	—	21,577	116
2	Splenectomized; 419 kg	9.3 L withdrawn in 28 min	Prebleeding	40	7.7	13.9	7.3	13,950	100
			0	38	7.2	12.3	6.85	10,752	77
			1	36	—	—	6.8	11,743	84
			4	33	6.65	11.5	6.7	13,018	93
			24	28	5.20	9.8	6.65	16,483	118

* Hemorrhage was produced in normal state in summer. Horses were splenectomized in the fall and the second blood loss trials were conducted in the following spring, when the horses were completely recovered.
† Volume of blood withdrawn was estimated to be approximately 30% of total blood volume.
‡ 0 hour represents the time at the end of blood withdrawal.
§ Predicted from Goldberg refractometer.

begin immediately after severe blood loss. The splenic reserve of erythrocytes is injected into the circulation in certain animals, particularly the horse, to increase oxygen transport. Simultaneously, oxygen delivery by the circulating red cells is increased by a shift in the oxygen dissociation curve. Extravascular fluid begins to move into the vascular space within minutes, but the plasma volume expands slowly. Replacement therapy must be instituted immediately to maintain adequate blood volume and prevent shock. Electrolyte solutions, plasma substitutes, or whole blood may be given, depending on need.

Changes in the Peripheral Blood

A blood sample taken within a few hours of blood loss often yields normal values for RBC count, PCV (packed cell volume), hemoglobin level, and total plasma protein concentration, despite the intravascular movement of fluid from an extravascular space. Thus, anemia is not evident during the early period of acute blood loss. The expansion of the plasma volume to a normal level is indicated by a diminishing total plasma protein concentration followed by decreases in red cell parameters. A slight decrease in plasma protein concentration may be evident as early as 1 hour after blood loss. Continuing hemodilution produces a significant fall in red cell parameters and plasma protein concentrations by 4 hours (Table 9–2). Remarkably, a blood sample collected 1 or 2 days after blood loss reveals a normocytic-normochromic anemia accompanied by hypoproteinemia (Table 9–4). A reticulocyte response is not evident for the first 3 days, so blood loss anemia at this stage might be mistaken for a depression anemia. The plasma protein concentration begins to increase in 2 to 3 days and is usually normal within 5 to 7 days, long before normal red cell parameters have been restored. A persistently low level of plasma proteins should suggest continuing blood loss

(Table 9–4). Plasma protein concentrations are usually within the normal range in patients with internal blood loss and hemolytic anemias.

The leukocyte number increases within hours because of the shift of neutrophils from the marginal pool and the bone marrow reserve. Similarly, platelet counts may increase as a result of mobilization of the splenic reserve. Immature leukocytes and nucleated red cells may also appear in blood, particularly in cases of severe blood loss accompanied by shock and tissue hypoxia. Neutrophilia with a left shift usually develops during response to anemia. The magnitude of the left shift may correlate with the intensity of the erythropoietic response. In acute hemolytic anemias, leukocytosis and pyrexia are to be anticipated and should not necessarily be interpreted as evidence of an infectious process.

Reticulocytes from intensified erythropoiesis begin to appear in the circulation 72 to 96 hours after onset of the blood loss or red cell destruction. Some "shift" (large) reticulocytes may appear in the blood as a result of erythropoietin-induced release from bone marrow, because enhanced secretion of erythropoietin may occur as early as 6 hours after blood loss. The increase in erythropoietin secretion varies with the severity of anemia and is associated with a gradual stimulation of erythropoiesis, which leads to reticulocytosis. Reticulocytes peak usually between the first and second weeks, followed by a gradual decline. During the peak response the blood profile is characterized by polychromatic macrocytes, nucleated erythrocytes, and erythrocytes with Howell-Jolly bodies (Plates XVI-3 and XII-9). Thus, the erythrocytic indices typically show a macrocytic-hypochromic anemia (Case 1, Table 9–5). The reticulocyte production index is usually elevated, which indicates a heightened erythropoietic response. The triad of anemia, hypoproteinemia, and reticulocytosis is therefore considered a hallmark of responsive acute blood loss anemia. A whole blood transfusion in an erythropoietically responding patient

Table 9–4. Erythrocyte Parameters and Plasma Protein Concentrations in Response to Repeated Blood Withdrawal from a 7-Month-Old Holstein-Frisian Bull

Day	Blood Withdrawn (liters)	RBC ($\times 10^6/\mu l$)	PCV (%)	Hb (g/dl)	MCV (fl)	MCHC (%)	MCH (pg)	Reticulocytes (%)	Nucleated RBC/100 WBC	Plasma Proteins (g/dl)
1	7.5	9.15	37.0	12.8	40.4	34.6	14.0	0	0	7.3
2	6.5	6.05	24.0	8.1	39.0	33.8	13.4	0	0	6.2
3	3.0	3.19	14.0	5.0	43.9	35.7	15.7	rare	0	4.8
4	—	2.90	13.0	4.2	44.8	32.3	14.5	2.8	0.5	5.0
5	—	3.14	15.0	4.8	47.8	32.0	15.3	3.9	2.0	5.4
6	—	3.11	17.0	5.2	54.7	30.6	16.7	8.4	1.0	5.5
7	5.0	3.01	17.0	5.5	56.5	32.3	18.3	12.8	3.5	5.5
8	3.5	2.70	16.0	4.9	59.2	30.6	18.1	19.6	4.0	5.5
9	2.5	1.83	14.0	3.9	76.5	27.8	21.3	21.8	3.0	4.9
15	—	2.39	14.0	4.0	58.6	28.6	16.7	10.6	1.0	4.6
20	—	3.90	20.0	6.5	51.3	32.5	16.6	4.4	3.0	5.2
28	—	6.95	27.0	9.0	38.8	33.3	12.9	0	0	6.2
48	—	9.00	33.0	10.5	36.7	31.8	11.7	0	0	7.1

From Schalm, O.W.: Differential diagnosis of anemias in cattle. Part I. Massive blood loss by repeated phlebotomies. Bovine Pract., 1:10, 1980.

Table 9–5. Hematologic Findings in Selected Cases of Acute and Chronic Blood Loss Anemias in the Dog

Parameter	Case 1: Ulcerated Leiomyoma of the Gut	Case 2: Ulcerative Colitis	Case 3: Heavy Blood-sucking Flea Infestation*	Case 4: Possible Nutritional Deficiency
RBC ($\times 10^6/\mu$l)	2.04	4.1	1.94	3.55
Hemoglobin (g/dl)	4.6	4.6	2.25	4.3
PCV (%)	17.0	18.0	9.0	18.0
MCV (fl)	83.3	43.9	46.4	50.7
MCHC (%)	27.1↑	25.5	25.0	23.8
MCH (pg)	22.5	11.2	11.6	12.1
ESR (mm/hr)	7 +	48 −	Diphasic	55 −
Reticulocytes (%)	32.0	7.3	2.3	17.0
nRBC/100 WBC	10.5	1.0	4.0	Rare
Anisocytosis	Moderate	Moderate	Prominent	Moderate
Hypochromasia	Moderate	Prominent	Prominent	Moderate
Polychromasia	Moderate	Moderate	Moderate	Slight
Poikilocytosis	—	Moderate	—	Slight
Leptocytosis	Marked	Marked	—	Marked
Howell-Jolly bodies	Few	None	—	—
II (units)	2	2	—	2
Plasma proteins (g/dl)	6.4	5.6	—	6.0
Fibrinogen (mg/dl)	700	—	—	400
WBC/μl	17,800	17,500	25,650	14,000
Bands	356	0	1,540	0
Neutrophils	12,282	13,038	20,520	12,460
Lymphocytes	1,513	2,100	1,795	770
Monocytes	3,204	1,487	1,795	490
Eosinophils	445	787	0	280
Basophils	0	0	0	0
Unclassified cells	—	88	—	—
Platelets/μl	—	—	—	828,000
M:E ratio	—	0.84:1	0.59:1	—

* Echidnophaga gallinacea.

rapidly curtails reticulocyte release into the peripheral blood, probably because of the inhibition of erythropoietin synthesis as the tissue hypoxia is alleviated (see Fig. 22–3).

The degree of reticulocytosis generally varies with the magnitude of blood loss, the period over which blood loss has occurred, the species, and concurrent disease. Dogs and cats exhibit the most commonly observed picture of a regenerative blood loss anemia. Even in these animals, the peak erythropoietic response to acute blood loss is usually less than that in hemolytic anemias. In the cat, aggregate reticulocytes disappear earlier than punctate reticulocytes; thus, the presence of many punctate reticulocytes suggests that blood loss or a hemolytic episode has occurred. Horses responding to acute blood loss of any magnitude show no reticulocytosis in their blood. They may manifest no obvious changes in erythrocyte morphology, occasionally exhibit moderate to marked anisocytosis or rarely, show macrocytosis based on an increased mean corpuscular volume (MCV; Table 9–6). Thus, red cell indices, even in the most responsive anemia in the

Table 9–6. Serial Hemograms on a 7-Year-Old Crossbred Horse Responding to a Massive Blood Loss Anemia That Developed 2 Weeks After Surgery

Parameter	Feb. 6	Days Posthemorrhage							
		1	3	4	6	8	10	14	20
Erythrocytes ($\times 10^6/\mu$l)	7.75	2.25	2.06	2.64	3.0	3.15	32.71	4.20	4.90
Hemoglobin (g/dl)	13.7	3.7	3.7	4.9	5.8	7.4	6.9	9.6	9.0
PCV (%)	38.0	11.5	11.5	15.0	18.0	21.0	20.0	25.0	28.0
MCV (fl)	49.0	51.1	55.8	56.8	60.0	66.6	53.9	59.5	57.1
MCHC (%)	36.0	32.2	32.2	32.7	32.2	35.2	34.5	38.4	32.1
MCH (pg)	17.8	16.4	17.9	18.5	19.3	23.5	18.6	22.8	18.3
Erythrocyte morphology	On the first day following hemorrhage, the erythrocytes were few in number in the stained blood film. Many red blood cells presented punched-out centers, meaning that the cell had retained the bowl shape assumed during circulation through the smallest capillaries. Beginning with the third day and increasing in prominence thereafter, macrocytic-normochromic erythrocytes were present in peripheral blood. This was the only evidence of increased erythropoiesis and release of new erythrocytes to the circulation in response to the blood loss. By the twentieth day, most erythrocytes appeared macrocytic. No polychromasia, nucleated erythrocytes, or reticulocytes were seen. Howell-Jolly bodies were few in number.								
WBC/μl	7,400	13,700	8,300	8,500	10,500	7,500	6,600	7,100	10,600

horse, usually reflect macrocytic-normochromic erythrocyte morphology rather than macrocytic-hypochromic features common to the dog, cat, and cow. However, red cell distribution width and erythrogram can provide useful information in evaluating erythrocytic response to acute blood loss and hemolytic anemias in the horse (Easley, 1985). Basophilic stippling is a characteristic finding during vigorous erythrogenesis in ruminants and may precede macrocytosis. The reticulocyte response of ruminants, however, depends on the degree of blood loss and may vary with the age of the animal.

Changes in Bone Marrow

The hematopoietic potential of the bone marrow can be stimulated as much as six- to eight-fold under appropriate circumstances. Some stimulation of granulopoiesis and thrombopoiesis may also be evident, depending on the magnitude of overall hematopoietic stimulation by various cytokines that may be produced in response to the conditions provoking the blood loss. The hypoxic state created by the acute blood loss stimulates erythropoietin production, which then stimulates erythropoiesis. During this period, the myeloid:erythroid ratio generally diminishes. For an optimal response, adequate supplies of nutrients essential to erythrogenesis, particularly iron, must be available, and the functional ability of the marrow should not be compromised. The presence of an inflammatory state and/or chronic renal disease can dampen the erythropoietic response.

CHRONIC BLOOD LOSS ANEMIA

The chronic loss of a small quantity of blood, such as from a bleeding gastrointestinal tumor, can lead to anemia. This becomes evident from the fact that 1 ml of blood contains about 0.5 mg of iron, and normally about 1 mg of iron is absorbed and excreted daily. Thus, an iron deficiency state can gradually manifest when the iron balance is tilted in favor of increased loss. This anemia is typically recognized as that of iron deficiency.

Iron Deficiency Anemia

Iron deficiency is rare among domestic animals. It commonly results from chronic blood loss (Table 9–3). The major portion of iron in the body (about two-thirds) is in the form of hemoglobin, but a substantial amount exists as nonhemoglobin iron. The iron balance in an individual is primarily maintained by the rate of iron absorption and to a lesser extent by the rate of iron loss. A small amount of iron is lost in the feces because of the exfoliation of epithelial cells of the gastrointestinal tract and the excretion of bile, and

a minor portion is lost in the skin, nails, hair, and urine. Women and primates lose iron from blood loss during menstruation.

Normally, iron loss is balanced by the absorption of an equivalent amount of iron from the diet. Iron deficiency from a reduced intake of iron develops in baby pigs reared in a sanitary environment (concrete floors), puppies, kittens, and lambs raised on milk, and ruminants grazing on iron-deficient pastures. A congenital iron deficiency anemia may occur in dairy calves, probably as a result of impaired in utero transfer of iron from the dam to the fetus. A failure in the transport mechanism of iron from the mother to the fetus is an important cause of low iron reserves in piglets at birth (Calvo et al., 1989). Foals at 2 weeks to 4 months of age have lower serum ferritin and iron concentrations, higher total iron-binding capacity, and a lower transferrin saturation percentage than adults. Most foals, however, have sufficient body iron stores at birth and adequate iron intake to meet their iron requirements during early postnatal life (Kohm et al., 1990).

ABSORPTION AND TRANSPORT OF IRON

Iron is absorbed from the gut in the bivalent or ferrous form, but it occurs in nature in the ferric form in organic complexes (e.g., phytates, oxalates, phosphates). Hydrochloric acid in the stomach releases the iron from the organic complex and a reducing substance in the alkaline medium of the duodenum (ascorbic acid) aids in converting the ferric iron into its ferrous form. A high phosphorous level in the diet binds the iron so that it is not available for absorption.

Iron absorption by mucosal cells occurs mainly in the upper duodenum. It is an energy-dependent mechanism and involves the binding of iron to specific receptors on the cell surface. Iron at this location is bound by a mucosal transferrin, a protein with properties similar to those of plasma transferrin (Williams et al., 1990). The mucosal cell either releases the ferrous iron into the plasma for transport to other parts of the body or converts it back to the ferric form for storage as ferritin, which may be reused or lost into the gut when the cell exfoliates. The extent of each of these mechanisms regulates the body's iron metabolism. The transfer of iron from the mucosal cell to the plasma transport protein (transferrin) is promoted by ATP, citrate, and ceruloplasmin. Transferrin (MW, 76,000) is a glycoprotein primarily synthesized by the liver. It is normally one-third saturated with iron and its major function is the transport of iron. A congenital deficiency of transferrin in humans is associated with a hypochromic anemia of iron deficiency.

The iron needed for heme synthesis mainly comes from the storage compartment, which is replenished by iron conserved after the degradation of hemoglobin molecules and by dietary sources. Iron is stored mainly in two forms, ferritin and hemosiderin, and the latter is more stable and less reusable. The major storage

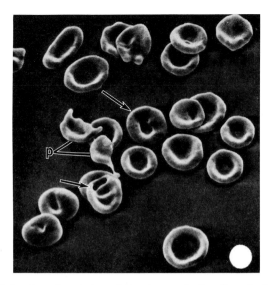

Fig. 9–1.   Scanning electron photomicrograph of erythrocytes from a dog with microcytic hypochromic anemia. Hypochromic erythrocytes with markedly enlarged concavity, poikilocytes (p), and erythrocytes with membrane defects (arrows) are apparent ($\times$ 2200). (From Jain, N. C.: Schalm's Veterinary Hematology. 4th Ed. Philadelphia, Lea & Febiger, 1986, p. 583.)

organs are the liver, spleen, and bone marrow. Macrophages in the bone marrow serve as a great reserve of recycled iron. Macrophages, however, primarily supply iron to the plasma transferrin; this process is aided by ceruloplasmin and ascorbate. Erythroid cells in the bone marrow can extract up to 85% of the transferrin iron presented to them. Transferrin donates iron on the cell surface or after internalization through attachment to specific surface receptors. The process of iron intake by developing erythroid cells is known as ropheocytosis. About 80 to 90% of the iron taken in by the erythroid cell is used for heme synthesis and the remainder is mostly converted to ferritin for temporary storage or ultimate excretion. Cytoplasmic accumulations of ferritin in erythroid cells constitute siderosomes and form the basis for the recognition of sideroblasts and siderocytes in bone marrow and blood films stained with Prussian blue (Plates XII-10 and XV-5).

Species variations are noted in regard to dietary requirements of iron. Generally, dietary need is low in adults and high in growing children and animals. Iron needs are increased during pregnancy, particularly in the last trimester. Iron requirements of cattle, horses, and pigs are higher than those for dogs, sheep, and cats. Women and female primates require more iron than males because of blood loss from menstrual bleeding.

CLINICAL AND LABORATORY FINDINGS

Hematologic and serum iron studies have been carried out on growing dogs and animals with iron deficiency anemias (Smith, 1989; Weeks et al., 1990). Iron deficiency occurs gradually, so changes observed in the blood depend on the extent of iron depletion. Changes in iron metabolism precede morphologic abnormalities. The anemia in early stages is normocytic-normochromic, whereas a microcytic-hypochromic anemia characterizes the blood picture of fully expressed iron deficiency (Cases 2 to 4, Table 9–5; Plates XVI-1, XVI-2 and XVIII-8). In iron deficiency, hemoglobin synthesis is slower than the rate of erythropoiesis; thus, microcytosis precedes hypochromasia. Microcytosis and hypochromasia are evident in Wintrobe indices only when most of the erythrocytes are so affected. The anemia is usually nonresponsive, although some reticulocytosis may be observed. The poorly structured red cells break apart in circulation, often producing poikilocytes (Fig. 9–1). The red cell life span is moderately shortened, probably because of reduced red cell deformability. Thrombocytosis of inexplicable origin is a common finding in iron deficiency anemia. Free erythropoietic protoporphyrin is increased several fold, even before anemia becomes apparent.

Rhesus monkeys subjected to repeated phlebotomies that involved the removal of 5 to 10% of their blood volume weekly for up to 10 weeks developed an iron deficiency anemia characterized by a reduced serum iron level, decreased percentage of transferrin saturation, increased free erythrocyte porphyrin concentration, and microcytic-hypochromic red cell morphology (Mandell and George, 1991). Hypochromasia from iron deficiency is also evident in oval red cells of llama and alpaca (Plates XVIII-5 and XVIII-7).

The bone marrow cytology is characterized by a predominance of late rubricytes and metarubricytes. These nucleated red cells often exhibit scanty, irregularly stained cytoplasm and ragged cell boundaries. The marrow macrophage iron is depleted and sideroblasts are reduced in number (Table 9–7).

The iron status of a patient can be assessed by measuring the serum iron (SI) and total iron binding capacity (TIBC, a measure of serum transferrin level) and calculating the percentage saturation of transferrin (100 $\times$ SI/TIBC). Species variations occur in SI and TIBC values (Table 9–8). The transferrin saturation may vary from 20 to 60%. Generally, normal animals and humans have an average SI level of approximately 100 μg/dl, a TIBC of 300 μg/dl, and a transferrin saturation of 33%. In humans with iron deficiency, the SI and transferrin saturation values are generally reduced and the TIBC is increased (Table 9–7). Dogs with iron deficiency, however, have a decreased SI and transferrin saturation but show no significant changes in TIBC values. The serum iron level and TIBC may be affected by various conditions unrelated to the iron status of the animal because the iron transport protein transferrin acts as an acute phase protein. Thus, increases in these values may occur during inflammatory conditions and after corticosteroid therapy and may also be affected by the age and hypothyroid state of the animal. In inflammatory conditions, iron remains sequestered in iron

Table 9–7. Comparative Features of Iron Deficiency Anemia and Anemia of Chronic Disease

Feature	Iron Deficiency Anemia	Anemia of Inflammatory Disease
Iron absorption		
Intestinal absorption of iron	Increased	Decreased
Serum measurements		
Iron level	Normal to decreased	Normal to decreased
TIBC*	Normal to increased	Decreased
TIBC, saturation (%)	Decreased	Decreased
Copper, zinc, and ceruloplasmin levels	—	Increased
Ferritin level	Decreased	Normal or increased
Erythrocyte measurements		
Erythrocyte parameters	Moderate to marked, nonresponsive anemia	Mild to moderate, nonresponsive anemia
Free RBC protoporphyrin	Increased	Increased
RBC life span	Slightly decreased	Slightly decreased
Bone marrow measurements		
Erythropoiesis	Normal or impaired	Impaired
Marrow macrophage iron	Decreased	Normal or increased
Marrow sideroblasts	Decreased	Decreased
Hepatic measurements		
Superoxide dismutase	?	Decreased

* TIBC, total iron-binding capacity or transferrin concentration.

storage pools and gastrointestinal iron absorption is decreased. Hypoferremia of inflammatory origin may be an important nonspecific host defense against bacterial infection as iron is an essential nutrient for bacterial growth.

A small amount of ferritin is found in plasma in a concentration proportional to that of iron stores in the body. Such a correlation has been observed in humans, certain birds, horses, dogs, rats, and pigs. Consequently, the measurement of serum ferritin levels is considered useful for the detection of iron deficiency (Calvo et al., 1989; Smith et al., 1986; Weeks et al., 1989). The plasma ferritin level is considered to be a reliable indicator of the status of iron stores in pigs. In newborn piglets, plasma ferritin levels and TIBC values are negatively correlated. A similar correlation is found in foals at birth to 6 months of age. Increasing numbers of microcytes are found in foals as their PCV decreases gradually from birth to a minimum at 3 months of age (Harvey et al., 1987).

The treatment of iron deficiency varies with the primary cause. Neonates should be provided sufficient dietary iron by using iron supplementation or admin-

istering iron compounds. Chronic blood loss as a cause of iron deficiency requires treatment of the condition responsible for blood loss first, and then providing adequate iron supplementation.

Anemias Associated with Parasitism

Bloodsucking parasites produce blood loss anemia. Examples include the sticktight flea Echidnophaga gallinacea, the hookworm Ancylostoma caninum, and coccidia in the dog; the bloodsucking louse Haematopinus eurysternus and the stomach worm Haemon-

Table 9–8. Serum Iron Values in Animals

Species	Serum Iron (μg/dl)	TIBC (μg/dl)*	UBIC (μg/dl)*	Ferritin (ng/ml)
Dog	86.4 ± 30.8	322 ± 44	200	76.7 ± 40.3
Cat	140	290	150	—
Cattle	97 ± 29	230 ± 65	131 ± 36	—
Horse	111 ± 11	330 ± 32	218 ± 21	152 ± 54.6
Sheep	193 ± 7	334 ± 18	—	—
Pig	121 ± 33	417 ± 72	196 ± 39	10 ± 9.4

Data from Kaneko, J.J.: Clinical Biochemistry of Domestic Animals. 4th Ed. San Diego, Academic Press, 1989, pp. 264, 888, 894.
* TIBC, total iron-binding capacity; UBIC, unbound iron-binding capacity.

Table 9–9. Hemogram of a 1-Year-Old Male Suffolk Sheep Infected with Haemonchus contortus

Parameter	Values	
Erythrocytes ($\times 10^6$/μl)	3.3	
Hemoglobin (g/dl)	2.9	
PCV (%)	11.5	
MCV (fl)	34.7	
MCHC (%)	25.2	
Icterus index units	<5	
Reticulocyte count (%)	5.7	
Nucleated erythrocytes	1/100 WBC	
Anisocytosis	Moderate to marked	
Poikilocytosis	Moderate to marked	
Hypchromasia	Moderate to marked	
Basophilic stippling	Marked	
Polychromasia	Moderate to marked	
Howell-Jolly bodies	Occasional	
Leukocytes/μl	7,100	%
Bands	71	1.0
Neutrophils	2,968	38.0
Lymphocytes	3,905	55.0
Monocytes	177	2.5
Eosinophils	213	3.0
Degenerated cells	35	0.5

Fecal examination: McMaster count—84,000 eggs per gram, most of which were Haemonchus contortus

Table 9–10.   Hemogram of a 1½-Year-Old Hereford Steer having Trichostrongyloidosis

Parameter			Plasma Protein Analysis	
Erythrocytes ($\times 10^6/\mu$l)	2.5			
Hemoglobin (g/dl)	3.7		Total protein (g/dl)	2.8
PCV (%)	14.0		Albumin (A)	1.8
MCV (fl)	56.2		Globulin (G)	1.0
MCHC (%)	26.4		α	0.3
Anisocytosis	moderate		β	0.6
Hypochromasia	moderate		γ	0.1
Leukocytes/μl	15,500	%	A:G ratio	1.8:1.0
Bands	155	1.0		
Neutrophils	7,750	50.0		
Lymphocytes	6,200	40.0	Fecal examination	
Monocytes	1,240	8.0	Flotation: Trichostrongyles, 5/low power field	
Eosinophils	155	1.0	Fecal count: Trichostrongyles, 500/g	

chus placei in cattle; and the stomach worm Haemonchus contortus in sheep. In acute hookworm disease, the blood picture is one of acute blood loss, whereas in the more chronic disease, the anemia may be microcytic-hypochromic. A severe microcytic-hypochromic anemia may develop in the dog from a heavy infection with the bloodsucking flea E. gallinacea (e.g., in a 2-year-old male springer spaniel: PCV, 9%; MCV, 46.4 fl; MCHC, 25%; reticulocytes, 2.5%; and myeloid: erythroid ratio, 0.59:1).

Anemia and hypoproteinemia are observed in acute and chronic helminthiases in cattle and sheep. Although the pathogenesis of anemia has not been definitively established, blood loss is believed to be primarily responsible for the anemia associated with bloodsucking worms such as Haemonchus contortus in sheep and H. placei in cattle, whereas impaired erythropoiesis is thought to be involved in anemias caused by nonbloodsucking parasites such as Trichostrongylus, Ostertagia, and Cooperia spp. In addition, a shortened red cell life span may contribute to the anemia from both chronic blood loss and impaired erythropoiesis. Hypoproteinemia in helminthiasis is primarily a result of hypoalbuminemia developing because of protein-losing gastroenteropathy, with anorexia and malabsorption somewhat accentuating the problem. Edema of the lips and intermandibular space (bottle jaw) may develop in animals with severe hypoproteinemia.

Heavy infestations with Haemonchus contortus in sheep present a blood picture of acute blood loss—macrocytic-hypochromic anemia. In chronic hemonchosis, the anemia gradually becomes well advanced and may appear as normocytic-normochromic or microcytic-normochromic, with little or no evidence of reticulocytosis. A normocytic-hypochromic anemia may also be seen, probably as a transitional phase from acute to chronic blood loss in which iron deficiency is setting in with a diminution of erythropoiesis (Table 9–9). Normocytic-normochromic anemia is common in trichostrongyloidosis in cattle (Table 9–10). Experimental schistosomiasis (Schistosoma matthei infection)

in sheep was found to cause blood loss anemia and hypoalbuminemia. The liver fluke, Fasciola hepatica, produces a blood loss anemia in cattle and sheep when large numbers of adult flukes are present in the liver. The anemia is accompanied by hypoalbuminemia and hypergammaglobulinemia. Experimental infection of sheep with F. gigantica has produced a marked anemia between 10 and 14 weeks of infection.

REFERENCES

Calvo, J.J., Allue, J.R., Escudero, A., et al.: Plasma ferritin of sows during pregnancy and lactation. Cornell Vet., 79:273, 1989.

Clarke, L.L., Argenzio, R.A. and Roberts, M.C.: Effect of meal feeding on plasma volume and urinary electrolyte clearance in ponies. Am. J. Vet. Res., 51:571, 1990.

Easley, J.R.: Erythrogram and red cell distribution width of equidae with experimentally induced anemia. Am. J. Vet. Res., 46:2378, 1985.

Harvey, J.W., Asquith, R.L., Sussman, W.A., et al.: Serum ferritin, serum iron, and erythrocyte values in foals. Am. J. Vet. Res., 48:1348, 1987.

Kohn, C.W., Jacobs, R.M., Knight, D., et al.: Microcytosis, hypoferremia, hypoferritemia, and hypertransferrinemia in Standardbred foals from birth to 4 months of age. Am. J. Vet. Res., 51:1198, 1990.

Mandell, C.P. and George, J.W.: Effect of repeated phlebotomy on iron status of rhesus monkeys (Maccaca mulata). Am. J. Vet. Res., 52:728, 1991.

Smith, J.E.: Iron metabolism and its diseases. In: Kaneko, J.J. (eds.), Clinical Biochemistry of Domestic Animals, San Diego, Academic Press, pp. 256–273, 1989.

Smith, J.E., Cipriano, J.E., DeBowes, R., et al.: Iron deficiency and pseudo-iron deficiency in hospitalized horses. J. Am. Vet. Med. Assoc., 188:285, 1986.

Torrington, K.G., McNeil, J.S., Phillips, Y.Y., et al.: Blood volume determinations in sheep before and after splenectomy. Lab. Anim. Sci., 39:598, 1989.

Weeks, B.R., Smith, J.E., and Northrop, J.K.: Relationship of serum ferritin and iron concentrations and serum total iron-binding capacity to nonheme iron stores in dogs. Am. J. Vet. Res., 50:198, 1989.

Williams, W.J., Beutler, E., Erslev, A.J., et al.: Hematology. 4th ed. New York, McGraw-Hill, 1990.

Yamoto, O. and Maede, Y.: Susceptibility to onion-induced hemolysis in dogs with hereditary high erythrocyte reduced glutathione and potassium concentrations. Am. J. Vet. Res., 53:134, 1992.

Chapter 10

Hemolytic Anemias Associated with Some Infectious Agents

Hemolytic anemias result primarily from increased erythrocyte destruction, whether intravascular or extravascular. An uncompensated hemolytic anemia is said to exist when the rate of red cell destruction exceeds the capability of the bone marrow for enhanced erythropoiesis and delivery of young erythrocytes to the circulation. A compensated hemolytic disorder exists when both red cell destruction and marrow erythropoiesis increase and red cell values are within the normal range. The red cell life span is reduced in either case.

Hemolytic anemias have numerous causes (Table 10–1) and involve several pathophysiologic mechanisms, one or more of which may be operative in a particular instance. Red cell destruction may occur because of membrane abnormalities, physical damage, osmotic changes, immune-mediated lysis, and phagocytosis by macrophages in the spleen, liver, and bone marrow. Although a particular disease may produce certain specific clinicopathologic changes, some clinical and laboratory findings are common to hemolytic anemias of various causes.

Clinical signs may vary with the specific cause and degree of the anemia. The onset may be sudden or progressive. Signs of anemia such as pale mucous membranes, weakness, fatigue, and tachycardia may be present, depending on the severity of the anemia. Rarely, mucous membranes may be discolored—reddened as the result of an intense hemolytic process. Hemoglobinuria may occur in an occasional patient and icterus may be evident in some cases. The former indicates an acute hemolytic episode and the latter denotes significant, persistent red cell destruction. Fever of a variable degree, constant or intermittent, may be present and is related partly to the hemolytic process. Disseminated intravascular coagulation (DIC) may occur as a sequel to the lysis of a large number of erythrocytes.

Various abnormalities may be found in blood values, bone marrow cytology, serum analytes, and urinalysis (Table 10–2). The extent of changes observed depends on the severity and duration of anemia and on the nature of the inciting cause. Some important diseases or conditions associated with hemolytic anemia in various animal species are discussed briefly in this chapter. Additional information can be found in the references cited.

PARASITIC AND RICKETTSIAL INFECTIONS

Anaplasmosis

Anaplasmosis is an infectious disease of cattle, sheep, goats, and some wild ruminants caused by organisms of the Anaplasma and Paranaplasma genera. The

Table 10–1. Some Causes of Hemolytic Anemia in Various Animal Species

Blood parasites and rickettsial agents
  Anaplasmosis in cattle, sheep, and goats
  Babesiosis in cattle, dogs, horses, sheep, and goats
  Haemobartonellosis in cats, dogs and cattle
  Eperythrozoonosis in cattle (splenectomized), sheep, and pigs
  Cytauxzoonosis in cats
  Trypanosomiasis in cattle
  Theileriasis in cattle
  Ehrlichiosis in dogs and horses
Bacterial infections
  Leptospirosis in cattle, sheep, and dogs
  Bacillary hemoglobinuria in cattle and sheep
  Staphylococcus pyogenes infection (gangrenous mastitis in cows)
Viral infections
  Equine infectious anemia

organisms are obligate intraerythrocytic rickettsia and are extremely host-specific. Causative agents of anaplasmosis in cattle are Anaplasma marginale, A. centrale, Paranaplasma caudatum, and P. discoides and, in sheep and goats, A. ovis. In cattle, A. marginale is the most pathogenic, A. centrale causes a mild clinical disease, and A. ovis is nonpathogenic.

Anaplasmosis is enzootic in certain areas of California and the southern and western areas of the United States and in most tropical areas of the world. The disease may occur in an acute, subacute, or chronic form during any season. A marked parasitemia is present during the acute phase of the disease and a low-grade infection, lasting from months to years, may be detected during the carrier state. Transplacental infection to fetus may occur during the second and third trimester of pregnancy in cows and sheep (Zaugg, 1985, 1987). Hypomagnesemic cattle are resistant to experimental clinical infection by A. marginale (Brown et al., 1986).

Table 10–2. Abnormal Blood, Bone Marrow, Urine, and Serum Biochemical Findings in Hemolytic Anemias of Varied Cause

Anemia of variable degree
Hemoparasites—depending on cause of anemia
Hemoglobinemia of variable degree
Hemoglobinuria—infrequent
Macrocytic-hypochromic RBC indices during remission in most species
Morphologic evidence of response to anemia—increased anisocytosis, polychromasia, Howell-Jolly bodies
Normoblastemia
Red cell abnormalities—Heinz bodies, acanthocytes, schistocytes, spherocytes, leptocytes, and other poikilocytes, depending on pathogenesis
Reticulocytosis—in blood in most species, in bone marrow in horses
Myeloid:erythroid ratio—usually decreased
Leukocytosis
Neutrophilia with left shift
Hyperbilirubinemia of variable degree
Icterus index—normal or increased
Plasma protein concentration—usually normal
Serum lactic dehydrogenase level—increased
Serum haptoglobin level—decreased during acute hemolytic crisis
Unconjugated bilirubin level > conjugated bilirubin level

CLINICAL AND HEMATOLOGIC FINDINGS

Anaplasmosis is characterized by fever, marked hemolytic anemia without hemoglobinuria, icterus, and splenomegaly. Hematologic findings in natural cases of anaplasmosis and an experimental infection are presented in Tables 10–3 and 10–4. The natural disease may be difficult to diagnose if blood studies are delayed many days beyond the hemolytic crisis. The Anaplasma bodies increase in number during the incubation period, which varies from 15 to 45 days. Clinical signs of the disease appear suddenly, within 2 to 21 days of establishment of the parasitemia. The parasitized erythrocytes may be removed within a few days and the mass of circulating red cells may decrease as much as 50 to 80%. Within 4 to 5 days, Anaplasma bodies may be too few to permit a definitive diagnosis. By this time the anemia is in remission, and reticulocytosis, polychromasia, anisocytosis with macrocytosis, and basophilic stippling are in evidence (Plates XVII-7 and XVII-10; Table 10–4). The anemia during regenerative phase is classified as macrocytic-hypochromic (Table 10–3). Leukocytosis caused primarily by neutrophilia may be seen in some cattle. Erythrophagocytosis and evidence of increased erythropoiesis are found in the bone marrow. Convalescence usually lasts for 1 to 2 months, but may take 3 or more months. It is followed by the carrier state.

PATHOGENESIS

The anemia in anaplasmosis results largely from the extravascular destruction of parasitized erythrocytes. Erythrophagocytosis by macrophages in the spleen and bone marrow results in marked icterus without hemoglobinemia and hemoglobinuria. Hence, com-

Table 10–3. Ranges, Means, and Standard Deviations in Hematologic Data of 38 Cattle with Natural Infection Caused by Anaplasma marginale

Parameter	Range	Mean ± 1 SD
Erythrocytes ($\times 10^6/\mu l$)	0.85–5.6	2.26 ± 1.18
Hemoglobin (g/dl)	2.30–8.2	4.42 ± 1.59
PCV (%)	7.0–25.0	14.86 ± 4.89
MCV (fl)	41.7–110.0	71.71 ± 17.25
MCHC (%)	23.1–35.8	29.73 ± 2.86
MCH (pg)	13.6–34.4	21.11 ± 4.71
Icterus index units	0–100	20 ± 24
Plasma proteins (g/dl)	6.0–9.4	7.71 ± 0.75
Fibrinogen (g/dl)	0.20–0.90	0.65 ± 0.17
Reticulocytes (%)	0–31.8	8.4 ± 7.6
WBC/μl	2,900–38,800	12,744 ± 6,743
Band neutrophils	0–1,900	319 ± 387
Mature neutrophils	377–20,370	4,520 ± 3,727
Lymphocytes	1,960–16,464	6,299 ± 3,102
Monocytes	0–2,190	924 ± 787
Eosinophils	0–2,000	288 ± 397
Basophils	0–194	21 ± 44
WBC (%)		
Band neutrophils	0–18.0	2.5 ± 3.2
Mature neutrophils	7.0–75.5	33.5 ± 15.1
Lymphocytes	15.0–83.0	52.9 ± 15.9
Monocytes	0.0–20.0	7.3 ± 5.2
Eosinophils	0.0–10.0	2.0 ± 2.3
Basophils	0.0–1.0	0.2 ± 0.3

Table 10–4. Clinical and Hematologic Changes in a Guernsey Heifer Given 10 ml Blood Subcutaneously from a Carrier of Anaplasma marginale

Parameter	Postinoculation day													
	17	*21*	*25*	*26*	*27*	*30*	*31*	*32*	*33*	*35*	*37*	*39*	*45*	*66*
Erythrocytes (×10⁶/μl)	—	—	7.25	6.55	6.15	3.16	2.58	2.12	1.67	1.24	1.11	1.41	2.42	4.88
Hemoglobin (g/dl)	12.0	11.4	13.0	10.7	9.7	4.4	3.8	3.4	3.4	3.4	3.4	3.8	5.0	7.9
PCV (%)	34.0	32.5	36.5	30.5	28.0	13.0	12.0	11.0	12.0	12.0	13.0	14.0	18.5	24.0
MCV (fl)	—	—	50.3	46.6	45.5	41.1	46.5	51.8	71.8	96.7	117.1	99.3	76.4	49.2
MCH (pg)	—	—	17.9	16.3	15.8	13.9	14.7	16.0	20.4	27.4	30.6	26.9	20.6	16.2
MCHC (%)	35.3	35.1	35.6	35.1	34.6	33.8	31.7	30.9	28.3	28.3	26.1	27.1	27.0	32.9
RBC morphology	—	—	—	—	30% AB*	—	50% AB*	—	Many polychromatophilic macrocytes			Basophilic stippling		
Leukocytes (μl)	—	—	8,000	6,900	7,500	9,600	11,000	16,550	31,829	—	—	—	11,000	10,300
Physical condition	Normal (N)	N	N	N	N	Marked depression, anorexia, constipation, and icterus			Down, emaciated, labored breathing			Up, eating a little		
Temperature (°F)	101.8	101.8	101.8	101.2	101.0	104.9	101.8	100.4	92.0	100.0	—	101.6	106.2	101.8
Pulse/min	80	84	80	76	84	132	144	152	120	100	—	96	88	80
Respiration/min	Normal	N	N	N	N	56	N	16	20	20	—	20	20	44

* AB, Anaplasma marginale bodies (Plate XVIII-7).

mon necropsy findings include splenomegaly, an enlarged and friable liver, and a distended gallbladder. The degree of anemia is often disproportionate to the prevailing parasitemia because of the immune-mediated destruction of nonparasitized erythrocytes, in addition to that of parasitized erythrocytes. The antibodies involved (IgG and IgM) are directed against the Anaplasma organism as well as against the erythrocytes. Only the antierythrocyte antibodies are implicated in the causation of anemia. The direct Coombs test may be positive and autoagglutinins may be found during the acute and convalescent stages of the disease. In addition, red cell destruction may also occur through a T-cell–mediated antibody-independent mechanism. Spherocytes, accompanied by increased osmotic fragility and a positive direct Coombs test, may be found in cows with anaplasmosis (Swenson and Jacobs, 1986).

ORGANISM MORPHOLOGY

The morphology of the Anaplasma and Paranaplasma organisms may vary with the geographic location of the disease. In blood films stained by Ro-manowsky stains, ring, tailed, matchstick, comet, and dumbbell forms of the parasite may be seen. The proportions of tailed and nontailed organisms may vary markedly with the animal and stage of the disease. Tails and loop-like appendages are readily demonstrable by staining unfixed blood films with new methylene blue stain (Fig. 10–1). The organism of A. centrale appears more frequently near the center of the erythrocyte in contrast to A. marginale, which usually appears as a densely stained, purplish coccoid body near the cell margin (Plates XVII-4, XVII-5, and XVII-7). The parasites with appendages are distinct from A. marginale and may be present in blood in combination with A. marginale. The name Paranaplasma caudatum is applied to the tailed form and Paranaplasma discoides to the dumbbell form (Fig. 10–2). These organisms show prominent differences in antigenicity and species infectivity.

DIAGNOSIS

The diagnosis of anaplasmosis is based on the history, clinical findings, and blood examination for evidence of anemia with or without remission and,

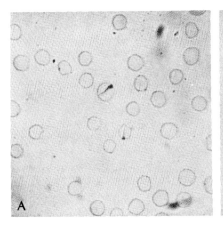
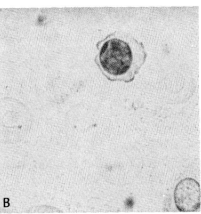

Fig. 10–1. Appendages associated with marginal bodies in anaplasmosis of cattle as demonstrated with new methylene blue vital staining technique. (From Jain, N. C.: Schalm's Veterinary Hematology. 4th Ed. Philadelphia, Lea & Febiger, 1986, p. 593.)

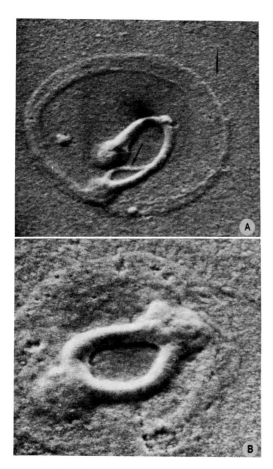

Fig. 10–2. Scanning electron micrographs of hemolyzed red cells parasitized with Paranaplasma organisms. *A,* Dumbbell form with two heads joined by a long, thin filament. Note the presence of a small, slender, secondary filament (*arrow*) (×5,775). *B,* Discoid form, two heads doubly joined by tails (×10,625). (From Keeton, K. S., and Jain, N. C.: Scanning electron microscopic studies of Paranaplasma sp. in erythrocytes of a cow. J. Parasitol., 59:331, 1973.)

most important, the presence of the organism. In Wright-stained blood films, Anaplasma marginale typically appears as a round, dark-staining inclusion, usually along the margin of the mature erythrocytes (Plate XVII-7). Immature (polychromatic) erythrocytes seem to be resistant to penetration by Anaplasma although, rarely, they may also be infected. Usually, one and infrequently two or three inclusion bodies are seen in a single erythrocyte. The tails and loops of Paranaplasma caudatum and P. discoides are evident only by special staining procedures (e.g., new methylene blue stain), because only the marginal body is seen in Wright-stained blood films. Detection of the carrier state may involve performing specific serologic tests such as the indirect immunofluorescence, complement fixation, capillary agglutination, or card agglutination test, or the inoculation of splenectomized calves to reproduce the disease.

THERAPY AND CONTROL

Acutely infected animals require rest and avoidance of undue excitement. Treatment consists of the ad-ministration of tetracycline and imidocarb. The carrier state can be eliminated by administering tetracycline mixed in feed, but these animals become susceptible to reinfection. Most carrier cows develop lifelong immunity and remain seropositive, but some may occasionally become seronegative and susceptible to reinfection (Lincoln et al., 1987). A blood transfusion may be given to severely anemic and to nonresponsive animals.

An age-related susceptibility of cattle to anaplasmosis seems to exist. Clinically, the disease is mild in calves up to 1 year of age, acute but rarely fatal in cattle up to 2 years of age, acute and occasionally fatal in cattle up to 3 years of age, and often peracute and fatal in cattle over 3 years of age. Calves, for some unknown reasons, are naturally resistant to Anaplasma infection. Immunization with an attenuated vaccine is possible, but neonatal isoerythrolysis may occur in calves born of vaccinated dams. Vector control and the elimination of natural reservoirs of infection are essential to limit spread of the disease. Several species of ticks (Boophilus and Dermacentor) and tabanids are important vectors, and deer and elk have been found as natural reservoirs of Anaplasma. Pronghorn antelope, bighorn sheep, and American bison have been experimentally infected with A. *marginale*. (Zaugg and Kuttler, 1985).

ANAPLASMOSIS IN SHEEP AND GOATS

Sheep do not become infected with Anaplasma marginale. A. ovis produces a mild subclinical disease in intact (nonsplenectomized) sheep, whereas carriers of A. ovis develop marked anemia after splenectomy. A. ovis morphologically resembles A. marginale and shows cross antigenicity. A. ovis generally does not infect cattle or produce any detectable immunity in cattle against A. marginale. Goats can be infected with A. ovis, however, and a transient infection of A. marginale into splenectomized goats may occur. Bighorn sheep experimentally infected with A. *ovis* develop a severe clinical disease, with a marked parasitemia, icterus, and anemia (Tibbitts et al., 1992).

Babesiosis (Piroplasmosis)

Protozoan parasites belonging to the family Babesiidae and the order Piroplasmoeda can infect vertebrate erythrocytes and cause a hemolytic anemia. The disease is transmitted by ixodid ticks. All domestic animal species are susceptible. Babesia are species-specific, though, and babesiosis does not normally spread among unrelated animal species. In cattle, babesiosis is caused by B. bigemina, B. bovis (synonymous with B. argentina), B. major, and B. divergens, the first two being economically more important, in sheep and goats, by B. ovis and B. motasi, in horses, by B. equi and B. caballi, in swine, by B. trautmanni and B. perroncitoi, in dogs, by B. canis, B. gibsoni, and B. vogeli and, in cats, by B. felis. B. bigemina is a large piroplasm (4.0 to 5.0 × 2.0 to 3.0 μm), whereas B. bovis is small (2.4 × 1.5 μm), but the disease caused by the latter is more serious and difficult to control than that caused by the former.

Historically, Babesia bigemina, the cause of Texas fever of cattle, was the first disease in which an arthropod was demonstrated to serve as an intermediate host and vector of the disease. Control of Texas fever through the destruction of the intermediate host (Boophilus annulatus) by the routine dipping of cattle in an insecticide led to the discovery of the means for controlling malaria and yellow fever in humans by eliminating the breeding areas of the mosquito vector.

CLINICAL SIGNS AND CLINICOPATHOLOGIC FINDINGS

The organisms (trophozoites) characteristically occur in the erythrocytes of the vertebrate host and present a round, ameboid, bizarre, rod-shaped, or typical pyriform morphology (Fig. 10–3). The pyriform organisms are connected at their narrow ends by a thin, filamentous structure and are usually arranged at an angle, forming a morphologic basis for distinguishing Babesia species. The organism divides by binary fission or a budding type of process within the erythrocyte and destroys the red cell intravascularly during escape from the cell. Thus, hemoglobinemia is often a prominent finding during the acute phase of the disease. The parasite may be removed from the red cells by the splenic macrophages through their pitting function.

The incubation period for babesiosis varies from 5 to 14 days, depending on the species of Babesia involved. Prominent clinical signs of acute infection include fever, anorexia, dehydration, anemia, hemoglobinuria, terminal icterus, and death. The anemia is usually regenerative and macrocytic-hypochromic. The degree of anemia is usually disproportionate to the degree of parasitemia, thereby indicating hemolysis not only of parasitized red cells but also of some unparasitized red cells, perhaps by an immune mechanism.

Prominent clinicopathologic findings include icterus, splenomegaly, reticuloendothelial cell hyperplasia with excessive hemosiderin, a swollen and dark liver, a distended urinary bladder with brownish-red urine, and enlarged red kidneys. A unique finding with Babesia bovis and B. canis infections is that autoagglutination of both parasitized and nonparasitized erythrocytes blocks the capillaries of the skin and brain. DIC may occur as a complication of hemolytic anemia from babesiosis.

DIAGNOSIS

Blood examination is essential to demonstrate babesiosis. If the organisms are not found in the peripheral blood, capillary blood from an ear should be obtained and examined, and the periphery of stained blood films should be given special attention to find for the protozoan. Babesia organisms may also be

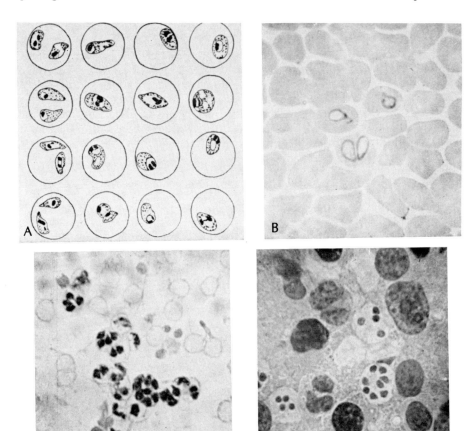

Fig. 10–3. Drawings (A) and photographs (B–D) of red cells parasitized with Babesia canis. Blood film stained with Wright stain (B) and blood (C) and bone marrow (D) films stained with new methylene blue. (From Jain, N. C.: Schalm's Veterinary Hematology. 4th Ed. Philadelphia, Lea & Febiger, 1986, p. 597.)

found in erythrocytes in the bone marrow, spleen, and liver. Because their specific gravity is lower, the infected cells tend to accumulate below the buffy coat in a hematocrit tube. A thick film of red cells from the top of the red cell column can be obtained and placed in Giemsa stain prepared in buffered, distilled water. The erythrocytes are lysed, leaving the protozoa intact. Diagnosis in some cases, especially during the chronic phase, may require transmission in a splenectomized animal. Serologic tests have been developed to detect carriers of infection; the complement fixation and indirect immunofluorescence tests are widely used.

TREATMENT AND CONTROL

Control of the disease involves treatment with babesiacidal drugs (e.g., imidocarb and acaprin), immunization, and vector control. In general, small Babesia organisms are more refractory to treatment than the large ones. Recovery from an acute infection is followed by the development of a carrier state. The carrier state in adult animals, however, is generally created by premunition as a result of infection while young. For some unknown reasons, young calves and horses are highly resistant to infection, whereas puppies are highly susceptible and newborn calves may develop the disease. Mild to marked relapses may occur following stress or splenectomy.

CANINE BABESIOSIS

Both Babesia canis and B. gibsoni have been found in North America (Conrad et al., 1991; Harvey et al., 1988; Taboada et al., 1992). B. canis is usually larger (2.5 to 3.0 × 5 μm) and pyriform (Plate XVII-6), whereas B. gibsoni is usually much smaller (1.0 to 2.5 μm) and appears spherical, ring-like, oval, elongate, ameboid, or rod-shaped, but rarely pyriform. Babesiosis in the dog may occur concurrently with infection by other blood parasites (e.g., Ehrlichia canis and Haemobartonella canis). Patients with dual infection become seriously ill and develop a severe normocytic-normochromic anemia. The anemia results from increased red cell destruction and from depressed erythropoiesis.

The acute disease is characterized by depression, anorexia, fever, hemolytic anemia, thrombocytopenia, hemoglobinuria, bilirubinuria, bilirubinemia, and icterus. Severe disease is more common in young pups than in adult dogs. Parasitemia may be detected on blood examination. The response to anemia is evident in polychromasia and reticulocytosis, with or without normoblastemia. Dogs infected with Babesia gibsoni become listless and anorectic and may develop an intermittent fever (Conrad et al., 1991). Splenomegaly is frequently seen and may accompany hepatomegaly. Icterus and hemoglobinuria are rare, but thrombocytopenia is common. The infection is more severe in splenectomized dogs in that parasitemia is greater and hemoglobinemia more frequent than in nonsplenectomized animals (Itoh et al., 1988). DIC may occur as

a complication during acute phase of the disease. B. canis, like B. bovis, may be associated with the agglutination of red cells in the blood and cerebral capillaries. In addition, metabolic acidosis may occur, in contrast to the alkalosis in calves with B. bovis infection.

The diagnosis of babesiosis involves the examination of well-stained blood films for the parasites. The identification of Babesia gibsoni can be facilitated by staining blood films with Giemsa or Field stain, because these parasites may be difficult to visualize with Wright stain. Diagnosing the chronic form is challenging and requires persistence. A low-grade or progressive anemia may be seen in such cases, but parsitemia is often undetectable. Serologic examination is particularly helpful in diagnosing such cases. An indirect immunofluorescence test may be performed to diagnose the disease. Lymphocytosis seems to be a feature in dogs chronically infected with B. canis. Dogs infected with B. gibsoni may show a positive Coombs test as a result of antierythrocyte antibodies formed because of alterations induced in erythrocyte surface antigens by the parasite. The disease can be transmitted to an intact or splenectomized dog, with parasitemia developing within a few days and death within a few weeks.

Treatment is difficult to carry out, particularly for Babesia gibsoni. Imidocarb dipropionate is commonly used to treat B. canis infections and infections with B. gibsoni have been treated with diminazene aceturate (3 mg/kg IM for 3 days), pentamidine isethionate, phenamidine isethionate, and metroniazide. Treatment may not completely eliminate the infection, particularly in splenectomized dogs, and adverse drug reactions may develop in some animals. Most dogs recovering from B. gibsoni become carriers and relapses may occur weeks or months later. Carrier dogs develop signs of infection when stressed and are a potential source of infection to other dogs. Transmission is commonly through ticks. The natural vector for B. gibsoni in Asia is Haemaphysalis bispinosa; a natural vector in the United States has not yet been established (Conrad et al., 1991).

FELINE BABESIOSIS

Infected cats become lethargic, anorectic, and anemic. Red cell parameters (PCV, hemoglobin, and RBC count) in experimental cases were found to decrease within 7 to 10 days and a marked anemia developed within 3 weeks of infection. The anemia was regenerative and macrocytic-hypochromic. Icterus was present only occasionally and fever was absent. The total plasma protein concentration did not change, but γ-globulin levels increased. Death occurred in all untreated cases.

EQUINE BABESIOSIS

Babesia equi and B. caballi infect horses, mules, donkeys, and zebras. B. caballi are most readily recognized in erythrocytes as paired pyriform bodies, with their pointed ends meeting at an acute angle. The trophozoites of B. equi are pleomorphic, with round, oval, and/or ring forms predominating. They are most readily distinguished when observed as small pyriform bodies in groups of four, with their pointed ends meeting to form a Maltese cross.

Equine piroplasmosis from Babesia caballi is considered endemic in certain parts of the United States. Acute cases usually display clinical signs of a progressive hemolytic anemia. Parasitemia is evident during febrile periods, but not in convalescing or carrier animals. The mortality rate may be as high as 20%. Dermacentor nitens is the principal vector of B. caballi, and transmission may occur through contaminated instruments. The incubation period in susceptible horses in endemic areas is 14 to 21 days. Experimental infection has been produced in intact and splenectomized horses and in donkeys. Infected animals developed fever, edema of limbs, anemia, icterus, and leukopenia or leukocytosis. Complement fixation and indirect fluorescent tests have been developed to detect infected horses. Horses experimentally infected with B. equi developed detectable paraistemia at an average of 30 days postinoculation and became seropositive within 23 to 30 days (Kuttler et al., 1986).

OVINE BABESIOSIS

Studies on the pathogenesis of Babesia motasi experimental infection in intact (nonsplenectomized) or splenectomized sheep showed that intact animals are refractory to infection, but splenectomized animals develop weight loss, fever, anorexia, lassitude, and a macrocytic hypochromic anemia, which coincides with the peak of parasitemia (Alani and Herbert, 1988). In splenectomized animals there was an initial leukocytosis, largely caused by a neutrophilia. The prepatent period following experimental infection was 2 to 3 days. Uncongugated and congugated (direct) bilirubin levels increased from pre-infection levels to peaks of 1.43 and 0.70 mg/100 ml of blood, respectively. Total serum protein levels increased temporarily and then returned to normal. Clinical infections, even in splenectomized sheep, were mild and of short duration, although recovered sheep remained carriers.

Haemobartonellosis

The blood parasites of the genus Haemobartonella are morphologically similar to Eperythrozoa. Haemobartonella organisms usually occur as small cocci, beaded bacilli, or rods on the surface of the erythrocyte, whereas Eperythrozoa organisms appear as small coccoid bodies or rings on or between the red cells.

HAEMOBARTONELLOSIS IN CATS

Haemobartonella felis is the cause of feline infectious anemia. The organism is highly pleomorphic. It may appear as a coccoid body, a delicate ring, or a small rod. The predominant form seen varies with the stage of the disease and the individual cat. Small, ring-like forms may be seen in large numbers on the surface

of erythrocytes at the height of parasitemia (Plates XVII-1 and XVII-2). The organisms may appear singly, in pairs, in a small group, or as short chains of coccoid bodies attached to the erythrocytes. The organism occupies an epicellular location. The erythrocyte membrane at the site of parasitic attachment is usually indented and may be partially eroded (Fig. 10–4). Usually, mature erythrocytes are parasitized. Rarely, the organisms may be observed in the plasma. The organism often detaches from erythrocytes in refrigerated anticoagulated blood and examination of fresh blood is therefore essential for diagnostic evaluation (Jain 1986).

The specific diagnosis of haemobartonellosis presents a problem, because infected cats may not be seen in the initial, acute stage of the disease, when the parasite is present in peripheral blood in large numbers. It is advisable to examine the blood at least on four occasions, generally on consecutive days, when the disease is suspected but the parasite has not been observed in the stained blood film. Blood films may be stained by Giemsa, acridine orange, and fluorescent-labelled antibody and examined to detect Haemobartonella felis.

Feline infectious anemia (FIA) is mostly a disease of male cats. A common presentation is a cat who had been in a fight and suffered bite wounds several weeks previously and has been lethargic and anorectic for 2 or more days. Variable clinical signs include weight loss, fever, dehydration, icterus, and enlarged lymphnodes and spleen. In addition, H. felis may reappear in the blood of carrier cats afflicted with a serious terminal or systemic disease, or after severe stress. Exogenous corticosteroids, however, did not induce a relapse in experimental carrier cats. Haemobartonellosis is associated with an increased incidence of feline leukemia virus (FeLV) infection.

The degree of anemia varies with the stage of the disease (Table 10–5). Cyclic bouts of parasitemia might lead to the more advanced stages of anemia (Fig. 10–5). The anemia is generally regenerative and macrocytic-hypochromic. A few cats, though, may not show evidence of remission of the anemia. The plasma protein concentration generally increases somewhat because of some hemoconcentration. Erythrocyte osmotic fragility is increased with the development of parasitemia and the loss of red cell membrane cholesterol and phospholipid. The direct Coombs test may be positive and red cell survival may be reduced. Cold agglutinins (IgM) may be detected in serum during the acute stage of the disease, when anemia is present (Zulty and Kociba, 1990). Sequestration of parasitized red cells occurs in the spleen, lungs, liver, and bone marrow, and erythrophagocytosis or removal of the parasite by macrophages and return of the pitted red cells to the circulation may occur. A bone marrow examination reveals a slight to marked increase in erythropoiesis and a decreased myeloid:erythroid ratio. Additional findings include leukopenia to leukocytosis with a regenerative left shift, variable icterus index, and absence of or low serum haptoglobin level.

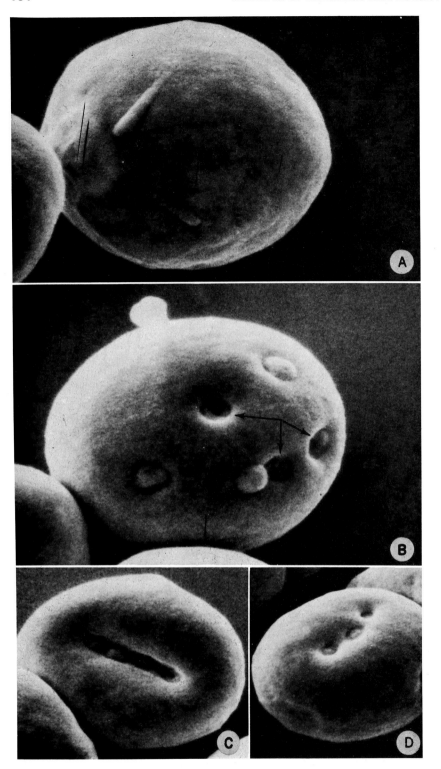

Fig. 10–4. Scanning electron photomicrographs of erythrocytes from a cat naturally infected with Haemobartonella felis. *A,* Erythrocyte with two rod-shaped organisms attached lengthwise (×16,600). *B,* Erythrocyte with coccoid bodies and surface lesions (*arrows*) apparently produced by parasitic adhesions and becoming evident after the parasite had become dislodged (×18,500). *C,* Erythrocyte with coccoid bodies and sites of parasitic attachment aligned in a rod-shaped groove that would appear as a short chain of Haemobartonella bodies under the light microscope (×12,500). *D,* Erythrocyte with three sites of parasitic attachment in the form of a short chain (×10,850). (From Jain, N. C., and Keeton, K. S.: Scanning electron microsopic features of Haemobartonella felis. Am. J. Vet. Res., 34:697, 1973.)

Table 10–5. Ranges, Means, and Standard Deviations in Hematologic Data of 30 Cats with Natural Infection Caused by Haemobartonella felis

Parameter	Range	Mean ± 1 SD
Erythrocytes ($\times 10^6/\mu l$)	0.63–5.60	2.32 ± 1.18
Hemoglobin (g/dl)	1.8–6.8	4.4 ± 1.5
PCV (%)	6.0–23.0	14.5 ± 4.6
MCV (fl)	33.9–109.9	70.8 ± 20.0
MCHC (%)	20.0–35.8	29.5 ± 4.0
MCH (pg)	12.1–28.8	20.8 ± 4.8
Plasma protein (g/dl)	5.7–10.9	7.9 ± 1.1
Icterus index units	0.0–75.0	8.0 ± 15.6
WBC/μl	2,300–49,000	12,660 ± 8,840
Band neutrophils	0–2,200	430 ± 490
Mature neutrophils	1,220–36,995	8,395 ± 7,365
Lymphocytes	560–5,984	2,828 ± 1,575
Monocytes	0–4,165	870 ± 869
Eosinophils	0–630	116 ± 179
Basophils	0–245	13 ± 47
WBC (%)		
Band neutrophils	0.0–8.0	3.0 ± 2.3
Mature neutrophils	35.0–93.0	61.9 ± 14.1
Lymphocytes	2.0–53.0	26.8 ± 12.3
Monocytes	0.0–22.0	7.0 ± 5.5
Eosinophils	0.0–5.0	1.0 ± 1.5
Basophils	0.0–1.0	0.1 ± 0.3

Haemobartonellosis may affect cats of all ages, with most cases seen in cats between 1 and 3 years of age. The mode of transmission of the parasite among cats under natural conditions is not known. Splenectomy does not influence the clinical course of the disease. The disease can be produced experimentally in normal, nonsplenectomized cats by the intravenous inoculation of a small amount of blood from natural cases (Fig. 10–5). Haemobartonella felis might be transmitted transplacentally or through the milk to kittens. Cats at risk include those with any of the following: anemia, FeLV-positive status, lack of vaccinations, history of cat bite abscesses and/or anemia, age 3 years or less, or outdoor-ranging status (Grindem et al., 1990).

The therapy of FIA varies with the clinical condition of the patient. A blood transfusion is recommended when the PCV is less than 12%, and fluids are to be given to dehydrated animals. Tetracycline is administered specifically to combat the infection. Corticosteroids have been found to be beneficial.

HAEMOBARTONELLOSIS IN DOGS

Haemobartonella canis can be found in normal dogs, but is seldom pathogenic for an intact (nonsplenectom-

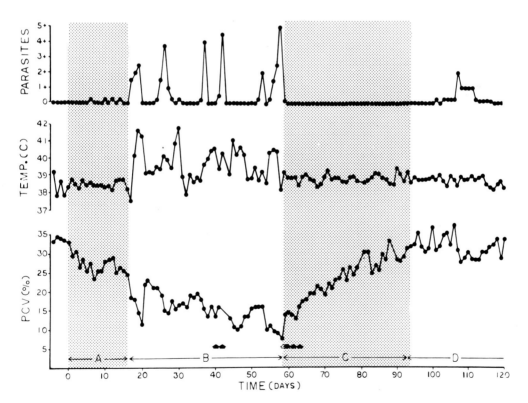

Fig. 10–5. Packed cell volume (PCV), rectal temperatures, and blood parasite values in a cat following intravenous inoculation with Haemobartonella felis-infected blood on day 0. Closed arrows indicate IV thiacetarsamide sodium (1 mg/kg) administration. Open arrow indicates a 25-ml IV whole blood transfusion. Phases of disease are indicated by letter and shading (A, preparasitemic phase; B, acute phase; C, recovery phase; D, carrier phase). (From Harvey, J. W., and Gaskin, J. M.: Experimental feline haemobartonellosis. J. Am. Anim. Hosp. Assoc., 13:28, 1977.)

ized) dog. Isolated incidences of anemia in intact dogs from this infection have been reported. Clinical anemia develops when a carrier dog is splenectomized for experimental or therapeutic purposes,when a carrier dog develops another disease, such as a bacterial or parasitic infection or lymphoma, or when a splenectomized dog is transfused with blood from a donor that is a carrier of H. canis. The incubation period in such cases is about 15 days. The infection can be transmitted experimentally in splenectomized dogs by the dog tick Rhipicephalus sanguineus.

Clinically affected dogs exhibit listlessness, episodes of fever, hemolytic anemia, icterus, and bilirubinemia. Hematologic findings are typical of a regenerative anemia. Leukocytosis from neutrophilia with a left shift may be seen in an occasional patient.

Haemobartonella canis differs in morphology from H. felis in that it more commonly forms chains that extend across the surface of affected erythrocytes,

although individual organisms appearing as small dots or rods can also be seen (Plate XVII-3). The degree of parasitemia is variable, staining is delicate, and a diligent search must be made to observe the organism when present in small numbers. The organism adheres to but does not penetrate the erythrocyte membrane. It is found singly, in small groups, or as chains on the surface of erythrocytes (Fig. 10–6). These observations indicate that the anemia in H. canis infection probably does not result from direct damage to the erythrocyte and may involve other mechanisms, such as immune-mediated red cell destruction (Jain, 1986).

HAEMOBARTONELLOSIS IN CATTLE

Haemobartonella bovis has been observed in cattle from some Asian, European, and African countries, but is rarely considered to cause anemia. It can also be found in association with other protozoan diseases.

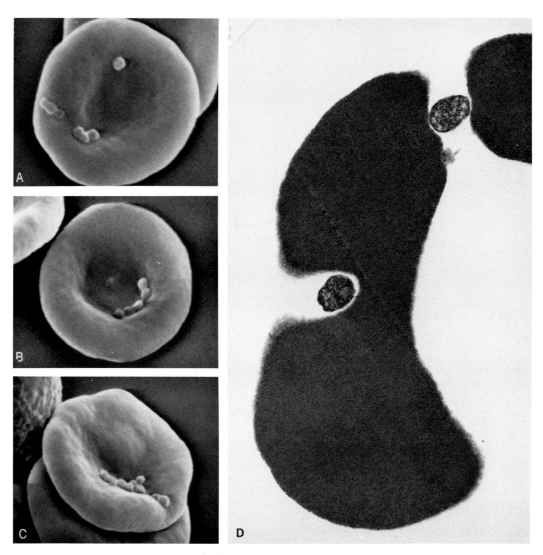

Fig. 10–6. Scanning (A–C) and transmission (D) electron photomicrographs of Haemobartonella canis. Single organisms as well as small groups and short chains are seen epicellularly on the erythrocytes, with surface indentations at some locations (A–C, ×6000; D, ×10,000). (From Jain, N. C.: Schalm's Veterinary Hematology. 4th Ed. Philadelphia, Lea & Febiger, 1986, p. 607.)

The parasite is either rod-shaped or ovoid, or in a chain form. Splenectomized calves develop anemia because of erythrophagocytosis in the liver, and not from hemolysis. A decrease in the PCV occurs at the peak of the parasitemia.

Eperythrozoonosis

EPERYTHROZOONOSIS IN CATTLE

Eperythrozoon wenyoni is a red cell parasite of cattle. The organisms appear as delicate ring, ovoid, comma, rod, dumbbell, and tennis racket forms in blood films stained with Wright stain (Plates XVII-4 and XVII-5). The parasites may be seen both epicellularly as solitary bodies and arranged in small chains, clusters, or pairs on erythrocytes (Fig. 10–7) and in the plasma. Coinfection with anaplasmosis may occur.

The erythrocyte surface at the site of parasitic adherence may sometimes be slightly depressed, but surface erosions and altered red cell morphology, as seen with Haemobartonella felis infection (Fig. 10–4), are not found (Fig. 10–7). The lack of notable eryth-

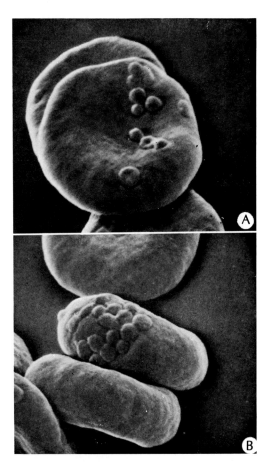

Fig. 10–7. Scanning electron micrographs of bovine erythrocytes parasitized with Eperythrozoon wenyoni (A, ×7840; B, ×8400). (From Keeton, K. S., and Jain, N. C.: Eperythrozoon wenyoni: A scanning electron microscope study. J. Parasitol., 59:867, 1973.)

rocyte membrane alterations is considered important because anemia is not a usual finding in Eperythrozoon wenyoni infection. The infection is typically latent, but is encountered clinically in splenectomized cattle or cattle severely ill from other causes. Hemolytic anemia has been encountered under experimental conditions, when calves carrying a latent infection were splenectomized for transmission trials with anaplasmosis. A regenerative anemia manifested in such cases within 8 to 10 days. The natural infection of cattle by E. wenyoni has been associated with a syndrome of swollen teats and distal portions of the hind limbs, prefemoral lymphadenopathy, transient fever, rough coat, decreased milk production, and subsequent weight loss and reproductive inefficiency. Experimental transmission of infection, however, did not induce these clinical signs (Smith et al., 1990).

EPERYTHROZOONOSIS IN SHEEP AND GOATS

Eperythrozoonosis in sheep differs from the disease in cattle in that Eperythrozoon ovis is more pathogenic and may produce a severe hemolytic anemia under natural and experimental conditions. The anemia is thought to result predominantly from intravascular hemolysis and partly from erythrophagocytosis. E. ovis is also an extracellular organism found on the surface of infected red cells (Martin et al., 1988). E. ovis can be transmitted to goats, which develop a lower degree of parasitemia than sheep and become chronic carriers. Sheep are not susceptible to E. wenyoni, even when splenectomized, although serologic cross-reactions may be seen.

EPERYTHROZOONOSIS IN PIGS

Eperythrozoon suis and E. parvum are blood parasites of swine in the United States. The former is more pathogenic—it can cause clinical anemia and icterus in young pigs under natural conditions. E. parvum is nonpathogenic for intact pigs, but can produce severe anemia in splenectomized pigs. The mechanism of anemia and icterus in acute eperythrozoonosis seems to be related to the formation of cold agglutinins (IgM) preceding massive parasitemia (Zachary and Smith, 1985).

The eperythrozoa of swine are similar in morphology to Eperythrozoon wenyoni and E. ovis but may be somewhat larger, averaging 0.8 to 1.0 μm in diameter, with an occasional form up to 2.5 μm. The organisms attach to the outer membrane of erythrocytes in infected swine (Zachary and Basgall, 1985). The parasite can be transmitted to susceptible pigs by the common hog louse, Haematopinus suis, and transplacentally. The eperythrozoon infection in swine is recognized by acute anemia and icterus without hemoglobinuria in stressed feeder pigs, delayed production gains, and reproduction losses in sows. Anemia and mild icterus are seen in newborn and weanling pigs. Hematologic abnormalities also include the spontaneous agglutination of red cells at room temperature, an increased erythrocyte sedimentation rate, and a transient thrombocytopenia. An ELISA test can be used for a rapid and effective diagnosis of *E. suis* infection in swine (Hsu et al., 1992).

An Eperythrozoon-like parasite was found to infect four llamas and cause a mild to moderate anemia (McLaughlin et al., 1990; Reagan et al., 1990). The organisms were coccoid or ring-shaped, measured about 0.5 to 1.0 μm in diameter, and epicellular, and caused no apparent deformations of the red cell membrane. The serum iron level decreased in all llamas, whereas the total iron binding capacity and percentage transferrin saturation were reduced in some. The serum albumin and β globulin levels were reduced in all llamas and γ globulins were decreased in some animals. The serologic antibody titer to E. suis was positive.

Cytauxzoonosis in Cats

The protozoan parasite Cytauxzoon felis is the cause of a fatal disease in domestic and wild cats known as cytauxzoonosis. Clinical signs of the disease in cats include lethargy, anorexia, pale and icteric mucous membranes, fever, and dehydration. Death usually occurs within a few days after clinical evidence of the disease. Parasitized erythrocytes show tiny densely stained or piroplasm-like organisms (Plate XVIII-9). The degree of red cell parasitization may vary from 1 to 25%. Parasitized erythrocytes usually contain a single, roundish organism, but occasionally up to four organisms may be present in a cell, and rarely they may form chains (Simpson et al., 1985). Sometimes elongated organisms may be found. Hemolytic anemia results from invasion of the erythrocytes by the parasites. Pathologic findings include icterus, petechial and ecchymotic hemorrhages over the surface of the heart and lungs, excessive clear yellow fluid in the pericardial sac, engorged abdominal vessels, splenomegaly, and swollen and hyperemic lymph nodes. In addition, large numbers of schizonts characteristic of Cytauxzoon are found in mononuclear phagocytes of the liver, lungs, spleen, and lymph nodes.

Theileriosis

Theileriosis is caused by a small protozoan parasite of the genus Theileria that infects the lymphocytes and erythrocytes of ruminants, especially cattle, sheep, and goats. The infection is spread by bloodsucking arthropods, particularly ticks of the family Ixodidae. Several species of Theileria are involved, but T. parva is the most important species economically because it is the cause of East Coast fever of cattle in East and Central Africa. The mortality rate is almost 100% in susceptible cattle, but some cattle have a high degree of innate resistance. Theileria mutans is the only protozoan of the family Theileridae to have been reported in cattle and deer in the United States, and it is mostly of academic interest.

Species of Theileria are distinguished on the basis of virulence and the nature of the immunity. The morphology of pathogenic and nonpathogenic forms (piroplasms) in the erythrocyte is similar. The organisms are pleomorphic and appear as rod-shaped, comma-shaped, oval, round, or Anaplasma-like. T. parva organisms are numerous in blood during the initial stage of infection, but not thereafter. T. mutans and T. annulata remain in cattle blood in small numbers for a long period, as do T. hirci and T. ovis in sheep and goat blood. Macroschizonts and microschizonts (Koch bodies) are found in the cytoplasm of lymphocytes in the peripheral blood and lymph nodes. These schizonts usually have a blue cytoplasm that contains numerous reddish-purple, dot-like granules. Infected lymphocytes often undergo blast transformation.

The incubation period of Theileria parva following tick transmission in susceptible animals is 8 to 25 days (mean, 13 to 14) and the duration of infection varies from 4 to 25 days (mean, 12 to 15). Experimental inoculations may take 3 to 7 days, weeks, or occasionally months to produce the disease.

Clinicopathologic changes vary with the severity of the disease. The disease is characterized by fever of variable duration, swelling of the superficial lymph nodes, anorexia, lacrimation and nasal discharge, depression, and diarrhea with bloody feces. Anemia might be significant in Theileria parva infection but leukopenia is marked, and slight bilirubinemia may be seen. In comparison, T. mutans usually produces only a slight anemia, but in severe cases anemia is marked and hemoglobinuria and icterus may occur. Anemia is inversely proportional to the degree of parasitemia and is regenerative. T. annulata induces a consistent anemia with bilirubinemia and bilirubinuria, occasional clinical icterus, rare hemoglobinuria, and, in contrast, leukocytosis. Sheep infected with T. hirci develop a variable degree of anemia and icterus. Red cell destruction in theileriosis may involve erythrophagocytosis from immune-mediated mechanisms.

The detection of carrier animals involves the use of various serologic tests; the indirect fluorescent antibody test is the most widely used, and an ELISA (enzyme-linked immunosorbent assay) test seems to be equally promising. Control of the disease involves immunization, limiting transport of cattle, and vector control. Therapy consists of the administration of oxytetracycline at the time of initial infection. The use of certain antimalarial and other drugs has been found to be highly effective against clinical theileriosis.

Trypanosomiasis

Trypanosomes are flaggellated protozoa that appear in the blood of all vertebrate classes; in some instances, they may invade the tissues. Most trypanosomes are nonpathogenic, but some are of great concern. Trypanosoma gambiense and T. rhodesiense cause African sleeping sickness of humans, which is spread by the tsetse fly (Glossina), whereas T. cruzi is implicated in Chagas disease of humans. Natural infection of dogs with T. cruzi produces an acute or chronic disease.

Many species of trypanosomes infect animals without any host specificity. Hence, a particular trypanosome may infect several animal species, and more than one species of trypanosomes may be found in the same animal. Some important trypanosomes of animals include Trypanosoma congolense (Nagana disease), T. vivax, T. brucei, and T. evansi (Surra disease), which infect cattle, T. suis, which infects pigs, and T. equiperdum (Dourine disease), which infects horses. Wild animals serve as a reservoir, e.g., common hosts for T. cruzi in North America include raccoons, opossums, armadillos, and skunks (Fox et al., 1986). Many modes of transmission have been described; the most important are insect and other arthropod vectors.

Trypanosomes are typically elongated organisms having a pointed, blunt, or round posterior end (Fig. 10–8). They possess a terminal, subterminal, or marginal kinetoplast and a poorly or well-defined undulating membrane. Various species of Trypanosoma in cattle can be distinguished by their morphology (Plate XVIII-10) and their behavior in wet preparations of fresh blood. Blood forms of T. theileria measure about 25 to 120 μm in length, whereas most other animal trypanosomes are relatively short. Although some overlap in size occurs, T. congolense is usually smaller, T. vivax is intermediate, and T. brucei is relatively larger in size. T. theleri is (Plate XVIII-10) generally nonpathogenic, but it may assume a pathogenic role under certain conditions of stress and concurrent infection (Hussain et al., 1985). Hematologic changes in human and animal trypanosomiasis have been reviewed (Anosa, 1988).

Clinical signs of trypanosomiasis include intermit-tent fever, enlarged superficial lymph nodes, tachycardia, progressively poor condition, stunted growth, and decreased fertility. Anemia manifests without hemoglobinuria. The incubation period in cattle varies from 3 to 20 days or more and clinical signs take about 2 to 4 weeks to appear; the disease may take an acute, subacute, or chronic form. An extremely acute infection, usually produced by Trypanosoma vivax, may assume a septicemic form with fever, marked parasitemia, and hemorrhagic diathesis with typical coagulation abnormalities.

Initially, a normocytic-normochromic anemia develops because of hemodilution from the expansion of plasma volume. A marked thrombocytopenia from reduced platelet survival may cause blood loss in some cases. A regenerative anemia then manifests for 3 to 4 months in response to erythrophagocytosis and a shortened red cell survival attributed to immune mechanisms. Anemia during the later stage of the disease also involves impaired erythropoiesis. Microcytic-hypochromic anemia develops when a concomitant iron deficiency is present. Bone marrow cytology during the acute phase of the disease indicates a regenerative anemia, whereas noticeable erythroid depression may be evident at later stages. A transient leukopenia develops because of both neutropenia and lymphopenia. Neutropenia is attributed to reduced myelopoiesis secondary to increased erythropoiesis and to the production of a circulating factor that inhibits granulopoieses. Acute hemorrhagic Trypanosoma vivax infection in calves causes dyserythropoiesis and dysgranulopoiesis which contribute, in part, to the developing anemia and neutropenia, respectively (Anosa et al., 1992). The leukopenia is later followed by leukocytosis associated with lymphocytosis. Dogs

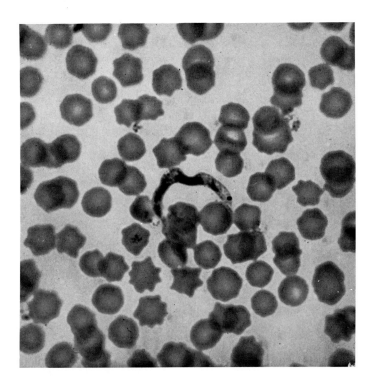

Fig. 10–8. Trypanosoma theileri (T. americanum, Crawley) in the blood of a cow in California (×1400). (From Jain, N. C.: Schalm's Veterinary Hematology. 4th Ed. Philadelphia, Lea & Febiger, 1986, p. 613.)

infected with Trypanosoma cruzi develop generalized lymphadenopathy and lymphocytosis between 14 and 17 day postinfection, when parasitemia is at its peak (Barr et al., 1991).

Diagnosis and control involve the parasitologic examination of ear vein or jugular blood, cerebrospinal fluid (CSF), lymph nodes, and material from lesions of the living or dead animal. The blood and CSF may be concentrated and buffy coat smears should be prepared to increase the chances of finding the organism. During the centrifugation of blood in a microhematocrit tube, trypanosomes settle at the interphase of the buffy coat and the plasma layer. The microhematocrit tube may be examined directly under the light microscope or the tube may be broken slightly above the buffy coat layer and its contents poured onto a clean glass slide for microscopic examination. Other diagnostic techniques include blood cultures in special media, inoculation of susceptible laboratory animals, and serologic diagnosis using complement fixation and indirect immunofluorescence tests. Various drugs have been used to treat trypanosomiasis and vector control has been attempted to prevent the spread of infection.

Sarcocystosis in Cattle and Sheep

A normocytic-normochromic anemia is found in natural and experimental cases of sarcocystosis in cattle and goats. The pathogenesis of the anemia remains undetermined, although a hemolytic origin was indicated by several findings, such as rapidity of onset, the presence of hyperbilirubinemia (primarily increased indirect bilirubin), and marked iron deposition in the liver. Hemoglobinuria was not a feature because of possible extravascular red cell destruction. Abnormalities of coagulation and platelet function may also be found.

BACTERIAL INFECTIONS

Leptospirosis

Hemolytic anemia in calves and lambs may be caused by Leptospira organisms. Over 100 serovars (serotypes) of leptospires are known, and more than one serovar may infect a particular animal species. The disease in cattle and swine is caused by L. pomona, L. grippotyphosa, L. icterohaemorrhagica, and L. canicola. In sheep it is caused by the first two and by L. hardjo, which may also cause a mild infection in cattle. Leptospires are shed in the urine and transmitted through contact with urine droplets.

Clinical signs are variable. Icterus and hemoglobinuria are frequent in cattle and sheep and occur in conjunction with fever at 4 to 8 days postinfection. Leptospirosis in sheep has been found to produce cold-reacting IgM antibody-mediated hemolytic anemia. The anemia is accompanied by an erythropoietic response in blood 7 to 10 days postinfection. Leukopenia resulting from lymphopenia and/or neutropenia occurs at 7 to 12 days postinfection. Thrombocytopenia is a constant feature of leptospirosis and other spirochetal infections, and is considered a useful diagnostic feature. Hemorrhagic diathesis is one of the most striking manifestations in acute leptospirosis.

Leptospirosis in the dog is caused primarily by L. canicola. and L. icterohaemorrhagica. Clinically inapparent but serologically detectable infections may occur from other serotypes. The disease is more severe from infection with L. icterohaemorrhagica than that from L. canicola. Clinical signs of leptospirosis in the dog vary according to the form of the disease and include fever, depression, anorexia, vomiting, and increased thirst. Hematologic and other laboratory findings vary with the severity of the disease. Moderate to marked anemia, icterus, and hemoglobinuria have been described, but often anemia may not be evident. Infection with L. canicola is not commonly associated with a hemolytic process, but, when the infection is caused by L. icterohaemorrhagica, a hemolytic crisis with hemoglobinuria may be anticipated. Hemoconcentration may be suggested by high total plasma protein values. The fibrinogen concentration and erythrocyte sedimentation rate are usually elevated. A modest leukocytosis (20,000 to 40,000/µl) resulting from neutrophilia with a left shift limited to band forms is a fairly constant finding. Other leukocyte numbers characteristically reveal a corticosteroid effect in old dogs. Lymphopenia is less obvious in dogs less than 1 year old, because the normal absolute lymphocyte number is generally high in young dogs (see Chap. 2). The blood urea nitrogen concentration generally increases, proteinuria may be a prominent finding, and glucosuria may occur.

The diagnosis of leptospirosis is based on demonstration of the organisms in urine and agglutinating antibody in serum. Urine may be inoculated intraperitoneally into hamsters or guinea pigs to propagate and demonstrate the presence of leptospires. Serologic testing involves the determination of increasing serum antibody titers in two samples taken 10 to 15 days apart during acute infection and of high titers in chronic infection.

Bacillary Hemoglobinuria in Cattle and Sheep

Bacillary hemoglobinuria is an infectious disease caused by Clostridium novyi, type D. It is characterized by a sudden onset, high fever, anorexia, depression, rapid hemolysis, a reddish nasal discharge, hemoglobinuria, and, sometimes, rapid death.

The organism produces a highly. lethal β toxin (phospholipase C) that degrades lecithin and causes marked intravascular destruction of erythrocytes; it also exerts a hepatotoxic effect. If the animal lives long enough for the anemia to enter a stage of remission, the blood picture is typical of a marked response, with polychromatic macrocytes, basophilic stippling, and the occurrence of nucleated erythrocytes. Leukocytosis with neutrophilia may accompany the erythropoietic response.

The mortality rate is high, with deaths occurring within 18 to 36 hours as a result of respiratory failure caused by a combination of hypoxia and toxemia. Necropsy findings are characteristic of anemia and icterus, in addition to specific lesions in the liver. The diagnosis requires a thorough history, necropsy, and examination of blood and impression smears of the liver lesions and spleen. An indirect immunofluorescence test can be performed to identify the causative organism. Treatment consists of antibiotic therapy, the administration of fluids, and blood transfusion. A vaccination can be administered to prevent future occurrences of bacillary hemoglobinuria.

VIRAL INFECTIONS

Equine Infectious Anemia

Equine infectious anemia (EIA) is a viral disease of the family Equidae. It occurs in acute and subacute forms in highly susceptible horses, but more commonly assumes a chronic course. The incubation period is 14 to 21 days and is characterized by cyclic occurrences of pyrexia, weakness, and anemia. Horses making an apparent recovery may remain carriers for months to years and, in some cases, for life. A severe relapse may occur as a result of intercurrent disease or stressful conditions.

Intermittent fever, debility, emaciation, pallor, icterus, and edema of dependent parts are signs suggestive of EIA. Additional clinical signs include petechial and ecchymotic hemorrhages in the mucous membranes and lymphadenopathy. Hematologic findings include moderate to marked anemia, leukopenia, and bilirubinemia. The red cell indices are those of a normocytic-normochromic anemia. The differential leukocyte count shows neutropenia and lymphopenia. Sideroleukocytes may be found in the blood (Plate XIV-11). Mild thrombocytopenia is common during early infection, prior to seroconversion and, rarely, a severe, immune-mediated thrombocytopenia may develop during the period of chronic infection (Cohen and Carter, 1991). The serum albumin level may decrease and levels of both β and γ globulin may increase. Liver-specific serum enzyme levels increase slightly.

Anemia in infected horses may be caused by immune-mediated hemolytic and reduced erythropoiesis. Evidence indicating that erythrocytes become coated with an autoantibody and complement support the concept of an immune-mediated hemolytic anemia in EIA. The antibodies involved may be IgG or IgM and autoagglutination of erythrocytes may occasionally occur. Evidence for reduced red cell production include impaired erythropoiesis as in anemia of chronic disease and selective suppression of erythroid progenitor cells, BFU-E and CFU-E (Swardson et al., 1992).

The diagnosis of EIA formerly required confirmation by reproducing the disease through inoculation of a susceptible horse with blood taken from a suspected case. Currently, the diagnosis is based on a positive agar gel immunodiffusion (Coggins) test. The test is 95% accurate for the diagnosis of EIA in acute, chronic, and inapparent forms.

The infection spreads principally through biting insects. Mechanical transmission from a carrier horse to a susceptible horse can occur through the action of horseflies or the use of contaminated needles, syringes, and/or surgical equipment. Infected horses may be isolated from normal horses to prevent spread of infection. No effective treatment is available. Corticosteroids may exacerbate the disease.

REFERENCES

Alani, A.J. and Herbert, I.V.: The pathogenesis of Babesia motasi (Wales) infection in sheep. Vet. Parasitol., 27:209, 1988.

Anosa, V.O., Logan-Henfrey, L.L. and Shaw, M.K.: A light and electron microscopic study of changes in blood and bone marrow in acute hemorrhagic Trypanosoma vivax infection in calves. Vet. Pathol., 29:33, 1992.

Barr, S.C., Gossett, K.A., and Klei, T.R.: Clinical, clinocopathologic, and parasitologic observations of trypanosomiasis in dogs infected with North American Trypanosoma cruzi isolates. Am. J. Vet. Res., 52:954, 1991.

Brown, J.E., Hidalgo, R.J., Jones, W., et al.: Blood magnesium values in healthy cattle and in cattle affected with anaplasmosis and eperythrozoonosis. Am. J. Vet. Res., 47:158, 1986.

Cohen, N.D. and Carter, G.K.: Persistent thrombocytopenia in a case of equine infectious anemia. J. Am. Vet. Med. Assoc., 199: 750, 1991.

Conrad, P., Thomford, J., Yamane, I., et al.: Hemolytic anemia caused by Babesia gibsoni infection in dogs. J. Am. Vet. Med. Assoc., 199:601, 1991.

Fox, J.O., Ewing, S.A., Buckner, R.G., et al.: Trypanosoma cruzi infection in a dog from Oklahoma. J. Am. Vet. Med. Assoc., 189:1583, 1986.

Grindem, C.B., Corbett, W.T., and Tomkins, M.T.: Risk factors for Haemobartonella felis infection in cats. J. Am. Vet. Med. Assoc., 196:96, 1990.

Harvey, J.W., Taboada, J., and Lewis, J.C.: Babesiosis in a litter of pups. J. Am. Vet. Med. Assoc., 192:1751, 1988.

Hsu, F.S., Liu, M.C., Chou, S.M., et al.: Evaluation of an enzyme-linked immunosorbent assay for detection of Epierythrozoon suis antibodies in swine. Am. J. Vet. Res., 53:352, 1992.

Hussain, K., Brodie, B., Ott, R.S., et al.: Prevalence of Trypanosoma theileri in cows and fetuses at slaughter. Am. J. Vet. Res., 46: 1256, 1985.

Itoh, N., Higuchi, S., and Kawamura, S.: The effect of diminazene aceturate on splenectomized dogs with Babesia gibsoni infection. Vet. Clin. Pathol., 17:94, 1988.

Jain, N.C.: Schalm's Veterinary Hematology. 4th ed. Philadelphia, Lea & Febiger, 1986, pp. 589–626.

John, D.T. and Hoppe, K.L.: Trypanosoma cruzi from wild raccoons in Oklahoma. Am. J. Vet. Res., 47:1056, 1986.

Kuttler, K.L., Gipson, C.A., Goff, W.L., et al.; Experimental Babesia equi infection in mature horses. Am. J. Vet. Res., 47:1668, 1986.

Lincoln, S.D., Zaugg, J.L., and Maas, J.: Bovine anaplasmosis: Susceptibility of seronegative cows from an infected herd to experimental infection with Anaplasma marginale. J. Am. Vet. Med. Assoc., 190:171, 1987.

Martin, B.J., Chrisp, C.E., Averill, D.R., Jr., et al.: The identification of Eperythrozoon ovis in anemic sheep. Lab. Anim. Sci., 38: 173, 1988.

McLaughlin, B.G., Evans, N., McLaughlin, P., et al.: An *Epierythrozoon*-like parasite of llamas. J. Am. Vet. Med. Assoc., 197:1170, 1990.

Reagan, W.J., Garry, F., Thrall, M.A., et al.: The clinicopathologic, light, and scanning electron microscopic features of eperythrozoonosis in four naturally infected llamas. Vet. pathol., 27:426, 1990.

Simpson, C.F., Harvey, J.W., and Carlisle, J.W.: Ultrastructure of the intraerythrocytic stage of *Cytauxzoon felis*. Am. J. Vet. Res., 46:1178, 1985.

Smith, J.A., Thrall, M.A., Smith, J.L., et al.: *Epierythrozoon wenyoni* infection in dairy cattle. J. Am. Vet. Med. Assoc., 196:1244, 1990.

Swardson, C.J., Kociba, G.J. and Perryman, L.E.: Effects of equine infectious anemia virus on hematopoietic progenitors in vitro. Am. J. Vet. Res., 53:1176, 1992.

Swenson, C. and Jacobs, R.: Spherocytosis associated with anaplasmosis in two cows. J. Am. Vet. Med. Assoc., 188:1061, 1986.

Taboada, J., Harvey, J.W., Levy, M.G., et al.: Seroprevalance of babesiosis in Greyhounds in Florida. J. Am. Vet. Med. Assoc., 200:47, 1992.

Tibbitts, T., Goff, W., Foreyt, W., et al.: Susceptibility of two Rocky Mountain bighorn sheep to experimental infection with Anaplasma ovis. J. Wildlife Dis., 28:125, 1992.

Zachary, J.F. and Basgall, E.J.: Erythrocyte membrane alterations associated with the attachment and replication of *Epierythrozoon suis*. Vet. Pathol., 22:164, 1985.

Zachary, J.F. and Smith, A.R.: Experimental porcine eperythrozoonosis: T-lymphocyte suppression and misdirected immune responses. Am. J. Vet. Res., 46:821, 1985.

Zaugg, J.L.: Bovine anaplasmosis: Transplacental transmission as it relates to stage of gestation. Am. J. Vet. Res., 46:570, 1985.

Zaugg, J.L.: Ovine anaplasmosis: In utero transmission as it relates to stage of gestation. Am. J. Vet. Res., 48:100, 1987.

Zaugg, J.L. and Kuttler, K.L.: *Anaplasma marginale* infections in American bison: Experimental infection and serologic study. Am. J. Vet. Res., 46:438, 1985.

Zulty, J.C. and Kociba, G.J.: Cold agglutinins in cats with haemobartonellosis. J. Am. Vet. Med. Assoc., 196:907, 1990.

Hemolytic Anemias of Noninfectious Origin

Hemolytic anemias associated with infectious agents (see Table 10–1) are described in Chapter 10. Hemolytic anemias associated with causes other than infectious agents (Table 11–1) are described in this chapter. For general comments on various hematologic abnormalities encountered in hemolytic anemias, see Chapter 10 and Table 10–2.

INTRAERYTHROCYTIC ABNORMALITIES

Many hereditary and acquired abnormalities of red cell skeletal proteins, membrane composition, globin chains, and enzymes in humans have been associated with hemolytic anemias (Williams et al., 1990). The prototype of red cell membrane skeletal protein defects that lead to hemolytic anemia is hereditary spherocytosis. In contrast, hereditary nonspherocytic anemias do not involve major abnormalities of red cell shape and may be caused by enzyme deficiencies, hemoglobinopathies, or red cell membrane defects. Red cell destruction in these instances may result from the depletion of ATP, abnormal deformability of red cells, and increased propensity for erythrophagocytosis by macrophages in the mononuclear phagocyte system (MPS), respectively. Major abnormalities of these types are briefly described here to provide background essential to search for such abnormalities in animal species. Some red cell abnormalities that have been described in dogs are also discussed.

Membrane Defects

HEREDITARY SPHEROCYTOSIS

Hereditary spherocytosis in humans is characterized by hemolytic anemia of varying severity, the formation of spherocytes and spherostomatocytes, and increased erythrocyte osmotic fragility (Williams et al., 1990). The mode of inheritance may be autosomal dominant or recessive. Abnormalities of red cell shape are related to a deficiency of the membrane skeletal proteins spectrin, ankyrin, and protein band 4.2, or to the formation of defective spectrin. Consequently, the lipid bilayer becomes destabilized and lipid is released from the membrane, leading to a reduction in surface area and to the formation of spherostomatocytes and spherocytes. Sequestration of poorly deformable spherocytic red cells within the spleen results in hemolytic anemia. Clinical improvement occurs after splenectomy.

A probable case of hereditary spherocytosis was recorded in a goat (see Fig. 7–10C), but anemia was not evident. The mode of inheritance and basis of cell shape were undetermined.

HEREDITARY ELLIPTOCYTOSIS

Hereditary elliptocytosis is characterized by the presence of primarily elliptic erythrocytes, although some poikilocytes representing other red cell shapes may be present. The shape change is related to abnormalities

Table 11–1. Some Causes of Hemolytic Anemias of Noninfectious Origin

Anemias associated with intrinsic abnormalities of erythrocytes
  Membrane defects
    Hereditary spherocytosis
    Hereditary elliptocytosis in dogs
    Hereditary stomatocytosis in dogs
    Acanthocytosis and stomatocytosis in dogs
  Enzyme deficiencies
    Pyruvate kinase deficiency in dogs
    Phosphofructokinase deficiency in dogs
    Congenital erythropoietic porphyria in cattle, cats, and pigs
    Methemoglobinemia in dogs, cats, and horses
  Globin abnormalities
    Hemoglobinopathies
Anemias associated with abnormalities extrinsic to erythrocytes
  Infectious agents (see Table 10–1)
  Chemicals and drugs
    Copper poisoning in sheep, cattle, and pigs
    Lead poisoning in dogs, horses, cattle, sheep, pigs, and cats
    Oxidants causing Heinz body formation (e.g., phenothiazine toxicosis in horses and sheep; methylene blue, acetaminophen, and DL-methionine toxicosis in cats; propylene glycol in cats; cephalosporins in dogs)
    Nitrate and nitrite poisoning in cattle, L-tryptophan and its metabolite indole in horses
    Phenol compounds, benzene and related compounds, naphthalene in mothballs
    Zinc toxicosis in cattle, sheep, and dogs
  Poisonous plants and venoms
    Onion toxicity in cattle, sheep, horses, dogs, and cats
    Rape and kale poisoning in cattle and sheep
    Castor been toxicity in cattle
    Other miscellaneous toxic plants
    Snake venom
  Antibody-mediated anemias
    Autoimmune hemolytic anemia caused by warm- and cold-reacting antibodies in dogs, cats, and horses
    Neonatal isoerythrolysis in cattle, horses and, possibly in cats
    Hemolytic transfusion reactions
  Metabolic disease
    Postparturient hemoglobinuria in cattle, severe hypophosphatemia in cats
  Mechanical factors
    Microangiopathic hemolytic anemia, hemolytic uremic-like syndrome in horses and cows
  Hyperactivity of the monocyte-macrophage system
    Hypersplenism
  Miscellaneous causes
    Water intoxication in cattle
    Heparin administration in horses

of the red cell membrane skeletal proteins—a deficiency of protein band 4.1 and glycophorin C, or the formation of defective spectrin and protein band 4.1 (Williams et al., 1990). These abnormalities of red cell membrane proteins may be associated with a mild to severe hemolytic anemia or may be asymptomatic (carrier state). The osmotic fragility of erythrocytes may be normal or increased.

Hereditary elliptocytosis in association with microcytosis has been described in a crossbred dog (Smith et al., 1983). Anemia was absent, but the reticulocyte count was about twice normal. The abnormal red cell shape was attributed to a deficiency of band 4.1 protein.

ACANTHOCYTOSIS AND STOMATOCYTOSIS

Acanthocytes and target cells are found in severe liver disease in humans and occasionally in dogs. These shape changes are presumably caused by an accumulation of cholesterol and phospholipids in the outer layer of the red cell membrane. This increase in membrane lipids causes an expansion of the red cell surface area relative to the contents, and reduces intravascular red cell life span. Acanthocytes and target cells may also be found in other diseases (see Table 7–5).

Hereditary stomatocytosis in humans is characterized by a sodium leak, which leads to increases in intracellular sodium and water content. Hemolytic anemia results from increased osmotic fragility of the erythrocytes.

Hereditary stomatocytosis as an autosomal recessive trait has been described in chondrodysplastic Alaskan malamute dogs with short-limb dwarfism (Pinkerton et al., 1974). The red cells retain increased amounts of water; consequently, the mean corpuscular volume (MCV) increases and the mean corpuscular hemoglobin concentration (MCHC) decreases. The red cells have an elevated intracellular sodium concentration and a decreased glutathione (GSH) content. A mild anemia is detected, based on the reduced hemoglobin concentration, because the PCV remains within the normal range because of the increased red cell size. The reticulocyte count increases slightly.

Enzyme Deficiencies

Deficiencies of many enzymes concerned with red cell metabolism have been found to cause hemolytic anemia in humans (Williams et al., 1990). The most common is the deficiency of glucose-6-phosphate dehydrogenase (G-6-PD) involved in aerobic glycolysis. Similar enzyme deficiencies have been incriminated as a cause of anemia in animals. In addition, some red cell enzyme deficiencies have been reported to occur without anemia and, in others, the cause of hemolytic anemia remains to be determined. Examples include a male dog with G-6-PD deficiency, γ-glutamylcysteine synthetase deficiency in sheep, and familial hemolytic anemia of undefined cause in poodles with myelofibrosis and osteosclerosis (Kaneko, 1987; Harvey, 1989; Williams et al., 1990).

PYRUVATE KINASE DEFICIENCY

A familial hemolytic anemia attributed to a deficiency of the erythrocytic enzyme pyruvate kinase (PK) has been reported in the basenji, beagle, West Highland white terrier, and Cairn terrier dogs (Giger et al., 1991; Harvey, 1989). The mode of inheritance in the basenji and beagles is autosomal recessive. The age at detection of the anemia is often less than 6 months, and usually less than 3 years. The two major types of PK are the R-type enzyme found in erythrocytes and the muscle-type enzymes M_1 (found in muscle) and

M_2 (found in the spleen, leukocytes, and platelets). The R-type enzyme closely resembles the L-type liver enzyme. Erythrocytes are deficient in the normal R-type PK isoenzyme, but contain a defective, heat-labile, M_2-type PK. The PK deficiency leads to impaired erythrocyte energy metabolism (decreased glucose utilization and ATP formation) and consequently to premature red cell destruction. Phosphoenol pyruvate, the substrate for PK, is significantly increased in erythrocytes of the affected animals and, similarly, enzymes of the glycolytic cycle and phosphorylated glycolytic intermediates are also elevated (Harvey et al., 1990a). The red cell content of 2,3-diphosphoglycerate (2,3-DPG) is increased, and, as a result, the whole blood oxygen saturation (P_{50}) is higher than normal. Affected dogs may show a higher than normal PK activity in vitro, but a functional erythrocyte PK deficiency may be found. Thus, a definitive diagnosis requires the following, in addition to a simple assay of PK activity: (1) the measurement of glycolytic substrates that accumulate in red cells; and (2) enzyme stability and immunologic or electrophoretic studies of erythrocyte PK (Giger and Noble, 1991).

Affected basenji dogs are less tolerant of exercise than normal littermates. Common clinical findings include pale mucous membranes and splenomegaly. Splenectomy is not associated with substantial clinical improvement. Moderate to marked anemia (PCV, 15 to 25%) is accompanied by a persistently high reticulocyte count (15 to 50%) associated with macrocytic-hypochromic erythrocytic indices (Table 11–2). Spherocytes are absent and various tests for autoantibody to erythrocytes yield negative results. The myeloid:erythroid ratio is below 1, reflecting intense erythrogenesis. Myelofibrosis and osteosclerosis are common sequels. Death occurs before 4 years of age as a result of the anemia and hepatic hemosiderosis. Similar findings have been seen in PK-deficient dogs of other breeds.

PHOSPHOFRUCTOKINASE DEFICIENCY

English Springer spaniel dogs were found to develop a persistent hemolytic anemia because of an autosomal recessive deficiency of phosphofructokinase (PFK) (Giger et al., 1985; Giger and Harvey, 1987). Canine PFK is composed of muscle (M), liver (L), and platelet (P) subunits. Normal canine red cells contain predominantly M and some P subunits, whereas red cells of dogs with PFK deficiency lack the M form.

Dogs homozygous for PFK deficiency exhibit a persistent compensated hemolytic anemia, because their PCV is generally normal or low normal and reticulocyte counts are elevated (7 to 23%). Hemolytic anemia and hemoglobinuria are evident during periodic episodes of hemolytic crisis, however, as a result of hyperventilation-induced alkalemia. Red cells of these dogs show a marked alkaline fragility as their intracellular pH increases because of the decreased synthesis of 2,3-DPG. The reduction in 2,3-DPG also increases the oxygen affinity of hemoglobin. Aged dogs develop a severe progressive myopathy and associated abnormal polysaccharide deposits (type VII glycogen storage disease) in skeletal muscle (Harvey et al., 1990b).

CONGENITAL ERYTHROPOIETIC PORPHYRIA

Congenital erythropoietic porphyria (porphyria erythropoietica, or congenital porphyria), commonly called "pink tooth," is an infrequently encountered inborn error of metabolism in cattle. The disease

Table 11–2. Congenital Hemolytic Anemia (Pyruvate Kinase Deficiency) in the Basenji Dog*

Parameter	Dog Number				
	1	2	3	4	5
Number of hemograms	17	14	14	13	8
Sex	F	M	M	M	F
Age range (mo)	18–24	5–30	5–11	5–26	10–18
RBC ($\times 10^6/\mu l$)	2.0 ± 0.2	3.1 ± 0.5	2.6 ± 0.4	2.3 ± 0.3	2.9 ± 0.4
Hb (g/dl)	5.2 ± 0.5	6.9 ± 1.1	6.2 ± 0.8	5.3 ± 0.7	7.0 ± 0.7
PCV (%)	18.5 ± 1.9	24.7 ± 3.7	22.4 ± 2.7	19.6 ± 2.6	24.5 ± 3.5
MCV (fl)	92.5 ± 6.5	80.2 ± 5.4	86.0 ± 5.8	85.1 ± 6.5	85.0 ± 2.9
MCH (pg)	26.1 ± 1.6	22.1 ± 1.5	23.8 ± 1.7	23.2 ± 1.4	24.3 ± 1.4
MCHC (%)	27.4 ± 2.9	27.7 ± 1.8	27.7 ± 1.8	27.5 ± 2.3	28.6 ± 1.3
Reticulocytes (%)	27.6 ± 6.0	30.9 ± 9.8	45.7 ± 8.4	41.1 ± 10.2	36.1 ± 9.0
Icterus index units	2.7 ± 1.3	4.6 ± 2.2	5.3 ± 1.7	2.5 ± 1.1	2.8 ± 1.3
Protein (g/dl)	6.7 ± 0.4	6.6 ± 0.3	6.7 ± 0.2	6.7 ± 0.4	6.7 ± 0.4
Fibrinogen (g/dl)	0.17 ± 0.07	0.245 ± 0.13	0.211 ± 0.08	0.2 ± 0.08	0.188 ± 0.08
WBC ($\times 10^3/\mu l$)	17.3 ± 1.3	17.3 ± 2.8	21.8 ± 3.9	25.6 ± 6.4	19.3 ± 2.8
WBC (%)					
Bands	0.9 ± 0.8	0.5 ± 0.5	1.0 ± 0.9	1.0 ± 0.9	1.3 ± 1.1
Segmenters	46.5 ± 5.3	59.8 ± 5.2	61.0 ± 6.8	61.8 ± 8.4	61.5 ± 3.1
Lymphocytes	40.7 ± 6.5	24.7 ± 6.4	23.6 ± 6.8	23.7 ± 8.9	24.9 ± 5.1
Monocytes	10.3 ± 3.7	11.5 ± 2.9	13.0 ± 5.0	12.5 ± 3.8	8.9 ± 2.4
Eosinophils	1.5 ± 1.2	3.4 ± 1.8	1.2 ± 1.1	0.8 ± 1.1	3.2 ± 2.5
Basophils	0.0	0.0	0.0	0.0	0.0

* Mean ± 1 SD.

mainly occurs in Holstein cattle, but other breeds may also be involved. Bovine congenital erythropoietic porphyria results from an autosomal recessive deficiency of the enzyme uroporphyrinogen (UROgen) III cosynthetase. Carrier animals show intermediate levels of the UROgen III cosynthetase. Because of a failure to form adequate amounts of protoporphyrin III for hemoglobin synthesis, abnormal quantities of the useless uroporphyrin and coproporphyrin accumulate in the bones, teeth, tissues, and organs, and produce the clinical syndrome (Jain, 1986; Kaneko, 1989).

Porphyric cattle may show varying intensity of anemia, depending on the degree of the enzyme defect. The principal defect is an inability to produce normal amounts of hemoglobin. Marrow erythropoiesis is intensified, as expressed by the presence of macrocytic erythrocytes, basophilic strippling, nucleated erythrocytes, polychromasia, and reticulocytes in blood. Erythrocyte survival is markedly shortened; this varies with the erythrocyte coproporphyrin and protoporphyrin concentrations. Porphyrins induce hemolysis and delay the maturation of reticulocytes and metarubricytes.

Calves with congenital porphyria fail to grow at a normal rate, and the white parts of their bodies are photosensitive when exposed to sunlight. Consequently, affected animals develop photophobia and dermatitis. The urine is pigmented with the brownish-red uroporphyrin. The teeth are reddish-brown; this is why the disease is called pink tooth. The teeth and bones produce a pink fluorescence when exposed to ultraviolet light. Bones become weak and spontaneous fractures may occur. A definitive diagnosis involves the detection of excessive porphyrins in various tissues and body fluids (e.g., bone marrow, urine, erythrocytes, and plasma). Animals protected from sunlight may mature, reproduce, and live for years.

At birth, calves homozygous for porphyria erythropoietica have exhibited many nucleated erythrocytes and marked poikilocytosis, along with anisocytosis, polychromasia, reticulocytes, and basophilic stippling of red cells in blood. The myeloid:erythroid ratio is decreased as a result of the intensified erythropoiesis. The nucleated erythrocytes and basophilic stippling tend to disappear by the end of the first week, but a slight to moderate poikilocytosis may persist.

Congenital porphyria has been reported in pigs and cats with an autosomal dominant inheritance pattern. Affected pigs do not show photosensitization, but discoloration and fluorescence of teeth may be observed. Porphyrinuria is observed in the most severely affected pigs. The disorder in cats produces fluorescence of the teeth and urine, but anemia is not seen.

METHEMOGLOBINEMIA

Oxygen binding to the ferrous iron (Fe^{2+}) in the hemoglobin molecule results in the formation of oxyhemoglobin with iron in the ferric state (Fe^{3+}) and the generation of a heme-bound superoxide anion. Delivery of oxygen to the tissues normally reverses the reaction with the formation of native (deoxy-) hemoglobin. During the normal process of oxygen binding to the hemoglobin, however, a small amount (0.5 to 3% in humans) of methemoglobin (MetHb) is produced. The iron in the MetHb is in the nonfunctional ferric state, whereas that in the native hemoglobin is in the functional ferrous form. Methemoglobin is also produced by the direct action of superoxide anion and hydrogen peroxide, both of which are also generated within the red cells. Methemoglobinemia results when the formation of MetHb exceeds the ability of the erythrocyte to reduce it back to the native state. Oxidative damage to erythrocytes also includes the oxidation of membrane sulfhydryl groups and denaturation of the globin moiety, which results in Heinz body formation. These abnormalities of red cells not only reduce oxygen transport but may also be accompanied by hemolytic anemia and sometimes death.

The oxidative denaturation of hemoglobin is prevented by methemoglobin reductase, superoxide dismutase (SOD), glutathione peroxidase, and catalase. MetHb in red cells in nonenzymatically reduced by ascorbic acid and GSH and (most important) enzymatically, either by NADH (generated by glucose metabolism through the Embden-Meyerhof pathway) or NADPH (generated through the pentose phosphate pathway) as electron donors. The predominant mechanism under normal conditions is a reaction involving NADH and the enzyme NADH-methemoglobin reductase (also known as NADH diaphorase, or cytochrome b_5 reductase). The enzyme NADPH diaphorase or NADPH-methemoglobin reductase is of minor importance under normal conditions but becomes highly functional in the presence of redox dyes, such as methylene blue, and various flavins, such as riboflavin. This forms the basis of methylene blue and riboflavin therapy for methemoglobinemia from various causes. The NADPH-dependent diaphorase reduces methylene blue to leukomethylene blue, which in turn reduces MetHb to native hemoglobin and becomes converted back to methylene blue to be reused.

Superoxide dismutase, a copper-zinc enzyme, catalyzes the dismutation of superoxide to oxygen and hydrogen peroxide (H_2O_2). Hydrogen peroxide is degraded through a reaction involving glutathione peroxidase, a selenium-containing enzyme, and reduced GSH. During this process, oxidized GSH (GSSH) is formed. The supply of reduced GSH is maintained either by the de novo synthesis of GSH by the erythrocytes, or by the rapid reduction of GSSH to GSH by a reaction involving glutathione reductase and NADPH (see Fig. 7–13). GSH is not only essential for detoxifying H_2O_2, but also for preventing the oxidation of hemoglobin and sulfhydryl groups in the red cell membrane and, in turn, for ensuring erythrocyte survival. Thus, inadequacies of GSH are usually associated with Heinz body formation. Catalase is of minor significance in the degradation of H_2O_2 in the red cell.

Several situations are known to cause methemoglobinemia (with varying frequency) in animals; these include acetaminophen toxicity in cats and dogs (Harvey et al., 1986), nitrite poisoning in cows and pigs, cats anesthetized with ketamine, horses who feed on red maple (Acer rubrum) leaves, and diminished red cell GSH and decreased glutathione reductase in horses (Jain, 1986). A congenital deficiency of NADH-methemoglobin reductase has been reported in dogs of several breeds (Harvey et al., 1991). Benzocaine induced methemoglobinemia has been described in a cat (Wilkie and Kirby, 1988).

Animals with methemoglobinemia exhibit weakness, lethargy, anorexia, exercise intolerance, dyspnea, tachycardia and, most important, muddy brown cyanotic-appearing mucous membranes and chocolate brown blood. Anemia is absent. The arterial P_{O_2} is generally normal and venous blood samples remain dark, with a brownish tinge, even when exposed to air. The quantitation of the hemoglobin concentration by the cyanmethemoglobin method measures all forms of hemoglobin in blood, whereas that using the oxyhemoglobin method measures only oxyhemoglobin and not other forms, including MetHb. Therefore, hemoglobin values obtained by the two methods are incongruous for blood samples, containing excessive amounts of MetHb. In fact, this provides a means of quantifying MetHb. Hemoglobin can be measured by the cyanmethemoglobin method as well as by the oxyhemoglobin method, and the difference between the two values provides a good estimate of the MetHb present in that blood sample. A chemical procedure is also available for the measurement of MetHb. Normal values of MetHb are dogs, 0.0 to 1.1% (mean 0.3%), and cows, 0.0 to 1.0% of normal hemoglobin concentration. Dogs with NADH-methemoglobin reductase deficiency had 18 to 41% MetHb. Methemoglobinemia of 70% or above is critical, and often fatal.

Globin Abnormalities or Hemoglobinopathies

SICKLE CELL DISEASE

Hereditary abnormalities of globin chain synthesis in humans have been associated with hemolytic anemias resulting from decreased red cell survival and decreased oxygen binding of the aberrant hemoglobin (Hb). Abnormal hemoglobins such as HbS, HbC, and HbD have been associated with sickle cell disease. Red cells of individuals homozygous for these hemoglobins develop abnormalities of red cell shapes when blood becomes deoxygenated in the tissues. Consequently, red cell deformability is reduced and intravascular survival is shortened. Hemolytic anemia and clinical manifestations of sickle cell disease ensue.

Sickle cell anemia results from excessive synthesis of HbS and reduced intravascular survival of irreversibly sickled cells. The anemia is generally normocytic-normochromic, despite a reticulocytosis. In HbS, the sixth glutamic acid residue in the β-globin chain is replaced by valine. This single amino acid substitution causes the aggregation of HbS on deoxygenation in the form of longitudinal tubules, which confer the sickle shape to the afflicted red cells. Repeated sickling and unsickling produces irreversibly sickled red cells. The susceptibility of red cells to sickle varies with the concentration of HbS within a red cell; this is less than 50% in the red cells of individuals with benign sickle cell trait. Sickle cells occur in oxygenated deer blood, and spindle-shaped and fusiform erythrocytes occur in goats, particularly of the Angora breed. These animals, however, are not anemic.

In HbC, the sixth-glutamic acid residue in the β-globin chain is replaced by lysine. Target cells comprise the prominent red cell shape abnormality and occasional erythrocytes show a large hemoglobin crystal (see Fig. 7–19L). Deformability of these cells is also reduced, leading to their reduced circulating life span. Occasional hemoglobin crystals have been found in the red cells of cats, dogs, and camels, but an association with hemolytic anemia remains to be shown.

THALASSEMIAS

Normal human hemoglobins contain two pairs of globin chains; two α chains are found in association with two β chains in HbA, two δ chains in HbA_2 with two γ chains in HbF. Thalassemias result from an inherited abnormality of globin production, and are named after the defective globin chain. Thus α-, β-, and δ-thalassemia, respectively, result from a complete or partial absence of the α-, β-, and δ-globin chains. A mixed deficiency may also occur; for example, δ-β–thalassemia results from the absence of both the δ and β chains. The incidence of thalassemia varies with the geographic location and human populations. Thalassemia has not been diagnosed in animals.

In thalassemias, defective hemoglobin synthesis results in hypochromasia and the excess globin chains precipitate as intracellular inclusion bodies, which are often visible on light microscopy. Red cell inclusions become more prominent after splenectomy or when splenic function has been compromised. These inclusions are more common in β-thalassemia than in α-thalassemia. Thalassemic individuals show varying degrees of anemia from hemolysis of defective red cells and from ineffective erythropoiesis, depending on the type of thalassemia. Anemia in thalassemia major (homozygous state) is microcytic-normochromic or microcytic-hypochromic. Anisocytosis, poikilocytosis, target cells, and basophilic stippling may be observed, along with increased numbers of reticulocytes and nucleated red cells. Red cells in thalassemia minor (heterozygous state) are microcytic, but anemia is not seen.

Miscellaneous Abnormalities

HEREDITARY NONSPHEROCYTIC HEMOLYTIC ANEMIA

A nonspherocytic hemolytic anemia with an autosomal dominant mode of inheritance has been described in poodles (Randolph et al., 1986). A mild to marked anemia (PCV, 13 to 31%) with reticulocytosis and macrocytic-hypochromic red cell morphology was present in the affected dogs. Necropsy findings included myelofibrosis, osteosclerosis, and hemosiderosis (excessive iron) in hepatocytes and macrophages. Although the clinicopathologic findings resembled those seen in dogs with PK deficiency, the basic defect was undetermined.

Three beagles from a large breeding colony were found to have a chronic anemia (PCV, 30 to 39%; reference range, 46 to 56%) with reticulocytosis (Maggio-Price et al., 1988). The dogs appeared clinically healthy, except for a splenomegaly. Bone marrow aspirates revealed erythroid hyperplasia. The red cell life span was reduced; the survival of ^{51}Cr-labelled red cells was 7.2 to 15.4 days in anemic dogs, compared to 22.2 to 25.2 days in control dogs. Erythrocyte osmotic fragility was altered. The breeding of two anemic dogs resulted in offspring with anemia and reticulocytosis. The basic defect remained unknown, because the red cells had normal glycolytic enzyme activities, no evidence of abnormal or unstable hemoglobin, and no abnormalities of membrane cytoskeletal proteins.

INTRINSIC RED CELL DEFECTS UNACCOMPANIED BY ANEMIA

An inherited (autosomal recessive) high Na^+, K^+-ATPase activity has been found in some mongrel and Japanese Shiba and Akita dogs (Maede and Inaba, 1987; Maede et al., 1991). The red cells of these animals had high potassium (HK), compared to low potassium (LK) concentration found in normal canine red cells. Their GSH concentration was markedly elevated, glycolytic rate about twice normal, and osmotic fragility increased. Changes in red cell indices (increased MCV, decreased MCHC, and normal MCH) indicated an increase in cell water. Although anemia was not evident, their red cell life span was shortened and a slight increase in reticulocyte count could be seen in some dogs. These findings might be considered suggestive of a compensatory hemolytic state.

The presence of an abnormal hemoglobin was associated with diminished exercise tolerance in the absence of anemia in a dog (Jones and Hinton, 1978).

ABNORMALITIES EXTRINSIC TO ERYTHROCYTES

Chemicals and Drugs

Many chemicals and drugs can induce hemolytic anemia, including copper, lead, zinc, phenothiazine, methylene blue, saponins, and naphthalene, and drugs such as acetanilid, nitrofurantoin, neoarsphenamine, phenacetin, and some sulfanilamides. The mechanism of hemolysis in these cases may involve a toxic insult of an undefined nature to the red cell membrane, oxidative damage to the cell membrane and hemoglo-

bin, inactivation of red cell enzymes, and/or immune mechanisms. A summary of some hematologic abnormalities associated with copper and lead poisoning is presented here.

COPPER POISONING

Copper accumulates in the liver of animals receiving copper from drenches, feeding on copper-contaminated forage, plants with a high copper content, or grains containing copper but little or no molybdenum, or drinking water from water containing copper algicides. Copper toxicosis in ruminants is common when the copper:molybdenum ratio in forage is greater than 10:1, either because of excessive copper or a deficiency of molybdenum. Physiologic requirements for copper, molybdenum, and sulfate are in delicate balance, particularly in sheep.

Cattle can tolerate high concentrations of copper and low concentrations of molybdenum in their diet, but sheep accumulate large amounts of copper in their liver over several weeks to months, without any apparent problem. A precipitous release of copper from the liver in sheep under stress triggers an intravascular hemolytic crisis. The stresses involved may vary and include strenous exercise, handling, hauling, or weather changes. Growing lambs are most susceptible. Liver damage precedes an increase in the blood copper level. An acute hemolytic crisis with hemoglobinemia and hemoglobinuria is an outstanding finding. Heinz bodies may be found (Kerr and McGavin, 1991). The condition is usually fatal, with death occurring within 24 to 48 hours. If the individual sheep lives long enough, the sclera becomes icteric and the blood picture is one of marked bone marrow response to acute hemolysis. The diagnosis is based on clinical signs and the demonstration of high levels of copper in liver and kidney specimens and in the forage. Ceruloplasmin activity correlates more closely with serum or plasma copper values than liver copper levels in cattle and sheep (Blakley and Hamilton, 1985). Treatment with ammonium molybdate (50 to 500 mg/day) and with sodium thiosulfate (300 to 1000 mg/day) for 3 weeks can have beneficial results (Kerr and McGavin, 1991).

Hemolytic anemia from copper poisoning occurs also in swine, calves, and chickens. Chronic copper toxicosis in growing pigs can manifest as iron deficiency anemia, probably as a result of impaired iron absorption from the gastrointestinal tract. Horses are relatively tolerant to copper accumulation in the liver.

An inherited (autosomal recessive) copper toxicosis with progressive hepatopathy has been described in Bedlington terriers, but acute hemolytic anemia was seen only in a small number of such dogs. The disease resembles Wilson's disease of humans in many respects, and was found to have a similar metabolic defect of impaired biliary excretion of copper.

The mechanism of hemolysis from copper toxicity is not well known. The primary cytotoxic effects are from the interaction of copper with the sulfhydryl groups of red cell membrane proteins and membrane lipid peroxidation. Additional mechanisms include inhibition of important red cell enzymes, such as glutathione reductase, G-6-PD, and pyruvate kinase, depletion of GSH, and increased MetHb formation.

LEAD POISONING

Lead poisoning may be acute or chronic, but anemia is evident only if it is chronic. Dogs are highly sensitive, cattle, horses, and sheep are less susceptible, and pigs, water buffaloes, and camels are relatively resistant to lead poisoning (Abdel-Azis et al., 1988; Jain, 1986). Lead poisoning has also been reported for cats, birds, rabbits, a chinchilla, and a raccoon (Morgan et al., 1991). A positive diagnosis of lead poisoning was made on the basis of blood lead levels of 40 µg/dl (0.4 ppm) or higher.

Lead poisoning should be suspected when the blood examination reveals polychromatic erythrocytes and normoblastemia (nucleated erythrocytes in blood) disproportionate to the PCV, which may be within the normal range. Both nucleated and non-nucleated erythrocytes should be examined for evidence of basophilic stippling (Plates XVII–11 and XVII–12). The basophilic stippling may be in the form of distinct granules (punctate) or, more commonly, of fibrillar material (reticulated). The stippling is attributed to an unusual clumping of ribosomes resulting from a lead-induced acquired deficiency of pyrimidine-5'-nucleotidase (P5N) in the red cells. This enzyme normally degrades ribosomal RNA in maturing reticulocytes.

The anemia of chronic lead poisoning varies in degree and appears to result both from decreased erythropoiesis, because of impaired formation of heme, and shortened red cell survival. The latter forms the basis of hemolytic anemia. Lead inhibits several enzymes of heme synthesis (e.g., δ-aminolevulinic acid (ALA) dehydrase, ALA synthetase, coproporphyrinogen oxidase, and heme synthetase) (Fig. 7–21). Hence, concentrations of free protoporphyrins in erythrocytes are elevated and the urinary excretion of δ-ALA and coproporphyrin is increased. The anemia is usually normocytic-normochromic, with a tendency to be slightly on the microcytic-hypochromic side, and some reticulocytosis may be present. Erythrocyte osmotic fragility is reduced, but mechanical fragility is increased. Synthesis of α- and β-globin chains may also be defective in cases of lead poisoning and contribute to the anemia. Bone marrow examination reveals erythroid hyperplasia, along with some ineffective erythropoiesis. Biochemical abnormalities become evident before anemia and serve as early biochemical indices of lead toxicity.

Canine Plumbism. Clinical signs of lead poisoning in the dog and cat are similar and are referable to the gastrointestinal and central nervous system disorders. Although lead poisoning may occur at any age, it is common in dogs 5 years of age or younger. Lead poisoning is particularly likely to develop in dogs 1 year of age or younger because of their feeding habits

and propensity to accumulate lead (Jain, 1986). Poodles and German shepherd's are the most frequently affected breeds (Morgan et al., 1991).

Mild or borderline anemia, basophilic stippling, and normoblastemia unaccompanied by an appropriate reticulocyte response are prominent findings in dogs with lead poisoning. The finding of more than 15 red cells with basophilic stippling/10,000 erythrocytes in the dog is suggestive, and more than 40/10,000 is almost pathognomonic, of lead poisoning. Some basophilic stippling may be seen in dogs and cats during an intense erythropoietic response to anemia (e.g., polychromasia and reticulocytosis) from causes other than lead poisoning. A firm diagnosis of lead poisoning must be based on the demonstration of an excessive lead concentration in the body. Lead levels increase in blood and urine when poisoning exists. Therapy is based on the chelation of lead by administering calcium EDTA.

Equine Plumbism. Clinical signs of chronic lead poisoning in horses include harsh hair coat, muscular weakness, stiffness of joints, dyspnea with roaring on exercise, and foreign body pneumonia as a sequel to pharyngeal paralysis. A "lead line" on the gums may be present in some horses. Blood lead levels of 0.35 ppm or more are considered significant, particularly in the presence of clinical signs. A modest anemia with PCV values between 21 and 28% has occurred in some horses exhibiting chronic lead poisoning. Basophilic stippling of erythrocytes or the presence of large numbers of nucleated erythrocytes in blood is not characteristic. An occasional stippled erythrocyte or stippled metarubricyte may be seen (Plate XVII–12), but only on careful search of the blood film.

Bovine Plumbism. Lead poisoning in calves and cows is usually an acute disease caused by an apparent craving for lead and the uncanny ability of cattle to locate sources of lead. Common clinical signs are those of central nervous system involvement—blindness, grinding of teeth, and depression. Ruminal stasis is also common. Marked elevations of free protoporphyrins in erythrocytes, basophilic stippling, and nucleated erythrocytes have been seen in chronic lead poisoning in calves. The increased basophilic stippling was attributed to a decrease in erythrocyte P5N activity.

Ovine Plumbism. Sheep may develop chronic lead poisoning. It can be detected by measuring erythrocyte δ-ALA dehydrase activity, which was found to be strongly inhibited by relatively low doses of lead. Urinary porphyrins and basophilic stippling are not sensitive indicators, whereas the urinary lead level and δ-ALA activity can vary greatly. The blood lead concentration parallels the degree of lead exposure.

Swine Plumbism. Pigs seem to be highly tolerant to lead toxicosis. Blood lead concentrations of up to 290 µg/dl were associated with only mild clinical signs, but a marked decrease in δ-ALA dehydrase activity was seen, along with a moderate anemia. Basophilic stippling was evident in the erythrocytes of affected animals.

Feline Plumbism. Little is known about lead poisoning in cats. Occasional nucleated red cells and basophilic stippling of erythrocytes may be seen in cats with lead poisoning (serum lead, ≥0.4 ppm; normal, <0.4 ppm).

ZINC TOXICOSIS

Zinc toxicosis has been found to cause hemolytic anemia in cattle, sheep, and dogs (Latimer et al., 1989; Torrence and Fulton, 1987). The mechanism of hemolytic anemia remains unknown, although oxidative damage to erythrocyte hemoglobin and cell membrane proteins may be involved (Luttgen et al., 1990).

OXIDANTS CAUSING HEINZ BODY FORMATION

In 1890, Heinz described the occurrence of inclusions within the erythrocytes of humans and animals following exposure to certain coal tar drugs, which resulted in the hemolytic destruction of the involved cells. These inclusions, now referred to as Heinz bodies, were described as round, oval, or serrated highly refractile granules, usually located near the margin of the cell or protruding from the cell (Plate XVIII–2). Heinz bodies are best demonstrated with vital stains such as crystal violet, brilliant crysal blue, or new methylene blue (NMB) applied to an unfixed blood film (Fig. 11–1; Plates XVIII–3 and XVIII–4). Heinz bodies can be visualized as bluish-green structures with the stain routinely employed for making reticulocyte counts (Plate XVII–8). In Wright-stained films, Heinz bodies stain poorly and may occasionally appear as a whitish spot within the erythrocyte or near the cell margin, or as a hemoglobinized mass projecting from the cell surface (Fig. 11–2; Plate XVIII–1).

Mechanisms of Heinz Body Formation and Associated Anemia. Heinz bodies are formed by the irreversible precipitation of oxidatively denatured hemoglobin. The administration of an oxidant such as methylene blue or acetaminophen to cats and phenothiazine to horses (Case 1, Table 11–3) and sheep, or the ingestion

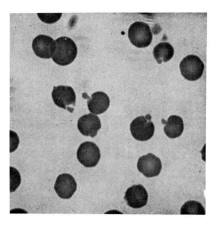

Fig. 11–2. Heinz bodies in phenothiazine toxicosis in the horse (Wright-Leishman stain; × 1000). (From Jain, N.C.: Schalm's Veterinary Hematology. 4th Ed. Philadelphia, Lea & Fibiger, 1986, p. 632.)

of an oxidant or plant materials containing an oxidant (see below) results in Heinz body formation and hemolytic anemia. Heinz body formation occurs in calves and dogs given phenylhydrazine. Heinz body formation resulting from the production of hydroxylamine in the rumen has been associated with postparturient hemoglobinuria in cattle. Finnish Landrace sheep with a deficiency of red cell GSH, because of inherited defective amino acid transport into red cells, are susceptible to oxidant injury and may develop Heinz body-induced anemia (Tucker et al., 1981). A Heinz body mediated hemolytic anemia developed in dogs treated with cephalosporins (cefoperazone and dihydroxy phenol cephalosporin) (Batchelor et al., 1992).

The presence of Heinz bodies reduces the deformability of the erythrocytes. This impedes passage of the erythrocytes through the microcirculation of the spleen. Sequestration within the spleen leads to erythrophagocytosis or hemolysis of the more severely dam-

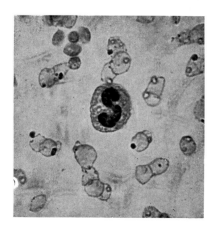

Fig. 11–1. Heinz bodies in phenothiazine toxicosis in the horse. New methylene blue stain applied to the dry, unfixed blood film (× 1000). (From Jain, N.C.: Schalm's Veterinary Hematology. 4th Ed. Philadelphia, Lea & Febiger, 1986, p. 632.)

Table 11–3. Hematologic Findings in Hemolytic Anemia in the Horse

Parameter	Case 1: Phenothiazine Toxicosis in a 2½-Year-Old Horse	Case 2: Neonatal Isoerythrolysis in a 3-Day-Old Foal
RBC (×10⁶/μl)	2.05	3.86
Hemoglobin (g/dl)	4.3	5.7
PCV (%)	13.0	16.0
MCV (fl)	63.4	41.5
MCHC (%)	33.1	35.6
MCH (pg)	21.0	14.8
Reticulocytes (%)	0.0	0.0
nRBC/100 WBC	0.0	0.0
Heinz bodies	Few	—
Macrocytosis	3+	—
Anisocytosis	Moderate	Slight
Icterus index (units)	25	>100
WBC/μl	16,300	12,500*
Plasma proteins (g/dl)	—	5.7
Total bilirubin (mg/dl)	—	28.8

* Rare monocyte with phagocytosed RBC.

aged erythrocytes within the splenic pulp. Thus, hemolytic anemia with or without bilirubinemia manifests in patients with significant Heinz body formation. Heinz bodies begin to appear in small numbers of red cells after splenectomy in humans and horses, and similar observations have been made in other species. Similarly, the suppression of splenic function by corticosteroids may permit the formation of Heinz bodies. Oxidant-induced Heinz body formation, their removal by the MPS, and associated structural damage to red cells may produce aberrant morphologic forms such as echinocytes, acanthocytes, and schistocytes (Akuzawa et al., 1989).

Heinz Bodies in Cats. Heinz bodies, also known as Schmauch or "erythrocyte refractile" bodies, have been found in normal cats (Jain, 1986; Schalm and Smith,

1963). The routine application of NMB stain to dry, unfixed blood films led to the observation that almost all normal domestic cats, as well as other members of the family Felidae, have a small but variable number of erythrocytes that contain a single small to medium-sized refractile body at the margin of the cell (Plates XVIII-1 to 4). Heinz bodies vary in size, shape, and position in the red cell. More commonly, however, the larger inclusions are irregular in shape and are located at the margin of the erythrocyte (Fig. 11–3). Heinz bodies have been found in as many as 96% of the erythrocytes of clinically normal domestic cats. No relationship to the age of the cats nor any association with a specific disease or hemolytic anemia has been found, even in cats in which most of the erythrocytes contained the inclusions.

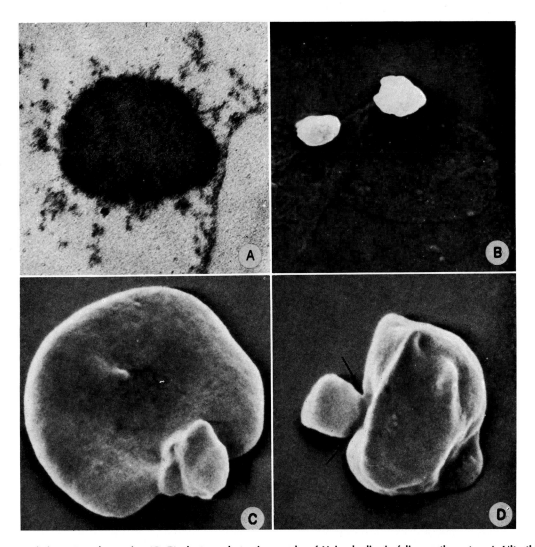

Fig. 11–3. Transmission (*A*) and scanning (*B–D*) electron photomicrographs of Heinz bodies in feline erythrocytes. *A*, Ultrathin section of a large Heinz body within a portion of an erythrocyte ghost. The Heinz body is composed of a highly electron-dense mass; strands of reticular material of an electron density similar to that seen elsewhere within the plasma membrane of the empty ghost are attached to the periphery (×42,000). *B*, Erythrocyte ghosts containing Heinz bodies, (×6,800). *C*, Intact erythrocyte with marginal Heinz body (×11,700). *D*, Side view of an erythrocyte showing a protruding Heinz body. Note the constriction of the cell membrane at the base of the Heinz body (*arrows*) (×11,700). (*A* from Jain, N.C.: Demonstration of Heinz bodies in erythrocytes of the Cat. Bull. Am. Soc. Vet. Clin. Pathol., 2:13, 1973; *B* and *C* from Jain, N.C.: Schalm's Veterinary Hematology. 4th Ed. Philadelphia, Lea & Febiger, 1986, p. 635; *D* Courtesy of N.C. Jain and K.S. Keeton.)

Some studies have suggested that Heinz body formation in normal cats may be caused by the consumption of certain diets (Bauer et al., 1991; Hickman et al., 1990; Weiss et al., 1990). Among the commercial diets examined, fish-based diets induced Heinz body formation most consistently. The incidence of Heinz bodies in the blood of kittens (4 to 5 months of age) consuming a purified diet was less than 1%. All kittens fed diets containing 5 or 10% propylene glycol (PG) developed Heinz bodies. The maximum number of Heinz bodies developed after the diet was given for 5 to 6 weeks, and the proportion of Heinz bodies varied with the amount of PG in the diet—20% in kittens fed a 5% PG diet, and 28% in kittens fed a 10% PG diet. After discontinuation of the PG diet, Heinz bodies gradually diminished to control levels over a period of 6 to 8 weeks. Anemia and methemoglobinemia did not develop, but the erythrocyte life span was reduced. The erythrocyte half-life of ^{51}Cr-labelled cells was 8.3 days for kittens fed PG compared to 12.6 days for the control group. Cats fed 41%, but not 12% PG, became anemic. It appears that red cells from cats fed PG-containing diets are highly susceptible to oxidative stress (Weiss et al., 1990). PG-containing diets cause a dose dependent increase in Heinz body formation, erythrocyte destruction, and reticulocyte numbers (Christopher et al., 1989).

The spleen plays a minor role in the removal of Heinz bodies in the cat, unlike that in the dog and the horse. This conclusion is based on the following: (1) splenectomy in a cat having a high but declining Heinz body number did not prevent a further reduction in the number of Heinz bodies; (2) splenectomy was unassociated with a significant elevation of Heinz body number over a period of several weeks; and (3) transfused Heinz body-containing erythrocytes were removed from the blood of an intact (nonsplenectomized) or splenectomized cat at similar rates. Furthermore, in the splenectomized cat, transfused Heinz bodies were removed at the same rate recorded for her own erythrocytes containing Heinz bodies when the cat was intact.

The propensity of feline red cells to develop Heinz bodies seems to be related, at least in part, to their hemoglobin structure. The indications are that the hemoglobin of the family Felidae is highly susceptible to oxidation because of its eight sulfhydryl (SH) reactive groups, as compared to about two SH groups in other species. This makes feline hemoglobin remarkably unstable and subject to denaturation by oxidation under various circumstances that are not deleterious to other species' erythrocytes. The oxidation of hemoglobin is also accelerated by a marked propensity of cats to form methemoglobin because of the low rate of methemoglobin reductase activity compared to that in other species. Endogenous factors that enhance Heinz body formation remain unknown. An increased incidence of Heinz body formation, however, has been observed in cats with diabetes mellitus, hyperthyroidism, and lymphoma (Christopher, 1989). In some cats, a significant inverse correlation was found between the percentage of Heinz bodies and PCV, or erythrocyte GSH. DL-methionine, used to prevent feline urologic syndrome, fed to cats (2–3 g daily for about 3 weeks) induced a significant increase of methemoglobin and Heinz bodies leading to hemolytic anemia (Maede et al., 1987).

It is intriguing that natural Heinz body formation in cats is not associated with anemia, whereas anemia follows Heinz body formation from an oxidant drug. It is possible that such drugs, in addition to the formation of Heinz bodies, may induce oxidative damage to the erythrocyte membrane, which then signals the MPS for erythrophagocytosis. Healthy cats with naturally occurring Heinz bodies might not develop anemia because the undefined oxidant largely induces Heinz body formation without significant oxidative damage to the erythrocyte membrane.

NITRATE AND NITRITE POISONING

Nitrate poisoning is a serious problem in ruminants, particularly cattle. It may occur from drinking contaminated water, but a common cause is the consumption of feeds rich in nitrates (e.g., Sudan grass, Sorghum vulgare, var. sudanensis). Clinical signs of acute toxicity include dyspnea, cyanosis, weak pulse, and muscular weakness. Nitrite, produced from the reduction of nitrate by rumen bacteria, is highly toxic because of its oxidative action. It oxidizes hemoglobin to produce methemoglobinemia. Blood appears chocolate brown when about 30 to 40% of the total hemoglobin is in the form of methemoglobin, and death occurs when its level reaches about 80 to 90%. Dairy cows may have 6 to 7% methemoglobin (attributable to the nitrate in feed) without any signs of illness (Lebeda and Prikrylova, 1985).

The diagnosis of nitrate poisoning involves the consideration of clinical signs, characteristic color of blood, increased levels of methemoglobin, and determination of nitrate and nitrite levels in feed, water, intestinal contents, plasma or serum, and urine. Treatment consists of the administration of methylene blue (1 to 4.4 mg/kg body weight intravenously in the form of a 2 to 4% solution) to induce reduction of methemoglobin (ferric iron) to deoxyhemoglobin (ferrous iron). This paradoxic action of methylene blue depends on the activation of the NADPH-dependent methemoglobin reductase system (Fig. 7–13). The dosage of methylene blue is crucial, because an excess could induce a life-threatening methemoglobinemia.

Toxic Plants and Plant Products

The excessive ingestion of a wide variety of plants or their products has been found, on rare occasions, to cause hemolytic anemia in animals. These materials include castor beans, oak shoots, frosted turnips, broom, ranunculus, convolvulus, colchicum, ash, privet, hornbeam, hazel, hellebore, wild onions, and plants of the Brassica family (e.g., rape and kale).

Castor bean consumption in a 14-month-old short-horn heifer was found to cause a severe hemolytic anemia, with hemoglobinemia and hemoglobinuria. Ricins in the beans were incriminated as causing the erythrocyte destruction.

Kale causes Heinz body-induced hemolytic anemia in cattle, sheep, and goats. Sheep with low GSH levels are more prone to develop anemia than those with high levels. Heinz body formation in humans also occurs as a result of a deficiency of GSH or of enzymatic defects of GSH metabolism and the pentose phosphate pathway. Kale contains *S*-methyl cysteine and its sulf-oxide, which give rise to methanethiol and dimethyl disulfide in the rumen. The latter product, after absorption, interacts with reduced GSH in the erythrocytes and induces Heinz body formation. Disulfides were found to produce hemolytic anemia experimentally in goats and dogs.

Onions, when consumed in excess, cause Heinz body-induced anemia in cattle, sheep, horses, dogs, and cats (Table 11–4). Cattle are more susceptible; horses and dogs are intermediate; and sheep and goats are more resistant to onion toxicosis compared to other domestic animals (Lincoln et al., 1992). Onions contain *n*-propyl disulfide, which decreases glucose-6-phosphate dehydrogenase activity in erythrocytes. This curtails the regeneration of reduced glutathione, which is needed to prevent oxidative denaturation of hemoglobin, leading to Heinz body production. Eryth-

rocytes of dogs with inherited high concentrations of potassium and reduced GSH are, for some unknown reasons, more susceptible to Heinz body and methemoglobin formation than erythrocytes of normal dogs (Yamoto and Maede, 1992). Some of these dogs develop a severe hemolytic anemia after eating onions.

Horses ingesting red maple (Acer rubrum) leaves develop Heinz body-associated acute hemolytic anemia from an oxidant present in the leaves. The oral administration of L-tryptophan and its major metabolite, indole, in ponies caused a Heinz-body hemolytic anemia with hemoglobinemia, hemoglobinuria, and hyperbilirubinemia (Paradis et al., 1991a, 1991b). It was suggested that this may be of clinical relevance because tryptophan is found in high concentrations in green pasture, and equine intestinal microflora can convert tryptophan to indole. The oral and intravenous administration of L-tryptophan to cattle did not cause significant hemolysis.

Immune Mechanisms

AUTOIMMUNE HEMOLYTIC ANEMIA

Autoimmune hemolytic anemia (AIHA) is a consequence of accelerated red cell destruction by an autoantibody directed against mature erythrocytes. AIHA occurs in humans, dogs, and cats, and, rarely,

Table 11–4. Hemograms in Onion Poisoning (Heinz Body Hemolytic Anemia) in Cattle

	Steer Number and Breed			
Parameter	1 Holstein	2 Angus	3 Angus	4 Angus
RBC ($\times 10^6$/μl)	6.39	2.76	1.39	1.42
Hb (g/dl)	8.9	5.3	3.3	3.5
PCV (%)	25.0	18.0	11.0	13.0
MCV (fl)	39.1	65.2	79.0	91.5
MCHC (%)	35.6	29.4	30.0	27.1
MCH (pg)	13.9	19.2	23.7	25.7
Icterus index units	15	15	20	15
Plasma proteins (g/dl)	6.6	7.1	7.3	6.7
Fibrinogen (g/dl)	0.6	0.6	0.6	0.5
Reticulocytes (%)	0	10.2	20.0	26.8
Nucleated RBC/100 WBC	0	5	37	18
WBC/μl	9,300	7,200	17,000	8,700
WBC corrected for nucleated RBC	9,300	6,900	12,500	7,400
Band neutrophils	93 (1.0%)	0 0	1,000 (8.0%)	74 (1.0%)
Segmenters	1,488 (16.0%)	3,864 (56.0%)	4,812 (38.5%)	2,146 (29.0%)
Lymphocytes	7,440 (80.0%)	2,484 (36.0%)	6,062 (48.5%)	5,032 (68.0%)
Monocytes	279 (3.0%)	207 (3.0%)	62 (0.5%)	148 (2.0%)
Eosinophils	0 0	345 (5.0%)	500 (4.0%)	0 0
Basophils	0 0	0 0	62 (0.5%)	0 0
Anisocytosis	Slight	Moderate	Marked	Marked
Polychromasia	—	Moderate	Marked	Marked
Basophilic stippling	—	Few	—	Moderate
Heinz bodies	Many	Many	Few	Few

in horses and cattle. A hereditary AIHA is known to occur in the NZB strain of mice. AIHA associated with immune-mediated thrombocytopenia is called Evans syndrome.

Autoimmune hemolytic anemia may be a primary (idiopathic) disorder or may be secondary to other diseases or conditions, such as bacterial, viral, rickettsial, or protozoan infections, hepatopathy, and other autoimmune disorders. In the dog, most cases of AIHA are primary and may occur at any age. The disorder is slightly more common in females with a possibility of some familial predisposition. Clinical signs are related to the primary disease and/or to the amount and nature of the autoantibody. Clinical findings may reflect anemia, hemolysis, thrombocytopenia, and cold agglutinin disease (agglutination of erythrocytes in the peripheral circulation, as in the extremities). The hemolytic anemia may have a peracute or acute onset or, more commonly, may be chronic, with one or more relapses occurring over weeks to months.

Antibodies associated with AIHA are generally categorized as warm-reactive (mostly at 37°C) or cold-reactive (usually at <30 to 32°C) antibodies and are principally of the IgG and IgM types, respectively. Most cases of AIHA are a result of warm-reactive IgG but a few involve cold-reactive IgM (cold agglutinin), the latter usually occurring in association with the former. Low levels of cold agglutinins may occur in some normal dogs and horses and are inconsequential, as in most people. The basis of autoantibody formation remains speculative. Autoantibodies reacting with red cells may be produced because of a change in the antigenic structure of the self-erythrocytes, the formation of cross-reactive antibodies, and/or a change in the immune status of the patient. In humans, cold-agglutinins are usually directed to I/i antigens in red cells, whereas a cold-reactive nonagglutinating IgG antibody (Donath-Landsteiner) is directed to a P-blood group antigen. Warm-type IgG autoantibodies bind to epitopes on red cell membrane band 3 glycoprotein (Victoria et al., 1990).

The IgG antibody reacting with red cells in AIHA does not cause the agglutination of sensitized erythrocytes. The presence of antibody on erythrocytes can be demonstrated by adding a species-specific antiglobulin reagent to a saline-washed suspension of the patient's erythrocytes, a serologic procedure called direct Coombs test. Agglutination results if the erythrocytes are coated with the autoantibody. The IgG antibody does not promote agglutination by itself because negative charges on the cell surface repel the erythrocytes beyond the span of the two Fab portions of the IgG molecule. In contrast, the IgM antibody, being a larger molecule, can bind to different red cells and promote agglutination directly. A broad-spectrum Coombs reagent consists of anti-IgG, anticomplement, and even anti-IgM. Anticomplement detects complement-coated erythrocytes in both warm- and cold-antibody mediated AIHA.

In the indirect Coombs test, the patient's serum is tested to detect free autoantibody. In this test, normal homologous erythrocytes are first exposed to the patient's serum and then to the antiglobulin reagent to induce agglutination. The IgG autoantibody reacts with antigens present on normal red cells; enzyme-treated red cells are more sensitive to agglutinate than untreated cells. Binding of a minimum of 300 to 400 IgG molecules or 60 to 115 C3 molecules to human red cells has been found essential to yield a weak positive Coombs test.

The primary mechanism of red cell destruction in AIHA is erythrophagocytosis by the MPS as a result of coating the erythrocytes by IgG autoantibody and/or the fixation of complement component C3 (Fig. 11–4). Red cell destruction occurs primarily in the spleen and, to some extent, in the liver and bone marrow. The macrophages have surface receptors for the Fc portion of the IgG and for complement components C3b and C3bi (inactivated C3b). Partial erythrophagocytosis by macrophages is believed to result in the formation of spherocytes. On rare occasions, erythrophagocytosis may also be detected in blood. Spherocytes, the hallmark of AIHA, are typically small and densely stained cells (Plate XVI–4) and exhibit increased osmotic fragility (see Figs. 7–15B and 22–2). Spherocytes are difficult to detect in the blood of species other than the dog, but careful examination has revealed their presence in some feline and equine patients with AIHA. The rapid inactivation of C3b to C3d by complement inhibitors in the blood results in the circulation of C3d-coated red cells. These red cells have a normal life span and are detected by anticomplement in the Coombs reagent. Vigorous complement fixation by IgG or IgM autoantibody, leading to the formation of a membrane attack complex (C5 through C9), can result in direct intravascular hemolysis, hemoglobinemia, and hemoglobinuria.

Cold autoantibody is deleterious only when it is in high titer and the patient is exposed to cold. Cold agglutinins activate and bind complement components to the red cells at low body temperature (<30 to 32°C, optimally at 20 to 25°C). The antibody dissociates at higher temperatures, but activated complement remains adhered to the red cells. The complement-mediated destruction of red cells occurs by direct lysis or through erythrophagocytosis, as discussed above.

Hematologic findings in AIHA vary with the stage of the disease at presentation (Table 11–5). Hemolysis is indicated by hemoglobinemia, hemoglobinuria, or a high icterus index from hyperbilirubinemia (mainly unconjugated). The urinary excretion of urobilinogen may also be increased. The plasma concentration of haptoglobin is reduced during acute hemolytic episodes. In cases involving cold-reactive IgM antibody, red cell agglutination may be seen in Wright-stained films (Plate XVI–5) and, occasionally, may be visible grossly in vials containing anticoagulated blood (Fig. 11–5). Such agglutination can be enhanced by placing the blood at 4°C and reversed by warming to 37°C. Stained blood films often reveal spherocytosis. Reticulocyte counts indicate a regenerative anemia and erythrocyte indices are typically those of a macrocytic-

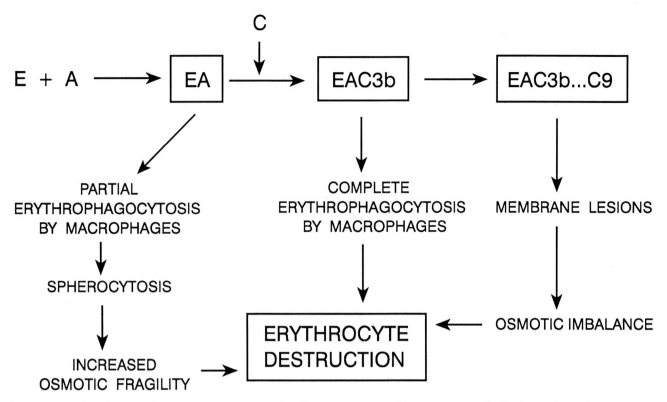

Fig. 11–4. Outline of red cell destruction in autoimmune hemolytic anemia, (E, erythrocyte; A, autoantibody, C, complement).

hypochromic red cell morphology. Bone marrow examination reveals a decreased myeloid:erythroid ratio as a result of increased erythropoiesis. In rare cases, reticulocytopenia may be ascribed to antibody directed against reticulocytes or erythroid precursors in the bone marrow.

Total leukocyte counts vary but tend to increase as the anemia enters a stage of remission. A neutrophilia with a modest left shift is a common finding, as is a monocytosis. The mechanism of this regenerative left shift is unknown, but it may probably be the result of the concomitant release of colony-stimulating factors

Table 11–5. Representative Hemograms of Autoimmune Hemolytic Anemia in the Dog

Parameter	Dog Number					
	1	2	3	4	5	6
Sex	XF	XF	XF	M	F	M
Age (yr)	7	6	8	2	1	7
Days sick to date of admission	2	4	12	77	96	180
PCV (%)	18	20	18	25	23	31
MCV (fl)	70.9	98.5*	125.9	109.6*	117.0	72.6
MCHC (%)	32.8	35.5	22.2	29.2	25.7	32.9
Icterus index units	50	Free hemoglobin	7.5	2	.2	7.5
Reticulocytes (%)	4.0	7.6	39.4	54.0†	36.0	20.8
Erythrocyte fragility at 0.85% saline	—	35.0%	—	92.5%	—	10%
Anisocytosis‡	+	+ +	+ + + +	+ +	+ + + +	+ +
Polychromasia‡	+	+ +	+ + + +	+ +	+ + + +	+ +
Spherocytosis‡	+ + + +	+ + + +	+	+ + + +	+	+ + + +
Agglutination of erythrocytes‡	+ + + +	+ + + +	None	+ +	None	None
Nucleated RBC/100 WBC	0	25.5	707	28.5	34	84
Thrombocytes/µl	245,000	55,000	519,000	461,000	38,000	18,000
WBC/µl (corrected)	15,000	21,600	15,800	34,000	25,400	25,800
Coombs' test‡	+ + +	+ + + +	+ + +	+	+	+ + + +

* Not valid; greater than actual RBC size as a result of erythrocyte hemolysis, leading to error in MCV.
† Not valid because lysis of spherocytes left reticulocytes out of proportion to their actual number.
‡ +, occasional; + +, slight; + + +, moderate; + + + +, marked.

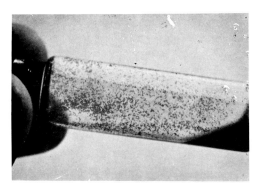

Fig. 11–5. Spontaneous agglutination of erythrocytes in drawn blood as seen in a dog with autoimmune hemolytic anemia. (From Jain, N.C.: Schalm's Veterinary Hematology. 4th Ed. Philadelphia, Lea & Febiger, 1986, p. 649.)

(GM-CSF and G-CSF) from the macrophages engaged in active erythrophagocytosis. A variable thrombocytopenia may be found in some dogs, possibly also because of the formation of autoantibody to platelets.

Corticosteroid therapy is the treatment of choice in AIHA. High-dose corticosteroid therapy is initiated and then gradually tapered with clinical improvement. Corticosteroids are generally beneficial primarily because they decrease antibody production, reduce the binding of antibody to the red cells, and diminish the receptor concentration on macrophages. Consequently, increased survival of red cells is noted. Adequate steroid therapy and follow-up are essential for the successful management of AIHA. Occasionally, a dog fails to respond to corticosteroid therapy. In such cases, chemotherapy with immunosuppressive drugs such as azathioprine and cyclophosphamide may be instituted in combination with prednisolone. Splenectomy may be beneficial, as judged from experience in humans with AIHA and limited observations on dogs with AIHA and immune-mediated thrombocytopenia. (See Chapter 22 for details.)

Blood transfusions should be withheld as long as the PCV exceeds 12% and evidence of an erythropoietic response to anemia is present. Blood transfusions should not be instituted, except in life-threatening situations, because it is extremely difficult to find a compatible donor. In addition, the recipient may have circulating antibody that could react rapidly with transfused red cells and lyse them. Plasmapheresis can be tried to reduce the concentration of circulating antibody and increase red cell survival.

Cold agglutinin disease generally does not respond to corticosteroid therapy. Symptomatic treatment consists of keeping the patient warm and avoiding cold exposure.

NEONATAL ISOERYTHROLYSIS

Neonatal isoerythrolysis or hemolytic disease of the newborn has been reported in mule foals, horse foals, piglets, calves and, rarely, in puppies and kittens (Cain and Suzuki, 1985; Jain, 1986). The young is normal at birth, but hemolysis begins within hours of the ingestion of colostrum. Anemia, icterus, and hemoglobinuria develop within a few days (Case 2, Table 11–3). Antibody-coated red cells are presumably destroyed from erythrophagocytosis in the MPS and from complement-mediated lysis in the circulation. A positive direct Coombs test may be obtained with appropriate anti-IgG and/or anti-C reagent. If death does not occur, the bone marrow response is typical of a hemolytic anemia.

The problem arises when the dam is bred more than once to the same sire, so that antigens of the male's erythrocytes are transmitted to the erythrocytes of the fetus. The dam develops antibodies against the fetal red cells when she becomes sensitized to them as a result of transfer across the placental membranes from spontaneous minor bleeds during pregnancy. Similar exposure also occurs at the time of delivery. In addition, the vaccination of females with tissue vaccines containing erythrocytes may sensitize them to red cell antigens that might later appear in the erythrocytes of the newborn (e.g., vaccination of cows with an anaplasmosis vaccine of bovine blood origin). Consequently, the colostrum contains antibodies against the erythrocytes of the neonate.

Hemolytic disease in newborn pups may develop when the bitch is blood group A-negative and has become sensitized to A-positive red blood cells because of mating to an A-positive male. Pups inheriting the A-positive factor experience hemolytic destruction of their red cells after receiving anti-A antibody produced by the dam and passed into the colostrum. The degree of anemia in affected pups varies widely, with the PCV falling as low as 10%. Spherocytosis, reticulocytosis, and nucleated erythrocytes may be seen in severely anemic pups. Erythrocyte osmotic fragility is increased.

DRUG-INDUCED HEMOLYTIC ANEMIAS

Drug-induced immune-mediated hemolytic anemias are described in Chapter 22.

Postparturient Hemoglobinuria

Postparturient hemoglobinuria in cattle is characterized by hemoglobinuria following intravascular hemolysis. The disease usually occurs within 2 or 3 weeks after calving, but may occur as long as 42 days after parturition. It may be a sporadic or a herd problem. The visible mucous membranes first become pale and later icteric. The anemia is regenerative and macrocytic-hypochromic. The mechanism of red cell destruction is not definitively known, although phosphorus and copper deficiencies are suspected as a direct or indirect cause. The red cells of phosphorus-deficient cattle have decreased ATP and GSH concentrations, increased methemoglobin levels, and enhanced osmotic fragility. ATP production is hampered because of disturbance of reactions at the glyceraldehyde 3-phosphate dehydrogenase step (Ogawa et al., 1987, 1989).

Postparturient hemoglobinuria is also seen in water buffaloes, sheep, and goats. Hypophosphatemia is a prominent finding in hemoglobinuric water buffaloes (inorganic phosphate concentration, 2.68 ± 0.16 mg/dl; normal, 5.40 ± 0.24 mg/dl) (Singari et al., 1989). Red cell membrane phospholipid levels were found to be reduced in water buffaloes with postparturient hemoglobinuria (1.83 ± 0.42 mg/ml) compared to healthy animals (2.86 ± 0.39 mg/ml) (Rana and Bhardwaj, 1990b). Glutathione reductase levels increase in hemoglobinuric water buffaloes, probably as a compensatory response to decreased levels of G-6-PD, glutathione peroxidase, and reduced GSH (Rana and Bhardwaj, 1990a). Dietary phosphorus deficiency has been reported to cause reductions in anaerobic glycolysis, ATP, and 2,3-DPG levels, and may cause a decrease in the synthesis of GSH, NAD, and NADP. Thus, phosphorus deficiency may predispose metabolically compromised red cells to the deleterious effects of a plant hemolysin (e.g., saponins from sugar beets or alfalfa) or an oxidant. Copper deficiency may decrease superoxide dismutase levels in red cells, compromising their ability to withstand oxidative damage and rendering them vulnerable to Heinz body formation as a result of feeding on poisonous plants. Hemolytic anemia and hemoglobinemia were found in a diabetic cat with severe hypophosphatemia (serum phosphorus, 0.8 mg/dl), but not in six diabetic dogs with severe hypophosphatemia (serum phosphorus, 1-2 mg/dl) (Willard et al., 1987).

Specific treatment consists of administering sodium acid phosphate and copper glycerate to cases associated with phosphorus and copper deficiencies, respectively.

Microangiopathic Hemolytic Anemia

Microangiopathic hemolytic anemia (MHA) in humans is characterized by the fragmentation of circulating erythrocytes passing through abnormal arterioles or an intravascular fibrin clot. Poikilocytes and schistocytes are formed when red cells contact the fibrin strands or an abnormal arteriolar surface. MHA occurs in various conditions. As a primary disorder, it is seen in thrombotic thrombocytopenic purpura in adults and in hemolytic uremic syndrome in children. Secondarily, it may occur in association with immunologic diseases, malignancies, drug therapy, radiation therapy, and disseminated intravascular coagulation (DIC). Characteristic findings in MHA include schistocytes in blood films and laboratory abnormalities of DIC. Therapy is directed toward management of the disease process causing the MHA.

A case of postpartum hemolytic-uremic syndrome was described in cow (Roby et al., 1987). The cow with a history of dystocia had delivered a dead calf 6 days ago. Hematologic findings included a mildly responsive anemia (PCV 16%, reticulocytes 1.3%), normoblastemia, thrombocytopenia, hyperfibrinogenemia, and neutrophilia with left shift. Marked poikilocytosis with extensive red cell fragmentation, keratocytosis, anisocytosis, with a few unusually large, sometimes basophilic, stippled red cells were present in blood films. Trypanosomes were frequently found in blood films. Bone marrow examination revealed granulocytic hyperplasia with some toxic changes and dysmyelopoiesis, mild erythroid hypoplasia, and increased numbers of megakaryocytes. Prothrombin time and partial thromboplastin time were greater than normal, but fibrinogen degradation products were not found. Prominent necropsy findings included extensive hemorrhages and edema of many tissues, necrotizing endometritis and vaginitis, fibrin thrombi in glomerular capillaries, and a large thrombus in a uterine vessel. A hemolytic uremic syndrome with clinicopathologic evidence of intravascular hemolysis, renal microangiopathy, and intravascular coagulation was described in two horses (Morris et al., 1987).

Hypersplenism

Hypersplenism is characterized by an inappropriate increase in the phagocytic activity of the splenic macrophages, leading to cytopenias especially anemia and thrombocytopenia. This is generally associated with splenomegaly and compensatory bone marrow hyperplasia. Splenomegaly may have various causes, but hypersplenism should be suspected when a concomitant cytopenia with marrow hyperplasia is present. The enlarged spleen sequesters increased numbers of red cells, platelets, and neutrophils, and destroys them prematurely. Splenectomy is generally beneficial. Hypersplenism in a dog was associated with a severe nonresponsive anemia, poikilocytosis with schistocytes and dacryocytes, normoblastemia, mild thrombocytopenia, hypocellular marrow, extramedullary hematopoiesis in a moderately enlarged spleen, and recovery following splenectomy (Kuehn and Guant, 1986).

Miscellaneous Causes

WATER INTOXICOSIS

Cattle, particularly 2- to 10-month-old calves, may develop hemoglobinuria from an excessive intake of water. Water-loaded calves have died within 2 hours, although most such calves survive with no permanent ill effects and recover after 2 days. Hematologic findings include hemolytic anemia, decreased total plasma protein, serum sodium, and chloride levels, and decreased osmolality. Clinical signs of water intoxication are convulsions, coma, respiratory distress, hemoglobinuria, and death. The urine's specific gravity is low. The most common necropsy lesion is edema of the lungs. Decreased blood electrolyte concentrations induce the osmotic destruction of erythrocytes. Hemolysis with attendant hemoglobinuria in some calves may be related to the fact that the osmotic fragility of erythrocytes in calves is greatest at 4 to 5 months of age. Treatment consists of administering hypertonic fluid (2.5% sodium chloride and 10% dextran) and diuretics (e.g., mannitol), along with other appropriate therapy.

HEPARIN ADMINISTRATION

Administration of heparin in large doses in ponies was found to enhance phagocytosis of erythrocytes by the mononuclear phagocyte system, leading to a reduced hematocrit and hemoglobin concentration, as well as an increased plasma bilirubin concentration and biliary bilirubin excretion (Engelking and Mariner, 1985).

REFERENCES

Abdel-Aziz, S.A., Soliman, M.M., Ahmed, A.A., et al.: Delta-aminolevulinic acid dehydratase activity in blood of Egyptian camel and buffalo. Arch. Exp. Vet. Med., 42:854, 1988.

Akuzawa, M., Matumoto, M., Okamoto, K., et al.: Hematological, osmotic, and scanning electron microscopic study of erythrocytes of dogs given β-acetylphenylhydrazine. Vet. Pathol., 26:70, 1989.

Batchelor, J., Fuller, J., and Woodman, D.D.: An in vitro comparison of the oxdiative effects of two structurally related cephalosporins on normal canine and human haemolysate. Comp. Haematol. Int., 2:24, 1992.

Bauer, M.C., Weiss, D.J., and Perman, V.: Hematologic alterations in adult cats fed 6 or 12% propylene glycol. Am. J. Vet. Res., 53:69, 1991.

Blakley, B.R. and Hamilton, D.L.: Ceruloplasmin as an indicator of copper status in cattle and sheep. J. Comp. Med., 49:405, 1985.

Cain, G.R., and Suzuki, Y.: Presumptive neonatal isoerythrolysis in cats. J. Am. Vet. Med. Assoc., 187:46, 1985.

Christopher, M.M.: Relation of endogenous Heinz bodies to disease and anemia in cats: 120 cases (1978–1987). J. Am. Vet. Med. Assoc., 194:1089, 1989.

Christopher, M.M., Perman, V., and Eaton, J.W.: Contribution of propylene glycol-induced Heinz body formation to anemia in cats. J. Am. Vet. Med. Assoc., 194:1045, 1989.

Engelking, L.H. and Mariner, J.C.: Enhanced biliary bilirubin excretion after heparin-induced erythrocyte mass depletion. Am. J. Vet. Res., 46:2175, 1985.

Giger, U. and Harvey, J.W.: Hemolysis caused by phosphofructokinase deficiency in English Springer Spaniels: Seven cases (1983–1986). J. Am. Vet. Med. Assoc., 191:453, 1987.

Giger, U., Harvey, J.W., Yamaguchi, R.A., et al.: Inherited phosphofructokinase deficiency in dogs with hyperventilation induced hemolysis. Increased in vitro and in vivo alkaline fragility of erythrocytes. Blood, 65:345, 1985.

Giger, U., Mason, G.D. and Wang, P.: Inherited erythrocyte pyruvate kinase deficiency in a beagle dog. Vet. Clin. Pathol., 20:83, 1991.

Giger, U. and Noble, N.A.: Determination of erythrocyte pyruvate kinase deficiency in Basenjis with chronic hemolytic anemia. J. Am. Vet. Med. Assoc., 198:1755, 1991.

Harvey, J.W.: Erythrocyte metabolism. In: Kaneko, J. J. (eds), Clinical Biochemistry of Domestic Animals. San Diego, Academic Press, p. 185, 1989.

Harvey, J.W., French, T.W., and Senior, D.F.: Hematologic abnormalities associated with chronic acetaminophen administration in a dog. J. Am. Vet. Med. Assoc., 189:1334, 1986.

Harvey, J.W., King, R.R., Berry, C.R., et al.: Methemoglobin reductase deficiency in dogs. Comp. Haematol. Int., 1:55, 1991.

Harvey, J.W., Kociba, G.J., and Peteya, D.J.: Utilization of an enzyme heat stability test and erythrocyte glycolytic intermediate assays to assist in the diagnosis of canine pyruvate kinase deficiency. Vet. Clin. Pathol., 19:55, 1990a.

Harvey, J.W. Mays, M.B.C., Gropp, K.E., et al.: Polysaccharide storage myopathy in canine phosphofructokinase deficiency (type VII glycogen storage disease). Vet. Pathol., 27:1, 1990b.

Hickman, M.A., Rogers, O.R., and Morris, J.G.: Effect of diet on Heinz body formation in kittens. Am. J. Vet. Res., 51:475, 1990.

Jain, N. C.: Schalm's Veterinary Hematology. 4th Ed. Philadelphia, Lea & Febiger, 1986, pp. 627–654.

Jones, D.R.E. and Hinton, M.: Reduced exercise tolerance in a dog associated with an abnormal hemoglobin. Vet. Rec., 102:105, 1978.

Kaneko, J.J.: Animal models of inherited hematologic disease. Clin. Chim. Acta, 165:1, 1987.

Kaneko, J.J.: Clinical Biochemistry of Domestic Animals. 4th ed. San Diego, Academic Press, 1989, pp. 235–255.

Kerr, L.A. and McGavin, H.D.: Chronic copper poisoning in sheep grazing pastures fertilized with swine manure. J. Am. Vet. Med. Assoc. 198:99, 1991.

Kuehn, N.F. and Gaunt, S.D.: Hypocellular marrow and extramedullary hematopoiesis in a dog: Hematologic recovery after splenectomy. J. Am. Vet. Med. Assoc., 188:1313, 1986.

Latimer, K.S., Jain, A.V., Inglesby, H.B., et al.: Zinc-induced hemolytic anemia caused by ingestion of pennies by a pup. J. Am. Vet. Med. Assoc., 195:77, 1989.

Lebeda, M. and Prikrylova, J.: Observation on methemoglobinemia in dairy cows during four years. Acta. Vet. Brno, 54:157, 1985.

Lincoln, S.D., Howell, M.E., Combs, J.J., et al.: Hematologic effects and feeding performance in cattle fed cull domestic onions (Alium cepa). J. Am. Vet. Med. Assoc., 200:1090, 1992.

Luttgen, P.J., Whitney, M.S., Wolf, A.M., et al.: Heinz body hemolytic anemia associated with high plasma zinc concentration in a dog. J. Am. Vet. Med. Assoc., 197:1347, 1990.

Maede, Y., Amano, Y., Nishida, A., et al.: Hereditary high-potassium erythrocytes with high Na, K-ATPase activity in Japanese Shiba dogs. Res. Vet. Sci., 50:123, 1991.

Maede, Y., Hoshino, T., Inaba, M., et al.: Methionine toxicosis in cats. Am. J. Vet. Res., 48:289, 1987.

Maede, Y. and Inaba, M.: Energy metabolism in canine erythrocytes associated with inherited high Na$^+$- and K$^+$-stimulated adenosine triphosphate activity. Am. J. Vet. Res., 48:114, 1987.

Maggio-Price, L., Emerson, C.L., Hinds, T.R., et al.: Hereditary nonspherocytic hemolytic anemia in beagles. Am. J. Vet. Res, 49:1020, 1988.

Morgan, R.V., Moore, F.M., Pearce, L.K., et al.: Clinical and laboratory findings in small companion animals with lead poisoning: 347 cases (1977–1986). J. Am. Vet. Med. Assoc. 199: 93, 1991.

Morris, C.F., Robertson, J.L., Mann, P.C., et al.: Hemolytic uremic-like syndrome in two horses. J. Am. Vet. Med. Assoc., 191: 1453, 1987.

Ogawa, E., Kobayashi, K., Yoshiura, N., et al.: Bovine postparturient hemoglobinemia: Hypophosphatemia and metabolic disorder in red blood cells. Am. J. Vet. Res., 48:1300, 1987.

Ogawa, E., Kobayashi, K., Yoshiura, N., et al.: Hemolytic anemia and red cell metabolic disorder attributable to low phosphorus intake in cows. Am. J. Vet. Res., 50:388, 1989.

Paradis, M.R., Breeze, R.G. and Bayly, W.M.: Acute hemolytic anemia after oral administration of L-tryptophan in ponies. Am. J. Vet. Res., 53:742, 1991a.

Paradis, M.R., Breeze, R.G., Laegreid, W.W., et al.: Acute hemolytic anemia induced by oral administration of indole in ponies. Am. J. Vet. Res., 52:748, 1991b.

Pinkerton, P.H., Fletch, S.M., Brueckner, P.J., et al.: Hereditary stomatocytosis with hemolytic anemia in the dog. Blood, 44: 557, 1974.

Rana, J.P. and Bhardwaj, R.M.: Glutathione reductase: Role and status in healthy and haemoglobinuric buffaloes. Indian Vet. J., 67:261, 1990a.

Rana, J.P. and Bhardwaj, R.M.: Role of erythrocyte membrane phospholipids in pathogenesis of post-parturient haemoglobinemia. Indian Vet. J., 67:308, 1990b.

Randolph, J.F., Center, S.A., Kallfelz, F.A., et al.: Familial nonspherocytic hemolytic anemia in poodles. Am. J. Vet. Res., 47:687, 1986.

Roby, K.A., Bloom, J.C., and Becht, J.L.: Postpartum hemolytic-uremic syndrome in a cow. J. Am. Vet. Med. Assoc., 190:187, 1987.

Schalm, O.W., and Smith, R.: Some unique aspects of feline hematology in disease. Small Anim. Clin., 3:311, 1963.

Singari, N.A., Bhardwaj, R.M. and Mata, M.M.: Effect of hypophosphatemia on erythrocytic metabolism in postparturient haemoglobinuria of buffaloes. Ind. J. Ani. Sci., 59:1235, 1989.

Smith, J.E., Moore, K., Arens, M., et al.: Hereditary elliptocytosis with protein band 4.1 deficiency in the dog. Blood, 61:373, 1983.

Torrance, A.G. and Fulton, R.B.: Zinc-induced hemolytic anemia in a dog. J. Am. Vet. Med. Assoc., 191:443, 1987.

Tucker, E.M., Young, J.D. and Crowley, C.: Red cell glutathione deficiency: Clinical and biochemical investigations using sheep as an experimental model system. Br. J. Haematol., 48:403, 1981.

Victoria, E.J., Pierce, S.W., Branks, M.J., et al.: IgG red blood cell autoantibodies in autoimmune hemolytic anemia bind to epitopes on red blood cell membrane band 3 glycoprotein. J. Lab. Clin. Med., 115:74, 1990.

Weiss, D.J., McClay, C.B., Christopher, M.M., et al.: Effects of propylene glycol-containing diets on acetaminophen-induced methemoglobinemia in cats. J. Am. Vet. Med. Assoc., 196:1816, 1990.

Wilkie, D.A. and Kirby, R.: Methemoglobinemia associated with dermal application of benzocaine cream in a cat. J. Am. Vet. Med. Assoc., 192:85, 1988.

Willard, M.D., Zerbe, C.A., Schall, W.D., et al.: Severe hypophosphatemia associated with diabetes mellitus in six dogs and one cat. J. Am. Vet. Med. Assoc., 190:1007, 1987.

Williams, W.J., Beutler, E., Erslev, A.J., et al.: Hematology. 4th ed. New York, McGraw-Hill, 1990.

Yamoto, O. and Maede, Y.: Susceptibility to onion-induced hemolysis in dogs with hereditary high erythrocyte reduced glutathione and potassium concentrations. Am. J. Vet. Res., 53:134, 1992.

Depression or Hypoproliferative Anemias

Anemias primarily associated with reduced erythropoiesis may result from a limited supply or defective utilization of nutrients essential for red cell production or from anatomic disruption, functional impairment, or lack of stimulation of hematopoietic tissue (Table 12–1). An important distinction exists between anemias of nutritional deficiencies and anemias secondary to chemical or drug toxicity and organic diseases. In the former, the bone marrow is fully capable of resuming normal erythropoietic activity as soon as adequate nutrients have been supplied. In contrast, in the latter, the bone marrow's ability to produce red cells is often compromised, so that anemia ensues despite the presence of adequate essential nutrients. Bone marrow damage in such cases may be reversible or permanent. In most cases of marrow suppression secondary to drugs, chemicals, or organic disease, the anemia is normocytic-normochromic. A microcytic or macrocytic anemia, however, may occur following a deficiency of iron or vitamin B$_{12}$, respectively.

NUTRITIONAL DEFICIENCY ANEMIAS

Prolonged nutritional deficiencies of protein and several vitamins and minerals essential for erythrocyte production lead to anemia in humans and animals (Jain, 1986; Williams et al., 1990). The type of anemia varies with the nutrient lacking and the species involved. The most experimental work in this regard has been done with pigs (Table 12–2). In this species, a mild to modest normocytic anemia develops after deficiencies of protein and vitamins such as niacin, riboflavin, and pantothenic acid. A marked normocytic anemia with bone marrow abnormalities develops in cases of vitamin E deficiency. Severe microcytic anemia is characteristic of iron, copper, and pyridoxine deficiencies. Vitamin B$_{12}$ deficiency causes only a slight normocytic anemia, but macrocytic anemia results from a deficiency of folate or both folate and vitamin B$_{12}$. A macrocytic-normochromic anemia occurs in cobalt deficiency in cattle. A normocytic-normochromic anemia is seen in copper deficiency in the dog.

Vitamin Deficiencies

VITAMIN A

Chronic vitamin A deficiency in humans results in a microcytic-hypochromic anemia similar to that seen in iron deficiency. The serum iron level is low, but the marrow iron stores are increased. The serum transferrin level is usually normal or decreased. The anemia is corrected by vitamin A supplementation, but not by iron. Experimental vitamin A deficiency in rats results in a "masked" anemia accompanied by hemoconcentration and marrow hypoplasia and fibrosis.

Table 12–1. Depression or Hypoproliferative Anemias and Some of Their Causes in Various Animal Species

Nutritional deficiency anemias
   Protein deficiency
   Mineral deficiencies: iron, copper, cobalt, and selenium
   Vitamin deficiencies; B_{12}, folic acid, niacin, pyridoxine, thiamine, pantothenic acid, riboflavin, ascorbic acid, and vitamins A and E
Anemia of chronic or inflammatory disease
Anemias associated with organic or tissue disorders
   Nephritis with uremia in the dog
   Malignancies
   Endocrine disorders such as hypothyroidism and hypoadrenocorticism in the dog
   Liver disease
Anemias associated with parasitic diseases
   Tichostrongylosis in sheep and cattle
Aplastic or hypoplastic anemias
   Irradiation
   Bracken fern poisoning in cattle and sheep
   Trichloroethylene-extracted soybean meal toxicity in cattle
   Estrogen toxicity in the dog
Anemias associated with myeloproliferative disorders

VITAMIN B_6

Vitamin B_6 (pyridoxine) is needed for erythropoiesis, mainly because it serves as a cofactor for the synthesis of δ-aminolevulinic acid (ALA) and is probably required for the optimal synthesis of heme from iron and protoporphyrin (Fig. 7–21). An experimental deficiency of vitamin B_6 causes microcytic-hypochromic anemia, iron overload, and neurologic abnormalities in various animal species, including the dog, cat, mouse, rat, and pig.

Humans receiving isoniazid, an antituberculous agent, occasionally develop a microcytic anemia from interference with vitamin B_6 metabolism. Drugs that reduce the pyridoxine concentration in blood and decrease the δ-ALA activity of erythroid cells, can induce a sideroblastic anemia in humans. The bone marrow is characterized by ineffective erythropoiesis, the presence of large numbers of ringed sideroblasts, and increased iron stores. Sideroblasts are erythroid cells containing iron-loaded mitochondria arranged in the form of a perinuclear ring. Sideroblastic anemia may also occur as a myelodysplastic syndrome and, rarely, as an X-linked hereditary disorder in humans.

VITAMIN B_{12} AND FOLIC ACID

Vitamin B_{12} and folic acid (folate) are essential for normal erythropoiesis. Characteristic hematologic findings in humans with deficiency of these vitamins include the following: (1) a macrocytic-normochromic anemia, hypersegmented neutrophils, ovalocytes, megalocytes, and multiple Howell-Jolly bodies in blood; and (2) megaloblastic erythroid cells, abnormal granulocytes (giant bands, metamyelocytes, and neutrophils) and, rarely, large megakaryocytes and increased mitotic figures in bone marrow. Megalocytes are macrocytic red cells, and megaloblasts are large, nucleated erythroid cells. The reticulocyte count is lower than normal and basophilic stippling may be present. Platelets vary in size; this is more noticeable from the measurement of platelet distribution width using electronic counters than on light microscopy of blood films (see Chapter 6). Anemia results from ineffective erythropoiesis and reduced life span of erythrocytes. Ineffective granulopoiesis and thrombopoiesis may occur. In addition, because of the defective synthesis of myelin, neurologic signs are seen in those with vitamin B_{12} deficiency but not with folate deficiency.

Deficiency of vitamin B_{12} and folate in humans may develop for several reasons, including dietary lack, malabsorption, increased physiologic need (e.g., during pregnancy and the neonatal period), liver disease, therapy for malignant diseases, and administration of

Table 12–2. Hematologic Characteristics of Experimental Nutritional Deficiencies in Swine

Deficiency	Anemia* Type	Anemia* Severity	Leukopenia	Plasma Iron	Serum Copper	EP†	Bone Marrow Morphology
Protein	N	+	None	Normal	Low	Normal	Normoblastic
Lysine	N	+	None	Normal	Normal	—	Normoblastic
Tryptophan	N	+ +	Present	Normal	—	Normal	Normoblastic
Iron	MH	+ + + +	None	Low	Normal	Normal	Normoblastic
Copper	MH	+ + + +	Present	Low	Low	Normal	Normoblastic
Pyridoxine	Mi	+ + + +	None	High	Normal	Low	Normoblastic
Niacin plus protein	N	+ +	None	Normal	Low	Normal	Normoblastic
Riboflavin	N	+	None	—	—	—	Normoblastic
Pantothenic acid	N	+ +	None	—	—	—	Normoblastic
Folate	Ma	+ + + +	Present	High	Normal	Low	Macronormoblastic
B_{12}	N	+	None	—	—	—	Normoblastic
Folate plus B_{12}	Ma	+ + + +	Present	—	—	—	Macronormoblastic with a few megaloblasts
Vitamin E	N	+ + + +	None	Normal	—	—	Abnormal‡

From Wintrobe, M. M., Lee, G. R., Boggs, D. R., et al.: Clinical Hematology, 8th Ed. Philadelphia, Lea & Febiger, 1981.
* Types of anemia: N, normocytic; MH, microcytic hypochromic; Mi, microcytic; Ma, macrocytic.
† EP, free erythrocyte protoporphyrin.
‡ Hyperplasia with multinucleated cells.

certain drugs. Drugs that cause megaloblastic anemia include anticonvulsive agents such as diphenylhydantoin, primidone, and phenobarbital, purine analogues such as 6-mercaptopurine and azathioprine, pyrimidine analogues such as 5-fluorouracil, and inhibitors of ribonucleotide reductase such as cytosine arabinoside and hydroxyurea. It takes several years for vitamin B_{12} deficiency caused by dietary lack to manifest because body stores of vitamin B_{12} are high, whereas folate deficiency appears within 2 to 4 months because of a relatively smaller body reserve. The liver is the principal storage site. In contrast, deficiency from impaired metabolism of these vitamins manifests early. Vitamin B_{12} deficiency commonly develops from malabsorption, whereas folate deficiency occurs from dietary deficiency. Vitamin B_{12} in the plasma is transported bound to transcobalamins, principally transcobalamin II, which is produced by the liver, macrophages, and granulocytes. A congenital deficiency of transcobalamin II in humans is associated with megaloblastic anemia.

Vitamin B_{12} of dietary origin is prepared for absorption from the gut by an intrinsic factor produced in the stomach. When this factor is lacking, pernicious anemia develops. It is attributed mainly to antibody-mediated destruction of the gastric mucosa and a genetic predisposition is suspected.

An important function of folic acid and vitamin B_{12} is in DNA synthesis (Fig. 12–1). In the body, folic acid is first converted to dihydrofolate (DHF) and then to tetrahydrofolate (THF); the latter conversion occurs under the influence of the enzyme DHF reductase in the presence of NADPH. Folate in plasma is found as free or protein-bound 5-methyl THF, which is produced in the intestinal mucosal cells and the liver. THF serves as a source of 5,10-methylene THF, a folate coenzyme involved in the conversion of deoxyuridylate to thymidylate under the influence of thymidylate synthetase. Thymidylate is subsequently used for DNA synthesis. It is conjectured that folate deficiency can express in a lack of the folate coenzyme, resulting in deranged DNA synthesis. Folate antagonists, such as methotrexate, aminopterin, and trimethoprim, inhibit DHF reductase and deprive the cell of reduced folate. Vitamin B_{12} deficiency leads to the depletion of the folate coenzyme as a consequence of the defective interaction between vitamin B_{12} and folate metabolism. According to the "methyl tetrahydrofolate trap" hypothesis, vitamin B_{12} in the form of methyl cobalamin is needed as a coenzyme for the metabolic conversion of homocysteine to methionine. During this process, 5-methyl THF, an inactive storage form of folate, is converted to THF. Most of the vitamin B_{12} in plasma is in the form of methyl cobalamin. Vitamin B_{12} deficiency leads to impaired conversion of homocysteine and to the trapping of folate as unusable 5-methyl THF; this results in the unavailability of 5,10-methylene THF, which is required for the synthesis of DNA.

Vitamin B_{12} is needed for the formation of stroma in the prorubricyte and basophilic rubricytes. In the absence of vitamin B_{12}, the S phase and the intermitotic

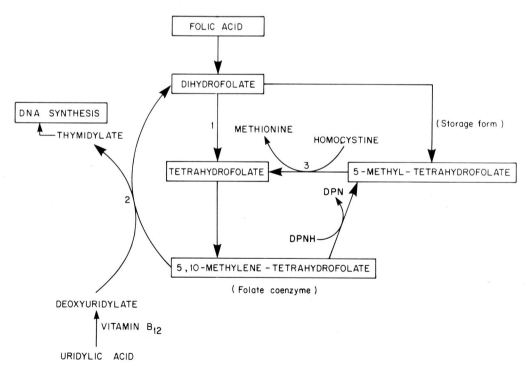

Fig. 12–1.   Interaction of folic acid and vitamin B_{12} in DNA synthesis. Sites of some enzyme interactions are also shown: 1, site of dihydrofolate reductase action + NADPH; 2, site of thymidylate synthetase action; 3, site of methyl B_{12} (cobalamin), a vitamin B_{12} coenzyme, action. (From Jain, N.C.: Schalm's Veterinary Hematology. 4th Ed. Philadelphia, Lea & Febiger, 1986, p. 658.)

period are prolonged and a maturation arrest occurs at the prorubricyte and basophilic rubricyte stages, causing these cells to be larger in size and more numerous in the bone marrow. A stained film from a dog or cat presumed to have vitamin B_{12} and/or folate deficiency presents an unusual number of large cells of varying sizes. The nuclei of these cells appear somewhat deficient in chromatin, because more parachromatin seems to be separating clumps of chromatin (Plate XXII–1). Although mitosis is delayed or slowed from impaired DNA synthesis, hemoglobin synthesis continues unabated, leading to an asynchrony of maturation and the production of some larger than normal erythroid cells (megaloblasts) and, finally, large mature erythrocytes (megalocytes or macrocytic red cells).

Spontaneous folate deficiency has been found to occur in the dog, although the dog can obtain folate from intestinal bacterial action. In the few instances of anemia in the dog and cat in which a vitamin B_{12} deficiency was suspected, a macrocytic-normochromic anemia was not found. These animals had a normocytic-normochromic anemia, although occasional macrocytes were found in the blood and macrocytes and megaloblastoid rubricytes were seen in bone marrow films. In an investigation of the hepatic effects in dogs of the long-term administration of phenytoin alone (or in combination with primidone), erythrocyte macrocytosis, neutropenia, neutrophil hypersegmentation, and thrombocytopenia were observed (Bunch et al., 1985). Such abnormalities were observed most often in dogs given phenytoin, and resembled those known to be attributable to folate deficiency in humans treated with phenytoin for epilepsy. Such abnormalities were not found, however, in a subsequent study involving the long-term administration of phenytoin to dogs (Bunch et al., 1990).

Vitamin B_{12} deficiency develops in cattle and sheep on cobalt-deficient pastures. A number of vitamin B_{12} analogues are produced in the rumen by bacterial fermentation. Cobalt is essential in the molecular structure of vitamin B_{12} so the term "cobalamins" is used to refer to this vitamin and its analogues. Cobalt-deficient areas have been reported in northern Michigan, northeastern Wisconsin, Florida, the British Isles, Australia, New Zealand, and Kenya. Prominent clinical signs and hematologic changes in cobalt deficiency of cattle and sheep include unthriftiness, progressive wasting, marked macrocytic or normocytic anemia, and hemosiderosis. Neurologic abnormalities are not found. Horses on cobalt-deficient pasture do not develop signs of cobalt deficiency, probably because the mature horse does not have a dietary requirement for vitamin B_{12}. In the horse, it is produced by bacterial action and is absorbed from the lower gastrointestinal tract.

An inherited (autosomal recessive) selective intestinal malabsorption of cobalamin was observed in a family of giant schnauzer dogs (Fyfe et al., 1991). Affected puppies exhibited chronic inappetence and failure to thrive beginning between 6 and 12 weeks of age. Neutropenia with hypersegmentation, anemia with anisocytosis and poikilocytosis, and megaloblastic changes of the bone marrow were present. Serum cobalamin concentrations were low, and methylmalonic aciduria and homocysteinemia were present. Parenteral, but not oral, cyanocobalamin administration rapidly eliminated all signs of cobalamin deficiency except for low serum cobalamin concentrations. Cobalamin malabsorption in affected dogs was documented by oral administration of ^{57}Co-cyanocobalamin with or without simultaneous oral administration of intrinsic factor or normal dog gastric juice. Quantitation and function studies of intrinsic factor and transcobalamin-II from affected dogs revealed no abnormality. Other gastrointestinal functions and ileal morphology were normal, indicating a selective defect of cobalamin absorption at the level of the ileal enterocyte. Immunoelectron microscopy of ileal biopsies showed that the receptor for intrinsic factor-cobalamin complex was absent from the apical brush border microvillus pits of affected dogs. This canine disorder resembles inherited selective intestinal cobalamin malabsorption (Imerslund-Gräsbeck syndrome) in humans, and is a spontaneously occurring animal model of early onset cobalamin deficiency

NIACIN

Dogs on experimental nicotinic acid-deficient diets have developed a severe macrocytic anemia with leukopenia. In contrast, a lack of niacin in pigs was associated with the development of a moderately severe normocytic anemia without leukopenia.

PANTOTHENIC ACID

Experimental pantothenic acid deficiency in swine resulted in a moderate normocytic anemia, a severe sensory neuron degeneration, and an extensive colitis.

RIBOFLAVIN

Riboflavin deficiency results in reduced glutathione reductase activity in the erythrocyte, because this enzyme requires flavin adenine dinucleotide for activation. Experimental dietary deficiencies of riboflavin in rats, baboons, monkeys, and pigs have resulted in a normocytic-normochromic anemia from reduced erythropoiesis. In contrast, experimental riboflavin deficiency in dogs has led to a microcytic-hypochromic anemia. Riboflavin deficiency in growing pigs failed to produce anemia, but a marked increase in neutrophilic granulocytes developed. Humans on riboflavin-deficient diets develop pure red cell aplasia.

VITAMIN C

Ascorbic acid (vitamin C) is normally synthesized by all mammals, except for primates and guinea pigs. A megaloblastic anemia develops in monkeys fed milk diets deficient in ascorbic acid. Severe deficiency in humans results in scurvy; this is characterized by hemorrhagic manifestations, particularly bleeding in the gums and skin. Many patients develop a mild to moderate normocytic-normochromic anemia, accompanied by moderate numbers of reticulocytes. A microcytic-hypochromic or macrocytic anemia may develop in some cases from abnormal iron and folate metabolism, respectively. Vitamin C facilitates the intestinal absorption of iron and it is required for the maintenance of DHF reductase in its active form to generate 5,10-methylene THF (Fig. 12–1).

VITAMIN E

Vitamin E deficiency rarely causes anemia in humans. In monkeys, it produces a normocytic-normochromic anemia after 1 to 2 years, depending on the breed. In contrast, growing pigs develop a severe anemia within 6 to 8 weeks. The bone marrow in both species shows erythroid hyperplasia, ineffective erythropoiesis, and characteristically multinucleated rubricytes. The erythrocyte life span is reduced and red cells are highly sensitive to hemolysis by H_2O_2 in vitro. Sheep on a vitamin E-deficient diet develop degenerative changes in their bone marrow.

POODLE MACROCYTOSIS SIMULATING VITAMIN B_{12} DEFICIENCY

An unusual bone marrow dyscrasia, the cytology of which appears to simulate that of vitamin B_{12}-folate deficiency in humans, is encountered infrequently in poodles, particularly in the miniature and toy breeds. The erythrocytes are distinctly macrocytic and nor-

mochromic (MCV, 85 to 95 fl; MCHC, 33 to 36%), but anemia is absent. Because of the large size of the erythrocytes, the hemoglobin concentration is high normal and the PCV is elevated (usually 50% or greater), disproportionate to the RBC count. Stained blood films reveal occasional erythrocytes with multiple Howell-Jolly bodies or larger nuclear fragments (Fig. 12-2D), large polychromatic erythrocytes, and occasional hypersegmented neutrophils (Fig. 12-2B). The bone marrow contains abnormal mitoses in erythroid cells, megaloblastic metarubricytes with fragmented nuclei (Fig. 12–2C), polychromatic red cells with multiple Howell-Jolly bodies, and occasional giant metamyelocytes and hypersegmented or bizarre neutrophils (Fig. 12-2A). Rare megaloblastic erythroid cells may also be found in blood in some cases. The cause of this blood dyscrasia in poodles remains unknown. It is generally detected as an incidental finding.

Mineral Deficiencies

Iron, copper, and cobalt are the primary minerals that can become deficient in certain animals and lead to anemia.

COBALT

The importance of cobalt to ruminants for the synthesis of vitamin B_{12} and erythropoiesis is discussed above (see Vitamin B_{12} and Folic Acid).

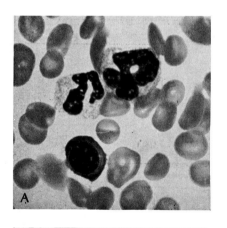
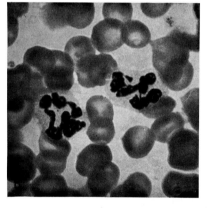
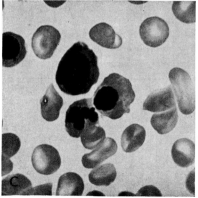
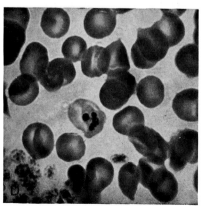

Fig. 12–2. Examples of abnormal maturation of erythrocytes and neutrophils in a poodle with a bone marrow dyscrasia simulating vitamin B_{12} deficiency. A, C, Bone marrow. B, D, peripheral blood, (×1400). (From Jain, N.C.: Schalm's Veterinary Hematology. 4th Ed. Philadelphia, Lea & Febiger, 1986, p. 661.)

COPPER

Copper is an essential trace metal for humans and animals. It is a constituent of several important enzymes, such as superoxide dismutase, δ-aminolevulinic acid dehydrase, and cytochrome c oxidase. Many of the clinical abnormalities associated with copper deficiency in humans and animals can be traced to reduced activities of cupric enzymes. Copper plays an important role in hematopoiesis. Copper deficiency interferes with iron metabolism, including impaired absorption, defective transfer from macrophages and hepatocytes to the plasma, and inability of rubricytes to use intracellular iron for hemoglobin synthesis. Thus, in copper deficiency, a microcytic-hypochromic anemia similar to that of iron deficiency is a prominent feature in some animals. For example, copper deficiency anemia in swine is morphologically similar to iron deficiency anemia, but in dogs it is normocytic-normochromic. Sideroblasts are found in increased numbers in the bone marrow and red cell life span is reduced. Copper deficiency has also been implicated as a cause of postparturient hemoglobinuria in cattle through its role in maintaining red cell integrity.

Copper in plasma is largely bound (90 to 95%) to ceruloplasmin, a blue glycoprotein (MW, 151,000) found in the α_2-globulin fraction of plasma and, to a small extent (5 to 10%), it is loosely bound to albumin and certain amino acids. Ceruloplasmin binds six to eight atoms of copper per mole. It functions in the transport of copper from the liver to other tissues as a donor of copper to cupric enzymes. Ceruloplasmin also regulates the rate at which ferrous iron is released from storage cells and is converted to ferric iron bound to transferrin. Copper deficiency can be diagnosed by the finding of a below-normal ceruloplasmin or copper level in blood.

The highest concentrations of copper are found in the liver, brain, and bone marrow. The liver plays the key role in copper metabolism. The interaction of copper with certain other trace elements affects its metabolism. High levels of dietary zinc, iron, cadmium, and molybdenum inhibit copper absorption, reduce plasma levels of ceruloplasmin, and affect the cellular activity of cupric enzymes. Zinc and iron protect swine from the adverse effects of copper, and conversely zinc and iron deficiencies accentuate copper deficiency. In cattle and sheep, the inhibitory effect of molybdenum on the absorption of copper is potentiated by dietary inorganic sulfate or sulfur amino acids. Dietary molybdate reacts with sulfides in the rumen to produce thiomolybdates, which then interfere with copper absorption.

Thus, a primary or secondary copper deficiency may occur. Primary copper deficiency develops in animals fed on milk or on pastures deficient in copper. Copper-deficient areas are known in the United States and other parts of the world. Secondary copper deficiency in cattle and sheep occurs when these animals are pastured on soil with a high molybdenum content. Such soils are found in the United States (in California, Oregon, Nevada, and Florida), England, Ireland, New Zealand, and Holland. Hematologic findings in calves affected with molybdenum poisoning include normocytic-normochromic anemia, a moderate to marked anisocytosis, and a marked crenation of smaller (mature) red cells. Serum ceruloplasmin concentration is markedly reduced. Molybdenum contamination of fodder can cause secondary copper deficiency in cattle grazing on such a pasture (Sas, 1989).

IRON

Iron deficiency is discussed in Chapter 9.

SELENIUM

Selenium is an essential component of the enzyme glutathione peroxidase (GSHPx) present in the erythrocytes. Hence, erythrocyte GSHPx correlates directly with selenium deficiency in cattle, horses, pigs, sheep, goats, and humans. The measurement of GSHPx concentration can be used as a diagnostic test to detect selenium deficiency. In the erythrocyte, GSHPx protects hemoglobin from oxidation by hydrogen peroxide (II_2O_2) (see Fig. 7–13).

Protein Deficiency

An anemia of protein deficiency in rats was associated with decreased erythropoiesis, maturation arrest, and a slight decrease in erythroid progenitor cells. Protein deficiency in children (kwashiorkor) results in a normocytic-normochromic, nonresponsive anemia from erythroid hypoplasia.

APLASTIC AND HYPOPLASTIC ANEMIAS

Aplastic anemia is characterized by pancytopenia and depressed hematopoiesis as a result of hypoplastic or aplastic fatty marrow. Pancytopenia is characterized by a reduction in all three components of the formed elements of blood. Bone marrow depression may also be expressed as unicytopenia or bicytopenia. Unicytopenia involves a reduction in a single component (e.g., pure red cell aplasia), whereas a reduction in two components denotes bicytopenia (e.g., anemia and thrombocytopenia). Such changes usually signify an impending pancytopenia.

Aplastic Anemia

Pancytopenia is the hallmark of aplastic anemia in humans. The magnitude of leukopenia, particularly neutropenia, and thrombocytopenia varies. The red cells are usually normochromic and moderately macrocytic. The reticulocyte count is below normal and nucleated red cells may be found in the blood. Bone marrow aspirates are usually difficult to obtain and yield poorly cellular preparations. The diagnosis requires obtaining a bone marrow biopsy and demonstrating markedly hypoplastic and fatty marrow.

Aplastic anemia in humans is usually an acquired disorder, but it may also be inherited. Inherited disorders of this type in children include constitutional aplastic anemia with physical abnormalities (Fanconi's anemia) or without physical abnormalities (Estren-Dameshek anemia), Diamond-Blackfan anemia (see below), and congenital dyserythropoietic anemia. Acquired hypoplasia or aplasia of the bone marrow may develop from various causes such as viral and bacterial infections, exposure to radiation, chemicals (e.g., benzene), drugs such as alkylating agents, and antimetabolites, metabolic diseases such as pancreatitis, and immunologic injury. It may also occur as a myelodysplastic syndrome or be idiopathic. Spontaneous hemorrhage caused by thrombocytopenia and terminal infection as a result of granulocytopenia are common sequelae.

A syndrome of congenital anemia, dyskeratosis, and progressive alopecia has been described in polled Hereford calves (Steffen et al., 1991). The anemia present at birth was nonprogressive and was classified as normocytic-normochromic to macrocytic-normochromic. Reticulocytosis was absent, but the bone marrow was markedly hyperplastic. Nuclear cytoplasmic asynchrony of the rubricyte and metarubricyte stages occurred in the bone marrow. Abnormal rubricyte nuclei and maturation arrest at the late rubricyte stage were common. Cytologic features of the erythrocyte series were similar to those of type I congenital dyserythropoietic anemia in humans. The defect seems to be hereditary, but the inheritance pattern remains to be determined.

Acquired aplastic anemia has been reported in the horse, dog, and cat (Lavoie et al., 1987; Riedel et al., 1988; Rottman et al., 1991; Weiss and Christopher, 1985; Weiss and Klausner, 1990). In the dog, drug-induced aplastic anemia is most frequent and includes causes such as estrogen and diethylstilbestrol injections, hyperestrogenism caused by Sertoli's cell tumors, and the administration of phenylbutazone, meclofenamic acid, trimethoprim-sulfadiazine, fenbendazole, and quinidine (Weiss and Christopher, 1985; Weiss and Klausner, 1990). Rarely, it may be idiopathic. The fungistatic agent griseofulvin has been incriminated as a cause of bone marrow hypoplasia in a cat (Rottman et al., 1991). Spontaneous recovery may occur in some cases of drug-induced marrow hypoplasia after drug withdrawal. Chloramphenicol administration in dogs and cats causes reversible bone marrow hypoplasia and nonregenerative anemia, partly through the inhibition of ferrochelatase.

Marrow hypoplasia in dogs may also develop from myelofibrosis, cancer chemotherapy, chronic ehrlichiosis, bone marrow necrosis, and hypersplenism. Bone marrow necrosis is characterized by nonregenerative anemia with or without leukopenia and thrombocytopenia (Weiss et al., 1986). Hypersplenism in a dog was associated with severe nonregenerative anemia with macrocytic hypochromic erythrocytic indices, poikilocytosis with schistocytes and dacryocytes, normoblastemia, and mild thrombocytopenia (Kuehn and Gaunt,

1986). Extramedullary granulopoiesis and erythropoiesis were evident in a splenic aspirate and marrow hypoplasia was found in a bone marrow core biopsy. Splenectomy was associated with an increase in erythropoiesis and thrombopoiesis leading to recovery from anemia and thrombocytopenia, respectively. Infection with Haemobartonella canis occurred following splenectomy, but was successfully treated with tetracycline.

Sensitivity of the bone marrow to damage by drugs and chemicals varies among individuals and bone marrow suppression may be reversible or irreversible. Some drugs can cause selective depression of a particular cell line, whereas others can induce a generalized hypoplasia or aplasia. For example, chloramphenicol produces a reversible marrow suppression primarily of the erythroid series in about 50% of humans receiving the drug, whereas a severe nonregenerative bone marrow depression occurs in the remainder. Bone marrow failure in aplastic anemia could result from qualitative or quantitative abnormalities of hematopoietic stem cells, abnormal cellular or humoral control of hematopoiesis, and abnormalities of hematopoietic microenvironment. The erythropoietin concentration, however, is usually elevated. Because of its general nonresponsiveness to various modes of therapy, aplastic anemia has also been referred to as refractory anemia.

Therapy is aimed at eliminating the causative agents, providing supportive care, and attempting marrow transplantation to restore normal hematopoiesis and effect a cure. Immunosuppressive therapy has been reported to result in complete remission in many cases, and splenectomy has been adjunctive. Myelostimulatory agents such as androgens and, more recently, hematopoietic growth factors (e.g., erythropoietin, GM-CSF, and interleukin-3) may be used to stimulate hematopoiesis specifically. Recovery from estrogen-induced aplastic anemia has been observed in dogs treated with anabolic steroid nandrolone decanote and methyltestosterone (Van Kruiningen and Friedland, 1987). The usefulness of recombinant cytokines in the treatment of aplastic anemia, however, remains to be definitively established.

Pure Red Cell Aplasia

Pure red cell aplasia in humans is an acquired or congenital disorder characterized by erythroid hypoplasia that leads to a normocytic-normochromic, nonresponsive anemia. The red cell life span is normal. Granulocytopenia and thrombocytopenia may be present in some cases, but neutrophil and platelet counts are usually normal or even elevated. The bone marrow typically shows depressed erythropoiesis and, occasionally, megaloblastic erythroid cells.

Pure red cell aplasia in humans may occur as an acute or chronic disorder. Acute pure red cell aplasia is a self-limited disorder in which marked erythroid hypoplasia of short duration is followed by a spontaneous recovery with an erythroid hyperplasia. Often

Table 12–3. Clinical Signs and Pathologic Changes in the Dog Following Total Body X-Irradiation

Time After Irradiation	Period	Clinical Pathologic Features
1–24 hours	Peracute	Nausea
1–7 days		Period of well-being
7–21 days		Acute symptoms: anorexia, weight loss, depression, vomiting, and diarrhea followed by death or survival
25–40 days	Subacute	Anemia and infertility
Over period of months	Chronic	Obesity, lethargy, decreased efficiency
Years later	Latent	Neoplasia, leukemia, cataract, shortened life span

it is caused by a parvovirus infection or drug toxicity of the erythroid progenitor cells. Chronic pure red cell aplasia may be acquired or congenital (Diamond-Blackfan anemia).

The acquired disease occurs mostly in adults and is frequently associated with thymic tumors and immune-mediated disorders. Immune suppression of erythropoiesis or erythropoietin synthesis is suspected as the cause of the anemia. It responds to corticosteroids and other immunosuppressive therapy. Thymectomy is performed in cases with thymic enlargement. The congenital disease occurs in early childhood and is caused by a defective stem cell whose committed erythroid progenies, BFU-E and CFU-E, are insensi-

tive to erythropoietin response. Therapy with corticosteroids and androgens has been beneficial.

Radiation Syndrome

Clinical signs and other events in the dog following total body x-irradiation may be divided into several periods (Table 12–3). Hematologic changes develop rapidly. Lymphopenia develops within hours and granulocytopenia is evident within a week (Fig. 12–3). If the WBC count falls below 1000/µl, few dogs survive. Thrombocytopenia combined with vascular fragility leads to petechial and ecchymotic hemorrhages along the gastrointestinal tract and in the musculature. If the dog survives, the radioresistant hematopoietic stem cells of the bone marrow and progenitor cells in the spleen and lymph nodes give rise to granulocytes and lymphocytes, which begin to appear in the blood by 15 to 20 days. At this time, the maturation arrest induced in erythropoiesis begins to be expressed as a normocytic-normochromic anemia from which the animal also later recovers. Similar trends of lymphopenia, neutropenia, and anemia have been observed in newborn pigs given whole body γ-irradiation.

Death is thought to occur because of leukopenia and damage to the gastrointestinal tract, which leads to septicemia. If bacterial infection is controlled, death can be delayed for several days. Animals surviving for 25 days have a good chance of recovering from the acute radiation syndrome, but may later develop tissue abnormalities as a result of the exposure.

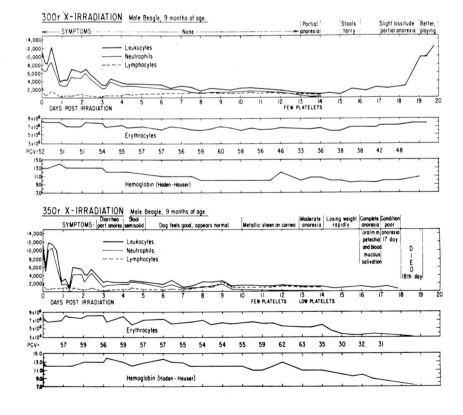

Fig. 12–3. Signs and symptoms and blood value changes in a beagle surviving a minimum lethal dose of x-ray exposure, compared to values seen in a lethal exposure. (From Andersen, A.C.: Effects of ionizing radiations on blood. In Veterinary Hematology, 2nd Ed. by O.W. Schalm. Philadelphia, Lea and Febiger, 1965, Chap. 10.)

Bracken Fern Poisoning

Bracken fern poisoning is a disease of cattle that follows the prolonged consumption of bracken fern when other forage is in short supply. A high temperature, depression, anorexia, bleeding from body openings, and high mortality characterize the disease. Bracken fern contains active carcinogens that are excreted in the urine. In natural and experimental situations, fern-fed cattle develop tumors in the urinary bladder and gastrointestinal tract. Hematuria manifests as a prominent sign in such cattle, so the syndrome has been called "chronic enzootic hematuria" or "bovine enzootic hematuria." Hematuria may develop as early as 2 months after commencement of fern feeding and anemia and pancytopenia develop in later stages from severe damage to the bone marrow. Bracken fern poisoning has been produced in sheep experimentally.

Extracted Soybean Meal Toxicity

Cattle fed extracted soybean meal develop aplastic anemia as a result of the formation of a toxic factor (dichlorovinylcysteine). This is produced because of the interaction of the trichloroethylene used to extract the oil and the cysteine present in the beans.

ANEMIAS SECONDARY TO ERYTHROID HYPOPLASIA

A normocytic-normochromic anemia, usually unaccompanied by an adequate reticulocyte response, is seen in various conditions of diverse cause. The findings of anemia in such patients is usually incidental and of secondary importance. Although an acute blood loss or hemolytic anemia within the first 3 days of its occurrence may manifest as a nonresponsive, normocytic-normochromic anemia, such anemias are to be excluded from consideration under anemias resulting from erythroid hypoplasia.

Two broad categories of secondary anemias have been recognized: (1) those without an obvious intrinsic marrow disease (e.g., chronic renal failure, liver disease, endocrine disorders, and deficiency or impaired utilization of iron); and (2) those with marrow abnormality (e.g., marrow hypoplasia or aplasia, marrow infiltration by metastatic tumors or leukemic cells, and dyserythropoiesis). Dyserythropoiesis has been described in the dog; it may occur as a manifestation of poodle macrocytosis or myelodysplastic syndrome (see above). Idiopathic dyserythropoiesis in the dog may occur in association with increased sideroblasts in bone marrow and siderocytes in blood, or as a chronic, normocytic-normochromic, nonregenerative anemia with cellular marrow and abnormal morphology of erythroid precursors (Weiss and Reidarson, 1989).

Anemia of Chronic Disease

A normocytic-normochromic, nonresponsive anemia is commonly found in association with chronic infections, chronic noninfectious inflammatory conditions, and some types of malignancies. These types of anemias are grouped under a common category, anemia of chronic disorder or disease (ACD) or anemia of inflammatory disease (AID). In natural cases, the anemia develops slowly, usually over a period of weeks or months, and then becomes stabilized. The degree of anemia varies with the nature of the disease process, but is usually mild to modest. ACD should be distinguished from hypoplastic anemias with a specific cause such as drug therapy, iron deficiency, renal disease, and myelophthisis.

Although the anemia is typically normocytic-normochromic, in rare instances it may become microcytic-hypochromic, as in true iron deficiency. The reticulocyte count is normal or slightly elevated. Iron metabolism and erythropoiesis are abnormal in patients with ACD (see Table 9–7). The major abnormalities include decreases in serum iron level, total iron-binding capacity (serum transferrin), percentage transferrin saturation, erythropoiesis, and marrow sideroblasts, an increased marrow macrophage iron store, and a normal or increased serum ferritin level. Corticosteroid administration and an endogenous increase in serum cortisol levels in dogs result in increased serum iron concentrations and may mask the hypoferremia of iron deficiency (Harvey et al., 1987). Similarly, exogenous corticosteroids cause hyperferremia in horses, but a hypoferremia manifests in cattle (Weeks et al., 1989). A microcytic-hypochromic anemia was found in two horses with intra-abdominal neoplasms and abscesses (Zicker et al., 1990).

Experiments in dogs and cats have shown that the formation of sterile abscesses is associated with reductions in red cell parameters by as much as 30% within 2 weeks, although a frank anemia was not evident. Red cell indices and reticulocyte counts indicated a normocytic-normochromic and nonregenerative erythrocytic response. The depressed erythropoiesis was characterized by reduced levels of serum iron, decreased total iron-binding capacity (serum transferrin), reduced percentage saturation of transferrin, and decreased numbers of sideroblasts in the bone marrow. Free protoporphyrin concentration within red cells was increased and, similarly, serum levels of copper, zinc, and ceruloplasmin were elevated. Bone marrow macrophage iron and hepatic nonheme iron levels were increased. Ferrokinetic studies indicated effective but inadequate erythropoietic response of the bone marrow, limited mainly by the amount of iron available for this purpose. Iron stored in marrow macrophages seemed to be in a form that could not be readily mobilized by injecting deferoxamine, an iron-chelating agent. Other abnormalities included elevations of free erythrocyte porphyrin levels and increased excretion of coproporphyrin I and III.

Anemia of inflammatory disease has been attributed

to various causes such as impaired erythropoiesis, defective iron metabolism, and slightly shortened red cell survival. Inadequate erythropoiesis may be attributed to several mechanisms: (1) the sequestration of iron in marrow macrophages so that it is unavailable for compensatory erythropoietic response; (2) decreased erythropoietin production; (3) reduced erythropoietin response of the erythroid progenitor cells; and (4) the production of inhibitors of erythropoiesis such as prostaglandins, acidic isoferritins, interferons, and tumor necrosis factor. An immune mechanism may be involved in the shortened red cell survival, as indicated by observations that the erythrocytes of cats who developed sterile abscesses became increasingly coated with IgG and their phagocytosis by macrophages in vitro was significantly increased (Weiss and McClay, 1988). Serum from dogs with anemia secondary to infection, malignancy, and chronic renal failure was found to inhibit in vitro erythropoiesis, although serum inhibition did not correlate with decreased PCV (Weiss, 1986).

The administration of iron to treat ACD is uneventful; the cause must be traced and alleviated to stimulate compensatory erythropoiesis. The effectiveness of recombinant erythropoietin administration in stimulating erythropoiesis in ACD in humans is under investigation.

Chronic Renal Disease with Uremia

Chronic renal disease or end-stage kidney disease in the dog is generally associated with a normocytic-normochromic, nonresponsive anemia. In addition, the hemogram is usually characterized by a high corrected erythrocyte sedimentation rate (ESR), hyperfibrinogenemia, and marked lymphopenia (Table 12–4). The PCV is usually about 20 to 30%. In dogs that survive for many months, the anemia may be progressive and the PCV may fall as low as 10%. Anemia may be masked by dehydration from renal loss of water, in which case it becomes apparent from

hyperproteinemia or after hydration. Highly crenated erythrocytes (burr cells) are found in humans with uremia, but this has not been our experience with the dog. Schistocytes and spiculated red cells are found in humans with hemolytic uremic syndrome. Bone marrow cytology reveals hypoplasia of the erythrocytic series, leading to an elevated M:E ratio (see Table 1–8). Granulopoiesis is generally not affected, although increased neutrophil production and a few abnormal cells may be seen in some cases as a response to inflammation.

Common hematologic findings in 74 cats with chronic renal disease included nonregenerative anemia, lymphopenia, and hyperproteinemia (DiBartola et al., 1987). In a similar study on 59 dogs with renal amyloidosis, common hematologic findings included leukocytosis, lymphopenia, and nonregenerative anemia (DiBartola et al., 1989).

The anemia of renal disease is primarily the result of inadequate erythrocyte production. Proposed pathogenetic mechanisms include the following: (1) decreased production of erythropoietin; (2) production of a factor or factors inhibiting erythropoietic activity (e.g., guanidinosuccinic acid, phenols, and urea); (3) decreased erythrocyte survival because of extracellular (mechanical fragmentation) and intracellular (reduced activities of the hexose monophosphate shunt and the Na^+-K^+ pump) defects; and (4) in some cases, a defective response of bone marrow to erythropoietin. Neutrophil and immune functions may also be compromised because patients with renal disease are prone to infection. Functional abnormalities of platelets may be found.

Therapeutic approaches to the management of anemia in humans with kidney disease have varied, ranging from no therapy in mild cases to hemodialysis, the administration of cobalt, androgens, and erythropoietin to stimulate erythropoiesis, and kidney transplantation in severe cases. Cobalt stimulates erythropoiesis from inducing tissue hypoxia, which then stimulates erythropoietin production. Androgens have been shown to stimulate erythropoiesis by increasing eryth-

Table 12–4. Biochemistry and Hematology of Chronic Renal Failure in the Dog

Age (yr)	Sex	Clinical Type*	Urine		Plasma or Serum (mg/dl)				Plasma		ESR (cor)	PCV (%)	Differential Leukocyte Count in Absolute Numbers/μl						
			Specific Gravity	Protein	BUN	Creatinine	Ca	P	Fibrinogen (g/dl)	Protein (g/dl)			WBC/μl	Band	Neutrophils	Lymphocytes	Monocytes	Eosinophils	Basophils
1	F	P	1.009	1+	120	—	12.1	10.2	0.8	8.4	27+	25	30,300	0	21,059	2,575	6,060	606	0
1	M	I	1.004	2+	157	—	11.6	11.4	1.0	8.0	33+	38	10,800	0	8,748	810	810	378	54
2	F	PG	1.008	2+	141	6.4	13.3	14.0	0.7	6.8	27+	23	12,100	0	8,470	2,057	726	847	0
3	F	PO	1.012	1+	360	13.0	8.2	21.0	0.7	9.4	27+	21	7,700	38	6,699	423	539	0	0
4	M	IO	1.009	1+	103	—	10.8	5.9	0.7	7.2	33+	24	16,300	81	11,247	1,304	3,260	245	163
5	M	G	1.008	1+	144	6.0	4.6	18.8	0.7	6.1	9+	10	18,400	0	17,204	184	920	92	0
5	M	I	1.013	—	156	28.0	6.9	28.0	0.5	8.7	42+	36	9,000	0	8,190	495	315	0	0
6	F	G	1.017	4+	177	3.8	7.9	17.6	0.7	5.2	1+	37	10,900	109	9,374	545	763	109	0
7	M	P	1.011	2+	204	—	13.0	14.2	0.7	10.9	24+	44	31,100	0	27,213	311	3,577	0	0
7	M	IO	1.013	4+	282	4.4	6.2	20.8	0.6	7.3	—	22	8,300	83	7,262	83	830	41	0
8	M	IO	1.013	2+	136	—	10.9	11.2	0.8	8.5	25+	28	16,500	0	13,860	165	2,475	0	0
8	F	I	1.010	2+	277	15.6	4.5	30.0	0.7	8.1	35+	29	21,800	0	19,838	872	981	109	0
9	F	G	1.013	3+	205	—	—	—	0.9	8.4	27+	43	15,800	395	13,746	395	1,264	0	0
10	F	PG	1.011	2+	150	7.7	—	15.3	0.4	7.9	16+	26	9,500	142	7,362	522	1,377	95	0
11	F	G	1.013	4+	265	—	6.6	17.8	1.3	7.5	34+	39	18,700	0	16,082	281	1,963	374	0
15	M	G	1.010	2+	169	—	—	—	0.3	9.0	8+	50	14,300	429	11,011	858	1,215	787	0

* P, pyelonephritis; I, interstitial nephritis; G, glomerulonephritis; O, osteodystrophy fibrosa.

ropoietin production (5β-H isomer) or the marrow responsiveness of erythroid cells to erythropoietin (5α-H isomer). Erythropoietin administration is now feasible because of the commercial availability of a recombinant erythropoietin. Such therapy has been successfully tried in some dogs and cats with chronic renal disease and further investigations are underway to develop specific recommendations (Cowgill, 1991).

Endocrine Disease

A mild to moderate anemia has been observed in humans with endocrine disorders of the thyroid, adrenals, gonads, pituitary, and parathyroids. These endocrine disorders include hypothyroidism, Addison's disease, hypogonadism in males, hypopituitarism, and primary hyperparathyroidism. Most of these disorders result in suppressed erythropoietin production. Hypothyroidism may be complicated by iron deficiency anemia or vitamin B_{12} and folate deficiency anemia, in which case a microcytic or macrocytic anemia, respectively, may be seen. Goats with goiter induced by feeding thiourea develop a reversible anemia.

Hypothyroidism in the dog may be associated with normocytic-normochromic anemia. The anemia is commonly borderline, with the PCV ranging between 30 and 37%, although in some instances it may fall below 30% (Table 12–5). The erythrocyte morphology is characteristic of a depression anemia. The reticulocyte numbers remain low, with lack of polychromasia. Orthochromatic leptocytes are prominent and their presence may cause a diphasic ESR. A significantly positive ESR is seen in many cases, probably because of pathologic changes in the blood vessel walls and skin of hypothyroid dogs. The leukocytic response in hypothyroid dogs would suggest a response to changes in the devitalized skin as a result of infection (Table 12–5).

Liver Disease

A normocytic-normochromic anemia is seen in humans with cirrhosis and other uncomplicated liver diseases. Prominent findings include the presence of target cells, thin macrocytes (erythrocytes with increased diameter but normal MCV), and acanthocytes (see Figs. 7–10D, 7–17C, and 7–19E). The reticulocyte count and leukocyte response are variable. A mild thrombocytopenia may be present. Bone marrow erythropoietic activity is reduced for the degree of anemia.

Anemia is believed to result primarily from decreased erythrocyte survival and partly from an impaired marrow response. Other contributing mechanisms include chronic blood loss from the gastrointestinal tract and iron and folic acid deficiencies. Decreased erythrocyte survival may be a consequence of characteristic changes observed in erythrocyte membrane lipids because of decreased plasma LCAT (lysolecithin cholesterol acyltransferase) activity, increased plasma levels of bile salts, and an increased plasma free cholesterol:phospholipid ratio. An increased membrane rigidity promoting red cell lysis was also thought to result from a decrease in the intraerythrocytic ATP concentration, probably secondary to the hypophosphatemia common to hepatic disease. Inadequate erythroid response of the bone marrow may be the result of impaired mobilization of hepatic iron or diminished hepatic function in erythropoietin production.

Anemia associated with liver disease is observed in animals, but remains to be characterized fully. Acute intravascular hemolysis with hemoglobinemia and hemoglobinuria has been observed in some horses with fulminating hepatic failure, but its precise mechanism remains unknown.

Myelophthisis and Myelofibrosis

Anemia associated with bone marrow infiltration by foreign cells is called myelophthistic anemia. This anemia is mild to severe and may be accompanied by leukopenia and thrombocytopenia. The anemia is typically normocytic-normochromic and nonresponsive. Morphologic abnormalities of erythrocytes include poikilocytes, particularly teardrop forms. Nucleated red

Table 12–5. Hemogram in Hypothyroidism in the Dog

Dog No.	Sex	Age (yr)	Thyroid Function Tests*	Cholesterol (mg/dl)	RBC (×10⁶/μl)	Hb (g/dl)	PCV (%)	MCV (fl)	MCHC (%)	ESR (cor.)	WBC/μl	Neutrophils Band	Neutrophils Mature	Lymphocyte	Monocyte	Eosinophil
1	F	2	$T_4 = 0$	—	4.08	8.5	27	66.1	31.5	28+	13,300	133	10,308	864	1,724	266
2	F	4	^{131}I = 0%	300	6.0	12.5	37	61.7	33.8	5–	8,900	0	6,185	2,047	489	178
3	XF	5	Atrophy	470	5.7	10.2	31	54.4	32.9	21+	8,650	0	6,055	1,816	788	0
4	M	5	Atrophy	1454	4.6	9.8	30	65.2	32.7	37+	8,300	0	5,810	1,909	498	83
5	F	5	Atrophy	446	5.0	13.3	40	80.0	33.2	—	9,000	45	5,850	2,160	765	180
6	F	5	Atrophy	740	4.2	10.0	30	71.4	33.3	Diphasic 20+	14,250	0	7,339	4,346	1,211	1,354
7	XM	6	Atrophy	400	4.6	10.2	32	69.6	31.0	26+	6,900	0	5,072	1,587	138	103
8	F	7	Atrophy	322	5.2	11.8	35	67.3	33.7	2+	21,050	105	14,630	4,210	1,579	526
9	F	8	^{131}I = 1.0%	508	5.2	13.5	41	79.8	32.0	0	22,200	222	15,762	2,664	1,110	2,442
10	F	9	^{131}I = 1.0%	260	6.1	15.0	41	67.2	36.6	27+	28,100	422	25,009	842	1,545	281
11	XM	10	Atrophy	262	3.2	8.8	24	75.0	36.7	29+	36,500	1,643	29,747	2,190	2,555	365

Differential Leukocytes, Absolute Numbers/μl

(From Jain, N.C.: Schalm's Veterinary Hematology. 4th Ed. Philadelphia, Lea & Febiger, 1986, p. 1065.)
* T_4 normal, 0.6–3.6 μg/dl; ^{131}I normal uptake, 10 to 40%.

cells and immature neutrophils may be found in blood, constituting the leukoerythroblastic reaction. Bone marrow infiltration may occur from metastatic neoplasms such as carcinoma and melanoma, hematopoietic neoplasms such as myeloproliferative and lymphoproliferative disease, infections, or granulomatous inflammatory diseases, and myelofibrosis. Anemia results from decreased erythropoiesis and increased hemolysis of defective red cells. A leukoerythroblastic response develops primarily because of the release of immature cells into the blood from disturbed marrow architecture, and perhaps also partly from extramedullary hematopoiesis.

Myelofibrosis is associated with a nonresponsive anemia, thrombocytopenia, and leukopenia from neutropenia. Myelofibrosis has been observed in dogs, cats, and goats (Blue, 1988; Jain 1986; English et al., 1988). Myelofibrosis may be a terminal event in myeloproliferative diseases, secondary to bone marrow damage or malignancies (mammary, prostrate, or stomach carcinoma), or it may be idiopathic. Plateletderived growth factor and serotonin released from megakaryocytes have been incriminated in myelofibrosis. Myelofibrosis may also occur as a consequence of prolonged erythropoietic response to pyruvate kinase deficiency anemia in dogs.

Neoplasia

Neoplasia, especially when malignant, causes a selective depression of erythrogenesis. Various mechanisms may be involved but, more frequently, the anemia is caused by marrow suppression, blood loss, autoantibody production, and hematopoietic dysplasias. Anemia may also occur as a result of cancer chemotherapy. The normocytic-normochromic, nonresponsive anemia associated with feline leukemia virus infection in cats is attributed to diminished erythropoiesis.

Parasitism in Sheep and Cattle

The trichostrongyloid parasites of cattle and sheep (excluding Haemonchus contortus) may produce a severe normocytic-normochromic anemia because of the depression of erythropoiesis. (See Chapter 9 for a discussion of blood loss anemias associated with parasitism.)

REFERENCES

Blue, J.T.: Myelofibrosis in cats with myelodysplastic syndrome and acute myelogenous leukemia. Vet Pathol., 25:154, 1988.
Bunch, S.E., Castleman, W.L., Baldwin, B.H., et al.: Effects of longterm primidone and phenytoin administration on canine hepatic function and morphology. Am. J. Vet. Res., 46:105, 1985.
Bunch, S.E., Easley, J.R., and Cullen, J.M.: Hematologic values and plasma and tissue folate concentrations in dogs given phenytoin on a long-term basis. Am. J. Vet. Res., 51:1865, 1990.
Cowgill, L. D.: Clinical experience and use of recombinant human erythropoietin in uremic dogs and cats. Proceedings of the 9th ACVIM Forum, 147, 1991.
DiBartola, S.P., Rutgers, H.C., Zack, P.M., et al.: Clinicopathologic findings associated with chronic renal disease in cats: 74 cases (1973–1984). J. Am. Vet. Med. Assoc., 190:1196, 1987.
DiBartola, S.P., Tarr, M.J., Parker, A.T., et al.: Clinicopathologic findings in dogs with renal amyloidosis: 59 cases (1976–1986). J. Am. Vet. Med. Assoc. 195:358, 1989.
English, R.V., Breitschwerdt, E. B., Grindem., C. B., et al.: Zollinger-Ellison syndrome and myelofibrosis in a dog. J. Am. Vet. Med. Assoc., 192:1430, 1988.
Fyfe, J.C., Giger, U., Hall, C.A., et al.: Inherited selective intestinal cobalamin malabsorption and cobalamin deficiency in dogs. Pediatr. Res., 29:24, 1991.
Harvey, J.W., Levin, D.E., and Chen, C.L.: Potential effects of glucocorticoids on serum iron concentration in dogs. Vet. Clin. Pathol., 16:46, 1987.
Jain, N.C.: Schalm's Veterinary Hematology. 4th ed. Philadelphia, Lea & Febiger, 1986, pp. 655–675.
Kuehn, N.F. and Gaunt, S.D.: Hypocellular marrow and extramedullary hematopoiesis in a dog: Hematologic recovery after splenectomy. J. Am. Vet. Med. Assoc., 188:1313, 1986.
Lavoie, J.-P., Morris, D.D., Zinkl, J.G., et al.: Pancytopenia caused by bone marrow aplasia in a horse. J. Am. Vet. Med. Assoc., 191:1462, 1987.
Riedel, N., Hoover, E.A., Dornsife, R.E., et al.: Pathogenic and host range determinants of the feline aplastic anemia retrovirus. Proc Natl Acad Sci, 85:2758, 1988.
Rottman, J.B., English, R.V., Breitschwerdt, E.B., et al.: Bone marrow hypoplasia in a cat treated with griseofulvin. J. Am. Vet. Med. Assoc., 198:429, 1991.
Sas, B.: Secondary copper deficiency in cattle caused by molybdenum contamination of fodder: A case history. Vet. Human. Toxic., 31:29, 1989.
Steffen, D.J., Leipold, H.W., Gibb, J., et al.: Congenital anemia, dyskeratosis, and progressive alopecia in Polled hereford calves. Vet. Pathol., 28:234, 1991.
Van Kruiningen, H.J. and Friedland, T.B.: Responsive estrogen-induced aplastic anemia in a dog. J. Am. Vet. Med. Assoc., 191:91, 1987.
Weeks, B.R., Smith, J.E., BeBowes, R.M., et al.: Decreased serum iron and zinc concentrations in cattle receiving intravenous dexamethasone. Vet. Pathol., 26:345, 1989.
Weiss, D.J.: Potential role of serum inhibitors of erythropoiesis in the anemia associated with infection, renal disease and malignancy in the dog. Vet. Clin. Pathol., 15:7, 1986.
Weiss, D.J., Armstrong, P.J., and Reimann, K.: Bone marrow necrosis in the dog. J. Am. Vet. Med. Assoc., 187:54, 1986.
Weiss, D.J., and Christopher, M.M.: Idiopathic aplastic anemia in a dog. Vet. Clin. Path., 14:23, 1985.
Weiss, D.J., and Klausner, J.S.: Drug-associated aplastic anemia in dogs: Eight cases (1984–1988). J. Am. Vet. Med. Assoc., 196:472, 1990.
Weiss, D.J. and McClay, C.B.: Studies on the pathogenesis of the erythrocyte destruction associated with the anemia of inflammatory disease. Vet. Clin. Pathol., 17:90, 1988.
Weiss, D.J. and Reidarson, T.H.: Idiopathic dyserythropoiesis in a dog. Vet. Clin. Pathol., 18:43, 1989.
Williams, W.J., Beutler, E., Erslev, A.J., et al.: Hematology. 4th ed. New York, McGraw-Hill, 1990, Chaps. 47, 48, and 53.
Zicker, S.C., Wilson, D. and Medearis, I.: Differentiation between intra-abdominal neoplasms and abscesses in horses, using clinical and laboratory data: 40 cases (1972–1988). J. Am. Vet. Med. Assoc., 196:1130, 1990.

The Neutrophils

Neutrophils form the first line of cellular defense against microbial infection. They are produced in the bone marrow and are delivered to the blood on maturation. Normally, this process of granulopoiesis is completed within a few days. After a brief intravascular sojourn, these cells enter the tissues and body cavities to execute their physiologic functions. A bone marrow reserve and an intravascular marginal pool of mature neutrophils remain in dynamic equilibrium with the neutrophils in circulation. Cells from both locations provide a physiologic means for meeting sudden demands for neutrophil participation in the body's defense. Subpopulations of neutrophils are being recognized in humans and cattle based on differences in their functional properties and cell surface antigens. Using recombinant hemotopoietic growth factors and cytokines, it is now possible to manipulate neutrophil numbers and functions to increase the host defense (Cairo, 1991; Steinbeck and Roth, 1989).

GRANULOPOIESIS AND RELEASE OF NEUTROPHILS FROM BONE MARROW TO BLOOD

Granulopoiesis, or granulocytopoiesis, involves the production of neutrophils, eosinophils, and basophils through an orderly process (Fig. 13–1). The traditional concept of granulopoiesis envisioned the formation of neutrophils, eosinophils, and basophils from a common precursor cell, the promyelocyte. Newer studies have shown, however, that each of the three granulocyte types can be identified as early as the promye-

locyte stage on the basis of granule ultrastructure and cytochemical reactions. Furthermore, the results of colony culture studies have suggested that a separate myeloblast probably exists for each cell series, although they cannot be distinguished morphologically (see Fig. 4–6).

Myeloid Stem Cells

In the bone marrow, under proper stimulus, the pluripotential stem cell gives rise to progenitor cells committed to producing various granulocytes (see Fig. 4–6). The cell concerned with the production of neutrophils and monocytes is known as the colony-forming unit–granulocyte-monocyte (CFU-GM) because, at this early stage, it is bipotential. Subsequently, under appropriate stimuli, the CFU-GM differentiates into unipotential cells, CFU-G and CFU-M, committed to producing a neutrophilic or monocytic precursor cell, respectively. Similarly, in vitro studies on granulopoiesis have provided evidence for the existence of separate progenitor cells for eosinophils (CFU-Eos) and basophils (CFU-Bas). The granulocytic unipotential cells give rise to morphologically identifiable precursors known as myeloblasts, which divide, differentiate, and mature to yield specific blood granulocytes. The morphologic maturation of neutrophils is associated with changes in various cellular components and properties such as cell surface carbohydrates, glycoproteins, glycolipids, histocompatibility antigens, surface charge and receptors, cytoskeletal elements, and functional attributes.

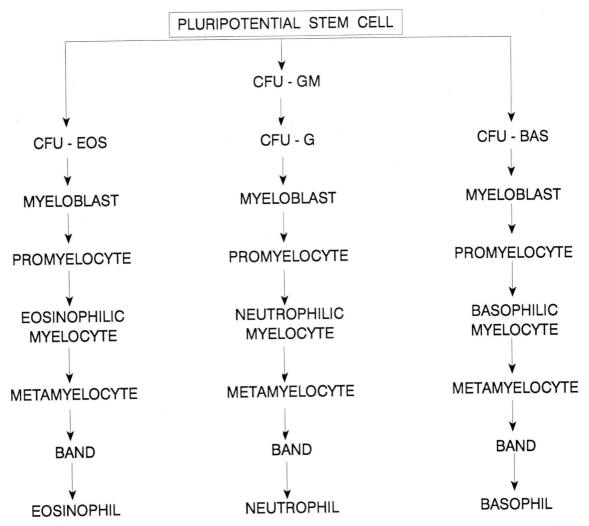

Fig. 13–1. Outline of sequential development of granulocytes. The pluripotential cell and the committed stem cells (CFU-GM, CFU-G, CFU-Eos, and CFU-Bas) are not recognizable by light microscopy. Their existence is demonstrable in colony culture assays. Myeloblasts and promyelocytes can be identified by light microscopy, but their lineage-specific features are found only on electron microscopy and ultrastructure cytochemistry. In Wright-Giemsa stained bone marrow films, myeloblasts of the three cell lines remain indistinguishable and promyelocytes almost invariably have similar features. Very rarely, an eosinophilic promyelocyte can be found to have larger azurophilic granules than those in the neutrophilic promyelocyte. The three cell lines can be readily identified from the myelocyte stage onwards because of the development of prominent specific granules which display unique tinctorial properties. A round nucleus with fine chromatin is present in myeloblasts and promyelocytes, and one or more distinct or indistinct nucleoli are present in the former and usually not in the latter cells. The myelocyte has a round nucleus with coarse or clumped chromatin and without nucleolus. The nucleus assumes a kidney-bean shape in metamyelocytes, horse-shoe shape in bands, and segmented form in all mature granulocytes.

Light Microscopic Features of Developing Granulocytes

Various sequential, morphologically recognizable cellular stages are shown in Figure 13–1. The morphologic identity of the early progenitor cells through myeloblasts remains uncertain.

The myeloblast is the most immature recognizable cell of the series (Plates V–3, V–5, and VI–1). It has a round nucleus with stippled chromatin and one or more nucleoli or indistinct nucleolar rings. Sometimes, a nucleolus or nucleolar ring may not be visible. The cytoplasm is modest to fairly abundant and stains moderately blue, in contrast to the deep blue cytoplasm of rubriblasts (Plates IV–1 and VI–5). The cytoplasm

is generally devoid of fine, reddish-purple azurophilic granules (type I myeloblast), but some granules (less than 15) may be present in an occasional cell (type II myeloblast; Plate VI–2).

The promyelocyte is often larger than the myeloblast, but its nuclear features are usually similar (Plates V–4). The cytoplasm is more abundant, stains lighter blue, and typically contains many small, reddish-purple azurophilic granules.

The myelocyte varies in size because it often divides twice before maturing into a metamyelocyte (Plates V–6 and XXIV–4). Its nucleus is round to slightly dented, lacks a nucleolus, and displays some chromatin aggregation. Its cytoplasm stains faintly blue, particularly along the periphery, and contains lineage-specific granules. Azurophilic granules are normally not seen at this and subsequent stages. The neutrophilic myelocyte has numerous barely visible pale granules, many large reddish granules decorate the eosinophilic myelocyte, and deep purplish-violet granules identify the basophilic myelocyte. Subsequent stages of the three granulocyte types are recognized according to their nuclear shape and granule colors.

The metamyelocyte may also vary in size. Its cytoplasmic features are similar to those of myelocytes, but the nucleus is indented, similar to a kidney bean, or is wide and elongated, with fat ends (Plates V–3 and V–6).

The band cell is about the size of the mature granulocyte, but has a slender, nonsegmented nucleus with scattered small clumps of chromatin, a smooth contour, and parallel-appearing sides (Plates V–6, VI–4, and XII–3). The cytoplasm may be clear, pale, or faintly blue, and contains specific granules.

The mature or segmented neutrophil, eosinophil, and basophil are distinguished by their segmented nuclei, clumped chromatin, irregular nuclear outline, and specific granules. Distinct nuclear lobes are less prominent in eosinophils and basophils than in neutrophils. A drumstick or club-shaped nuclear appendage (Barr body) may be seen in an occasional neutrophil of females (Plate XI-7). These appendages contain an inactivated X chromosome.

Ultrastructural and Cytochemical Features of Neutrophils

The most significant aspect of granulopoiesis is the formation of lysosomal granules in the developing neutrophils. Electron microscopic and cytochemical studies have revealed that, in most species, neutrophils and their precursors contain at least two types of granules, azurophilic (primary) and specific (secondary) granules (Figs. 13–2 and 13–3). A third type of granule, the tertiary granule, is found in the neutrophils of some species (humans and rabbits). These granules are smaller than the secondary granules, so they are visible only on electron microscopy. They are peroxidase-negative but contain acid hydrolases and sulfate. A third granule type that contained peroxidase, acid phosphatase, and vicinal-glycol-containing complex carbohydrates was found in feline neutrophils (Fittschen et al., 1988b).

In marrow films stained with Wright or Giemsa stain, azurophilic granules are seen only in type II myeloblasts and promyelocytes. They are also found with the electron microscope, although in reduced numbers, in the subsequent stages of neutrophil maturation. In mature neutrophils, the ratio of azurophilic to specific granules is usually 1:2. Such a distinction in granule types is unclear in eosinophils and basophils. In both these cells, granule maturation or transformation is more common than formation of distinctly different granules.

Azurophilic granules in mature neutrophils are not demonstrable by methods routinely employed to stain blood films because of a reduction in the granule content of glycosaminoglycans (mucopolysaccharides). They may be visualized in "toxic" neutrophils, however, because of retention of these chemicals. Primary granules stain positive for myeloperoxidase (MPO), but not for alkaline phosphatase (ALP). Specific granules appear at the myelocyte stage and remain abundant through the mature neutrophil stage. Specific granules lack MPO but contain ALP, except in the dog and cat (Jain, 1986). Although primary and secondary granules have an enriched content of enzymatic and nonenzymatic constituents (Table 13–1), the single most reliable marker of primary granules is MPO, whereas that of secondary granules is lactoferrin.

Azurophilic granules appear first (primary granules), and specific granules appear later (secondary

Table 13–1. Some Enzymatic and Nonenzymatic Constituents of Mature Neutrophils

Primary or azurophilic granules	Secondary or specific granules	Constituents of uncertain location
Peroxidase	Alkaline phosphatase	Leukin
Sulfated mucopolysaccharides	Lysozyme ($\frac{2}{3}$)	Procoagulant activity
Cationic proteins	Lactoferrin	Endogenous pyrogen
Defensins	Aminopeptidase	Histamine
Lysozyme ($\frac{1}{3}$)	Specific collagenase	Kinin-forming and kinin-destroying enzymes
Acid proteases: cathepsins B and D	C5-Inactivating factor	Aminopeptides
Neutral proteases	Phospholipase A_2	"Microbodies": catalase
Cathepsin G	Transcobalamin I	
Elastase	Leukocyte adhesion receptors (in membrane)	
Nonspecific collagenase	Plasminogen activators	
Proteinase 3	Histaminase	
Acid phosphatase	Receptors for FMLP, CR3, CR3bi, and laminin	
Arylsulfatase	cytochrome b_{558}	
Chloroacetate esterase	Tertiary granules	
Acid hydrolytic enzymes	Acid phosphatase	
β-Galactosidase	Arylsulfatase B	
β-Glucuronidase	β-Glycerophosphatase	
β-Glycerophosphatase	Acid mucosubstance	
5′-Nucleosidase	Cathepsins B and D	
α-Mannosidase	Gelatinase	

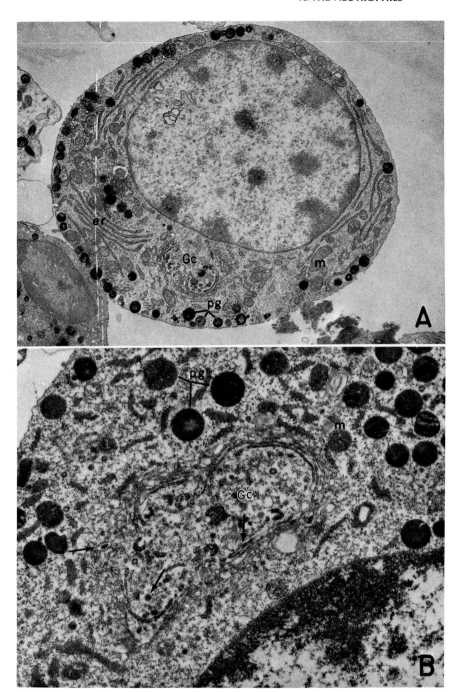

Fig. 13–2. Progranulocytes from canine bone marrow. These cells are characterized by the presence of numerous primary or azurophilic granules *(pg)*, which are peroxidase-positive, numerous mitochondria *(m)*, several profiles of prominent rough endoplasmic reticulum *(er)*, and abundant ribosomes and polyribosomes. The nucleus shows slight chromatin clumping, primarily along the nuclear membrane. The Golgi complex *(Gc)* is active and engaged in manufacturing primary granules. This is evident in *B*, in which tiny primary granules, vesicles containing condensing proteinaceous material and cisternae containing condensing material can be seen in the Golgi complex area *(arrows)* (transmission electron photomicrographs, peroxidase stain; *A*, ×6,300; *B*, ×21,600). (From Jain, N.C.: Schalm's Veterinary Hematology. 4th Ed. Philadelphia, Lea & Febiger, 1986, p. 680.)

granules; Figs. 13–2 and 13–3). The formation of primary granules is generally restricted to the promyelocyte stage, and that of secondary granules is thought to occur only at the myelocyte stage. Morphometric and cytochemical observations in the cat have indicated, however, that MPO-positive granules are also formed in late (nondividing neutrophils and that secondary granule genesis may extend into the metamyelocyte stage (Fittschen et al., 1988a). Primary granules are relatively large, more electron-dense, roundish, and less pleomorphic than secondary granules. Both granule types are produced by the Golgi apparatus and are often referred to as lysosomes. Tertiary granules also constitute lysosomes. Collectively, the three granule types contain many hydrolytic enzymes and antibacterial substances needed to kill and digest phagocytosed microorganisms (Williams et al., 1990).

Regulation of Granulopoiesis

The number of neutrophils entering and leaving the blood is kept constant under steady state conditions. Factors regulating granulopoiesis and the release

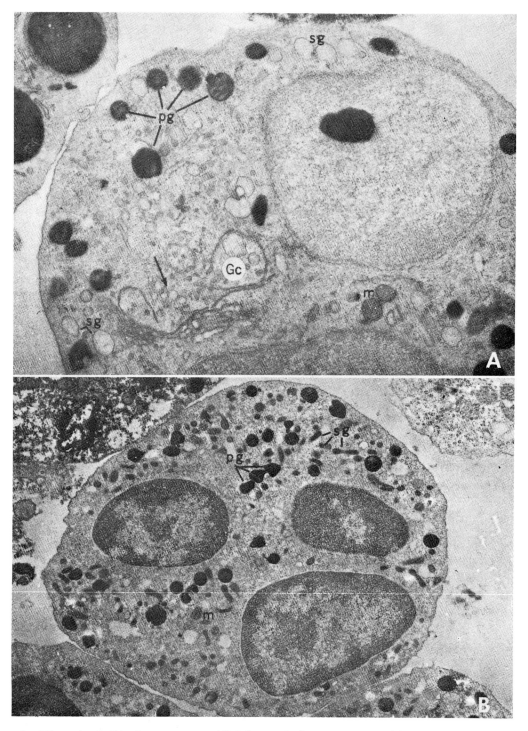

Fig. 13–3.   A neutrophilic myelocyte *(A)* and a mature neutrophil *(B)* from canine bone marrow stained for peroxidase. These cells are characterized by the presence of both primary granules *(pg)*, which are peroxidase-positive, and secondary granules *(sg)*, which are peroxidase-negative. *A*, In the myelocyte, note the presence of an active Golgi complex *(Gc)* engaged in manufacturing secondary granules. Many clear saccules *(arrow)* of varying sizes can be seen in the vicinity of the Golgi complex, and similar large granules *(sg)* are apparent scattered in the cytoplasm. A few mitochondria *(m)* are also present (×25,000). *B*, The mature neutrophil distinctly contains larger, round, peroxidase-positive primary granules *(pg)* and smaller, pleomorphic, peroxidase-negative secondary granules *(sg)*. Romanowsky staining of blood films ordinarily demonstrates only one granule population because the primary granules by this stage have lost their acid mucopolysaccharide, which is responsible for their azurophilic staining at the progranulocyte stage. Some mitochondria *(m)* are also present. The nuclear lobes show condensation of chromatin (transmission electron photomicrographs, ×12,000). (From Jain, N.C.: Schalm's Veterinary Hematology. 4th Ed. Philadelphia, Lea & Febiger, 1986, p. 681.)

of marrow neutrophils in blood are listed in Table 4–2 and discussed in Chapter 4. Briefly, the hematopoietic inductive microenvironment (HIM) is important in the early differentiation of pluripotential stem cells to committed progenitors. In addition, several specific humoral factors controlling the development of granulocytic precursors and the formation of mature neutrophils have been identified by in vivo and in vitro studies (Williams et al., 1990). These factors are broadly categorized as colony-stimulating and colony-inhibiting factors and as chalone and antichalone. Both represent a system of positive and negative feedback control of granulopoiesis. Abnormalities of such control mechanisms have been found in pathologic states, such as myeloid leukemias, and in neutropenias resulting from diminished production, such as cyclic hematopoiesis of gray collie dogs.

The production of neutrophils is regulated primarily by interleukin-3 (IL-3), GM-CSF, and G-CSF, and the production of eosinophils and basophils is chiefly promoted by IL-3 and GM-CSF. An increased supply of neutrophils to blood is affected by the following: (1) increase in the numbers of neutrophil-committed progenitors cells and myeloblasts; (2) increase in the number of mitoses at the myeloblast through myelocyte stages; (3) shortening of transit time through the mitotic and maturative pools; and (4) increased release of mature neutrophils into the peripheral blood (see Table 4–3 and Fig. 4–7).

Injection of human recombinant G-CSF into cows, cats, and dogs has been found to stimulate neutrophil production and induce a 3- to 5-fold elevation of neutrophil numbers in blood within 5 to 14 days (Cullor et al., 1990a, 1990b; Fulton et al., 1991; Zinkl et al., in press). Monocyte and lymphocyte counts also were significantly elevated in cats. Injection of recombinant murine, but not human, GM-CSF in rats caused leukocytosis associated with neutrophilia and monocytosis, peaking between 4 and 8 hours and returning to normal by 12 hours postinoculation (Ulrich et al., 1990). These changes were preceded by a transient neutropenia and monocytopenia, with a nadir at 15 minutes, and a mild lymphopenia between 2 to 8 hours postinoculation. A slight left-shifted myeloid hyperplasia was detected at 6 hours after inoculation.

CSFs also augment neutrophil functions (e.g., adhesion, chemotaxis, degranulation, oxidative metabolism, arachidonic acid metabolism, phagocytosis, bacterial kill, and cytotoxicity) directly or indirectly by priming the cells for enhanced activity in response to other agents (Reddy et al., 1990). Receptors for both G-CSF and GM-CSF are present on the neutrophils. Because of their broad effects on neutrophil production and functions, CSFs are finding increasing therapeutic uses, including the ablation of myeloid aplasias, mitigation of bone marrow toxicities resulting from drug therapy such as cancer chemotherapy, increasing host defenses, and treating neutrophil disorders (Cairo, 1991; Ganser et al., 1991; Morstyn and Sheridan, 1991). See Chap. 4 for additional information.

Tumor necrosis factor-alpha, interferon-gamma, and IL-1 have been found to similarly prime and stimulate several neutrophil functions (Chiang et al., 1991; Sample and Czuprynski, 1991; Sordillo and Babiuk, 1991; Thomsen and Thomsen, 1990). IL-1 and TNF are believed to be the major humoral factors involved in stimulating CSF secretion by responsive cells in the bone marrow as well as in other tissues. It has been suggested that CSFs secreted by bone marrow endothelial cells and fibroblasts may serve to stimulate the proliferation and differentiation of myeloid progenitor cells, whereas CSFs elaborated locally in areas of infection or inflammation most likely augment functions of various leukocytes (Cannistra and Griffin, 1988).

GRANULOKINETICS

Quantitative information about the production of granulocytes in bone marrow and their intravascular and tissue phases are considered under the term "granulokinetics." The information is derived from studies on blood and marrow granulocytes labelled with radioisotopes, such as tritiated thymidine (^{3}H-TdR), di-isopropyl fluorophosphate ($DF^{32}P$), radioactive sulfate (^{34}S), radiochromate (^{59}Cr) and, more recently, indium (^{111}In-oxine). The results have generally been obtained only for neutrophils, and mostly from studies on humans and only a few studies on animals (Jain, 1986; Williams et al., 1990). ^{111}In-labeled neutrophils have been used to aid in the detection of internal abscesses (Koblik et al., 1985).

Functional Compartments of Granulocytes in Bone Marrow

Three functional compartments of granulocytes are recognized in the bone marrow: (1) the proliferative or mitotic pool, consisting of myeloblasts, promyelocytes, and myelocytes; (2) the maturative or postmitotic pool consisting of metamyelocytes and band cells; and (3) the storage or reserve pool, primarily comprised of mature neutrophils and some band cells.

A neutrophil precursor in the mitotic pool generally undergoes four mitoses, one each at the myeloblast and promyelocyte stages and two at the myelocyte stage. Under certain circumstances, a mitosis may be skipped or additional mitoses may occur, giving a range of three to seven mitoses. Depending on the species, developing granulocytes spend a variable amount of time in various marrow pools before emerging into the blood (Table 13–2). Some "ineffective granulopoiesis" at the myelocyte stage (premature death of about 10% of the granulocytic precursors in the bone marrow) occurs in dogs and humans. Factors regulating granulopoiesis have been discussed (see above), and those influencing the release of marrow neutrophils into the blood are discussed here.

Table 13–2. Estimates of Various Phases of Bone Marrow Granulokinetics in Dogs and Humans

		Dogs		Humans	
Marrow Pools and Cellular Stages	*Estimated Number of Mitoses*	*Proportion of Cells (%)*	*Average Transit Time (hr)*	*Proportion of Cells (%)*	*Average Transit Time (hr)*
Proliferative pool					
Myeloblast	1	1.0	10	0.9	24
Promyelocyte	1	1.3	8	3.3	47
Myelocyte	2	13.6	30	12.7	87
Maturative pool					
Metamyelocytes	0	8.8	20	15.9	33
Band cells	0	11.9	26	12.4	58
Storage pool					
Mature neutrophils	0	6.0	50	7.4	59
Emergence time in blood					
Myeloblast to mature neutrophils			144		308
Last myelocyte to mature neutrophils			106		179

Neutrophil Release from Bone Marrow to Blood

Mature neutrophils normally emerge into the blood in about 7 to 11 days in humans, 3 to 5 days in the dog, and 4 to 6 days in the bovine. The marrow reserve of neutrophils is large enough to provide a 4- to 8-day supply in humans and about a 5-day supply in the dog. Cells from this reserve can be quickly mobilized on demand, and depletion of the reserve leads to neutropenia and a myeloid left shift in the bone marrow and possibly in the blood. For example, leukopenia induced by leukapheresis (continuous flow centrifugation of blood to obtain leukocyte-rich plasma) in dogs and horses is restored within 4 to 6 hours, primarily from the release of neutrophils from the bone marrow reserve (Gordon et al., 1986). Expansion of the mitotic pool, with increased effective granulopoiesis, leads to a sustained neutrophilia, but it manifests in about 3 to 4 days in the dog and takes longer in cattle and humans. The marrow neutrophil reserve in an animal can be estimated by injecting a minute amount of endotoxin intravenously or by administering corticosteroids and measuring the changes in neutrophil numbers in blood at specified intervals.

Neutrophil release into the blood is influenced by several factors, including marrow structure (microanatomy), anatomic location of the cells in the marrow, cell properties (e.g., cell age, deformability, and surface charge), marrow sinusoidal blood flow, cell-releasing factors, and neurohormonal factors. A specific humoral factor, the neutrophil-releasing factor or leukocytosis-promoting factor, has been found in the plasma of dogs injected intravenously with endotoxin. CSFs have been found to induce the release of marrow neutrophils into the blood. Mature neutrophils are the first to migrate because cellular deformability and motility increase with maturation and, simultaneously, the surface negative charge is reduced. Cells enter the marrow sinusoidal lumen through the endothelial cells, as opposed to passing through the intercellular junctions while traversing the vascular wall to enter the tissues.

Functional Compartments of Neutrophils in Blood Vasculature

Two functional compartments of neutrophils are recognized within the confines of the blood vessels: (1) the marginal pool, consisting of cells stuck to or rolling along the walls of small vessels; and (2) the circulating pool, consisting of cells freely circulating in the blood. The marginal pool is primarily located in the spleen, lungs, and splanchnic region, but some species differences are found. Species and age variations can occur in the size of these pools (Table 13–

Table 13–3. Blood Granulokinetic Data for Humans and Some Animals*

Species	*Label*	*TBGP*	*CGP*	*MGP*	*GTR*	*Half-Life (hr)*
Human	DF^{32}P	61	31	29	160	6.3
	^{3}H-TdR	40	22	17	87	7.6
Dog	DF^{32}P	90 ± 10	47 ± 8	43 ± 4	228 ± 40	5.2 ± 0.7
	^{3}H-TdR	75 ± 11	47 ± 8	23 ± 8	165 ± 22	7.6 ± 1.2
Cat	^{3}H-DFP	228 ± 108	78 ± 24	210 ± 91	650 ± 186	7.4 ± 1.8
Calves (aged, 187–380 days)	^{51}Cr	63 ± 15	29 ± 9	34 ± 7	124 ± 3	8.9 ± 2.9
Horse	^{51}Cr	56 ± 15	27 ± 7	29 ± 9	88 ± 15	10.5 ± 1.3

* Mean values (± 1 SD) are given for TBGP, total blood granulocyte pool ($\times 10^7$ cells/kg body weight); CGP, circulating granulocyte pool ($\times 10^7$ cells/kg body weight); MGP, marginal granulocyte pool ($\times 10^7$ cells/kg body weight); GTR, granulocyte turnover rate ($\times 10^7$ cells/kg/day).

3). In normal humans, only half of neutrophils are circulating freely, because about half are in the marginal pool. Such is also the case in dogs, calves, and horses, but in cats many more (about 2.5-fold) cells are found in the marginal pool than in the circulating pool. Neonatal calves (8 to 16 days old) have a larger total granulocyte pool than calves 6 months to 1 year old.

Neutrophils in the blood pools remain in a dynamic equilibrium. The marginal pool can be mobilized quickly under the influence of epinephrine and corticosteroids released into the circulation because of physiologic and pathologic stimuli (e.g., emotional stress, exercise, trauma, and infections). Factors involved in the margination of neutrophils include C5a, cyclic nucleotides, prostacyclin (PGI$_2$) produced by endothelial cells of the vessel wall and, more importantly, some neutrophil granule components, including leukocyte adhesion molecules. Epinephrine decreases adherence by increasing cyclic AMP production (see below, Mechanisms of Neutrophilias and Neutropenias, for additional comments). Complement-induced (C5a) adhesiveness and aggregation in vitro can be inhibited by nonsteroidal anti-inflammatory drugs (NSAIDs) (Slauson et al., 1987).

Neutrophils randomly disappear from the circulation to enter the tissues and body cavities, with an average intravascular life span of about 7 to 14 hours in different animal species and humans. This is in contrast to the long intravascular life span of erythrocytes (weeks to months) and the approximately 5- to 10-day survival of platelets, both of which normally leave the blood because of senescence. Once in tissues, neutrophils normally do not re-enter the blood to recirculate (i.e., from the marrow to blood to tissue is a one-way street). Leukemic neutrophils may, however, recirculate. With minor variations, similar observations

have been made on eosinophils, but no data are available for basophils. The tissue survival of neutrophils is normally about 2 to 3 days, but it may be considerably shorter under pathologic conditions.

Mechanisms of Neutrophilias and Neutropenias

It should be clear from this discussion that the blood neutrophil count obtained at any given time accounts only for freely circulating cells. The dynamics of production and release from the bone marrow, the intravascular distribution, and the egress from blood to tissues can influence the neutrophil count in conditions of health and disease. The blood neutrophil count is basically influenced by one or more of the following mechanisms: (1) the rate of granulopoiesis; (2) the inflow rate of cells from the bone marrow; (3) a shift of cells between the circulating and marginal pools; (4) the intravascular life span of cells; and (5) the outflow rate of cells from blood to tissues.

Thus, a neutrophilia results from an increased shift of cells from the marginal pool, a decreased migration of cells into tissues, and increased marrow release and production of neutrophils. Conversely, a neutropenia occurs from an increased shift of cells in the marginal pool, a decreased intravascular survival, accelerated migration into tissue, and reduced marrow release and production of neutrophils. Such changes may occur under various physiologic and pathologic conditions and manifest as acute or chronic neutrophilia and neutropenia (Table 13–4 and Fig. 13–4). Dysgranulopoiesis (morphologic abnormalities of neutrophils) may occur in conjunction with abnormalities of neutrophil production.

Epinephrine, released during various forms of acute physical and emotional stress, causes a transient neu-

Table 13–4. Neutrophil Kinetics in Certain Clinical and Experimental Situations*

| Cause | Blood Pools | | | Blood Half-Life | Marrow | |
	CGP	MGP	TBGP		Production	Release
Epinephrine	I	D	NC	NC	NC	NC
Etiocholanolone	I	I	I	NC	NC	I
Corticosteroids						
Acute	I	I	I	I	NC	I
Sustained	I	I	I	I	NC/I	NC/I
Endotoxin						
Early phase	D	I	NC	NC	NC	NC
Intermediate phase	I	I	I	NC	NC	I
Late phase	I	I	I	NC	I	I
Infection						
Initial phase	NC/D	I	NC	D	NC	NC
Intermediate phase	NC	I/NC	I	NC/I	NC	I
Established	I	I	I	NC/I	I	I
Chronic granulocytic leukemia	I	I	I	I	I	I
Hypersplenism						
Shift neutropenia	D	I	NC/I	NC/I	NC	NC/I
True neutropenia	D	I	D	NC/D (rare)	D	D
Immune-mediated neutropenia	D	D	D	D	NC/I	I

* CGP, circulating granulocyte pool; MGP, marginal granulocyte pool; TBGP, total blood granulocyte pool; I, increase; D, decrease; NC, no change. Peripheral blood neutrophilia is indicated by I in CGP and neutropenia by D in CGP.

MECHANISMS OF SOME NEUTROPHILIAS AND NEUTROPENIAS

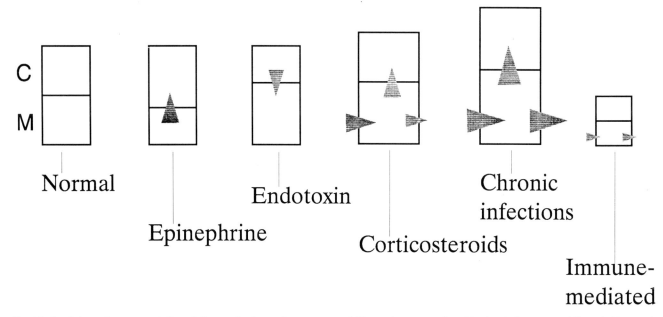

Fig. 13–4. Schematic representation of the mechanisms of some neutrophilias and neutropenias. (C, circulating neutrophil pool; M, marginal neutrophil pool). The arrowheads indicate the direction of cell movement and their size represents the relative magnitude of cell entry or exit. The arrows on the left side of the lower boxes represent entry of cells from the bone marrow, and those on the right side indicate cells leaving blood to enter tissues. See text for details of cell movements associated with the various examples shown.

trophilia by shifting cells from the marginal pool into the circulating pool. This response is mediated through the β-adrenergic effect of epinephrine, which causes the release of cyclic AMP from endothelial cells and thereby decreases neutrophil adherence to vessel walls. This demargination of neutrophils is often accompanied by lymphocytosis, and sometimes by monocytosis and eosinophilia. The epinephrine response is more common in young animals than in adults.

Glucocorticoids, endogenous or exogenous, cause neutrophilia primarily by inducing the increased release of neutrophils from the bone marrow reserve and decreasing the egress of neutrophils from the circulation, and partly by shifting cells from the marginal pool. Associated changes in the differential leukocyte count include lymphopenia, eosinopenia, and monocytopenia or monocytosis. These effects usually last for less than 24 hours, but continuous endogenous release or the long-term administration of corticosteroids results in sustained changes in leukocyte numbers, particularly eosinophilia and lymphopenia (Wong et al., 1992). The magnitude of the neutrophilia, however, is diminished in such cases.

The intravenous administration of endotoxin produces a marked neutropenia within minutes, followed by a rebound neutrophilia within a few hours (Table 13–5). "Toxic" changes such as cytoplasmic foaminess and vacuolation of neutrophils, lymphopenia, and

thrombocytopenia may also occur. The neutropenia results from cell margination and sequestration in the microvasculature, primarily in the lungs. Various mechanisms include the direct action of endotoxin (lipid A moiety of the lipopolysaccharide) on neutrophils and the release or generation of C5a, thromboxane (TxA$_2$), leukotriene B$_4$, plasma kallikrein, leukocyte adherence proteins, and lactoferrin. Studies have shown that the tumor necrosis factor is an early-acting pivotal mediator of the effects of endotoxin in humans and animals (MacKay et al., 1991; Morris and Moore, 1991; Waage et al., 1991). Similarly increased plasma levels of cathepsin G released from neutrophils may contribute to endotoxic shock (Bjork et al., 1991). The rebound neutrophilia, with or without left shift, results from the increased release of cells from the bone marrow pools mediated by a neutrophil-releasing factor. The magnitude of the left shift depends on the severity of the endotoxin insult. Subsequently, granulopoiesis is stimulated by the endotoxin-induced increased elaboration of GM-CSF and/or G-CSF and contributes to blood neutrophilia. Gram-negative bacterial infections produce severe neutropenia and neutrophilia, generally through similar mechanisms. An important additional contributory factor in such cases, however, is the local demand for neutrophils to combat infection.

Pseudoneutropenia results from a greater distribu-

Table 13–5. Changes in Peripheral Blood Leukocyte Numbers of Cows Given an Intravenous Injection of Escherichia coli Endotoxin

Endotoxin (μg)	Time (hr)	Cells/μl of Blood			
		Leukocyte Count	Immature Neutrophils*	Mature Neutrophils	Lymphocytes
5	0	7,200	0	2,376	3,924
	1	6,300	0	1,922	3,348
	2	5,500	0	2,117	3,080
	4	10,500	0	6,247	3,150
	6	10,500	0	5,652	3,780
	8	10,500	0	5,774	3,622
	10	8,100	0	3,888	3,280
	24	7,600	0	2,584	3,914
20	0	7,100	71 B	2,023	4,012
	1	6,000	0	1,920	3,600
	2	5,600	0	2,352	2,968
	4	7,600	0	3,876	2,850
	6	8,500	0	3,995	3,570
	8	8,600	0	3,569	4,042
	10	8,000	40 B	2,920	4,120
	24	6,800	0	1,530	4,352
50	0	8,100	0	3,078	4,212
	1	4,000	0	1,480	2,420
	2	2,300	58 B	402	1,610
	4	2,400	24 B	588	1,584
	6	3,500	70 B	1,015	2,152
	8	4,700	47 B	1,692	2,585
	10	5,300	26 B	1,404	3,418
	24	5,800	29 B	1,218	3,973
100	0	8,900	0	1,691	5,295
	1	1,700	0	68	1,496
	2	2,300	80 Mt	69	1,898
	4	1,600	16 B	80	1,336
	6	1,700	17 B	153	1,317
	8	3,900	468 Mt	643	2,281
	10	6,800	1632 Mt	1,088	3,366
	24	11,600	2088 Mt	3,422	5,104

From Jain, N.C., and Lasmanis, J.: Leucocytic changes in cows given intravenous injections of Escherichia coli endotoxin. Res. Vet. Sci., 24:386, 1978.
* Left shift involving B, band cells; Mt. metamyelocytes.

tion of cells in the marginal pool, rather than being present in the circulating pool. Consequently, a persistently low neutrophil count may be found, but generally without features of ill health. Neutropenia resulting from a disorder of neutrophil release from the bone marrow that contains abundant myeloid precursors and mature neutrophils is called myelokathexis.

Cyclic neutropenia in grey collie dogs results from a hereditary, defective regulation of the hematopoietic pluripotent stem cell (see Chapter 4). Treatment with G-CSF abrogated cyclic neutropenic episodes, but did not correct the cellular defects such as reduced myeloperoxidase activity in neutrophils and platelet functional defects (Pratt et al., 1990).

A genetic deficiency of neutrophil FcRIII-1 was found to be the cause of an isoimmune neutropenia in a human newborn because the mother had produced antibodies against neutrophil FcRIII during pregnancy (Huizinga et al., 1990).

LYSOSOMAL GRANULES OF NEUTROPHILS AND THEIR CONSTITUENTS

Neutrophil granules contain various biochemical substances of biologic importance (Table 13–1). The various enzymatic and nonenzymatic constituents might be located in different subpopulations of azurophilic and specific granules. Species differences in granule type, structure, and biochemical constituents have been found. For example, bovine neutrophils have little lysozyme and chicken neutrophils (heterophils) lack MPO and catalase. In the bovine, cationic proteins and lactoferrin are found in a large granule type that differs from both azurophilic and specific granules. Several functions have been ascribed to the granule contents. Various bactericidal substances can act synergistically, and species differences are found in the relative importance of various factors.

Myeloperoxidase, present in the primary granules, is of the utmost importance in bactericidal action (see below, Microbicidal Activity). Its color imparts a greenish hue to pus. Alkaline phosphatase is present in neutrophils of humans and many animal species, but absent from canine and feline neutrophils. Its functional significance is uncertain, but a diagnostic significance in myeloid leukemias has been established. Human neutrophils generally exhibit low ALP activity in chronic myelogenous leukemia, whereas increased enzyme activity occurs during leukocytosis from infections and sometimes also during the blast crisis of chronic myelogenous leukemia. Conversely, neutrophilic ALP activity is almost invariably increased in the dog and cat during acute and chronic myelogenous and myelomonocytic leukemias. The enzyme activity is usually found in blast cells and their progeny, but rarely in mature neutrophils.

Lysozyme is present in both primary and secondary granules. This enzyme exerts a lytic action, particularly on gram-negative bacteria, after the microorganisms have been acted on by specific antibodies and complement.

Several cationic proteins have been isolated from neutrophil granules; some of these proteins are bactericidal and some are involved in the initiation and maintenance of acute inflammation. The antimicrobial cationic proteins associated with azurophilic granules of human neutrophils include defensins, cathepsin G, azuocidin (MW 29,000 to 37,000 daltons), and a bacterial permeability increasing protein (Lehrer and Ganz, 1990; Spitznagal, 1990; Valore and Ganz, 1992). Defensins are a group of low molecular weight (MW 3,000 to 4,000 daltons) bactericidal peptides containing about 30 amino acids with broad antimicrobial, antiviral, and cytotoxic activities (Ganz et al., 1990). Bacterial permeability-increasing protein (MW 55,000 to 58,000 daltons) is bactericidal for certain gram-negative bacteria. Several bactericidal peptides have been found in bovine neutrophils (Selsted et al., 1992). Two highly cationic proteins, termed bactenecins, have been purified from the large granules of bovine neutrophils and shown to have a potent in vitro antimicrobial activity (Frank et al., 1990; Zanetti et al., 1990). The precise mechanism of action of these bactericidal proteins is unknown, but defensins may act by inserting into biological membranes, generating pores, and inducing injury to DNA (Gera and Litchtenstein, 1991; Litchtenstein, 1991).

Lactoferrin, present in specific granules, is generally bacteriostatic because it binds the iron necessary for bacterial growth, but it may sometimes be bactericidal. Lactoferrin also increases neutrophil adherence and inhibits granulopoiesis. Lactoferrin deficiency in a dog with chronic granulocytic leukemia was considered to enhance GM-CSF synthesis and in turn granulocytic and monocytic proliferation (Thomsen et al., 1991a).

Several neutral and acid proteases have been obtained from neutrophil granules; they have bactericidal activity and a tissue-destroying capability. Elastase and collagenase facilitate the migration of neutrophils through the extracellular matrix and cause tissue injury during inflammation.

Receptors for the chemotactic peptide formyl-methionyl-leucyl-phenylalanine (FMLP), C3b, C3bi, and laminin have been localized in the membranes of specific granules. Species differences exist with regard to the presence of FMLP receptors. For example, human, non-human primate, rabbit, and rat neutrophils have FMLP receptors, but those from cows, pigs, and dogs lack such receptors and neutrophils from horses have little or no FMLP receptors (Fletcher et al., 1990). These receptors can be translocated to the plasma membrane following degranulation and potentiate neutrophil chemotactic and phagocytic activities. Similarly, leukocyte adhesion molecules have been found in the membranes of specific and tertiary granules.

NEUTROPHIL FUNCTIONS

The primary function of neutrophils is phagocytosis and the killing of microorganisms. Thus, serious infections follow severe neutropenia or functional defects of neutrophils. Neutrophils have also been found to initiate and modify the magnitude and duration of acute inflammatory processes, as shown by observations on laboratory animals and experimental studies on coliform mastitis in cows (Jain, 1986). Neutrophils can also cause tissue damage and exert cytotoxic effects, such as antibody-mediated parasiticidal and tumoricidal activities. The release of endogenous bioactive substances or their production by neutrophils has been recognized (e.g., release of neutrophil endogenous pyrogen and leukocyte adhesion molecules). Activated neutrophils have been found to secrete cytokines like tumor necrosis factor, G-CSF, and M-CSF (Djeu et al., 1990). A role in coagulation (through the production of prostaglandins and TxA_2) and fibrinolysis (through the activation of plasminogen) has also been suggested.

The role of neutrophils in maintaining normal health can best be understood by following the sequence of events that can occur after local infection with staphylococci or coliform bacteria. Initially, bacterial toxins elaborated locally and chemical substances released from damaged tissues increase vascular permeability, leading to the leakage of plasma proteins and the accumulation of leukocytes, predominantly neutrophils, in the inflamed area. Subsequently, the release of chemical substances from damaged or dying neutrophils, as well as the generation of activated complement components, accentuate the inflammatory process. With time, the phagocytic and bactericidal activities of infiltrating neutrophils and monocytes and the actions of antibody and activated complement components control the bacterial growth. The reaction subsides and recovery follows.

Several steps are involved in the functional response of neutrophils to control infection; the same events generally occur when monocytes act similarly. These steps include adhesion, chemotaxis, opsonization, phagocytosis, degranulation, microbicidal action, and exocytosis. In vitro techniques are available for evaluating these steps. Specific defects at each of these steps, leading to functional abnormalities of neutrophils, have been recognized in humans and are being found in animals. Recurrent infections, particularly with otherwise saprophytic microorganisms, are common signs of neutrophil function defects in such patients (Williams et al., 1990; Zinkl, 1989).

Receptor-Ligand Interactions and Signal Transduction

Signal transduction mechanisms involve a series of complex biochemical processes that are initiated after receptor-ligand interactions or some other direct perturbation of the cell membrane (Fig. 13–5). These mechanisms constitute the initial step in the stimulation of neutrophils, leading to cell movement, secretion of lysosomal contents, or execution of various functions (Morel et al., 1991). The neutrophil plasma membrane contains guanine nucleotide-binding proteins, phospholipase C, adenylate cyclase, protein kinase C, and other components necessary for signal transduction. Binding of a specific ligand to the surface receptor leads to conformational changes in the receptor protein and to activation of the accompanying G protein. The activated G protein then activates phospholipase C to cleave endogenous phosphatidylinositol biphosphate (PIP_2), yielding diacylglycerol (DAC) and inositol triphosphate (IP_3). The IP_3 releases calcium from bound intracellular locations to raise the levels of intracellular free calcium. The latter increase is augmented by an influx of calcium from the extracellular space, an event also mediated by IP_3. DAC, in concert with elevated free calcium or calcium-calmodulin complex, activates protein kinase C. The activated protein kinase C then relocates in the plasma membrane to phosphorylate the proteins essential for functional activities. An elevation in the intracellular free calcium level can also induce a discharge of lysosomal contents into the extracellular space; this process is promoted

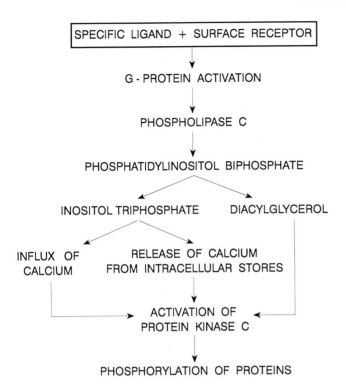

Fig. 13–5. Outline of receptor-ligand interaction and signal transduction mechanisms. See text for details.

by guanosine triphosphate (GTP). The tyrosine kinase signaling pathway is also involved in the activation of selective functional responses of neutrophils, e.g., chemotaxis and superoxide production (Naccache et al., 1990).

Inhibitors and promoters of signal transduction mechanisms acting at different levels of biochemical processes have been described (Krause and Lew, 1988). Interestingly, neonatal bovine neutrophils are deficient in respiratory burst activity because of the altered action of protein kinase C (Doré et al., 1991). Priming of neutrophils by GM-CSF for enhanced leukotriene synthesis by activation of a phospholipase A_2 appears to be mediated by action of protein kinase C (Schatz-Munding and Ullrich, 1992).

Adherence

The extravasation of neutrophils (diapedesis) begins shortly after microbial infection and is normally followed by chemotactic attraction toward the organism and its phagocytic destruction. During diapedesis, circulating neutrophils first adhere or marginate along the altered venular endothelial surface, emigrate through intracellular junctions, cross the basement membrane, and enter the tissue.

The adhesion of neutrophils to the vascular endothelium and extravasation are largely influenced by the integrin family of cell surface adhesion molecules (Arnaout, 1990; Suzuki et al., 1991; Yong and Khawja, 1990). Three major adhesion molecules have been recognized, LFA-1, Mac-1, and p150,95 (Fig. 13–6). Each of these proteins is a heterodimer containing a unique α subunit (CD11a, CD11b, and CD11c, respectively) complexed to a common β subunit (CD18). The membranes of specific and tertiary granules contain Mac-1 and possibly p150,95 molecules, which on degranulation can be transferred to the plasma membrane. A second class of adhesion protein, granule membrane protein 140 (gp100 or GMP-140) recognized by monoclonal antibody MEL-14, has been defined on human and murine neutrophils and lymphocytes (Berg and James, 1990). It is involved in initial adherence of neutrophils to endothelial cells in inflamed areas and in adherence of lymphocytes to high endothelial cells in lymph node venules. Rapid shedding of gp100 antigen during neutrophil activation appears to be necessary for neutrophil extravasation to inflammatory sites. The capacity of the endothelium to promote adhesion of neutrophils is increased by endotoxins and cytokines, such as tumor necrosis factor-alpha and IL-1, and is inhibited by another cytokine, transforming growth factor-beta (Gamble and Vadas, 1988).

A genetic absence of these adhesion molecules in Holstein cattle and Irish setters (see below, Functional Abnormalities) has been associated with reduced migration of neutrophils in tissues, defective neutrophil functions (adherence, chemotaxis, phagocytosis, and cytotoxicity), and a susceptibility to recurrent infections. Characteristic hematologic findings in leukocyte adhesion molecule deficiency include persistent neutrophilia, granulocytic hyperplasia in marrow, and paucity of neutrophils in inflammatory lesions.

Adherence is also promoted by many other factors, including cyclic nucleotides, divalent cations, prostaglandins and TxB_2, activated complement component C5a, fibronectin, platelet-activating factor, and substances released from the specific granules of neutrophils (e.g., lactoferrin). Neutrophils can synthesize or release stored fibronectin.

Chemotaxis

Chemotaxis is defined as a directional movement of the leukocyte toward a particulate target (e.g., bacteria) under the influence of a concentration gradient of chemotactic substances in the environment. In comparison, chemokinesis is defined as an enhanced, nondirectional (random) movement. Chemotaxis is an active process and involves the participation of cytoskeletal components such as microfilaments, microtubules, and perhaps other motility proteins, such as myosin. A motile neutrophil has a broad leading edge of cytoplasm (lamellipodium) that is almost devoid of lysosomal granules, and a knob-like uropod having many long, refractile filaments (Fig. 13–7). The nucleus is located toward the posterior end, whereas most of the cytoplasm and granules are in front of the nucleus but behind the lamellipodium. Chemotaxis involves the interaction of chemotactic factors with

ADHESION MOLECULES

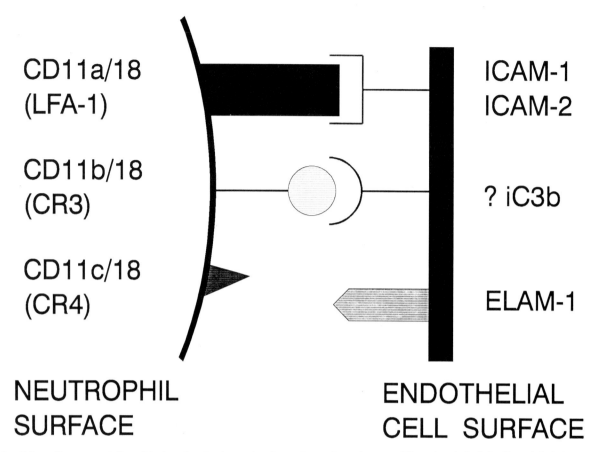

CD11a/18
(LFA-1)

CD11b/18
(CR3)

CD11c/18
(CR4)

ICAM-1
ICAM-2

? iC3b

ELAM-1

NEUTROPHIL
SURFACE

ENDOTHELIAL
CELL SURFACE

Fig. 13–6. Schematic representation of leukocyte adhesion molecules on the surface of neutrophils and endothelial cells and their interactions. The neutrophil surface has three major adhesion molecules, CD11a/18, CD11b/18, and CD11c/18. Functionally, these molecules are recognized as a lymphocyte function-associated antigen (LFA-1), complement receptor 3 (CR3 or Mac-1) and complement receptor 4 (CR4 or p150,95), respectively. Similarly, the endothelial surface presents a number of adhesion molecules. (ICAM-1, ICAM-2, intercellular adhesion molecules 1 and 2; iC3b, receptor for inactivated complement component C3b; ELAM-1, endothelial leukocyte adhesion molecule 1). The reciprocal interaction of two of the adhesion molecules is apparent.

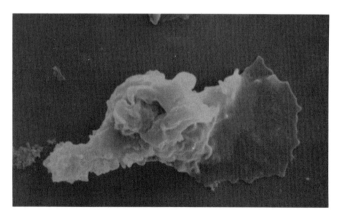

Fig. 13–7. Scanning electron photomicrograph of a motile equine neutrophil. The moving front end of the cell (lamellipodium) uniquely displays a wide zone of thinly spread agranular cytoplasm, and the tail end (uropod) is characterized by a knobby process with an irregular surface. The body of the cell has a highly ruffled surface membrane, with some scattered villous processes ($\times 9261$).

specific cell surface receptors, which induce signal transduction and lead to directional orientation and locomotion of the cell. Neutrophils with impaired deformability and abnormalities in cytoskeletal proteins show depressed chemotaxis.

Various chemotactic substances, referred to as cytotaxins, may be generated endogenously or exogenously (Harvath, 1991). These include plasma factors, particularly complement components (C5a and C567 complex) and kallikrein, bacterial products, particularly N-formyl methionyl peptides (FMLP) and toxins, viruses, arachidonic acid metabolites (prostaglandin Es and leukotriene B_4), some leukocyte and platelet products (lymphokines, platelet factor 4, and platelet-derived growth factor), mast cell products (platelet-activating factor), IgG and IgM fragments, and substances released from damaged tissues. Several types of cells, e.g., monocytes, produce a neutrophil activating peptide-1 (NAP-1), now termed IL-8, in response to inflammatory stimuli, which acts as a neutrophil attractant for extravasation of neutrophils during an inflammatory response (Baggiolini et al., 1989; Rot 1991). IL-8 activates most of the neutrophil functions in different species (Thomsen et al., 1991b). Species differences have been found in the chemotactic response to FMLP; human, non-human primate, rabbit, and rat neutrophils are chemotactically responsive, equine neutrophils may exhibit weak or no chemotaxis, and canine, feline, bovine, and porcine neutrophils do not respond (Fletcher et al., 1990; Stickle et al., 1985; Trowald-Wigh and Thoren-Tolling, 1990). A deficiency of chemotactic factors or the presence of substances interfering with chemotaxis can potentiate infection. Chemotactic factor inhibitors are found in plasma, or are produced locally by invading bacteria and tissue cells or infiltrating leukocytes. Drug-induced impairment of neutrophil motility may occur (e.g., by corticosteroids). In parturient cows, chemotactic activity is high at 2 weeks before parturition, highest on the day of parturition, and markedly decreased by the first week of parturition (Kehrli et al., 1989a; Romaniuka and Branicin, 1986). Lymphocyte function may also be impaired during the periparturient period (Kehrli et al., 1989b).

Phagocytosis and Degranulation

Phagocytosis is an active process of ingestion of a microscopic particle by the leukocyte through the extension of cytoplasmic pseudopods around the target. Pinocytosis refers to the internalization of a fluid vesicle by living cells. The two processes constitute endocytosis.

Neutrophils ingest rapidly dividing invasive or pyogenic bacteria, and mononuclear phagocytes ingest facultative or obligate intracellular microorganisms, such as Mycobacteria and Listeria. The phagocytosis of viruses, certain protozoa, and other cells by neutrophils has also been studied. Immature cells such as band neutrophils and metamyelocytes are phagocytically less active, whereas neutrophilic myelocytes and less mature precursors are almost nonfunctional in host defense.

Phagocytosis is influenced by various physical and chemical properties of both the phagocyte and particle, and it is also affected by environmental conditions. Functional heterogeneity of morphologically mature neutrophils is an important emerging concept, which holds that segmented neutrophils with similar cytomorphologic attributes may exhibit marked variations in antigenic expression and function (Jain et al., 1991b; Kabbur et al., 1991; Krause et al., 1986, 1990). Phagocytosis, like chemotaxis, is an active process that requires energy (ATP) generated through anaerobic glycolysis. It occurs rapidly and most efficiently at a pH of 6 to 8 and at a temperature of 37° to 40°C. Probably the most important and extensively studied promoters of phagocytosis are the plasma factors known as opsonins. Opsonins coat the surface of bacteria and other foreign particles, altering their surface properties and thereby rendering them more liable to undergo phagocytosis. Tuftsin, a strongly basic tetrapeptide fragment from the Fc region of IgG, similarly binds to the sialic acid residues on neutrophils, rather than particles, and enhances their phagocytic ability.

Opsonins may be specific (antibodies) or nonspecific (complement and α- and β-globulins). The phagocytosis of streptococci, smooth gram-negative bacteria, and capsulated bacteria such as pneumococci is limited in the absence of specific opsonins. Neutrophils, monocytes, and macrophages have surface receptors for IgG, C3b (CR1), and C3bi (CR3). Thus, particles coated with these substances are readily phagocytosed. Leukocytes may differ regarding the presence of these receptors. For example, bovine neutrophils, but not monocytes, have been found to have IgM receptors also, and IgG2 has been found to be the major opsonin in bovine serum, whereas IgG1 promotes neither neutrophil adherence nor phagocytosis in the cow (Miller et al, 1988). Serums and colostrums of cows vaccinated with E. coli J5 bacterin have higher opsonic activity, which correlates with higher serum IgM titer to E. coli J5 whole cell antigen (Hogan et al., 1992a). Corticosteroids inhibit phagocytosis by interfering with the binding of opsonized bacteria to C3b and/or Fc receptors. The phagocytic ability of bovine and equine uterine neutrophils is influenced by nonspecific opsonins present in the uterine fluid (Liu and Cheung, 1986; Watson, 1985).

Viable neutrophils recognize bacteria through differences in surface properties and/or their opsonic receptors. They instantaneously undergo metabolic stimulation, advance cytoplasmic processes (pseudopods) to entrap the bacteria, and then internalize them (Fig. 13–8). Fusion of the pseudopods around the bacterium results in the formation of a phagocytic vacuole or phagosome containing the organism. This restricted intracellular environment is created to destroy the engulfed pathogens selectively through the discharge of lysosomal contents and the generation of lethal oxygen metabolites within the confines of the phagosome (Figs. 13–9 and 13–10).

Phagocytic stimulation causes increases in aerobic and anaerobic glycolysis and oxygen consumption, a process referred to as the metabolic burst. This metabolic burst promotes activities necessary for destroying the ingested bacteria, particularly through the generation of oxygen metabolites—superoxide anions, hydrogen peroxide (H_2O_2), hydroxyl radicals, and singlet oxygen (Fig. 13–11). The production of oxygen metabolites can be measured by the nitro blue tetrazolium (NBT) reduction test and by detecting chemiluminescence (emission of light). Phagocytically active neutrophils convert yellow, soluble NBT to insoluble, blue-black deposits of formazan on the phagosomal membrane (Fig. 13–10).

Microbicidal Activity

Lysosomal granules in the vicinity of the phagocytic vacuoles fuse with the vacuolar membrane to form a

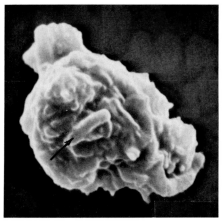 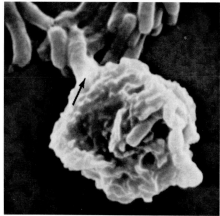

Fig. 13–8. Scanning electron photomicrographs of the phagocytosis of opsonized *Escherichia coli* by bovine blood neutrophils after 1 minute. Partially ingested bacteria are clearly visible. Note individual bacteria in the process of being ingested, as evident from a veil of cell cytoplasm *(arrows)* over the bacterial surface (× 6000). (From Jain, N.C.: Schalm's Veterinary Hematology. 4th Ed. Philadelphia, Lea & Febiger, 1986, p. 703.)

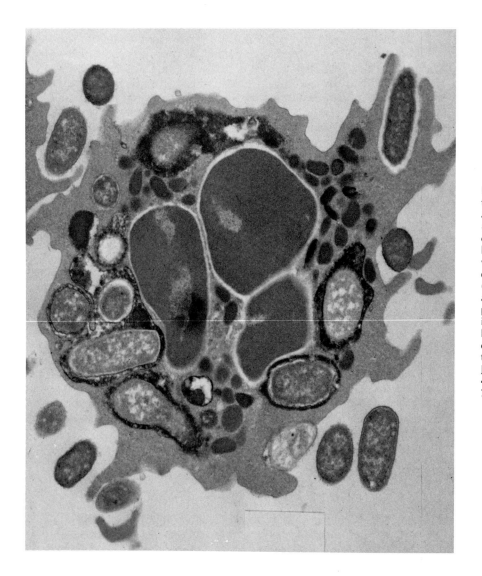

Fig. 13–9. Phagocytic and bactericidal activities of a bovine blood neutrophil that was allowed to interact with opsonized *Escherichia coli* for 1 minute. Active phagocytosis of extracellular bacteria as well as intracellular organisms are clearly evident. The cell was stained for peroxidase to delineate the degranulation of peroxidase-positive primary (dark-stained) granules and peroxidase-negative specific (light-stained) granules. The presence of dark-stained material surrounding several bacteria indicates the degranulation of primary granules within the confines of phagocytic vacuoles (transmission electron photomicrograph, × 16,800). (From Jain, N.C.: Schalm's Veterinary Hematology. 4th Ed. Philadelphia, Lea & Febiger, 1986, p. 704.)

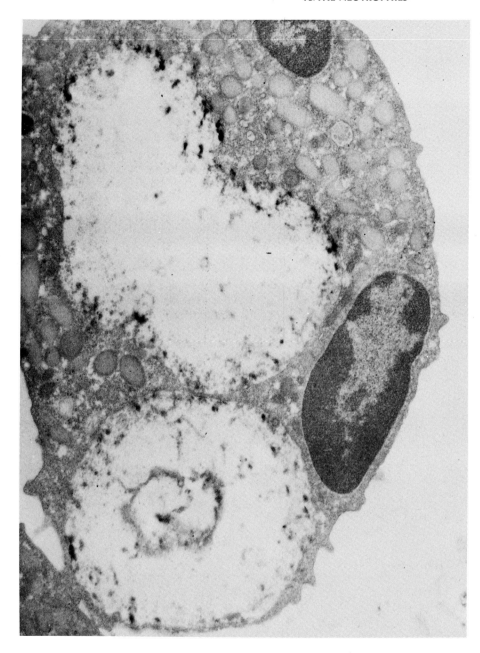

Fig. 13–10. Nitro blue tetrazolium (NBT) reduction in a bovine blood neutrophil that has phagocytized two opsonized zymogen particles. The sites of NBT reduction are evident as electron-dense, irregular specks, principally along the periphery of phagocytic vacuoles containing zymogen particles. Lysosomal granules are scattered throughout the cytoplasm of the cell (transmission electron photomicrograph, ×24,000). (From Jain, N.C.: Schalm's Veterinary Hematology. 4th Ed. Philadelphia, Lea & Febiger, 1986, p. 705.)

phagolysosome and release their contents therein to kill and digest the bacteria (Fig. 13–9). The specific and azurophilic granules undergo degranulation sequentially or randomly as soon as 5 seconds after the phagocytic event. Microtubules and microfilaments seem to be essential for the phagocytosis of larger particles (Escherichia coli), whereas only microfilaments are needed for the ingestion of smaller particles (Staphylococcus aureus and Streptococcus agalactiae) (Silva and Jain, 1989). Selective degranulation occurs with the ingestion of bacteria because it involves only granules coming in contact with the phagocytic vacuole, whereas generalized degranulation of the cell follows endocytosis of exotoxin or endotoxin.

Phagocytized bacteria are destroyed by neutrophils by different mechanisms that are broadly categorized as oxygen-independent or oxygen-dependent (Table 13–6). Both mechanisms act in concert to kill and destroy bacteria. Oxygen-independent microbicidal mechanisms include an acidic environment in the phagocytic vacuole and the presence of granule-associated substances such as cationic proteins, lactoferrin, lysozyme, and various proteases and other hydrolytic enzymes. Granule-associated substances are also operative under anaerobic conditions. The mechanisms of actions of some of these substances are briefly discussed (see the section on lysosomal granules of neutrophils and their constituents above).

Increased glucose utilization through the pentose phosphate pathway, enhanced respiratory activity, and the activation of membrane NADPH oxidase constitute the postphagocytic metabolic burst or respiratory

Table 13–6. Microbicidal Mechanisms in Neutrophils

Oxygen-dependent
    Myeloperoxidase-dependent: myeloperoxidase-H_2O_2-halide complex
Myeloperoxidase-independent
   H_2O_2
   Superoxide anion
   Hydroxyl radical
   Singlet oxygen
Oxygen-independent
   Acidity in phagosomes
   Lysosomal constitutents
      Cationic proteins—defensins, cathepsin G, azuocidin, bactenecins, "bacterial permeability increasing protein"
      Phagocytin and leukin
      Lysozyme
      Lactoferrin
      Proteases (cathepsins D, E)
      Phospholipase A_2

burst. Consequently, many oxygen metabolites with antibacterial activity are produced; these include the superoxide anion, H_2O_2, hydroxyl radicals, and singlet oxygen (Farber et al., 1990; Morel et al., 1991). The H_2O_2 complexes with MPO and a halide such as chloride to form a potent bactericidal system—the MPO-H_2O_2-halide (Fig. 13–11). This complex kills various bacteria, viruses, mycoplasmata, and fungi, and destroys antibody-coated red cells. Bacterial killing by the MPO-H_2O_2-halide complex is thought to occur through halogenation, deamination, and decarboxylation of the microbial proteins and nucleic acids. Singlet oxygen and hydroxyl radicals kill bacteria through lipid peroxidation, inner mitochondrial membrane damage, and oxidative damage to nucleic acid. Hypochloride, a reactive oxidant formed as an end product of the respiratory burst in activated neutrophils, is bactericidal and has been implicated in neutrophil-mediated tissue injury associated with the inflammatory process (Bernofsky et al., 1991).

Neutrophils and bacteria protect themselves against the toxic effects of various oxygen metabolites and other oxidants in several ways (Fig. 13–11). Superoxide dismutase prevents damage from superoxide anions, converting them to H_2O_2 at an accelerated rate. The glutathione system (reduced glutathione, glutathione peroxidase, and glutathione reductase) and catalase regulate the amount of intracellular H_2O_2 by converting it to water. Thus, catalase-positive bacteria are resistant to the killing effects of the MPO-H_2O_2-halide complex, but catalase-negative organisms are readily

Phagocytosis Stimulates Membrane Receptors

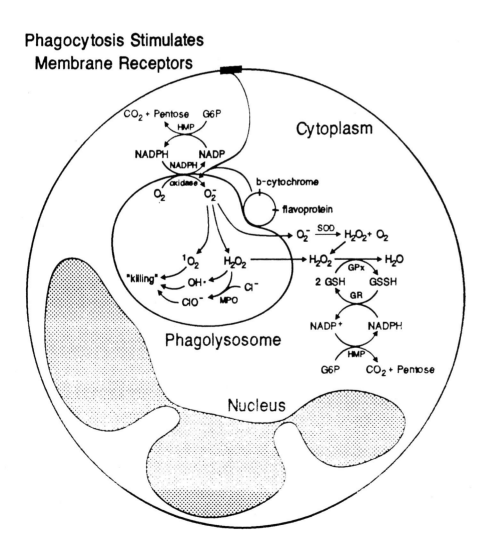

Fig. 13–11. Biochemical events associated with metabolic burst. (From Zinkl, J.G.: Leukocyte function. *In* Clinical Biochemistry of Domestic Animals. 4th Ed. Edited by J.J. Kaneko. San Diego, Academic Press, 1989, p. 321, Abbreviations used: ClO^-, hypochloride; G6P, glucose 6-phosphate; GPx, glutathione peroxidase; GR, glutathione reductase; GSH, reduced glutathione; GSSG, oxidized glutathione; H_2O_2, hydrogen peroxide; HMP, hexose monophosphate shunt; MPO, myeloperoxidase; NADP, nicotinamide adenine dinucleotide phosphate; NADPH, reduced nicotinamide adenine dinucleotide phosphate; O_2^-, superoxide anion; $^1O_2$, singlet oxygen; $OH\cdot$, hydroxyl radical; SOD, superoxide dismutase.

destroyed. Defensins are antibacterial, cytotoxic, and chemotactic and participate in host defense and inflammatory processes. In inflamed tissues, alpha$_2$-macroglobulin may act as a scavenger of defensins and other inflammatory peptides and may constitute an important mechanism for the regulation of inflammation (Panyutich and Ganz, 1991).

Different bactericidal systems may be active against different types of bacteria and some types of bacteria may escape destruction by neutrophils. In certain diseases, this function of the neutrophil and monocyte may be impaired, such as in chronic granulomatous disease and Chédiak-Higashi and granulocytopathy syndromes (see below, Functional Abnormalities).

Substances that would increase the phagocytic and/or bactericidal efficiency of neutrophils are being investigated. Various cytokines influence these and other neutrophil functions and appear to provide an upcoming mode of treatment to augment host defense against microbial infections. For example, injection of interferon-gamma increases bactericidal activity of neutrophils of some human patients with chronic granulomatous disease (Gallin and Malech, 1990). Neutrophils from cows injected with vitamin E showed greater intracellular killing of bacteria at calving than neutrophils from placebo-injected cows, although the degree of phagocytosis did not differ (Hogan et al., 1992b).

Exocytosis

Exocytosis refers to the extracellular discharge of cellular contents through the fusion of phagocytic vacuoles with the cell membrane. Killed bacteria, products of degraded bacteria, or neutrophil granules or their contents may be exocytosed. Discharge of granular contents into the environment may follow mere activation of the neutrophil membrane—that is, it can occur in the absence of phagocytosis. Neutrophils exposed to an antineutrophil antibody and complement become leaky, undergo osmotic swelling, and discharge granule contents to the exterior (Jain et al., 1991c).

Inflammation and Tissue Injury

Studies on acute inflammation have indicated that the early vascular response to a bacterial infection and other injuries is often biphasic. The initial increase in vascular permeability, which leads to edema, is mainly the result of the local release of one or more of the endogenous mediators—histamine, serotonin, bradykinin, kallikrein, and other less defined factors—depending on the animal species. In addition, a number of plasma-derived and cell-derived factors may be involved. The former group includes complement components, particularly C5a. The latter group includes factors from neutrophils (lysosomal constituents), lymphocytes (lymphokines), monocytes (mon-

okines), mast cells (platelet-activating factor), and platelets and endothelial cells (arachidonic acid metabolites).

Mechanisms for the delayed phase of increase in vascular permeability and leukocyte migration into tissue are complex and have not been clearly defined. Delayed vascular permeability may involve the continual production of many of the same stimuli incriminated in the initial phase of inflammation. Leukocyte emigration may involve other mechanisms, however, because factors such as histamine, serotonin, bradykinin, and kallikrein exert little or no such effect. Secretion of IL-8 by endothelial cells seems to be important in regulating the transvenular traffic of neutrophils during acute inflammatory process (Huber et al., 1991).

The local accumulation of neutrophils and the release of their products play an important part in initiating vascular permeability and other forms of tissue injury in acute inflammation (Anderson et al., 1991; Jain, 1986). Neutrophils are associated with the development of severe tissue injury as in the Schwartzman and Arthus phenomena; neutropenic animals fail to develop tissue injury compared to control animals. Similarly, compared to normal lactating cows, neutropenic lactating cows develop only a mild, acute inflammation in the mammary gland during the early phase of acute coliform mastitis. Severe inflammatory reaction and tissue injury develop during the later stage when neutropenia is no longer in existence and neutrophils migrate in increasing numbers into the inflamed mammary gland (Jain 1986). Furthermore, intact or lysed neutrophil granules and granular cationic proteins can produce a local increase in vascular permeability and/or leukocytosis (Fig. 13–12). Similar observations have been made in experiments with neutropenic laboratory animals. Neutrophils have been found to injure the lungs of animals with endotoxemia, embolism, and vascular thrombosis, e.g., neutrophils were required for the acute lung injury in-

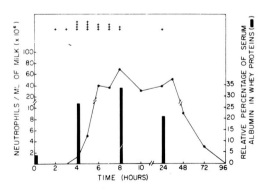

Fig. 13–12. **Response of Cow 1556 to intramammary inoculation of a lysosomal preparation.** Plus signs indicate degree of swelling of the gland: +, slight swelling or firmness; + +, slight swelling and firmness; + + +, moderate swelling and firmness; + + + +, marked swelling and firmness. (From Jain, N.C.: Leukocytes and tissue factors in the pathogenesis of bovine mastitis. Am. J. Vet. Res., 33:1137, 1972.)

duced by Pasteurella haemolytica as shown by studies in calves made neutropenic by hydroxyurea administration (Slocombe et al., 1985).

Neutrophils contain various substances that promote or inhibit inflammation, cause tissue injury, and induce antibody-dependent cellular cytotoxic (ADCC) effects. Monocytes, macrophages, neutrophils, and lymphocytes have been shown to function as effector cells in ADCC in different species. Neutrophil ADCC is important in host defense against viral infections because it can eliminate virus-infected cells. These types of injuries may be caused by nonoxidative and/or oxidative mechanisms. The degranulation of neutrophils, which leads to the extracellular release of lysosomal substances, can be caused by a number of mechanisms (e.g., cell death, phagocytosis, chemotaxis, secretion, and reversed endocytosis). Similar effects are produced by oxygen-derived free radicals generated after the metabolic burst of neutrophils engaged in phagocytosis or membrane perturbation (Hatherill et al., 1991). Substances promoting inflammation and tissue damage include various oxygen metabolites, lysosomal substances such as cationic proteins, histamine, and acid and neutral proteases such as collagenase, elastase, and cathepsins (Table 13–1), and products of arachidonic acid metabolism such as leukotrienes, prostaglandin E_2 (PGE$_2$), and TxA$_2$. Substances regulating the inflammatory process include superoxide dismutase, catalase, certain cationic proteins, prostaglandins, lysozyme, and protease inhibitors in plasma and neutrophil cytosol. Neutrophil-induced alteration of the erythrocyte membrane, through proteolytic cleavage and the generation of toxic oxygen radicals by activated neutrophils, is considered a potential cause of red cell destruction in anemias of inflammatory disease (Weiss et al., 1991). In addition, a neutrophil-induced antigenic alteration in the cell membrane results in IgG binding to the erythrocytes and makes such cells prone to removal by the phagocytic action of the mononuclear phagocyte system (Weiss and Murtaugh, 1990).

MORPHOLOGIC AND FUNCTIONAL ABNORMALITIES

It has been established that marked quantitative and qualitative changes in neutrophils may predispose to infection. Studies on the protective role of neutrophils in humans have shown that defective cellular activity may occur at various levels of functional execution. For example, interference with or defective adherence, migration, chemotaxis, ingestion, degranulation, metabolic stimulation, and microbicidal activity may contribute to a reduced resistance to infection, which can be fatal. Morphologic and functional abnormalities may manifest simultaneously. Morphologically abnormal neutrophils, however, may not necessarily be functionally so defective as to compromise the host defense and, conversely, morphologically normal neutrophils may have severe functional defects that can increase an animal's susceptibility to infection.

Morphologic Abnormalities

Morphologic abnormalities in neutrophils include aberrations of maturation, cell size, nuclear shape, granule characteristics, and cytoplasmic attributes (Table 13–7). Such changes may be acquired or hereditary and may be visible on light microscopy or demonstrable only by electron microscopy or cytochemical staining. Mature and immature neutrophils commonly display granular and cytoplasmic abnormalities referred to as toxic changes. These are seen in patients with severe bacterial infections, septicemia, acute inflammatory conditions, and extensive tissue destruction. Toxic neutrophils are functionally defective, because they have reduced chemotactic, phagocytic, and bactericidal activities. Bacterial toxins can induce lysosomal rupture or leakage of hydrolytic enzymes and autolytic changes leading to cytoplasmic foaminess and vacuolation. Toxic effects during granulopoiesis are reflected in cytoplasmic basophilia, the presence of "toxic" granules and Döhle bodies, hypersegmented nuclei, and the production of giant and bizarre neutrophils. Basophilia is the result of retained ribosomes and rough endoplasmic reticulum. Toxic granules are analogous to the reddish-purple azurophilic granules normally seen at the promyelocyte stage. They become visible in toxic neutrophilic myelocytes through mature neutrophils because of retained acid mucopolysaccharides. This may represent an adoptive phenomenon to increase host defense.

Döhle bodies are bluish cytoplasmic inclusions that result from the lamellar aggregation of rough endoplasmic reticulum (Plate IX-2; Fig. 13–13). They are more common in cats than in other animal species. Basophilic inclusions similar to Döhle bodies are found in granulocytes and monocytes of humans with hereditary May-Hegglin anomaly, and some large, lipid-containing vacuoles are found in leukocytes and plasma cells in humans with Jordon's anomaly.

Auer rods are intracytoplasmic structures commonly found in the myeloblasts and promyelocytes of some human patients with acute myelogenous leukemia. They are derived from azurophilic granules and are

Table 13–7. Morphologic Abnormalities of Neutrophils

Acquired Abnormalities	Hereditary Abnormalities
"Toxic" changes; cytoplasmic foaminess, vacuolation, and/or basophilia; "toxic" granules; Döhle bodies; bizarre giant forms	Hypersegmentation
	Macropolycytes
	Pelger-Huët anomaly
Hypersegmentation	May-Hegglin anomaly
Pseudo–Pelger-Huët anomaly	Alder-Reilly anomaly
Auer rods	Mucopolysaccharidosis
Asynchronous maturation	Chédiak-Higashi syndrome
Macropolycytes	Jordon's anomaly
Absence of primary or secondary granules	
Absence of peroxidase or alkaline phosphatase or other granule contents	

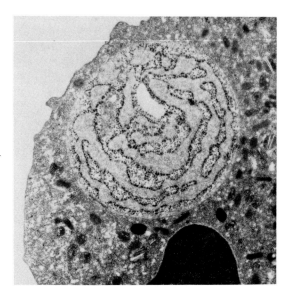

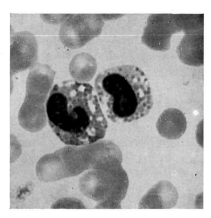

Fig. 13–14. Eosinophils from a dog with hereditary Pelger-Huët anomaly (× 1400). (From Jain, N.C.: Schalm's Veterinary Hematology. 4th Ed. Philadelphia, Lea & Febiger, 1986, p. 116.)

Fig. 13–13. Equine neutrophil with a whorl of rough endoplasmic reticulum. This structure would stain highly basophilic and appear as a Döhle body in blood films stained with a Romanowsky stain (transmission electron photomicrograph, × 14,400). (From Jain, N.C.: Schalm's Veterinary Hematology. 4th Ed. Philadelphia, Lea & Febiger, 1986, p. 716.)

best demonstrated in bone marrow films stained for MPO. They are not seen in blast cells in acute lymphocytic leukemia and reactive leukocytosis. Auer rods have not yet been found in leukemic animals, but Auer rod-like structures were seen in a cat with acute myelogenous leukemia (Jain et al., 1991a).

Hypersegmented neutrophils are found in poodles with macrocytic erythrocytes and in dogs on long-term corticosteroid therapy. They were found in a cat suspected of having a vitamin B_{12}-folate deficiency (Plate XI–7). Idiopathic hypersegmentation of neutrophils was observed in a horse. Animals with chronic neutrophilia, particularly the horse, may show occasional hypersegmented neutrophils in blood.

Pleokaryocytes are normal-sized neutrophils with increased (more than 5) nuclear lobes, whereas macropolycytes are giant neutrophils having a nucleus with or without increased nuclear lobes. These cells have been seen in humans as a hereditary abnormality or as an acquired defect in vitamin B_{12} or folate deficiency, in iron deficiency, after treatment with antimetabolites interfering with DNA synthesis (e.g., 6-mercaptopurine, cytosine arabinoside, and methotrexate), and in uremia. Such cells may occasionally be seen in the blood and bone marrow of cats with toxemic diseases.

Pelger-Huët anomaly is a hereditary disorder characterized by failure of the nucleus of granulocytes, especially the neutrophils, to undergo normal maturation to the segmented form (Plate IX-5; Figs. 13–14, and 13–15). Neutrophils generally have stunted unsegmented or round nuclei and relatively abundant cytoplasm. This nuclear hyposegmentation results in an apparent ("pseudo") left shift in neutrophils. The neutrophils are functionally normal with regard to

adherence, chemotaxis, phagocytosis, and bacterial killing (Latimer et al., 1989). The Pelger-Huët anomaly has been reported in humans, rabbits, dogs, and cats. In the rabbit, it is lethal when a homozygous state is produced by selective breeding. The homozygous rabbit tends to die in fetal life or, if it survives to parturition, usually dies within the first month of life. Surviving homozygous animals are stunted and present marked skeletal deformities. Humans, dogs, and cats with Pelger-Huët anomaly, however, appear to have no special health problems. Foxhounds with this anomaly may show an impaired antibody response and decreased neutrophil mobilization into the skin. Routine cytochemical examination of neutrophils from dogs with this anomaly reveal similarities to those of normal dogs (Latimer et al., 1987). Acquired hyposegmentation of the granulocyte nucleus is referred to as pseudo–Pelger-Huët anomaly. It may occur during disturbed granulopoiesis from severe infections, leukemias, or idiopathic causes. Such cells may occasionally be seen in dogs, cats, and other animal species (Plate IX-6).

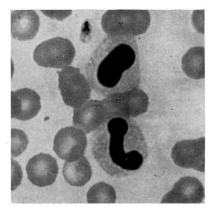

Fig. 13–15. Neutrophils from a dog with hereditary Pelger-Huët anomaly (× 1400). (From Jain, N.C.: Schalm's Veterinary Hematology. 4th Ed. Philadelphia, Lea & Febiger, 1986, p. 116.)

Chédiak-Higashi syndrome is characterized by partial ocular and cutaneous albinism, photophobia, a bleeding tendency, an increased susceptibility to infection, and morphologic and functional abnormalities of neutrophils. The platelets are also deficient in adenine nucleotides because of the absence of dense granules; thus, repeated hemorrhagic episodes are common. Chédiak-Higashi syndrome has been described in humans and several animal species, including Aleutian mink, Hereford cattle, Persian cats, a strain of beige mice, foxes, and killer whales (Plates IX-10, IX-11, IX-12). The primary defect is in the formation of giant lysosomal granules in various granule-containing cells such as granulocytes because of defective microtubule assembly and an inadequate production of cGMP. The defective formation of primary and secondary granules leads to granule fusion and the occurrence of irregular large granules in neutrophils. Enlarged granules are also found in eosinophils, basophils, melanocytes, and occasional monocytes. Such neutrophils can phagocytize bacteria, but they display defective chemotaxis, degranulation, and bacterial killing. Thus, Chédiak-Higashi animals die from recurrent infections. A pseudo–Chédiak-Higashi anomaly may be seen in acute or chronic myelogenous leukemia and other myeloproliferative disorders as a manifestation of the underlying abnormal granule formation.

Mucopolysaccharidosis (MPS) is characterized by the presence of coarse, large, intensely stained, azurophilic granules in mature neutrophils and bone and cartilage abnormalities. Similar granules may be found in other leukocytes and, more commonly, in bone marrow reticulum cells. The basic defect is an abnormality of mucopolysaccharide (glycosaminoglycan) catabolism caused by an enzyme deficiency that results in the accumulation of mucopolysaccharides and enlargement of leukocyte granules. Six genetic forms of specific enzyme deficiencies have been recognized in MPS in humans. Two genetic forms have been described in domestic cats: MPS I (Hurler's syndrome), associated with a deficiency of α-L-iduronidase, and MPS VI (Maroteaux-Lamy syndrome), caused by a deficiency of arylsulfatase B (N-acetylgalactosamine-4-sulfatase) activity. α-Mannosidosis (deficiency of α-mannosidase) is another lysosomal storage disease described in cats. In MPS VI, partially degraded glycosaminoglycans accumulate, whereas in α-mannosidosis N-linked oligosaccharides accumulate.

In cats with α-mannosidosis, vacuoles are seen in lymphocytes and monocytes on light microscopy, and electron microscopy also reveals vacuolation in neutrophils, eosinophils, and basophils. In cats with MPS VI, vacuoles containing metachromatic granules are seen in lymphocytes, neutrophils, eosinophils, and monocytes. Electron microscopy of these cells revealed an accumulation of fibrillar material often associated with lamellar membrane structures (Alroy et al., 1989). Allogeneic bone marrow transplantation has been found to correct MPS VI in some cats (Gasper et al., 1985) and neutrophil migration defect and platelet

storage pool deficiency in Chédiak-Higashi cats (Colgan et al., 1991). Dogs with MPS may show occasional leukocytes with abnormal granulation (Plates XIII-1 to XIII-4). A hereditary (autosomal recessive) anomaly of neutrophil granulation was found in purebred Birman cats (Hirsch and Cunningham, 1985). Neutrophils of the affected cats contained fine eosinophilic granules without any adverse influence on their phagocytic and bactericidal properties.

Functional Abnormalities

It has now been established that resistance to infection depends principally on an interaction of phagocytes, humoral factors (antibody and complement), and properties of the pathogen. Specific defects of phagocytes and immunologic deficiencies, in which the susceptibility to certain bacterial diseases is increased, have been demonstrated in humans (Table 13–8), and similar abnormalities are being recognized in animals. Patients with recurrent pyogenic infections should be investigated for abnormalities of neutrophil functions such as adherence, chemotaxis, phagocytosis, production of oxygen metabolites, degranulation, and bacterial kill (Rotrosen and Gallin, 1987; Sim and Goldman, 1991). In addition, the adequacy of plasma opsonins (immunoglobulins and complement) should be evaluated.

The neutrophil functions seem to be age-related in that human neonates and young foals and bovine calves have significantly reduced functional activity (Hauser et al., 1986; Martens et al., 1988). Neutrophils from patients with many infectious and noninfectious diseases have been found to have defects of adherence, chemotaxis, phagocytosis, degranulation, and bactericidal activity. For example, neutrophils from rhesus macaques with clinically confirmed simian acquired immunodeficiency syndrome are functionally deficient; their chemotactic, phagocytic, and bactericidal activities were reduced (Cheung and Gardner, 1991). Dexamethasone administration (50 μg/kg) in cows dampens the oxidative burst of neutrophils (Salgar et al., 1991). Dexamethasone-induced suppression of bovine neutrophil oxidative burst and ADCC were re-

---

Table 13–8. Disorders of Human Neutrophil Function

Defects of locomotion and chemotaxis
  Intrinsic cellular defects of locomotion: differences resulting from age of the individual or of the cells; acquired or hereditary defects
  Defective or inadequate generation of cytotaxins
  Chemotactic "deactivation" of neutrophils
  Cytotaxin inactivation or inhibition by serum and cell-derived inhibitors
Defective phagocytosis: acquired or hereditary cellular or humoral defects
Defective microbicidal activity: acquired or hereditary
  Abnormal degranulation or granular enzymes
  Defective metabolic activity
  Absence of peroxidase

versed by administration of ascorbic acid (Roth and Kaeberle, 1985). Impaired chemotaxis is found in dogs with pyoderma, disseminated prototothecosis, and hypophosphatemia. The chemiluminescence of neutrophils from persistently viremic feline leukemia virus-infected cats is diminished (Lafrado et al., 1990). Chemotactic activity of neutrophils from viremic, clinically affected cats is significantly lower than that in subclinically affected, viremic cats (Kiehl et al., 1987). Neutrophils from the uterus of mares considered susceptible to chronic uterine infections were functionally deficient in phagocytic and bactericidal activities compared to those from mares resistant to such infections (Liu and Cheung, 1986). Zinc deficiency is associated with an intrinsic neutrophil defect that specifically affects chemotaxis and is corrected with dietary zinc repletion (Vruwink et al., 1991).

Various drugs may influence the phagocytic property of neutrophils—for example, some NSAIDs (e.g., acetylsalicylic acid) enhanced phagocytosis, whereas some aminoglycosides, peptolids, tetracyclines, and β-lactams, as well as certain other NSAIDs (e.g., ibuprofen) decreased phagocytosis of Staphylococcus aureus by bovine neutrophils isolated from milk (Paape et al., 1991). Ingestion of milk fat and casein by neutrophils in milk reduces their phagocytic and chemiluminescence activities (Dulin et al., 1988).

A few hereditary functional defects have also been reported. The functional defects may be associated with morphologic defects, as in Chédiak-Higashi syndrome, or unassociated with morphologic abnormalities of neutrophils, as in chronic granulomatous disease and granulocytopathy syndrome (see below).

Chronic granulomatous disease in humans is a sex-linked recessive (in males) or autosomal recessive (in females) fatal disease of children, characterized by recurrent and chronic infections. Neutrophils from these patients engulf bacteria normally but cannot kill them. The basic defect is that the neutrophils cannot mount a respiratory burst and form H_2O_2 to produce the bactericidal MPO-H_2O_2-halide complex. Monocytes may also exhibit such a defect. This defect in the phagocytic cells is the result of gene mutations that lead to an absence or reduced synthesis of membrane NADPH-oxidase system (Curnutte 1992; Morel et al., 1991). The latter consists of NADPH oxidase, cytochrome b-558 (a heterodimer composed of two subunits of 22-KDa and 91-KDa), and two cytosolic factors (a 47-KDa and 65-KDa proteins). Both the NBT reduction test and chemiluminescence are consequently markedly reduced. Catalase-negative bacteria that produce H_2O_2, such as streptococci, can be readily killed by these neutrophils, whereas catalase-positive bacteria that do not produce H_2O_2, such as Staphylococcus aureus and Escherichia coli, are not destroyed. The latter class of organisms therefore proliferates, causing the premature death of affected children. In addition, fungal infections are frequent and extremely difficult to eradicate. Treatment has involved antibiotics, corticosteroids, neutrophil transfusions, marrow transplantation and, more recently, recombinant γ-

interferon (Gallin, 1991) and gene therapy (Gallin and Malech, 1990).

A disease with some similarity to chronic granulomatous disease or complement receptor deficiency in humans, was reported to occur in eight closely related Doberman Pinschers with chronic rhinitis and pneumonia. Neutrophils phagocytized bacteria normally, but had impaired bactericidal property probably because of a markedly reduced oxidative burst activity (Breitschwerdt et al., 1987).

Defective neutrophil bactericidal activity was found in male Irish setter dogs having a clinical history of recurrent, life-threatening bacterial infections, with associated peaks of pyrexia and marked neutrophilia. This condition was called canine granulocytopathy syndrome and appeared to have an autosomal recessive mode of inheritance. A granulocytopathy syndrome occurs in Holstein-Frisian cattle as an autosomal recessive trait. Clinical features include recurrent infection of soft tissues and delayed wound healing. Prominent laboratory findings include persistent and progressive neutrophilia, decreased neutrophilic infiltration of inflamed tissues, and impaired neutrophil chemotaxis, phagocytosis, and oxidative burst. The molecular basis of defective neutrophil functions in both species is the genetic deficiency of CD11/CD18 adhesion molecules, as reported for humans with similar disorders (Kehrli et al., 1990). Specifically, a calf with the granulocytopathy syndrome was severely deficiency in Mac-1 (CD11b/CD18). Leukocyte adhesion deficiencies have been reported in humans (Anderson and Springer, 1987).

Decreased glutathione peroxidase activity in phagocytic cells has been reported in selenium-deficient rats and cows and has been associated with reduced bactericidal activity of bovine neutrophils for pathogenic bacteria. Defective chemotactic migration and impaired bactericidal activity of neutrophils in selenium-deficient cows have been associated with more severe and prolonged coliform mastitis than in those given selenium supplementation (Erskine et al., 1989; Grasso et al., 1990). Decreased Fc-receptor expression and myeloperoxidase activity are found in neonatal calves compared to cows; such compromised neutrophil functions could potentially weaken the cellular host defense during the neonatal period (Zwahlen et al., 1992). A transient reduction in neutrophil chemotaxis and chemiluminescence was observed 1 day after a single bout of exercise-induced stress in horses (Wong et al., 1992).

REFERENCES

Alroy, J., Freden, G.O., Goyal, V., et al.: Morphology of leukocytes from cats affected with alpha-mannosidosis and mucopolysaccharidosis VI (MPS VI). Vet. Pathol., 26:294, 1989.
Anderson, B.O., Brown, J.M., and Harken, A.H.: Mechanisms of neutrophil-mediated tissue injury. J. Surg. Res, 51:170, 1991.
Anderson, D.C., and Springer, T.A.: Leukocyte adhesion deficiency: An inherited defect in the Mac-1. LFA-1, and p150,95 glycoproteins. Ann. Rev. Med., 38:175, 1987.

Arnaout, M.A.: Structure and function of the leukocyte adhesion molecules. Blood, 75:1037, 1990.

Baggiolini, M., Walz, A., and Kunkel, S.L.: Neutrophil-activating peptide-1/interleukin 8, a novel cytokine that activates neutrophils. J. Clin. Invest., 84:1045, 1989.

Berg, M., and James, S.P.: Human neutrophils release the Leu-8 lymph node homing receptor during cell activation. Blood, 76: 2381, 1990.

Bernofsky, C.: Nucleotide chloramines and neutrophil-mediated cytotoxicity. FASEB J., 5:295, 1991.

Bjork, P., Axelsson, L., and Ohlsson, K.: Release of dog polymorphonuclear leukocyte cathepsin G, normally and in endotoxin and pancreatitic shock. Isolation and partial characterization of dog polymorphonuclear leukocyte cathepsin G. Biol. Chem. Hoppe Seyler, 372:419, 1991.

Breitschwerdt, E.B., Brown T.T., De Buysscher, E.V., et al.: Rhinitis, pneumonia, and defective neutrophil function in the Doberman Pinscher. Am. J. Vet. Res., 48:1054, 1987.

Cairo, M.S.: Cytokines: a new immunotherapy. Clin. Perinatol., 18: 343, 1991.

Cannistra, S.A., and Griffin, J.D.: Regulation of the production and function of granulocytes and monocytes. Sem. Hematol., 25: 173, 1988.

Cheung, A.T.W. and Gardner, M.B.: Functional deficiency of polymorphonuclear leukocytes in simian acquired immunodeficiency syndrome. Am. J. Vet. Res., 52:1523, 1991.

Chiang, Y.W., Murata, H., and Roth, J.A.: Activation of bovine neutrophils by recombinant bovine tumor necrosis factor-alpha. Vet. Immunol. Immunopathol., 29:329, 1991.

Colgan, S.P., Hull-Thrall, M.A., Gasper, P.W., et al.: Restoration of neutrophil and platelet function in feline Chédiak-Higashi syndrome by bone marrow transplantation. Bone Marrow Transplant., 7:365, 1991.

Cullor, J.S., Fairley, N., Smith, W.L., et al.: Hemogram changes in lactating dairy cows given human recombinant granulocyte colony stimulating factor (r-MethuF-CSF). Vet. Pathol., 27:311, 1990a.

Cullor, J.S., Smith, W., Fairley, N., et al.: Effects of human recombinant granulocyte colony-stimulating factor (HR-GCSF) on hemogram of lactating dairy cattle. Vet. Clin. Pathol., 19:9, 1990b.

Curnutte, J.T.: Molecular basis of the autosomal recessive forms of chronic granulomatous disease. Immunodefic. Rev., 3:149, 1992.

Djeu, J.Y., Serbousek, D., and Blanchard, D.K.: Release of tumor necrosis factor by human polymorphonuclear leukocytes. Blood, 76:1405, 1990.

Dore, M., Slauson, D.O., and Neilsen, N.R.: Decreased respiratory burst activity in neonatal bovine neutrophil stimulated by protein kinase C agonists. Am. J. Vet. Res., 52:375, 1991.

Dulin, A.M., Paape, M.J., and Nickerson, S.C.: Comparison of phagocytosis and chemiluminescence by blood and mammary gland neutrophils from multiparous and nulliparous cows. Am. J. Vet. Res., 49:172, 1988.

Erskine, R.J., Eberhart, R.J., Grasso, P.J., et al.: Induction of *Escherichia coli* mastitis in cows fed selenium-deficient or selenium-supplemented diets. Am. J. Vet. Res., 50:2093, 1989.

Farber, J.L., Kyle, M.E., and Coleman, J.B.: Mechanisms of cell injury by activated oxygen species. Lab. Invest., 62:670, 1990.

Fittschen, C., Parmley, R.T., and Austin, R.L.: Ultrastructural cytochemistry of complex carbohydrates in developing feline neutrophils. Am. J. Anat., 181:149, 1988a.

Fittschen, C., Parmley, R.T., Bishop, S.P., et al.: Morphometry of feline neutrophil granule genesis. Am. J. Anat., 181:195, 1988b.

Fletcher, M.P., Stahl, G.L., and Longhurst, J.C.,: In vivo and in vitro assessment of porcine neutrophil activation responses to chemoattractants: Flow cytometric evidence for the selective absence of formyl peptide receptors. J. Leuk. Biol., 47:355, 1990.

Foster, A.P., Cunningham, F., and Lees, P.: The inflammatory effects of PAF in equine skin. Br. J. Pharm., 99:86P, 1990.

Frank, R.W., Gennaro, R., Schneider, K., et al.: Amino acid sequences of two proline-rich bactenecins. J. Biol. Chem., 265: 18871, 1990.

Fulton, R., Gasper, P.W., Ogilvie, G.K., et al.: Effect of recombinant human granulocyte colony-stimulating factor on hematopoiesis in normal cats. Exp. Hematol., 19:759, 1991.

Gallin, J.I.: Interferon-gamma in the treatment of the chronic granulomatous disease of childhood. Clin. Immunol. Immunopathol., 61:S100, 1991.

Gallin, J.I., and Malech, H.L.: Update on chronic granulomatous diseases of childhood. Immunotherapy and potential for gene therapy. J. Am. Med. Assoc., 263:1533, 1990.

Gamble, J.R. and Vadas, M.A.: Endothelial adhesiveness for blood neutrophils is inhibited by transforming growth factor-beta. Science, 242:97, 1988.

Ganser, A., Seipelt, G., and Hoelzer, D.: The role of GM-CSF, G-CSF, interleukin-3, and erythropoietin in myelodysplastic syndromes. Am. J. Clin. Oncol., 14 Suppl. 1:S34, 1991.

Ganz, T., Selsted, M.E., and Lehrer, R.I.: Defensins. Eur. J. Haematol., 44:1, 1990.

Gasper, P.W., Thrall, M.A., Wenger, D.A., et al.: Bone marrow transplantation for correction of feline arylsulfatase B deficiency (Mucopolysaccharidosis VI). Vet. Clin. Pathol., 14:13, 1985. (Abstract)

Gera, J.F., and Lichtenstein, A.: Human neutrophil peptide defensins induce single strand DNA breaks in target cells. Cell. Immunol., 138:108, 1991.

Gordon, B.J., Latimer, K.S., Murray, C.M., et al.: Evaluation of leukapheresis and thrombocytapheresis in the horse. Am. J. Vet. Res., 47:997, 1986.

Grasso, P.J., Scholz, R.W., Erskine, R.J., et al.: Phagocytosis, bactericidal activity, and oxidative metabolism of milk neutrophils from dairy cows fed selenium-supplemented and selenium-deficient diets. Am. J. Vet. Res., 51:269, 1990.

Harvath, L.: Neutrophil chemotactic factors. Experientia Suppl., 59: 35, 1991.

Hatherill, J.R., Till, G.O., and Ward, P.A.: Mechanisms of oxidant-induced changes in erythrocytes. Agents Actions, 32:351, 1991.

Hauser, M.A., Koob, M.D., and Roth, J.A.: Variation of neutrophil function with age in calves. Am. J. Vet. Res., 47:152, 1986.

Hirsch, V.M. and Cunningham, T.A.: Hereditary anomaly of neutrophil granulation in Birman cats. Vet. Clin. Pathol., 14:11, 1985. (Abstract)

Hogan, J.S., Todhunter, D.A., Tomita, G.M., et al.: Opsonic activity of bovine serum and mammary secretion after Escherichia coli J5 vaccination. J. Dairy Sci., 75:72, 1992a.

Hogan, J.S., Weiss, W.P., Todhunter, D.A., et al.: Bovine neutrophil responses to parenteral vitamin E. J. Dairy Sci., 75:399, 1992b.

Huber, A.R., Kunkel, S.L., Todd, R.F. III, et al.: Regulation of transendothelial neutrophil migration by endogenous interleukin-8. Science, 254:99, 1991.

Huizinga, T.W.J., Kuijpers, R.W.A.M., Kleijer, M., et al.: Maternal genomic neutrophil FcRIII deficiency leading to neonatal isoimmune neutropenia. Blood. 76:1927, 1990.

Jain, N.C.: Schalm's Veterinary Hematology. 4th ed. Philadelphia, Lea & Febiger, 1986, pp. 676–730.

Jain, N.C., Blue, J.T., Grindem, C.B., et al.: A report of the animal leukemia study group: Proposed criteria for classification of acute myeloid leukemia in dogs and cats. Vet. Clin. Pathol. 20: 63, 1991a.

Jain, N.C., Paape, M.J., Berning, L., et al.: Functional competence and monoclonal antibody reactivity of neutrophils from cows injected with Escherichia coli endotoxin. Comp. Haematol. Int., 1:10, 1991b.

Jain, N.C., Vegad, J.L., Dhawedkar, R.G., et al.: Ultrastructural and biochemical observations on antineutrophil antibody- and complement-induced immuno-injury to equine neutrophils. J. Comp. Pathol., 104:389, 1991c.

Kabbur, M.B., Jain, N.C., Zinkl, J.G., et al.: Heterogeneity in phagocytic and nitroblue tetrazolium reductive properties of neutrophils from cows. Am. J. Vet. Res., 52:2023, 1991.

Kehrli, M.E., Nonnecke, B.J., and Roth, J.A.: Alternations in bovine neutrophil function during the periparturient period. Am. J. Vet. Res., 50:207, 1989a.

Kehrli, M.E., Nonnecke, B.J. and Roth, J.A.: Alternations in bovine lymphocyte function during the periparturient period. Am. J. Vet. Res., 50:215, 1989b.

Kehrli, M.E., Schmalstieg, F.C., Anderson, D.C., et al.: Molecular definition of the bovine granulocytopathy syndrome: Identification of deficiency of the Mac-1 (CD11b/CD18) glycoprotein, Am. J. Vet. Res., 51:1826, 1990.

Kiehl, A.R., Fettman, M.J., Quackenbush, S.L., et al.: Effects of feline leukemia virus infection on neutrophil chemotaxis in vitro. Am. J. Vet. Res., 48:76, 1987.

Koblik, P.D., Lofstedt, J., Jakowski, R.M., et al.: Use of ^{111}In-labeled autologous leukocytes to image an abdominal abscess in a horse. J. Am. Vet. Med. Assoc., 186:1319, 1985.

Krause, K.-H. and Lew, D.P.: Bacterial toxins and neutrophil activation. Sem. Hematol., 25:112, 1988.

Krause, P.J., Malech, H.L., Kristie, J., et al.: Polymorphonuclear leukocyte heterogeneity in neonates and adults. Blood, 68:200, 1986.

Krause, P.J., Todd, M.B., Hancock, W.W., et al.: The role of cellular maturation in neutrophil heterogeneity. Blood, 76:1639, 1990.

Lafrado, L.J., Mathes, L.E., Zack, P.M., et al.: Biological effects of staphylococcal protein A immunotherapy in cats with induced feline leukemia virus infection. Am. J. Vet. Res., 51:482, 1990.

Latimer, K.S., Duncan, J.R. and Kircher, I.M.: Morphology and cytochemistry of canine Pelger-Huet blood cells. Vet. Clin. Pathol., 16:9, 1987. (Abstract)

Latimer, K.S., Kirchner, I.M., Lindl, P.A., et al.: Leukocyte function in Pelger-Huet Anomaly of Dogs. J. Leukoc. Biol., 45:301, 1989.

Lehrer, R.L., and Ganz, T.: Antimicrobial polypeptides of human neutrophils. Blood, 76:2169, 1990.

Lichtenstein, A.: Mechanism of mammalian cell lysis mediated by peptide defensins. Evidence for an initial alteration of the plasma membrane. J. Clin. Invest., 88:93, 1991.

Liu, I.K. and Cheung, A.T.: Immunoglobulin and neutrophil defense against uterine infection in mares resistant and susceptible to chronic endometritis: a review. J. Am. Vet. Med. Assoc., 189:700, 1986.

MacKay, R.J., Merritt, A.M., Zertuche, J.M., et al.: Tumor necrosis factor activity in the circulation of horses given endotoxin. Am. J. Vet. Res., 52:533, 1991.

Martens, J.G., Martens, R.J., and Renshaw, H.W.: Rhodococcus (Corynebacterium) equi: bactericidal capacity of neutrophils from neonatal and adult horses. Am. J. Vet. Res., 49:295, 1988.

Miller, R.H., Guidry, A.J., Paape, M.H., et al.: Relationship between immunoglobulin concentrations in milk and phagocytosis by bovine neutrophils. Am. J. Vet. Res., 49:42, 1988.

Moore, G.E., Mahaffey, E.A. and Hoeing, M.: Hematologic and serum biochemical effects of long-term administration of anti-inflammatory doses of prednisone in dogs. Am. J. Vet. Res., 53:1033, 1992.

Morel, F., Doussiere, J. and Vignais, P.V.: The superoxide-generating oxidase of phagocytic cells. Physiological, molecular and pathological aspects. Eur. J. Biochem., 201:523, 1991.

Morris, D.D. and Moore, J.N.: Tumor necrosis factor activity in serum from neonatal foals with presumed septicemia. J. Am. Vet. Med. Assoc., 199:1584, 1991.

Morstyn, G. and Sheridan, W.P.: The role of colony stimulating factors in cancer therapy. Cancer Chemother. Biol. Response Modif., 12:307, 1991.

Naccache, P.H., Gilbert, C., Caon, A.C., et al.: Selective inhibition of human neutrophil functional responsiveness by erbstatin, an inhibitor of tyrosine protein kinase. Blood, 10:2098, 1990.

Paape, M.J., Miller, R.H. and Ziv, G.: Pharmacologic enhancement or suppression of phagocytosis by bovine neutrophils. Am. J. Vet. Res., 52:363, 1991.

Panyutich, A. and Ganz, T.: Activated alpha 2-macroglobulin is a principal defensin-binding protein. Am. J. Resp. Cell Mol. Biol., 5:101, 1991.

Pratt, H.L., Carroll, R.C., McClendon, S., et al.: Effects of recombinant granulocyte colony-stimulating factor treatment on hematopoietic cycles and cellular defects associated with canine cyclic hematopoiesis. Exp. Hematol., 18:1199, 1990.

Reddy, P.G., McVey, D.S., Chengappa, M.M., et al.: Bovine recombinant granulocyte-macrophage colony stimulating factor enhancement of bovine neutrophil functions in vitro. Am. J. Vet. Res., 51:1395, 1990. (Abstract)

Romaniukowa, K. and Branicki, T.: Migration activity of leukocytes and some biochemical indices of the blood during peripartum period. Bull. Vet. Inst., Pulawy, 28/29:162, 1986.

Rot, A.: Chemotactic potency of recombinant human neutrophil attractant/activation protein-1 (interleukin-8) for polymorphonuclear leukocytes of different species. Cytokine, 3:21, 1991.

Roth, J.A. and Kaeberle, M.L.: In vivo effect of ascorbic acid on neutrophil function in healthy and dexamethasone-treated cattle. Am. J. Vet. Res., 46:2434, 1985.

Rotrosen, D. and Gallin, J.I.: Disorders of phagocyte function. Ann. Rev. Immunol., 5:127, 1987.

Salgar, S.K., Paape, M.J., Alston-Mills, B., et al.: Flow cytometric study of oxidative burst activity of bovine neutrophils. Am. J. Vet. Res., 52:1201, 1991. (Abstract)

Sample, A.K., and Czuprynski, C.J.: Priming and stimulation of bovine neutrophils by recombinant human interleukin-1 alpha and tumor necrosis factor alpha. J. Leuk. Biol., 49:107, 1991.

Schatz-Munding, M. and Ullrich, V.: Priming of human polymorphonuclear leukocytes with granulocyte-macrophage colony-stimulating factor involves protein kinase C rather than enhanced calcium mobilisation. Eur. J. Biochem., 204:705, 1992.

Selsted, M.E., Novotny, M.J., Morris, W.L., et al.: Indolicidin, a novel bactericidal tridecapeptide amide from neutrophils. J. Biol. Chem., 267:4292, 1992.

Silva, I. and Jain, N.C.: Effects of glycolytic and cytoskeletal inhibitors on phagocytic and nitroblue tetrazolium reductive activities of bovine neutrophils. Am J. Vet. Res., 50:1175, 1989.

Sim, T.C., and Goldman, A.S.: Defects in neutrophils: an overview. Allergy Proc., 12:31, 1991.

Slauson, D.O., Skrabalak, D.S., Neilsen, N.R., et al.: Complement-induced equine neutrophil adhesiveness and aggregation. Vet. Pathol., 24:239, 1987.

Slocombe, R.F., Ingersoll, M.R., Derksen, F.J., et al.: Importance of neutrophils in the pathogenesis of acute pneumonic pasteurellosis in calves. Am. J. Vet. Res., 46:2253, 1985.

Sordillo, L.M. and Babiuk, L.A.: Modulation of bovine mammary neutrophil function during the periparturient period following in vitro exposure to recombinant bovine interferon gamma. Vet. Immunol. Immunopathol., 27:393, 1991.

Spitznagel, J.K.: Antibiotic proteins of human neutrophils. J. Clin. Invest., 86:1381, 1990.

Steinbeck, M.J. and Roth, J.A.: Neutrophil activation by recombinant cytokines. Rev. Infect. Dis., 11:549, 1989.

Stickle, J.E., Kwan, D.K.-H. and Smith, W.: Neutrophil function in the dog: Shape change and response to a synthetic tripeptide. Am. J. Vet. Res., 46:225, 1985.

Suzuki, M., Asako, H., Kubes, P., et al.: Neutrophil-derived oxidants promote leukocyte adherence in postcapillary venules. Microvasc. Res., 42:125, 1991.

Thomsen, M.K., Jensen, A.L., Skak-Nielsen, T., et al.: Enhanced granulocyte function in a case of chronic granulocytic leukemia in a dog. Vet. Immunol. Immunopathol., 28:143, 1991a.

Thomsen, M.K., Larsen, C.G., Thomsen, H.K., et al.: Recombinant human interleukin-8 is a potent activator of canine neutrophil aggregation, migration, and leukotriene B4 biosynthesis. J. Invest. Dermatol., 96:260, 1991b.

Thomsen, M.K. and Thomsen, H.K.: Effects of interleukin-1 alpha on migration of canine neutrophils in vitro and in vivo. Vet. Immunol. Immunopathol., 26:385, 1990.

Trowald-Wigh, G. and Thoren-Tolling, K.: Chemiluminescence and chemotaxis assay of canine granulocytes: A methodological study. Acta Vet. Scand., 31:79, 1990.

Ulich, T.R., del Castillo, J., McNiece, I., et al.: Hematologic effects of recombinant murine granulocyte-macrophage colony-stimulating factor on the peripheral blood and bone marrow. Am. J. Pathol., 137:369, 1990.

Valore, E.V. and Ganz, T.: Posttranslational processing of defensins in immature human myeloid cells. Blood, 79:1538, 1992.

Vruwink, K.G., Fletcher, M.P., Keen, C.L., et al.: Moderate zinc deficiency in rhesus monkeys. An intrinsic defect of neutrophil chemotaxis corrected by zinc repletion. J. Immunol., 146:244, 1991.

Waage, A., Brandtzaeg, P., Espevik, T., et al.: Current understanding of the pathogenesis of gram-negative shock. Infect. Dis. Clin. North Am., 5:781, 1991.

Watson, E.D.: Opsonising ability of bovine uterine secretions during the oestrous cycle. Vet. Rec, 117:274, 1985.

Weiss, D.J., Murtaugh, M., and White, J.G.: Neutrophil-induced erythrocyte injury involves proteolytic cleavage of membrane proteins as well as oxidative damage. Vet. Clin. Pathol., 20:21, 1991.

Weiss, D.J. and Murtaugh, M.P.: Activated neutrophils induce erythrocyte immunoglobulin binding and membrane protein degradation. J. Leuk. Biol., 48:438, 1990.

Williams, W.J., Beutler, E., Erslev, A.J., et al.: Hematology. 4th ed. New York, McGraw-Hill, 1990.

Wong, C.W., Smith, S.E., Thong, T.H., et al.: Effects of exercise stress on various immune functions. Am. J. Vet. Res., 53:1414, 1992.

Yong, K. and Khwaja, A.: Leucocyte cellular adhesion molecules. Blood Rev., 4:211, 1990.

Zanetti, M., Litteri, L., Gennaro, R., et al.: Bactenecins, defense polypeptides of bovine neutrophils, are generated from precursor molecules stored in the large granules. J. Cell Biol., 111:1363, 1990.

Zinkl, J.G.: Leukocyte function. In: Kaneko, J.J. (eds), Clinical Biochemistry of Domestic Animals. San Diego, Academic Press, 1989, pp. 316–337.

Zinkl, J.G., Cain, G., Jain, N.C., et al.: Hematologic response of dogs to canine recombinant granulocyte colony stimulating factor (rcG-CSF). Comp. Haematol. Intl., (In Press).

Zwahlen, R.D., Wyder-Walther, M. and Roth, D.R.: Fc receptor expression, concanavalin A capping, and enzyme content of bovine neonatal neutrophils: a comparative study with adult cattle. J. Leuk. Biol., 51:264, 1992.

COLOR PLATES

Blood and bone marrow cells from coverslip films stained with Wright-Leishman stain unless otherwise noted.

PLATE I. CANINE AND FELINE BLOOD ABNORMALITIES IN THE WINTROBE HEMATOCRIT TUBE

1. Comparison of the Wintrobe hematocrit with the small capillary microhematocrit. The blood was taken from a case of chronic lymphocytic leukemia with a total leukocyte count of 87,000/μl. A borderline anemia existed, as shown by the PCV of 36%. The buffy coat of 5 mm reflects the high total leukocyte count. The reddish tinge to the buffy coat is imparted by the admixture of some red cells, particularly reticulocytes and/or leptocytes.

2. A diphasic erythrocyte sedimentation *(right)* is indicated by the reddish plasma, which clears on centrifugation *(center)*. The PCV of 29% reveals the existence of anemia, and the low icterus index as compared to the icterus index standard of 5 units *(left)* suggests an anemia of nonhemolytic origin.

3. Wintrobe hematocrit of a cat with polycythemia vera *(center,* PCV 67%) compared with hematocrits of two normal cats *(left,* PCV 32% and *right,* PCV 36%). A small buffy coat is evident above the red cell column in the left and right tubes; the top whitish layer was comprised primarily of platelets.

4. Buffy coat of an anemic cat (tube 2) compared with that of an anemic dog (tube 3) to illustrate differences in blood elements that may comprise a rather grossly similar buffy coat. The cream-colored buffy coat of about 9 mm in tube 2 is made up almost entirely of platelets (platelet count, 1.2 million/μl; WBC count, within normal range), whereas the reddish buffy coat of about 6 mm in tube 3 consists of primarily leukocytes (WBC count, 100,000/μl; platelet count, within normal range). The reddish tinge of the buffy coat in tube 3 is attributable to the admixture of young erythrocytes produced in response to anemia.

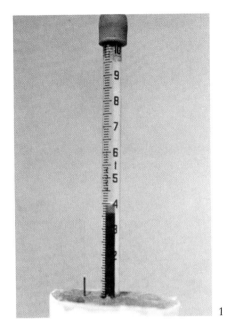

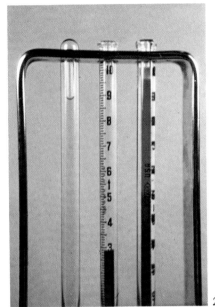

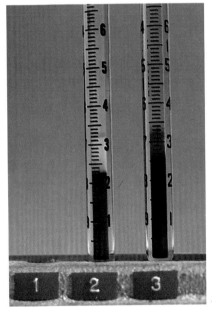

1

2

3

4

PLATE II. CANINE BLOOD ABNORMALITIES IN THE WINTROBE HEMATOCRIT TUBE

1. The left tube presents an icterus index value of 75 units caused by the retention of bilirubin from compression of the common bile duct in carcinoma of the pancreas. The blood in the center tube is typical of the anemia and low icterus index commonly observed in end-stage kidney disease with uremia. The blood on the right also has a colorless plasma. It is from a dog recently recovered from acute blood loss; the plasma is colorless because many of the erythrocytes are at the beginning of their life span. The daily destruction of overaged erythrocytes was too limited to contribute sufficient bilirubin to color the plasma.

2. Blood from two dogs with pyometra. The center tube is an icterus index standard of 5 units. The total leukocyte counts were 126,000/μl in the blood on the left and 82,500/μl in the blood on the right. These high leukocyte numbers are reflected in the buffy coats of 7 and 5 mm, respectively. The red tinge of these buffy coats is the result of the admixture of erythrocytes of low specific gravity (leptocytes) among the leukocytes. The PCV of each sample is 45%.

3. Lipemia is indicated in this hematocrit by the hazy plasma and the layer of neutral fat at the top of the plasma column. This hematocrit tube had been held overnight after centrifugation, which permitted a larger accumulation of fat at the top of the plasma column than had been present initially. The plasma is clear immediately above the buffy coat and is increasingly opaque toward the top. The chylomicra gradually rose to produce this effect.

4. Extreme lipemia. The hemolysis of erythrocytes, as shown by the red plasma that does not clear on centrifugation, often occurs with markedly lipemic blood. The hemolysis occurs after the blood has been withdrawn, and is enhanced by mechanical agitation of the sample or by forcing the blood from the syringe through the needle into the vial.

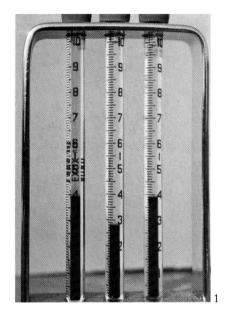

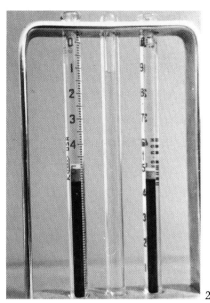

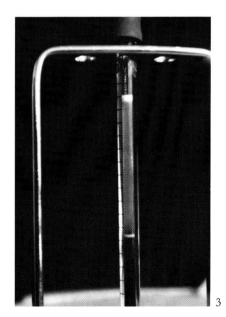

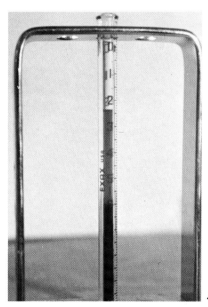

PLATE III. MEGAKARYOCYTOPOIESIS IN CANINE BONE MARROW

1. Megakaryoblast at the stage of first division of the nucleus from a dog with autoimmune hemolytic anemia and thrombocytopenia. Excessive cytoplasmic vacuolation is abnormal (×1800).

2. Promegakaryocyte in mitotic division without cell division endomitosis; (×1260).

3. Megakaryoblast with four nuclei from the same marrow as Plate III-1. Cells with one to four nuclei are regarded by some hematologists as megakaryoblasts (×1800).

4. Two promegakaryocytes (smaller cells) and two megakaryocytes (larger cells). The promegakaryocyte is distinguished from the megakaryoblast by the presence of a single mass of nuclear material with indistinct outline and larger cell size; it is distinguished from the megakaryocyte by its agranular blue cytoplasm (×800).

5. Megakaryocyte with a cytoplasmic process called a "proplatelet," which fragments into platelets (×1260; see Fig. 6).

6. Osteoclasts. Osteoclasts have irregular cell outlines and distinct multiple nuclei. Their cytoplasm may contain coarse reddish purple granules (not seen in this photograph) (×800).

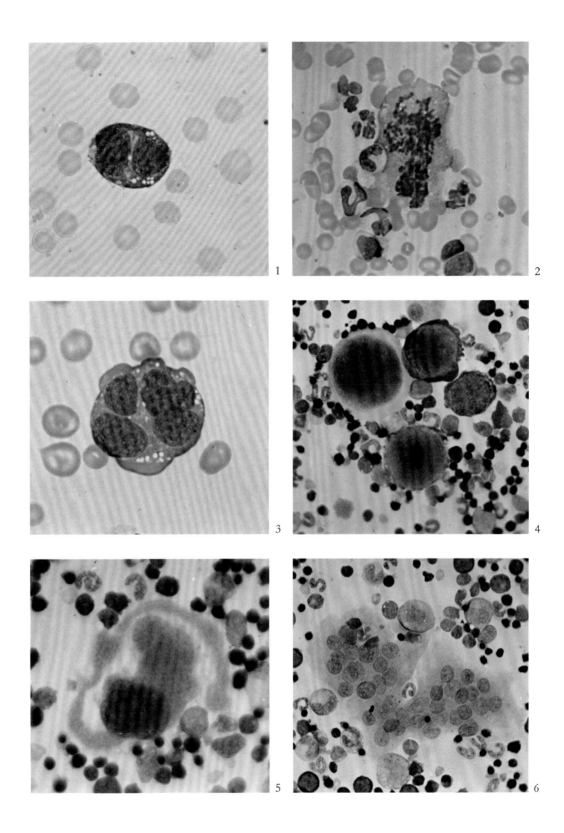

1

2

3

4

5

6

PLATE IV. ERYTHROPOIESIS IN CANINE AND FELINE BONE MARROW AND RETICULOCYTES IN FELINE BLOOD (×1800)

1. Canine bone marrow in hemangiosarcoma. The large cell in the center is a rubriblast with a prominent nucleolar ring, stippled chromatin, and deep blue cytoplasm. The ring of cells surrounding the rubriblast is comprised of polychromatic rubricytes in varying stages of hemoglobin synthesis and chromatin condensation. A portion of a naked nucleus of a reticuloendothelial cell is present in one corner.

2. Canine bone marrow in responsive anemia. A metarubricyte and a hematogone (free nucleus of a metarubricyte) are present above the eosinophil. Below the eosinophil are one prorubricyte and four polychromatic rubricytes at various stages of hemoglobin synthesis and maturity. The prorubricyte has blue cytoplasm and stippled nuclear chromatin, but no nucleolus. Two large polychromatic red cells are present among mature, discocytic red cells.

3. Canine bone marrow stained with new methylene blue. The large cell with two prominent nucleoli and deep blue cytoplasm is a rubriblast. The cell below the rubriblast with a lightly stained coarse chromatin and grayish blue cytoplasm is a polychromatic rubricyte. The small cell to the right of the rubriblast with a condensed nuclear chromatin and grayish cytoplasm is a late polychromatic rubricyte. Basophilic rubricytes (one above the rubriblast, one to the right of late polychromatic rubricyte, and one at the lower margin) have a relatively coarser nuclear chromatin and darker cytoplasm than the polychromatic rubricyte. The anuclear cell with bluish granular cytoplasmic material situated near the midright margin is a reticulocyte, and red cell ghosts are present in the background. The cell to the left of the reticulocyte is a polychromatic rubricyte.

4. Bone marrow from a normal cat. Shown here are two metarubricytes, two polychromatic rubricytes, a basophilic rubricyte, and a prorubricyte along with cells of the neutrophilic series. A neutrophilic myelocyte is present at the upper margin and a band neutrophil is at the lower margin of the photomicrograph.

5. Bone marrow from a cat with regenerative hemolytic anemia. Intensified erythropoiesis is indicated by the predominance of erythroid elements at various stages of maturation. Two rubriblasts, three polychromatic rubricytes, and three metarubricytes can be identified among the cells present.

6. Aggregate and punctate reticulocytes in the peripheral blood of a cat with regenerative hemolytic anemia. The large bluish objects near the margin of a few red cells are Heinz bodies (reticulocyte stain).

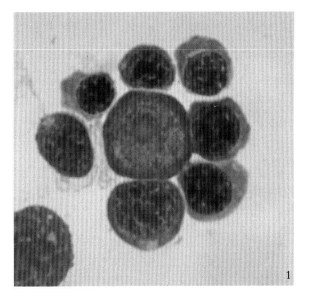

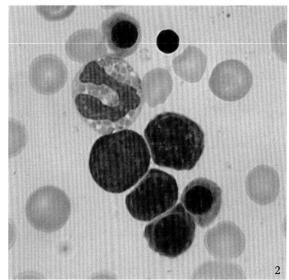

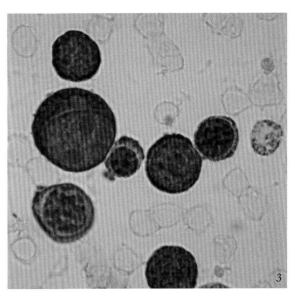

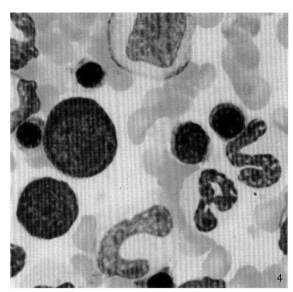

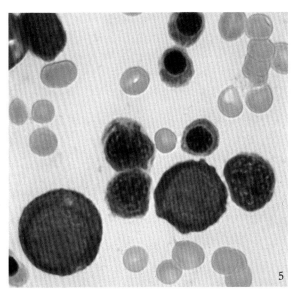

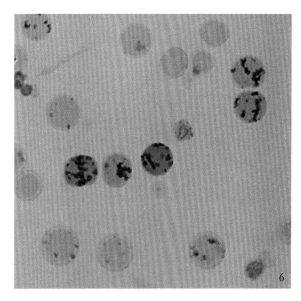

1. Intensified erythropoiesis in a horse responding to an anemia. All nucleated cells are of the erythrocytic maturation series. The cells, in descending order of size, are a rubriblast, two basophilic rubricytes, two polychromatophilic rubricytes, and five metarubricytes. Effective erythropoiesis is particularly indicated by the presence of large, polychromatophilic erythrocytes.

2. Cat bone marrow in feline infectious anemia (haemobartonellosis). The largest cell is a basophilic myelocyte exhibiting many small, lightly stained cytoplasmic granules and fewer large purple granules. The latter granules disappear as the basophil matures, leaving the lightly stained granules in a grayish cytoplasm as characteristic of the mature feline basophil (see Plate VII–6). The remaining nucleated cells are, in decreasing order of size, a basophilic rubricyte, polychromatophilic rubricytes, and metarubricytes. The amorphous pinkish mass is a degenerating nucleus. A few polychromatophilic erythrocytes can be seen.

3. Dog myeloblast (type I myeloblast) with three nucleolar rings and a neutrophilic metamyelocyte. A free lymphocyte nucleus is next to the latter cell.

4. A dog promyelocyte (progranulocyte) with azurophilic cytoplasmic granules. The nucleus presents a nucleolar ring, but the numerous azurophilic granules take precedence in classifying the cell.

5. Horse myeloblast (center) with several nucleolar rings, an eosinophilic myelocyte (largest cell), a basophilic metamyelocyte with purple granules, a degenerating neutrophilic metamyelocyte next to the basophil, and a small polychromatophilic rubricyte near the myeloblast.

6. Cluster of horse neutrophilic granulocytes. A myelocyte (cell with round nucleus), several metamyelocytes, one of which is abnormally large, and a band neutrophil (lower cell with V-shaped nucleus) can be seen. All cells with round, dark nuclei are either polychromatophilic rubricytes or metarubricytes.

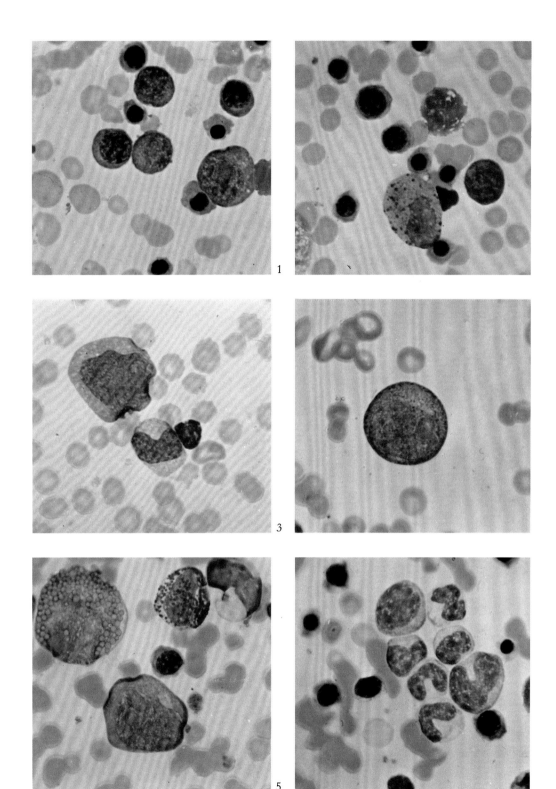

PLATE VI. ERYTHROPOIESIS AND GRANULOCYTOPOIESIS IN EQUINE BONE MARROW (×1800)

1. The lower large cell with a round nucleus with prominent nucleoli, finely stippled chromatin, and a moderately blue cytoplasm is a myeloblast. This cell may be termed a type II myeloblast because its cytoplasm contains some (less than 15) fine azurophilic granules. The upper large cell with a round nucleus with somewhat coarse chromatin, a pale blue cytoplasm, and some indistinct reddish granules is a late promyelocyte. A metarubricyte is present to the left of the myeloblast, and two polychromatic rubricytes with nuclei at different stages of chromatin condensation are present to the right of the myeloblast.

2. The large cell with a lightly stained, round nucleus and reddish-purple granules in the light blue cytoplasm is a promyelocyte. A basophilic rubricyte, three polychromatic rubricytes at various maturative stages, and two metarubricytes are present. A free nucleus, probably from a degenerated leukocyte, is present to the left of the promyelocyte.

3. A basophil myelocyte with prominent, large, reddish-purple granules somewhat masking the nucleus is present adjoining a neutrophilic metamyelocyte *(upper right)* and a mature monolobed neutrophil *(lower right)*.

4. The large cell with distinct nucleoli, somewhat clumpy nuclear chromatin, and a dark blue cytoplasm is a rubriblast. The nuclear chromatin in erythrocytic precursors, particularly rubriblasts and prorubricytes, is characteristically much coarser in the horse than in the dog and cat. An intermediate polychromatic rubricyte, two late polychromatic rubricytes, a neutrophilic metamyelocyte, and a neutrophilic band are present in the field.

5. Erythroid cells in various maturative stages in the bone marrow of a horse with lead poisoning. The largest cell is a prorubricyte and the two smaller cells with some clumpy chromatin and a bluish cytoplasm are basophilic rubricytes. Among five cells with grayish cytoplasm, the smallest one with fully condensed nucleus is a metarubricyte, whereas the remaining cells are polychromatic rubricytes with varying degrees of nuclear chromatin condensation.

6. Erythroid cells in various maturative stages from rubriblast to metarubricytes and two neutrophilic granulocytes in the bone marrow of a horse with responsive anemia.

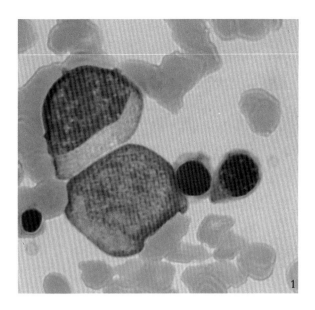

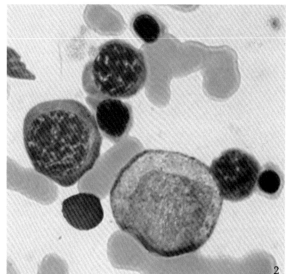

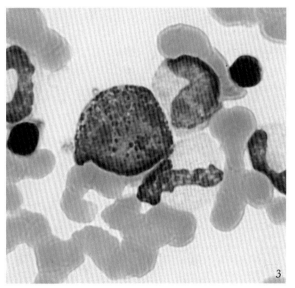

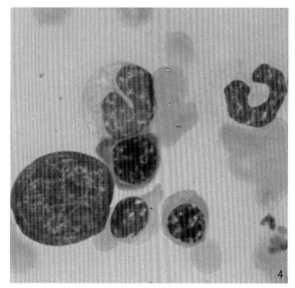

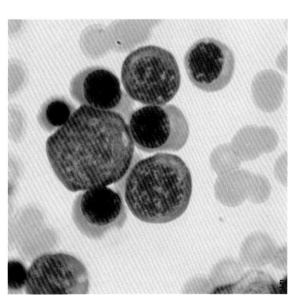

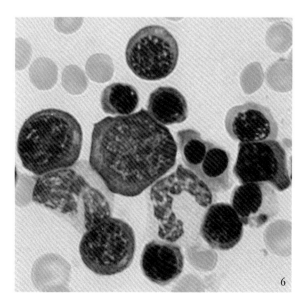

PLATE VII. LEUKOCYTES OF VARIOUS ANIMALS (×1800)

1. Mature bovine neutrophils. The rouleau formation of the erythrocytes is abnormal and represents a response to an inflammatory disease.

2. Bovine lymphocyte (cell with round nucleus) and monocyte.

3. Bovine monocyte and lymphocyte with azurophilic cytoplasmic granules.

4. Bovine eosinophil containing distinct reddish granules and a monocyte (from the same blood as Plate VII–1).

5. Bovine basophil. Intensely stained metachromatic cytoplasmic granules usually mask the nucleus in basophils.

6. Feline eosinophil and two basophils. The eosinophil has reddish, rod-like granules, whereas the basophils have faintly stained, round granules. The morphology of an immature basophil is shown in Plate XII–5.

7. Equine eosinophil and basophil.

8. Three mature equine neutrophils in a row and one band neutrophil on the left. Equine neutrophils often show more chromatin plaques than canine and feline neutrophils.

9. Mature neutrophil and an uncommon form of canine monocyte with a profuse number of reddish granules. The varied morphology of monocytes is shown in Plate VIII.

10. Three typical canine monocytes (also see Plate VIII).

11. Two monocytes of the Indian elephant. Others have classified the cells with round nuclei interconnected by a thin filament, as shown here, as lymphocytes, but they are peroxidase-positive (compare with Plate VII–12).

12. Peroxidase stain applied to leukocytes of the Indian elephant, a monocyte (left cell), and a neutrophil. Both are peroxidase-positive.

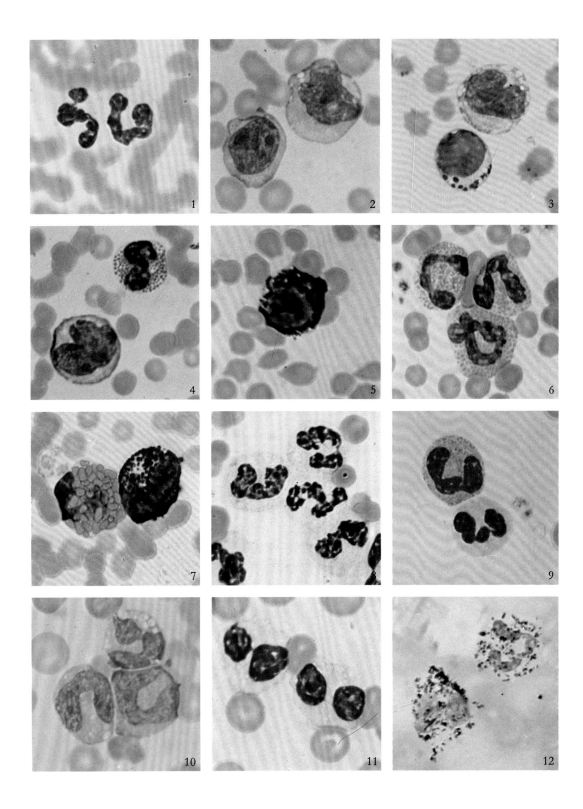

PLATE VIII. IMMATURE AND MATURE MONOCYTES, MACROPHAGES, AND TOXIC NEUTROPHILS IN CANINE BLOOD (×1800)

1. Monoblast with characteristic irregularly indented nucleus in the blood of a dog with leukemoid reaction (WBC count, 98,000 μl, with left shift to myeloblast). The cell has finely stippled nuclear chromatin, inconspicuous nucleolus, a moderately blue cytoplasm, and a high nucleus-to-cytoplasm ratio.

2. Monoblast and polyploid monocytoid cell in the blood of a dog with acute myelomonocytic leukemia. A platelet with distinct azurophilic granules is present above the two cells.

3. Promonocyte with an undulated nuclear outline, incipient chromatin condensation, and a moderate amount of vacuolated bluish cytoplasm.

4. Immature monocyte with round nucleus and a bluish vacuolated cytoplasm. The nuclear shape may be suggestive of a neutrophilic myelocyte, but the coarse, lacy nuclear chromatin and cytoplasmic features distinguish this cell as monocytoid.

5. Two young monocytes with oblong or indented nuclei, reticular nuclear chromatin, and distinctive cytoplasmic features. Cytoplasmic vacuolation is evident in only one cell.

6. Monocyte with a metamyelocyte-like nucleus but, unlike a neutrophilic metamyelocyte, it has blue and vacuolated cytoplasm. A neutrophil with clear cytoplasm is also present.

7. Monocyte with a band-like nucleus and a bluish cytoplasm tinged reddish with fine, indistinct azurophilic granules. The cytoplasmic features distinguish this cell from the nearby neutrophil.

8. More mature monocyte with pale blue, ground glass-like cytoplasm and a band-like nucleus is compared with two mature neutrophils having clear cytoplasm.

9. Typical mature monocyte with an ameboid nucleus and foamy blue, vacuolated cytoplasm (lower left) and a mature neutrophil.

10. Two macrophages with a highly vacuolated cytoplasm and an ameboid nucleus in the peripheral blood of a dog with bacterial endocarditis. Monocyte to macrophage activation may sometimes occur in the circulation, as in this patient. A medium-sized lymphocyte is present *(upper right)*.

11. Neutrophilic metamyelocyte and two neutrophilic bands with toxic foamy blue cytoplasm. The pattern of nuclear chromatin (coarsely granular but not lacy or reticular) and the cytoplasmic density and color (relatively clear and sky blue) distinguish these cells from the monocytoid cells in Plates VIII–7 and VIII–8, above.

12. Highly vacuolated toxic bands cells with partially folded nuclei. Note the nuclear and cytoplasmic features of these cells and those in Plate VIII–11 for differentiation from the macrophages in Plate VIII–10.

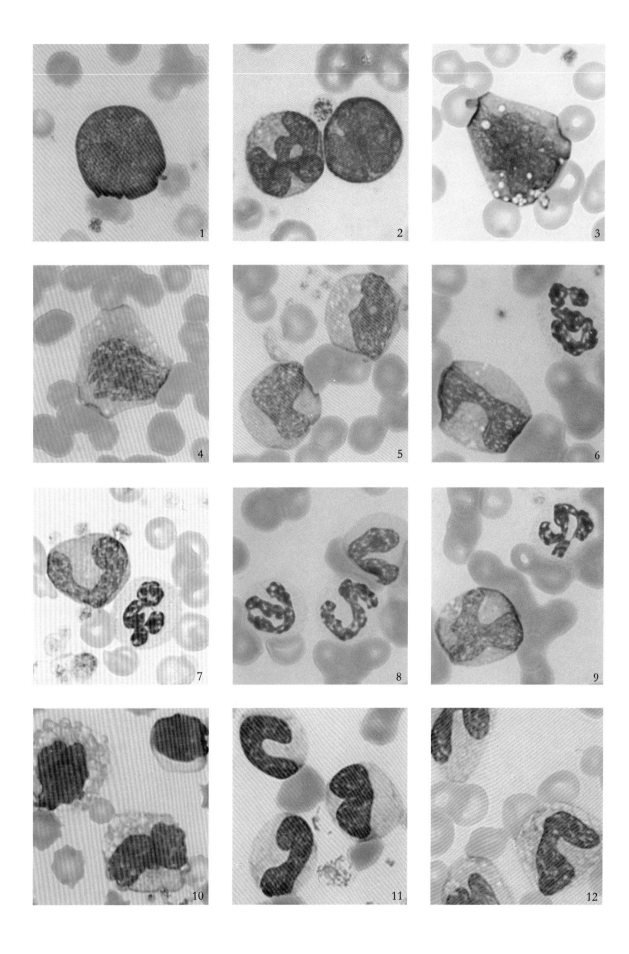

PLATE IX. LEUKOCYTE MORPHOLOGY IN TOXEMIC DISEASE, LYSOSOMAL STORAGE DISEASES, PELGER-HUËT ANOMALY, AND CHEDIAK-HIGASHI SYNDROME (×1800)

1. Eosinophil, lymphocyte, and three mature neutrophils with normal morphologic characteristics of feline leukocytes. Clusters of thrombocytes are also seen. Compare with Plates IX–2, 3, and 4.

2. Two mature feline neutrophils, slightly larger than normal. A Döhle body (blue spot) is present in the cytoplasm at one edge of one of the cells. Döhle bodies represent remnants of rough endoplasmic reticulum, resulting from a minor interference in the maturation of the cytoplasm.

3. Large feline neutrophils with a blue foamy cytoplasm. These cytologic features are signs of a defective maturation and characterize the cells as toxic neutrophils.

4. Giant neutrophils are seen in certain severe inflammatory diseases in the cat. One such giant neutrophil is shown here, along with neutrophils of normal morphology.

5. Neutrophil from an adult DSH male cat with hereditary Pelger-Huët anomaly. The cell has a band-like nucleus with condensed chromatin and relatively more abundant mature cytoplasm. (Blood film from a 1986 ASVCP slide review case submitted by Drs. K.S. Latimer and P.M. Rakich).

6. Neutrophil from a 5-year-old neutered male Collie dog with acquired Pelger-Huët anomaly secondary to inflammation or prolonged drug (primidone) administration. The cell has a metamyelocyte-like nucleus with condensed chromatin and relatively more abundant mature cytoplasm. (Blood film from a 1990 ASVCP slide review case submitted by Drs. K.S. Latimer and P.M. Rakich).

7. Two vacuolated lymphocytes from a 6-month-old Siamese female cat with GM_1 gangliosidosis. Such prominent cytoplasmic vacuoles were present in many lymphocytes and are common in lysosomal storage diseases such as fucosidosis, mannosidosis, mucopolysaccharidosis, and GM_1 gangliosidosis. The β-gangliosidase activity of leukocytes in this case was 0.40 nmoles/ml/hr compared to normal control value of 39.7 nmoles/ml/hr. (Blood film from a 1988 ASVCP slide review case submitted by Drs. S. Dial, M. A. Thrall, and P. Gasper).

8. Vacuolated lymphocyte from a 1-week-old female goat with β-mannosidosis. Several prominent cytoplasmic vacuoles or many small vacuoles were present in many lymphocytes of this goat. These vacuoles represent accumulation of material in lysosomes. (Blood film from a 1990 ASVCP slide review case submitted by Dr. W. Vernau).

9. Vacuolated eosinophils from a 5-year-old Sheltie dog. These cells resemble the atypical eosinophils common to Greyhounds. (Blood film from a 1986 ASVCP slide review case submitted by Drs. R. Raskin and H. Tvedten).

10. Neutrophil from a mink with aleutian disease or Chediak-Higashi syndrome. Many large densely stained cytoplasmic granules can be seen in the neutrophils from cases with Chediak-Higashi syndrome in humans and animals.

11. Neutrophil from a 3-year-old male DSH cat with Chediak-Higashi syndrome. The neutrophil contains few large pink granules in the pale cytoplasm. (Blood film from a 1987 ASVCP slide review case submitted by Drs. M. Menard and K. J. Wardrop).

12. Neutrophil from a 15-month-old Hereford heifer with Chediak-Higashi syndrome. The neutrophil contains several large pink granules in the pale cytoplasm. (Blood film from a 1987 ASVCP slide review case submitted by Drs. M. Menard and K. J. Wardrop).

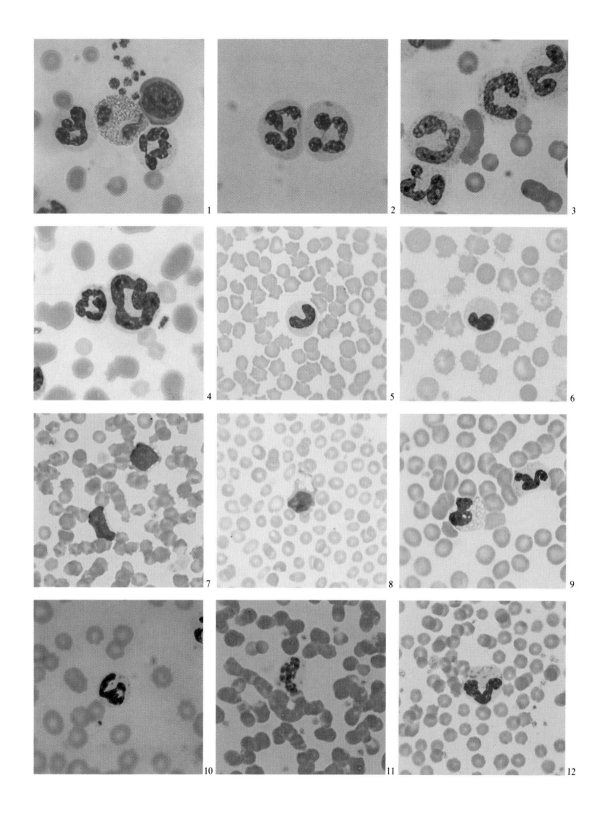

PLATE X. CYTOCHEMICAL REACTIONS OF BLOOD AND BONE MARROW CELLS (×1800)*

1. Two alkaline phosphatase-positive equine neutrophils (stained by the method of Kaplow;[1] naphthol AS-B1 phosphate was used as a substrate and fast red violet LB salt as the coupling agent).

2. Alkaline phosphatase activity in the intergranular cytoplasm of a canine eosinophil. Note the absence of enzyme activity in specific granules of the eosinophil and in the adjacent neutrophil (stained by the method of Kaplow,[1] as in Plate X–1 above).

3. Alkaline phosphatase activity in the intergranular cytoplasm of a feline basophil. Note the absence of enzyme activity in specific granules of the basophil and in the adjacent neutrophil (stained by the method of Kaplow[1]), as in Plate X–1 above.

4. Numerous peroxidase-positive orange granules in four canine neutrophils, (stained by the 3-amino-9-ethylcarbazol method of Graham et al.[2]).

5. Peroxidase-positive canine neutrophil with abundant orange granules and folded nucleus (right) is compared with a canine monocyte with sparse, similarly-stained cytoplasmic granules (left; stained by the 3-amino-9-ethylcarbazol method of Graham et al.[2]).

6. Monocyte with a few darkly stained, peroxidase-positive granules (left) compared with a neutrophil containing numerous intensely stained, peroxidase-positive granules (right; stained by the method of Kaplow;[1] benzidine dihydrochloride was used as the substrate).

7. Sudan black B-positive granules in a bovine neutrophil. Sudanophilia in neutrophils generally parallels their peroxidase activity, (stained by the method of Sheehan and Storey[3]).

8. Lipase-positive monocyte with diffuse reddish cytoplasmic reaction and a chloroacetate esterase-positive band neutrophil with bluish cytoplasmic granules in feline bone marrow (lipase staining by the method of Ansley and Ornstein[4] and chloroacetate esterase staining by the method of Yam et al.[5]; α-naphthyl outyrate was used as the substrate to demonstrate lipase activity and naphthol AS-D chloroacetate was used to demonstrate chloroacetate esterase activity).

9. Nonspecific esterase-positive monocyte with diffuse reddish cytoplasmic reaction (α-naphthyl acetate substrate) and a chloroacetate esterase-positive neutrophil with bluish cytoplasmic granules in human blood, (stained by the method of Yam et al.[5]).

10. Feline basophil exhibiting characteristic staining of its granules for naphthol AS-D chloroacetate esterase (stained by the method of Bauer-Sic[6]).

11. Periodic acid Schiff (PAS) reactivity of canine neutrophils indicated by diffuse magenta color in the cytoplasm. Methyl green was used as the nuclear stain (stained by a modified method of Bauer-Sic[6] and Hayhoe et al.[7]).

12. Methyl green pyronin staining of canine bone marrow cells. Distinctive pyroninophilia is evident in a typical plasma cell (stained by the method of Perry and Reynolds[8]).

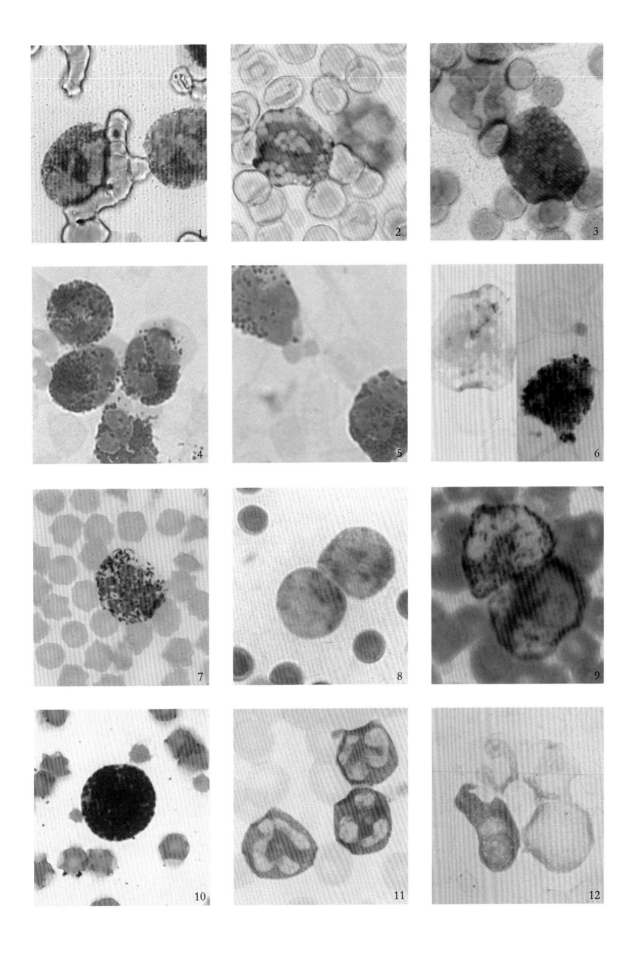

PLATE XI. CELLS IN NORMAL AND ABNORMAL BLOOD AND BONE MARROW (×1800)

1. Macrophage with phagocytosed iron particles and erythrocyte and nuclear debris from the bone marrow of a horse with anemia. Such a cell stains intensely for iron (see Plate XII–11).

2. Free nuclei of reticuloendothelial (RE) cells in bone marrow of a dog. The blue-staining nucleoli identify the structures as nuclei of RE cells. As the nucleus disintegrates, a net-like structure commonly referred to as a basket cell, is formed.

3. Neutrophil containing two circular masses of phagocytosed amorphous nuclear material typical of the lupus erythematosus (LE) cell from the bone marrow of a cat with a myeloproliferative disease.

4. Cluster of four plasma cells, a neutrophilic myelocyte, and a polychromatophilic rubricyte from the bone marrow of a dog with an idiopathic gammopathy.

5. A plasma cell filled with vesicles called Russell bodies (Mott cell) from the bone marrow of a dog. A neutrophilic myelocyte is also present.

6. Monocytoid cells in the peripheral blood of a dog with salmon poisoning.

7. *Top,* Neutrophil with a female sex chromatin lobe or drumstick from the peripheral blood of a dog. *Bottom,* Hypersegmented neutrophil in the peripheral blood of a cat with suspected vitamin B_{12}-folate deficiency.

8. Monocyte with azurophilic cytoplasmic granules and a macrocytic erythrocyte in the peripheral blood of a dog with suspected vitamin B_{12}-folate deficiency.

9. Two toxic metamyelocytes with foamy basophilic cytoplasm and a normal, small lymphocyte in the peripheral blood of a cow with acute coliform mastitis.

10. Toxic band neutrophils with foamy blue cytoplasm in the peripheral blood of a cat with empyema of the thoracic cavity.

11. Toxic neutrophils (metamyelocyte and band) in the blood of a foal with salmonellosis.

12. Neutrophils with toxic granulation in the blood of a horse with acute hepatitis.

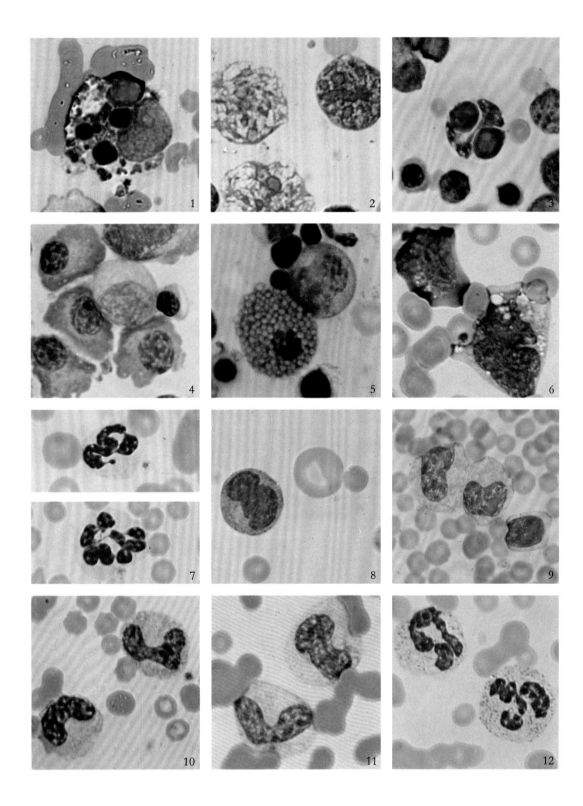

PLATE XII. BLOOD AND BONE MARROW CELLS OF VARIOUS ANIMALS IN HEALTH AND DISEASE (×1800)

1. Eosinophil and a basophil in the peripheral blood of a dog. The canine basophil characteristically contains sparse metachromatic granules in contrast to basophils in the horse and ruminants. Central pallor is evident in the mature red cells.

2. The canine eosinophil differs from the eosinophils of other domestic animals in that the granules may vary considerably in number and size, as shown by the two eosinophils from the blood of a dog with eosinophilia of undefined origin. A mature neutrophil is also present.

3. Canine eosinophilic promyelocyte with two types of cytoplasmic granules, some large azurophilic and many light pink specific granules. Such a cell is extremely rare in normal bone marrow, but it is sometimes found in bone marrow with increased eosinophilopoiesis. A band neutrophil is also present.

4. Bone marrow of a cat with mastocytoma. A mast cell *(upper right)* studded with metachromatic granules is compared with a basophil myelocyte *(lower right)* containing few metachromatic granules and many grayish specific granules.

5. Immature basophil in the peripheral blood of a cat. Note the presence of both large, metachromatic granules and round, grayish granules, as in the basophil myelocyte in the preceding photomicrograph. The reddish purple granules disappear with cell maturation. Compare this cell with the mature basophil in Plate VII–6.

6. Döhle bodies in the somewhat foamy cytoplasm of toxic band neutrophils in the peripheral blood of a dog with chronic peritonitis.

7. Leukergy (clumping of neutrophils) in the peripheral blood of a horse. The cause of this rare phenomenon is obscure, but it is more frequent in horses with severe inflammatory conditions.

8. Corynebacterium parvum in a clump of platelets in the blood of a dog given an intravenous injection of the bacteria to stimulate cytotoxic T-lymphocyte activity.

9. Three Howell-Jolly bodies (large, densely stained, marginal objects) and two Pappenheimer bodies (small, light blue, marginal structures) in the erythrocytes of a dog.

10. Siderocytes (red cells with dark blue specks) in the peripheral blood of a cat (Prussian blue stain for iron).

11. Macrophage with dense blue (4+) cytoplasmic iron in the bone marrow of a horse (Prussian blue stain for iron).

12. Brightly fluorescent (4+) megakaryocyte in the bone marrow of a dog with autoimmune thrombocytopenia. The bone marrow film was stained for direct immunofluorescence using anticanine IgG antibody.

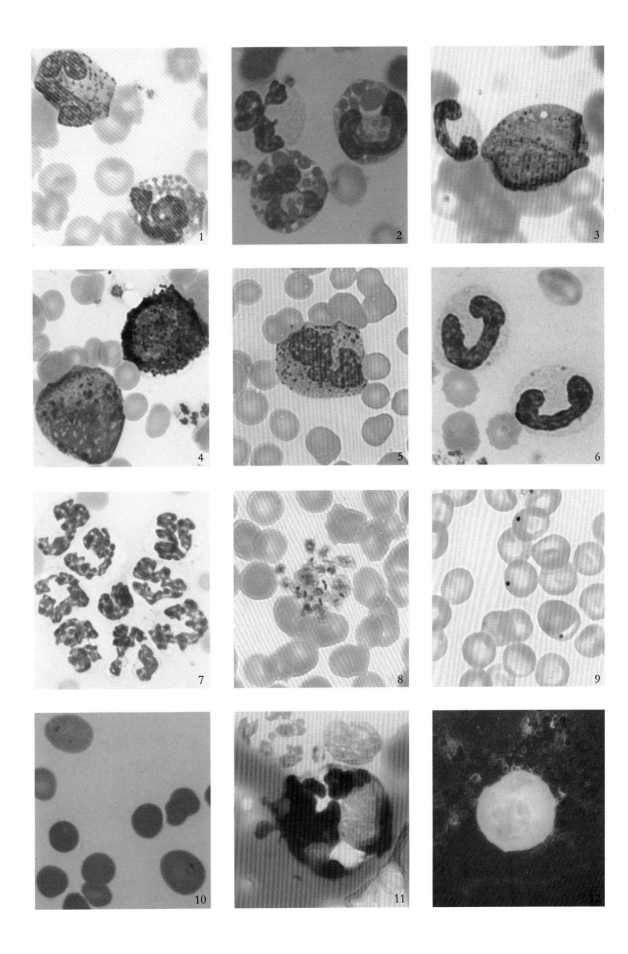

PLATE XIII. BLOOD AND BONE MARROW CELLS IN DISEASES OF THE DOG

1–4. Prominent, coarse, azurophilic granules in two lymphocytes *(1 and 2),* a monocyte *(3),* and a neutrophil *(4)* in the blood of a dog with mucopolysaccharidosis. Individual granules may appear to be within a clear vacuole or surrounded by a halo, as seen in the lymphocytes (×1800). (From Schalm, O.W.: Mucopolysoccharosis. Canine Pract., pp 28–32, Dec. 1977.)

5–6. Morulae of Ehrlichia canis in a lymphocyte *(5)* and a neutrophil *(6)* in the peripheral blood of a dog (×1800). (From Schalm, O.W., and Strombeck, D.R.: Pancytopenia in a dog due to *Ehrlichia canis.* Canine Pract., pp. 13–17, Nov.–Dec. 1974.)

7–9. Flame cells (plasma cells with abundant reddish cytoplasm) in the bone marrow of a dog with IgA myeloma *(7,* ×1400; *8* and *9,* × 800). (Courtesy of Dr. J.G. Zinkl.)

10–12. Macrophage with phagocytosed polychromatic red cell and rubricytes *(10),* macrophage with phagocytosed red cells and band neutrophil *(11)* in bone marrow smears, and erythrophagocytosis *(12)* in histologic section of the bone marrow from a dog with histiocytic medullary reticulosis or malignant histiocytosis *(10* and *11,* ×1800; *12,* ×1260). (From Schalm, O.W.: Histiocytic medullary reticulosis. Canine Pract., pp 42–45, Aug. 1978.)

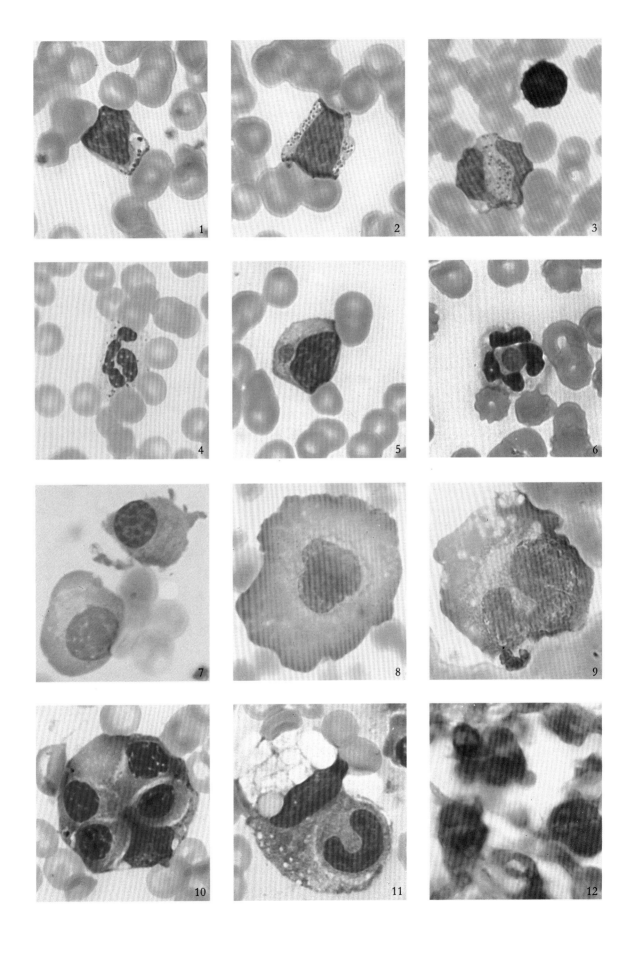

PLATE XIV. PARASITES AND ABNORMALITIES IN LEUKOCYTES OF VARIOUS ANIMALS (×1800)

1. Neutrophils in the blood of a horse. One neutrophil contains four morulae of Ehrlichia equi.

2. Two morulae of Ehrlichia equi in a band neutrophil in the blood of a horse.

3. Morula of Ehrlichia equi in a neutrophil of a horse (new methylene blue stain).

4. Morulae of Ehrlichia *(arrow)* in a monocytoid cell in the bone marrow of an experimentally infected dog.

5. Cytoplasmic inclusion with azurophilic granulation in the neutrophil of a cat with feline infectious peritonitis. The structure might be a Chlamydia occurring coincidentally with infectious peritonitis. (From Ward, J.M., Smith, R., and Schalm, O.W.: *Inclusions in neutrophils of cats with feline peritonitis.* J. Am. Vet. Med. Assoc., 158:348, 1970.)

6. Inclusion similar to that in Plate XIV–5 occurring in a mononuclear cell in the peripheral blood of a cat presented with an idiopathic anemia.

7. Inclusion in the cytoplasm of a lymphocyte in the peripheral blood of a young dog with distemper.

8. Blast cell with nuclear and cytoplasmic features suggestive of a rubriblast, containing a cyst of Toxoplasma gondii from the bone marrow of a cat in the terminal phase of erythroleukemia.

9. Trophozoites of Toxoplasma gondii in the same bone marrow as in the preceding photomicrograph.

10. Neutrophil containing phagocytosed staphylococci from the peripheral blood of a cat with staphylococcal septicemia.

11. Sideroleukocyte in the blood of a horse with an idiopathic anemia. The horse was negative for equine infectious anemia by the immunodiffusion test.

12. Lupus erythematosus cells in dog blood. A rosette of neutrophils surrounds amorphous nuclear material. Two of the neutrophils are typical LE cells, as shown by the filling of their cytoplasm with amorphous nuclear material *(arrow)*.

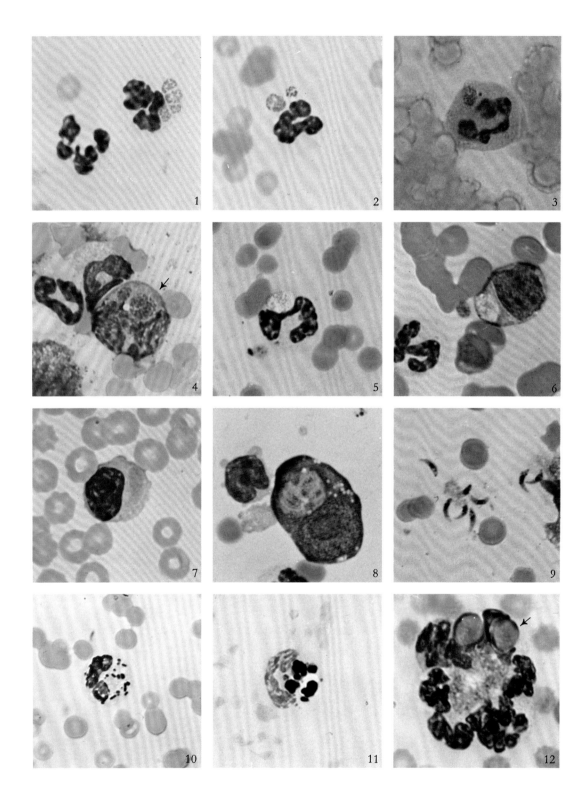

PLATE XV. ABNORMAL BLOOD AND BONE MARROW CELLS OF THE CAT (×1800)

1. Blast cell in the blood in acute undifferentiated myeloproliferative disorder (acute undifferentiated leukemia (AUL) previously termed reticuloendotheliosis).

2. Two unclassified cells in the blood in AUL. One cell has reddish cytoplasmic granules.

3. Unclassified cell with a pseudopod and cytoplasmic granules in the bone marrow in AUL.

4. Two megaloblastoid rubricytes in the bone marrow in erythremic myelosis. Note the difference in cytoplasmic maturation.

5. Megaloblastoid rubricyte with iron granules (sideroblast) in the bone marrow in erythremic myelosis (Prussian blue stain for iron).

6. Macrophage with two phagocytosed erythrocytes from the bone marrow of a cat with feline infectious anemia (haemobartonellosis). Erythrophagocytosis is a common finding in anemias of various causes in the cat. A lymphocyte and a metarubricyte are also seen.

7. Macrophage with a phagocytosed eosinophil from the bone marrow in a chronic disease associated with the development of an aplastic marrow.

8. Giant metamyelocyte, small lymphocyte, and polychromatic rubricyte in the bone marrow in panleukopenia. Maturation of the granulocyte has taken place directly from a primitive precursor cell without mitosis. Giant granulocytes with bizarre nuclear patterns are common in the bone marrow of the cat under conditions of depressed granulopoiesis.

9. Giant metamyelocyte in blood in depressed granulopoiesis.

10. Two giant toxic band neutrophils in blood of a cat convalescing from panleukopenia.

11. Abnormal maturation form of a granulocytic precursor cell (myelocyte) in the blood in staphylococcal septicemia (also see Plate XIV–10).

12. Reddish purple (toxic) granulation of neutrophils in the blood of a 3-month-old kitten with pneumonitis. Toxic granulation is not a common finding in feline neutrophils. See Plate XI–10 for the more commonly encountered toxic signs in the neutrophils of the cat.

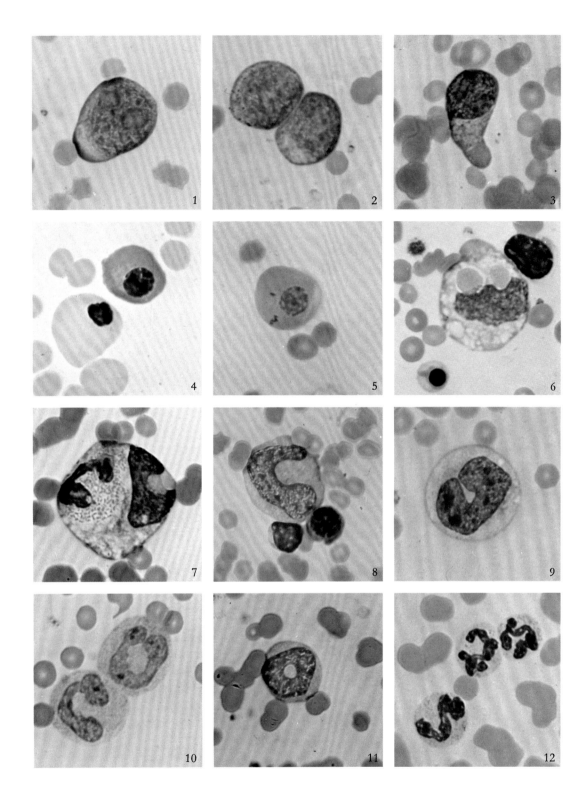

PLATE XVI. ERYTHROCYTES IN VARIOUS ANEMIAS (×1800)

1. Microcytic hypochromic anemia from chronic blood loss in a dog. A blood transfusion was given before the blood for this figure was taken. Normal transfused erythrocytes are more deeply stained and are larger than some of the microcytic hypochromic cells. Irregularly shaped erythrocytes (poikilocytes) represent fragments of poorly formed cells.

2. Bone marrow from the same dog represented in the preceding photomicrograph. A promyelocyte, two late rubricytes, and two metarubricytes are present.

3. Peripheral blood in anemia in remission in a dog. A metarubricyte, an erythrocyte with a Howell-Jolly body, and many polychromatophilic macrocytes are seen. Polychromatophilic red cells usually appear as reticulocytes when blood is stained with new methylene blue or a reticulocyte stain (see Plate IV–6).

4. Peripheral blood of a dog with autoimmune hemolytic anemia in remission. The small, densely stained erythrocytes are spherocytes. A metarubricyte is seen. Most of the lightly-stained cells are macrocytic erythrocytes, some of which present target cell patterns and may be polychromatophilic. Excessive surface membrane in relation to the inner contents produces target cell and bowl-shaped patterns in young red cells.

5. Blood in autoimmune hemolytic anemia in a cat. Note the cluster of agglutinated polychromatophilic erythrocytes. Polychromatophilic erythrocytes normally do not participate in the formation of clumps, and thus the phenomenon indicates the action of an antibody. A metarubricyte is seen.

6. Histologic section of a lymph node of a cat with a myeloproliferative disease. Cells of the mononuclear phagocyte system are engorged with erythrocytes *(arrow)* and hemosiderin. Extreme erythrophagocytosis, as seen in this figure, may lead to a rapid fall of the PCV.

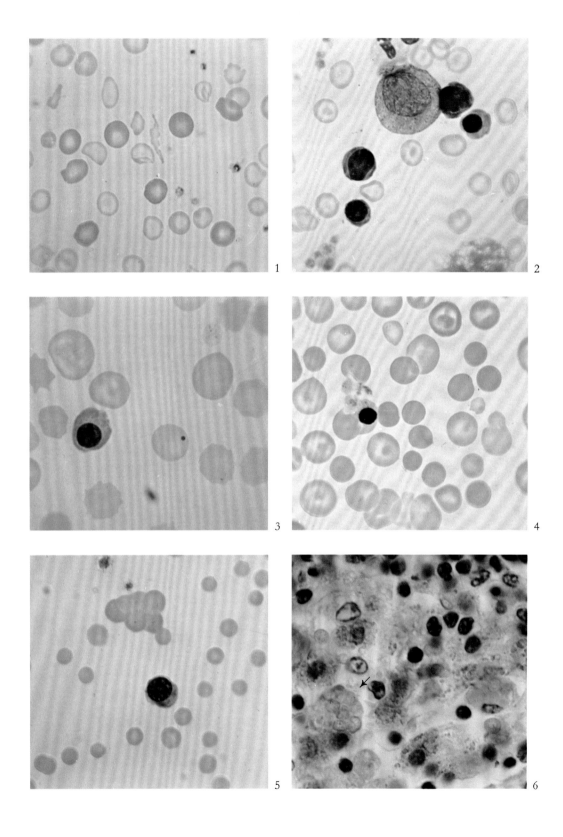

PLATE XVII. HEMOPARASITES AND ERYTHROCYTE ABNORMALITIES (×1800)

1. Blood in feline infectious anemia. One erythrocyte in the center area contains a round, deeply stained structure called a Howell-Jolly body. All other objects on the surface or at the margin of erythrocytes are Haemobartonella felis.

2. Blood in feline infectious anemia. H. felis appears as faintly stained spheres on the surface of erythrocytes and as more deeply stained specks and short rods on the outside margin (see also Fig. 10–4).

3. Blood from a splenectomized dog showing isolated dots and chains of H. canis on the surface of erythrocytes (see also Fig. 10–6).

4. Bovine blood with both Anaplasma marginale, appearing as round, deeply stained structures in an eccentric position in two erythrocytes *(arrow)*, and Eperythrozoon wenyoni, appearing as faintly stained objects on the surface or at the margin of several erythrocytes (see also Fig. 10–7)

5. Same blood as in the preceding photomicrograph, with a ring-like structure of E. wenyoni more clearly visible on the erythrocyte in the center *(arrow)*. The same erythrocyte has another E. wenyoni on its margin. Compare these structures with the more deeply stained and larger A. marginale located inside and at the margins of two erythrocytes.

6. Erythrocytes containing Babesia canis.

7. Bovine blood with many A. marginale in erythrocytes. A polychromatophilic rubricyte and a polychromatophilic erythrocyte are also present. The latter two cells indicate that the developing anemia is in a stage of beginning remission.

8. Heinz bodies in bovine erythrocytes in onion poisoning. Blood was stained with new methylene blue as for the routine reticulocyte count.

9. Canine distemper inclusions in erythrocytes. These inclusions vary in size and staining characteristics and occur in young erythrocytes. They are seen only infrequently in canine distemper. (See Fig. 18–2).

10. Basophilic stippling of a bovine erythrocyte. Stippled immature erythrocytes appear in the peripheral blood in response to blood loss or hemolytic anemia in ruminants.

11. Two stippled polychromatophilic erythrocytes in the blood of a dog with lead poisoning.

12. Metarubricyte with a few punctate granules in the peripheral blood of a horse with lead poisoning.

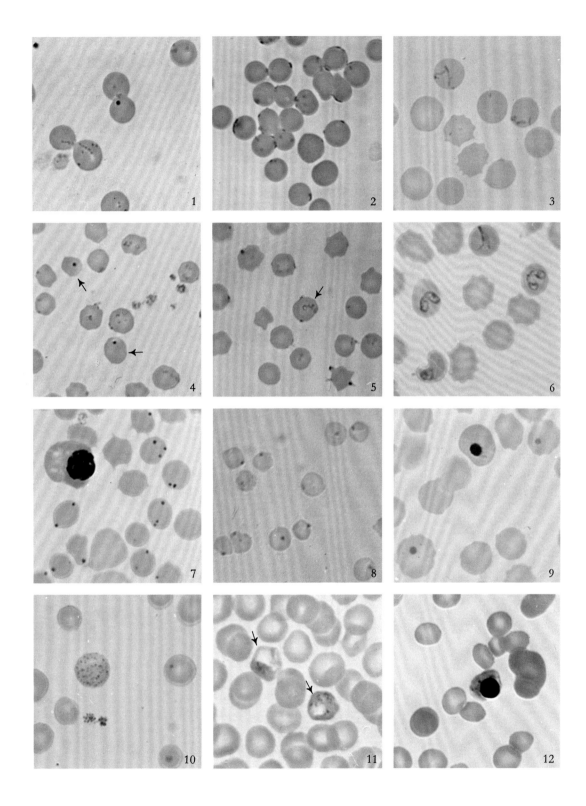

PLATE XVIII. HEINZ BODIES, ERYTHROCYTE ABNORMALITIES IN IRON DEFICIENCY ANEMIAS, AND HEMOPARASITES (×1800)

1. Anemia in remission in a cat. The large grayish erythrocytes and the two nucleated cells are young red cells released into the peripheral blood in response to anemia. Each small, mature red cell presents a pale structure near one edge that protrudes beyond the edge of some of the erythrocytes. These protruding structures are Heinz bodies. Destruction of Heinz-body-laden erythrocytes, mainly by the spleen, leads to hemolytic anemia.

2. Feline Heinz bodies in a dry, unfixed film. Several of the white protrusions have broken away from the erythrocytes and are free between the cells.

3. Same blood as in Plates XVIII–1 and –2 treated as a hanging drop stained with new methylene blue. The Heinz body in the red blood cell appears black (surface stain) when in focus and becomes refractile when the surface is out of focus. This characteristic suggested the name erythrocyte refractile or ER body.

4. Heinz bodies in a dry, unfixed feline blood film stained with new methylene blue. A metarubricyte and an unclassified cell are also present.

5. Iron deficiency anemia in an 18-month-old female llama. Oval erythrocytes, characteristic of the species, exhibit prominent hypochromasia (deficiency of hemoglobin), eccentrically placed hemoglobin, and poikilocytosis. Red cell fragments and a neutrophil are also present. (Blood film from a 1987 ASVCP slide review case submitted by Dr. J. S. Thomas.)

6. Erythrocytes from an adult female llama. Hemoglobin crystals, resembling hemoglobin C crystals in humans, were present in 1 to 2% of the red cells. The llama had chronic pneumonia and was nursing. Blood examination revealed anemia (PCV 18.5%) and leukocytosis (WBC 25,500μl). (Blood film from a 1987 ASVCP slide review case submitted by Dr. H. Tvedten.)

7. Abnormal erythrocyte morphology in an alpaca. Partially hypochromic erythrocytes and red cells with eccentrically placed hemoglobin are present among normal ovalocytes.

8. Blood film from a 13-year-old neutered female Siamese cat. Most of the erythrocytes show increased paleness of central area because of reduced hemoglobinization. The cat was found to have a microcytic hypochromic anemia associated with iron deficiency (decreased serum iron and reduced transferrin saturation) possibly from heavy flea infestation. (Blood film from a 1987 ASVCP slide review case submitted by Dr. J. Blue.)

9. Cytauxzoon felis in erythrocytes of a 1-year-old DSH cat. Signet ring-shaped piroplasma can be seen in some red cells. (Blood film from a 1987 ASVCP slide review case submitted by Dr. J. E. West.)

10. Trypanosoma theileri in blood film of a 3-day-old female Angus calf. (Blood film from a 1989 ASVCP slide review case submitted by Dr. H. Bender and coworkers.)

11. Spirochetes identified as Borrelia burgdorferi were present in a 2-year-old male Siberian Husky dog with fever and pancytopenia. Serologic results were positive for lyme disease and *Ehrlichia canis*. (Blood film from a 1986 ASVCP slide review case submitted by Dr. E. Wilson.)

12. Experimental Plasmodium berghei infection in a splenectomized mouse. Plasmodium trophozoites can be seen in polychromatic erythrocytes. Occasional mature erythrocytes also contained the parasites. (Blood film from a 1988 ASVCP slide review case submitted by Drs. N. Winjum, L. Senter, and S. Stockham.)

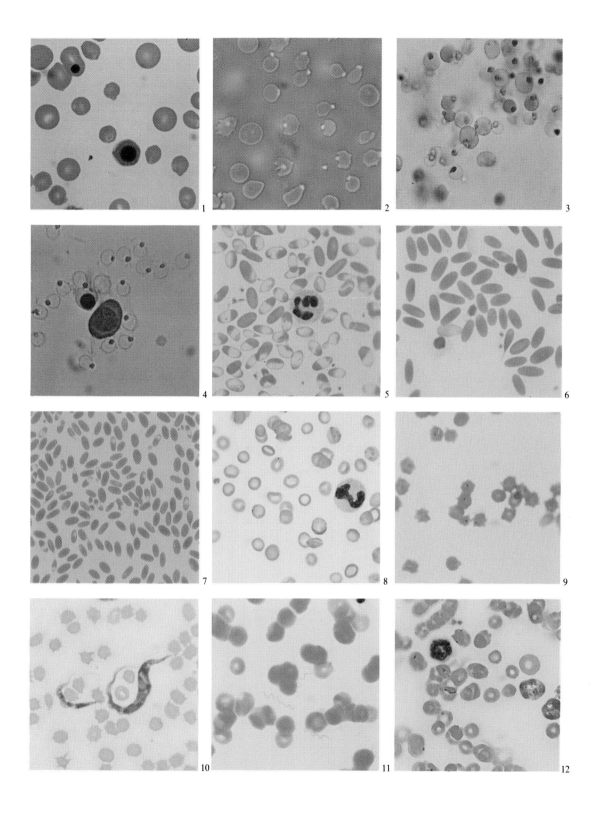

PLATE XIX. LYMPHOCYTIC LEUKEMIA IN THE DOG AND CAT ($\times 1800$)

1. Lymphoblasts and prolymphocytes in the peripheral blood of a dog with lymphoma. Note the single large nucleolus in the cell in center of field. Compare the nuclear morphology with that of the cells in Plate XIX–4.

2. Lymphoblasts in fluid aspirated from an enlarged lymph node of a dog with lymphoma.

3. Prolymphocytes (cells with smooth nuclear chromatin and no obvious nucleoli) in peripheral blood of a cat with lymphoma. Two neutrophils and a small mature lymphocyte are also present.

4. Bone marrow of a cat with lymphoma. A basophil myelocyte is near the center, but most of the cells are prolymphocytes. Cytoplasmic vacuolation in prolymphocytes is unusual.

5. Bone marrow of a cat with large, vacuolated lymphoid cells. The diagnosis at necropsy was lymphoma. Compare the cell size and morphology with Plate XIX–4.

6. Bone marrow from the same cat as in Plate XIX–5 stained for peroxidase. A peroxidase-positive granulocyte is in center of field. The vacuolated lymphoid cells are peroxidase-negative.

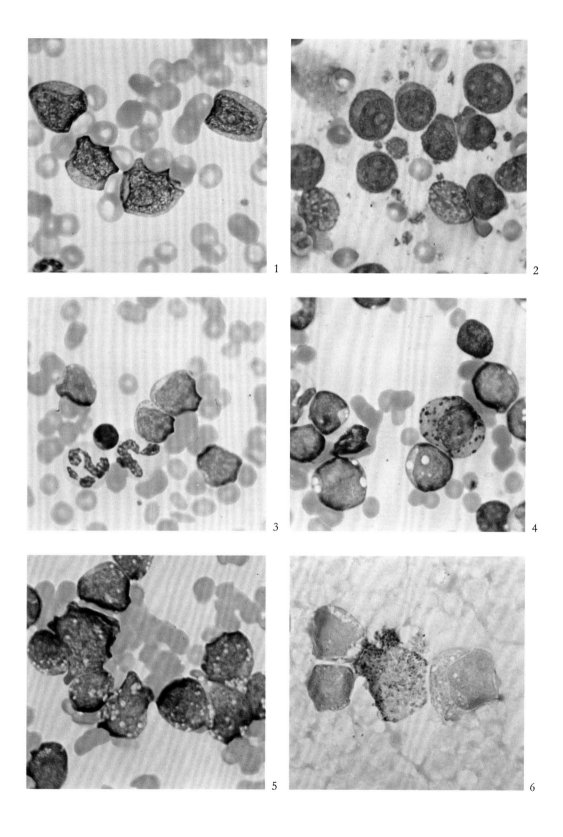

PLATE XX. BONE MARROW IN ACUTE MYELOID LEUKEMIAS IN THE
DOG AND CAT (×1800)

1. Acute myeloblastic leukemia without maturation (M1) in a cat. Blast cells with fine chromatin and distinct or indistinct nucleoli and a narrow rim of blue agranular cytoplasm predominate this form of AML. Granulocytic differentiation is minimal (<10%).

2. Acute myeloblastic leukemia with maturation (M2) in a dog. Increased numbers (>30% to <90%) of myeloblasts are found along with granulocytic differentiation in this form of AML. Myeloblasts with small to moderate amounts of cytoplasm and granulocytic differentiation to neutrophilic metamyelocytes is evident in this case.

3. Acute myelomonocytic leukemia (M4) in a dog. This form of AML is characterized by the presence of blast cells (>30%) with myeloblastic (nuclei with stippled chromatin and regular nuclear outline) and monoblastic (stippled to lacy chromatin and irregular to folded nuclear outline) features and differentiated granulocytic (>20%) and monocytic (>20%) cells. Myeloblasts with a moderate amount of cytoplasm and blast cells with some nuclear features of monoblasts are present in this case. Monocytic differentiation is evidenced by two cells with irregular nuclei and moderate blue cytoplasm. Neutrophilic metamyelocytes with pale blue cytoplasm indicate granulocytic differentiation.

4. Nonspecific esterase positive cells in a dog with acute myelomonocytic leukemia. Alpha-naphthyl butyrate was used as the substrate in this case. Diffuse reddish orange cytoplasmic staining is characteristic of monocytic cells, whereas granulocytic cells appear colorless.

5. Acute monoblastic leukemia (M5a) in a dog. Monoblasts and promonocytes, cells with undulated nuclear outline and/or folded nuclear membrane and chromatin, predominate (>80%) this form of AML. (From Jain N.C., et al.: Vet. Clin. Pathol. 20:63, 1991).

6. Acute monoblastic leukemia (M5b) in a dog. Prominent monocytic differentiation from monoblasts to monocytes is the main feature of this form of AML. Blast cell population is <80%, while monocytic differentiation is distinctive and granulocytic component is minimal (<20%). (From Jain N.C., et al.: Vet. Clin. Pathol. 20:63, 1991).

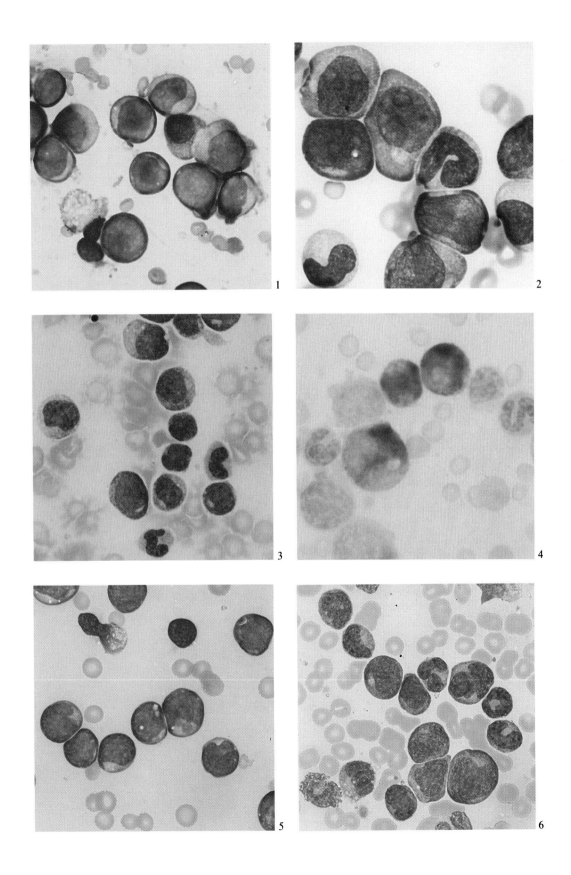

PLATE XXI. BLOOD AND BONE MARROW IN LEUKEMIAS AND MYELODYSPLASTIC SYNDROMES IN THE DOG AND CAT (×1800)

1. Bone marrow in erythroleukemia (M6) in a cat. Erythroid component is >50% and blast cell count is >30% of all nucleated cells in the marrow in this form of AML. A few myeloblasts, megaloblastic rubricytes, and mitotic erythroid cells can be seen in this field. (From Jain N.C., et al.: Vet. Clin. Pathol. 20: 63, 1991).

2. Bone marrow in myelodysplastic syndrome in a dog. Myeloblasts are <30% of all nucleated cells in the bone marrow in this condition. Neutrophilic differentiation is prominent in this case, but it is imbalanced because of a lack of immature forms, such as promyelocytes and myelocytes, while bands and segmented cells are more numerous.

3. Blood in acute megakaryocytic leukemia (M7) in a dog. Micromegkaryoblasts are cells with a small amount of blue cytoplasm and tiny surface blebs. Blast cells with smooth cell surfaces may be more primitive forms of megakaryoblasts, but their true identity, based only on morphologic features, remains uncertain. A few large and nongranular platelets are also present in this field.

4. Bone marrow in acute megakaryocytic leukemia (M7) in a dog (same case as shown in Plate XXI–3 above). This field has two micromegakaryoblasts with a narrow rim of blue cytoplasm and several small but prominent surface blebs.

5. Blood from a 12-year-old female Collie-cross dog with large granular lymphoma (LGL). A blast cell with smooth chromatin and distinct nucleolus is present along with lymphoid cells containing numerous large reddish purple cytoplasmic granules typical of LGL. The nuclear chromatin pattern of the lymphoid cells is similar to that of the blast cell. (Blood film from a 1989 ASVCP slide review case submitted by Drs. M. Wellman and G. Kociba.)

6. Blood from an 8-year-old neutered female DSH cat with large granular lymphoma (LGL). Two large lymphocytes with many prominent large reddish purple cytoplasmic granules and round nuclei with coarse chromatin are present. Most of the granules have a clear halo around them, unlike the LGL cells found in the case shown in Plate XXI–5. (Blood film from a 1989 ASVCP slide review case submitted by Drs. R. J. Sutherland, J. N. Mills, and S. A. Beetson.)

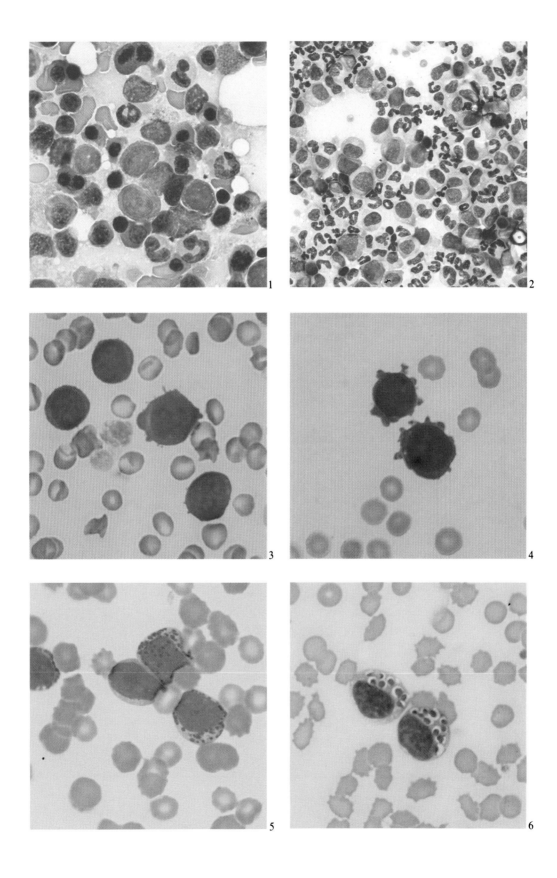

PLATE XXII. MYELOPROLIFERATIVE DISORDERS IN THE CAT (×1800)

1. Abnormal rubricytes in the bone marrow in suspected vitamin B_{12}-folate deficiency. Note the abnormal chromatin patterns of the two central cells.

2. Bone marrow cytology in a myeloproliferative disorder in which the primitive proliferating cells are of rubricytic origin. The nuclear chromatin patterns are similar to those of some cells seen in vitamin B_{12}-folate deficiency. Compare with Plate XXII–1.

3. Blood in erythremic myelosis exhibiting marked variation in size of fully hemoglobinized erythrocytes.

4. Blood in erythremic myelosis in which large numbers of nucleated erythrocytes are seen without accompanying anisocytosis or polychromasia. This pattern clearly indicates a myeloproliferative disorder involving the rubricytic series and leading to ineffective erythropoiesis.

5. Bone marrow of the same cat from which the blood was taken for Plate XXII–4. These are primitive unclassified cells, possibly rubricytic in origin, of which two have cytoplasmic, pseudopod-like projections. The more mature nucleated cells in the blood (Plate XXII–4) may have had their origin from extramedullary hematopoiesis in the greatly enlarged liver and spleen. See Plate XXIII–5 for liver histopathology.

6. Agglutinated polychromatophilic erythrocytes and metarubricytes in the bone marrow in a myeloproliferative disease. Also seen is a giant metarubricyte with two abnormal nuclei.

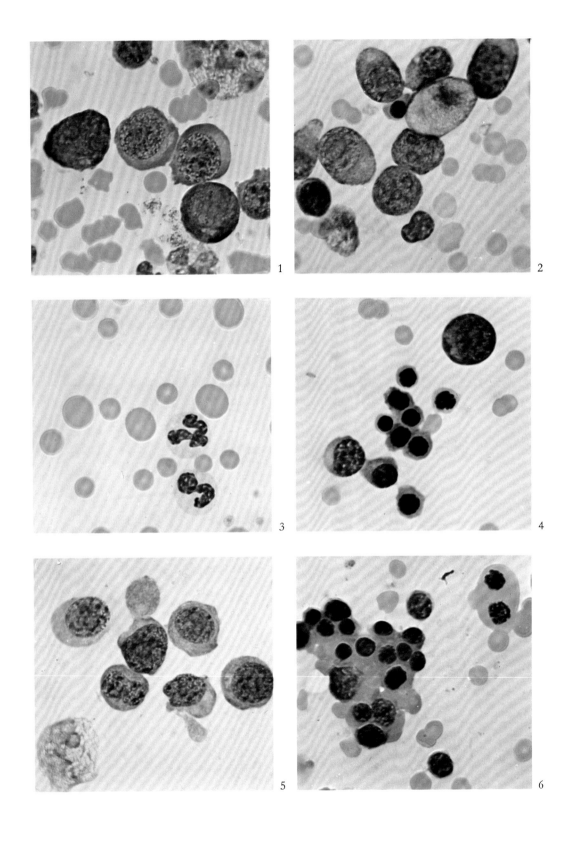

PLATE XXIII. MYELOPROLIFERATIVE DISORDERS IN THE CAT

1. Polyploidy involving polychromatophilic rubricytes in the bone marrow (×1800).

2. Erythrophagocytosis by a primitive cell of the bone marrow in erythremic myelosis (×1800). See Cat 4, Table 20–2.

3. Bone marrow cytology in erythroleukemia at a time when megaloblastoid rubricytes were prominent. Marked asynchronism is seen between the cytoplasm and nucleus of one rubricyte (×1800). See Cat 6, Table 20–2.

4. Bone marrow of the same cat as in Plate XXIII–3 taken 10 days later. Granulocytic precursor cells are predominant, suggesting a change in the direction of acute myelogenous leukemia. One giant polychromatophilic rubricyte is at the right border (× 1800).

5. Section of the liver in erythroleukemia demonstrating marked distention of sinusoids by proliferating hematopoietic cells. Two mitotic figures are seen in the central sinusoid (×1260).

6. Section of bone marrow demonstrating myelofibrosis, which may be a terminal event in myeloproliferative disease (×900).

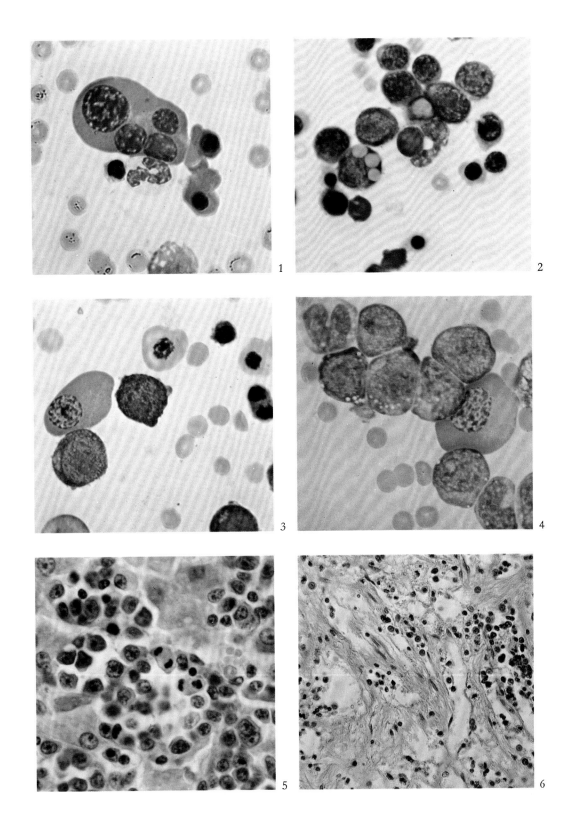

PLATE XXIV. MYELOGENOUS (GRANULOCYTIC) AND MAST CELL LEUKEMIAS IN THE CAT (×1800)

1. Blood in myelogenous leukemia in which the neoplastic cells are limited to myeloblasts, progranulocytes, and myelocytes. The total leukocyte count was 389,000/μl of blood.

2. Bone marrow from the same cat as in Plate XXIV–1. The many cytoplasmic azurophilic granules permit identification of the cells as of granulocytic origin, namely, promyelocytes.

3. Bone marrow in subleukemic myelogenous leukemia. Progranulocytes are present, as are bizarre nuclear forms in the more mature granulocytes.

4. Bone marrow in subleukemic myelogenous leukemia. The granulocytes are neutrophilic myelocytes and metamyelocytes. One megaloblastoid normochromic rubricyte is present. See Cat 8, Table 20–2.

5. Bone marrow in chronic eosinophilic leukemia. Two eosinophilic myelocytes and many band and segmented forms of eosinophils are present.

6. Bone marrow taken at necropsy from a cat with mast cell leukemia. The total leukocyte count in the blood was 30,000/μl, of which 35% were mast cells. The spleen was markedly enlarged.

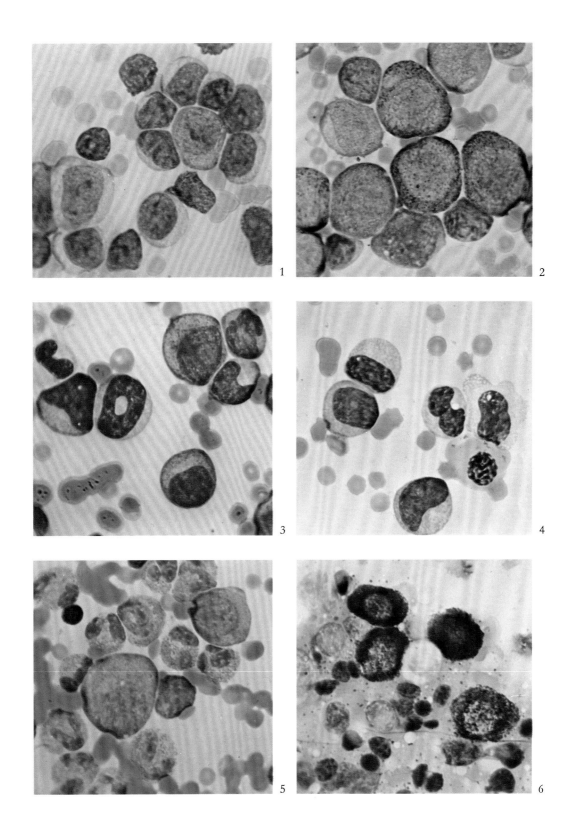

PLATE XXV. MYELOGENOUS (GRANULOCYTIC) LEUKEMIA IN THE DOG (×1800)

1. Blood in myelogenous leukemia (305,000 leukocytes/μl) with many myeloblasts and more advanced maturation forms. The myeloblasts present multiple nucleoli and finely stippled nuclear chromatin.

2. Blood in myelogenous leukemia (29,900 leukocytes/μl) with myeloblasts and myelocytes. See Table 20–7, 7-year-old Irish setter.

3. Bone marrow in myelogenous leukemia with giant, bizarre forms of neutrophilic granulocytes. See Table 20–7, 17-month-old German shepherd.

4. Bone marrow in myelogenous leukemia presenting myelocytes and metamyelocytes.

5. Blood with unclassified cells that were peroxidase-negative. The pathologist's study of gross and microscopic tissue changes led to a diagnosis of myelogenous leukemia. See comments for Plate XXV–6.

6. Bone marrow of the dog from which the blood of Plate XXV–5 was taken. One cell similar in morphology to the cells seen in the blood and another cell more typical of a bilobed granulocyte are shown to be positive for alkaline phosphatase. This reaction is interpreted as indicative of myelogenous leukemia in the dog. See Chapter 18 for a discussion of the alkaline phosphatase reaction in leukemic granulocytes.

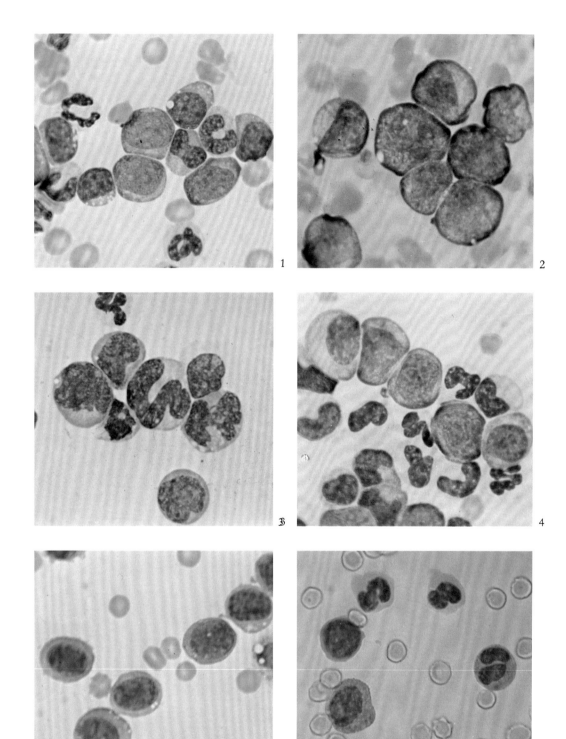

PLATE XXVI. ACUTE MYELOMONOCYTIC LEUKEMIA IN THE DOG (×1800)

1. Myeloblasts are recognized by their round or almost round nucleus and by other criteria of cell immaturity, such as stippled nuclear chromatin, indistinct nucleoli, and small amount of moderate blue cytoplasm, giving a high nucleus-to-cytoplasm ratio. The promyelocyte contains some small azurophilic granules (peripheral blood).

2. Myeloblast in the middle of two monoblasts. With the exception of an irregular or clefted nuclear outline, the monoblasts have morphologic features similar to those of myeloblasts (peripheral blood).

3. Monoblast, three promonocytes, and a polyploid monocyte. Progressive cellular maturity is indicated by increasing nuclear indentation, which produces a pattern of radiating petals of a flower (peripheral blood).

4. Bone marrow showing preponderance of immature monocytoid (cells with folded or indented nuclei) and myeloid (round cells with regular nuclear outline) precursors.

5. Bone marrow cells stained for alkaline phosphatase (ALP), a cytochemical marker of myeloid cells. A positive reaction is indicated by fine reddish-orange granules in the cytoplasm (stained by the method of Kaplow[1]).

6. Bone marrow cells stained for nonspecific esterase (NSE, α-naphthyl acetate substrate), a monocytic marker, and chloroacetate esterase (CAE), a myeloid marker. A positive reaction for NSE is indicated by localized, reddish-orange staining in the cytoplasm, whereas bluish granular staining is indicative of CAE activity. Abnormally increased numbers of both ALP-positive (Plate XXVI–6) and NSE-positive immature cells confirmed the morphologic diagnosis of acute myelomonocytic leukemia (stained by the method of Yam et al.[5]).

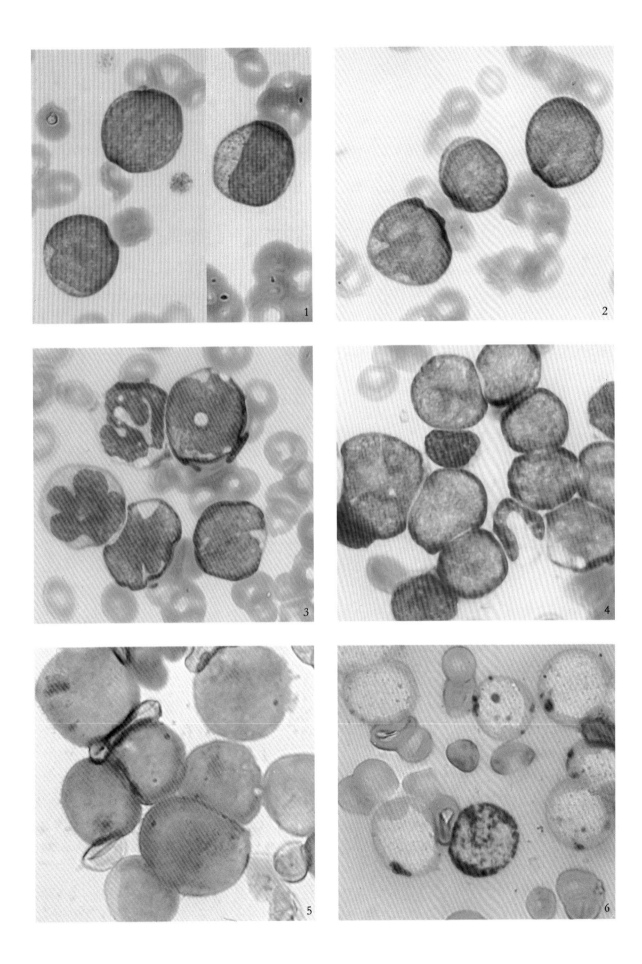

PLATE XXVII. BLOOD CELLS AND PARASITES OF BIRDS

1. Heterophil (left), basophil (right), and two thrombocytes in the blood of a tawny eagle, Aquila rapax (×1400).

2. Eosinophil in the blood of a barn owl, Tyro alba (×1400).

3. Heterophil and monocyte in the blood of a tawny eagle (×1400).

4. Lymphocyte (left) and thrombocyte (right) in the blood of a barn owl (×1400).

5. Reticulocytes in the blood of a hyacinth macaw, Anodorhynchus hyacinthus (new methylene blue stain; ×1400).

6. Microfilaria of an unidentified species in the blood of an umbrella-crested cockatoo, Kakatoe alba (×560).

7. Borrelia anserina in the blood of a domestic chicken (Gallus gallus) with spirochetosis (×1400).

8. Gametocyte of Haemoproteus sp. in an erythrocyte of a great horned owl (Bubo virginianus). Note the pigment and halter shape of the organism (×1400).

9. Immature gametocytes (trophozoites) of Plasmodium sp. in erythrocytes of a Swainson's hawk (Buteo swainsoni). Note the pigment and stained chromatin of the organisms (×1400).

10, 11. Gametocytes of Leucocytozoon sp. in leukocytes and immature gametocytes of Plasmodium sp. in erythrocytes of a Swainson's hawk (×1400).

12. Gametocytes of Leucocytozoon sp. in a leukocyte of a great horned owl. Note the marked displacement of the host cell nucleus (×1400).

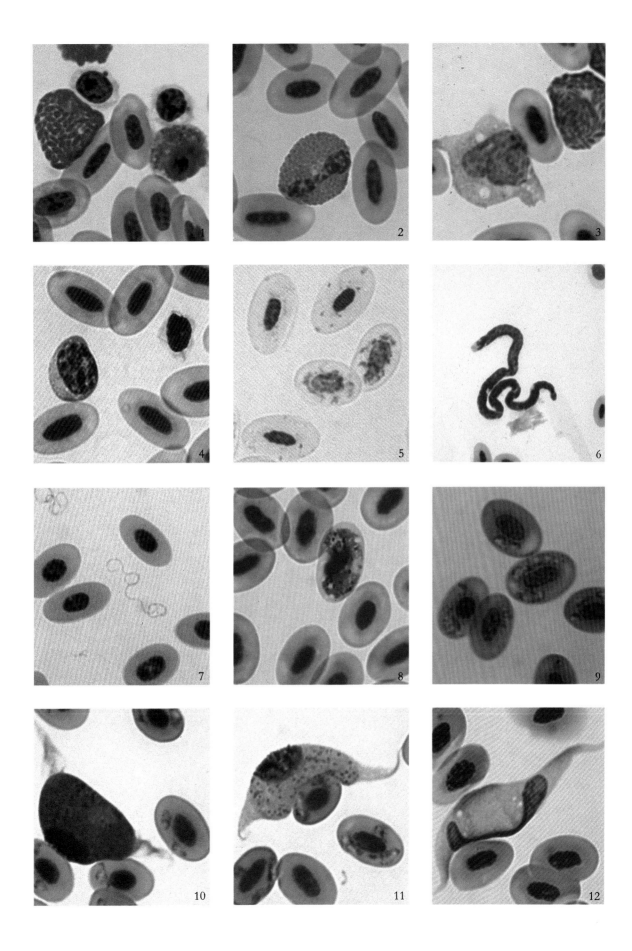

COLOR PLATE REFERENCES

1. Kaplow, L.S.: A histochemical procedure for localizing and evaluating leukocyte alkaline phosphatase activity in smears of blood and marrow. Blood, 10:1023, 1955.

2. Graham, R.C., Jr., Lundholm, U., Karnovsky, M.J., et al.: Cytochemical demonstration of peroxidase activity with 3-amino-9-ethylcarbazole. J. Histochem. Cytochem., 13:150, 1965.

3. Sheehan, H.L., and Storey, G.W.: An improved method of staining leucocyte granules with Sudan black B.: J. Pathol. Bacteriol., 59:336, 1947.

4. Ansley, H., and Ornstein, L.: Enzyme histochemistry and differential white cell counts on the Technicon Hemalog D: Advances in automated analysis. Technicon Int. Congress, 1:437, 1970.

5. Yam, L.T., Li, C.Y., Cromby, W.H., et al.: Cytochemical identification of monocytes and granulocytes. Am. J. Clin. Pathol., 55:283, 1971.

6. Bauer-Sic, P.: (Cytochemistry of bovine leucocytes in health and leucosis.) Zentralbl. Veterinärmed., 10:365, 1963.

7. Hayhoe, F.G.J., Quaglino, D., Flemans, R.J., et al.: Consecutive use of Romanowsky and periodic-acid-Schiff technique in the study of blood and bone marrow cells. Br. J. Haematol., 6:23, 1960.

8. Perry, S., and Reynolds, J.: Methyl-green-pyronin as a differential nucleic acid stain for peripheral blood smears. Blood, 11:1132, 1956.

The Eosinophils

Eosinophils have fascinated hematologists since 1879, when Paul Ehrlich first described them as leukocytes containing bright pinkish granules, but their biologic role remains mysterious. Eosinophils enter the circulation within a day or two after their production in the bone marrow and leave the vascular system shortly thereafter. Their physiologic and pathologic functions are being investigated. Research in the last two decades has elucidated possible mechanisms of eosinophilias commonly associated with parasitic and allergic diseases, regulation of eosinophil production, and immunobiology of eosinophils and their role in controlling helminthic parasites (Capron, 1991; Hartnell et al., 1990; Kay, 1991; Nutman, 1988a, 1988b, 1989a, 1989b; Thorne and Mazza, 1991; Weller, 1991). Eosinophils vary with regard to their granule morphology and composition in different species and they might be functionally heterogeneous, as are neutrophils and lymphocytes (Sorice and De Simone, 1986).

PRODUCTION AND RELEASE

The major site of eosinophilopoiesis (production of eosinophils) is the bone marrow, although a minor degree of eosinophil production occurs in other tissues (e.g., spleen, thymus, and cervical lymph nodes) in some laboratory animals. In general, eosinophils are produced over a period of 2 to 6 days and enter the peripheral blood about 2 days later. Their intravascular life span is estimated as 4 to 6 hours in humans and less than 1 hour in dogs. Eosinophils enter tissues randomly and remain there for several days (the rest of their lives); normally they do not re-enter the blood to circulate, although recirculation of eosinophils has been reported in hypereosinophilic human patients.

Eosinophilopoiesis

Eosinophil production in the bone marrow involves the multiplication and differentiation of the CFU-Eos (colony-forming unit–eosinophil), a committed progenitor cell derived from the pluripotential stem cell, to the myeloblast and promyelocyte destined to produce eosinophils (see Figs. 4–6 and 13–1). Mitotic, maturative, and reserve compartments of eosinophils, analogous to those of neutrophils, are recognized in the bone marrow.

A great reserve of eosinophils exists in the bone marrow of guinea pigs (blood:marrow ratio, 1:300), but species differences may exist, as evidenced by observations in humans (blood:marrow ratio, 1:3.4). Among common domestic animals, a low ratio may be anticipated, as in humans, except for cattle, which normally have relatively more eosinophils in the bone marrow. Eosinophils are found in large numbers in certain body tissues (e.g., the small intestine, lungs, skin, and uterus; blood:tissue ratio, 1:200 to 300). Their number in other tissues may be high, perhaps because of longer survival time in tissues (2 to 4 days) compared to blood (a few hours) and a preferential chemoattraction at such locations.

Regulation of Eosinophil Production and Release

In vitro and in vivo studies have shown that products from activated T lymphocytes and macrophages regulate eosinophil production (Bauman et al., 1992; Dvorak et al., 1989; Murata et al., 1992a; Warringa et al., 1992; Williams et al., 1990). The main substances are GM-CSF (granulocyte-macrophage colony stimulating factor), interleukin 3 (IL-3), and interleukin 5

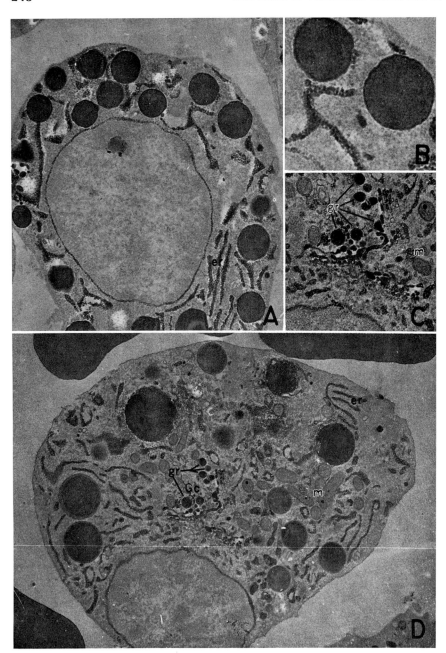

Fig. 14–1. Eosinophilic progranulocytes from canine bone marrow stained for peroxidase. An early progranulocyte *(A)* is characterized by the presence of many dense, homogeneous granules, whereas an intermediate or late progranulocyte *(D)* contains many condensing granules of varying morphology. *B* is an enlarged area of *A,* and *C* is an enlargement of the Golgi complex area of the cell in *D*. The Golgi complex *(C,D)* at this stage is very active in producing granules *(gr)*. The cytoplasm at this stage contains elaborate cisternae of rough endoplasmic reticulum *(er)* and numerous mitochondria *(m)*. In contrast to neutrophil progranulocytes, eosinophilic progranulocytes exhibit peroxidase activity in the rough endoplasmic reticulum, the Golgi complex, and along the outer nuclear membrane (*A*, ×10,080; *B*, ×18,900; *C*, ×14,280; *D*, ×10,080). (From Jain, N.C.: Schalm's Veterinary Hematology. 4th Ed. Philadelphia, Lea & Febiger, 1986, p. 732.)

(IL-5). Both GM-CSF and IL-3 stimulate the development of eosinophils and other leukocytes, while IL-5 promotes development and terminal differentiation of eosinophils. Interleukin-5 also activates eosinophils and may thereby influence eosinophil-mediated inflammatory response. Differentiation of the CFU-Eos is also influenced by a specific eosinophil colony-stimulating factor (Eo-CSF; MW, 50,000). Eosinophil growth-stimulating factor (Eo-GSF) or "eosinophilopoietin" (MW, 5,000) is a polypeptide of five to ten amino acid residues produced by activated T lymphocytes. It influences the proliferation of eosinophil precursors in the mitotic compartment and has some

effect on the CFU-Eos. An "eosinophil-releasing factor" promotes the release of eosinophils from the bone marrow to blood. Accelerated production and release of eosinophils occur in parasitic infections.

Intravenous injections of recombinant human interleukin-2 in cats caused an eosinophilia in blood preceded by a selective hyperplasia of eosinophil precursors in bone marrow (Tompkins et al., 1990). In addition, eosinophil activation was also induced as measured by a decrease in density and an increase in longevity of eosinophils in culture. No significant changes occurred in erythrocyte, neutrophil, and lymphocyte numbers.

Table 14–1.   Eosinophilia and Basophilia in the Dog and Cat

Number	Organ System or Disease Involvement	Eosinophils/μl		Basophils/μl	
		Mean ± 1 SD	Minimum–Maximum	Mean ± 1 SD	Minimum–Maximum
Dog					
143	Respiratory (lungs)	4,229 ± 3,786	1,330–15,958	356 ± 822	0–4,275
28	Skin	2,931 ± 1,931	1,536–12,627	91 ± 220	0–1,280
8	Ocular	2,841 ± 1,235	1,521–5,785	74 ± 104	0–292
20	GI tract	2,287 ± 1,447	1,424–7,812	93 ± 155	0–521
24	Bone and joint	2,649 ± 1,327	1,606–6,700	80 ± 164	0–750
24	Female genital	2,412 ± 1,337	1,379–7,275	56 ± 117	0–458
14	Urinary	2,250 ± 518	1,501–3,182	52 ± 158	0–612
22	Neurologic	2,294 ± 644	1,377–3,625	45 ± 133	0–522
7	Cardiac	1,918 ± 259	1,634–2,431	92 ± 123	0–344
28	Miscellaneous	3,931 ± 3,425	1,512–17,526	118 ± 211	0–968
7	Suppurative	3,598 ± 2,695	1,609–9,879	0	0
12	Neoplasia	2,149 ± 831	1,442–4,446	56 ± 117	0–458
Cat					
23	Skin	5,373 ± 4,408	1,500–22,230	111 ± 174	0–537
11	Respiratory (lungs)	3,322 ± 1,539	1,522–6,883	37 ± 41	0–166
13	GI tract	2,706 ± 1,190	1,674–6,341	114 ± 172	0–564
12	Suppurative	2,964 ± 1,614	1,522–7,375	156 ± 171	0–486
13	Miscellaneous	3,147 ± 1,647	1,642–7,832	132 ± 285	0–1,026

Migration of Eosinophils in Tissues

The entry of eosinophils into tissues is influenced by specific, local chemoattractants. Various substances are chemotactic for eosinophils, including antigen-antibody complexes involving primarily IgE, mast cell products such as histamine and eosinophil chemotactic factor of anaphylaxis (ECF-A), activated complement components (C5a, C567), arachidonic acid metabolites such as 12-hydroperoxyeicosatetraenoic acid (HETE), 12-hydroxylicosatetraenoic acid (HHT), and leukotriene B₄, at least two eosinophil-specific lymphokines, interleukin-2, fibrinogen and fibrin, and some undefined products from damaged tissues (Faccioli et al., 1991; Jain, 1986; Weller, 1992).

The central events in most situations involving eosinophils are the release of histamine from mast cells and the production of eosinophil-specific lymphokines. Therefore, tissue eosinophilia and consequently blood eosinophilia are to be anticipated in various conditions associated with the formation and release of eosinophil chemoattractants (Table 14–1). On the other hand, eosinopenia is seen in many stressful conditions, and is primarily attributed to the increased release of glucocorticoids and their neutralizing action on histamine. In addition, the lympholytic effects of glucocorticoids tend to diminish T-cell activity.

MORPHOLOGY, GRANULE STRUCTURE, AND BIOCHEMICAL CONSTITUENTS

Cell Morphology

Eosinophils characteristically have bright, pinkish-red, uniformly stained cytoplasmic granules and a polymorphic nucleus that is smoother and less segmented than that in mature neutrophils. The granules loosely pack the cell and their size and shape vary among different species, and sometimes within species. For example, granules in equine eosinophils are the largest among common domestic animals and feline eosinophil granules are usually rod-shaped (Plates VII–6 and VII–7). Canine eosinophils display a few partly vacuolated granules (Plate XII–1), and those of the greyhound are highly vacuolated (Plate IX–9). An occasional dog may have rare eosinophils with a few granules as big as the red cell (Plate XII–2). A rare eosinophil may contain a few small dark purplish-black granules, probably as a result of deranged eosinophil development under some toxic influence (Jain, 1986).

Granule Structure

The earliest morphologically identifiable precursor cell of the eosinophil is the promyelocyte. It is rarely seen in marrow films stained with Wright-Giemsa stain and is identified by its many large azurophilic granules (Plate XII–3), compared to the fine granules of the neutrophilic promyelocyte (Plate V–4). With the electron microscope, these granules appear spherical, homogenous, and dense (Fig. 14–1). These primary granules are elaborated by the Golgi complex. With cell maturation to the myelocyte through the mature eosinophil stage, the homogeneous granules either transform into crystalloid granules or remain homogeneous, but become more compact and assume lineage-specific characteristics (Jain, 1986).

Thus, two types of granules, homogeneous and crystalloid, characterize the eosinophils. Some species

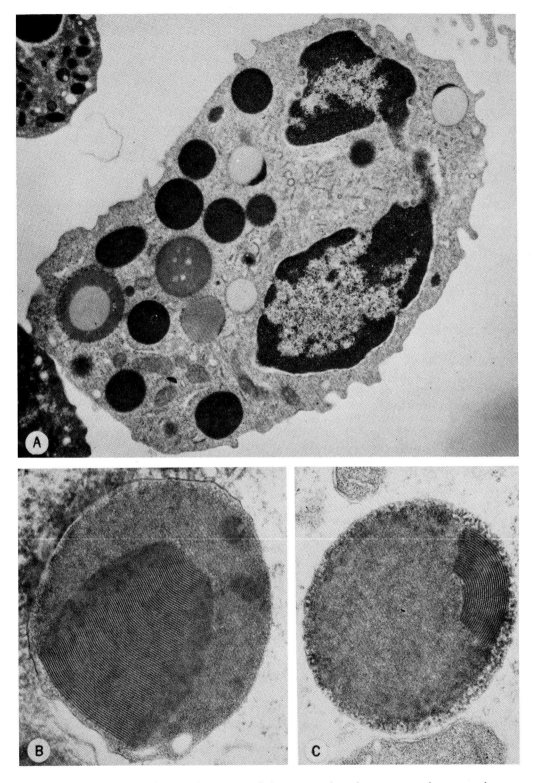

Fig. 14–2. *A,* Canine eosinophil containing granules of various morphology types—dense homogeneous, dense amorphous mass surrounded by a narrow rim of somewhat light matrix, and clear vesicles with a cap and/or rim of dense material. A few mitochondria are present in the lower portion of the cell, a few remnants of rough endoplasmic reticulum are scattered throughout the cell, and some "microgranules" are visible in the cytoplasmic area between the nuclear lobes (×32,000). *B, C,* Clearly defined "fingerprints" of portions of the crystalloid of two eosinophil granules (×62,500). (From Jain, N.C.: Schalm's Veterinary Hematology. 4th Ed. Philadelphia, Lea & Febiger, 1986, p. 733.)

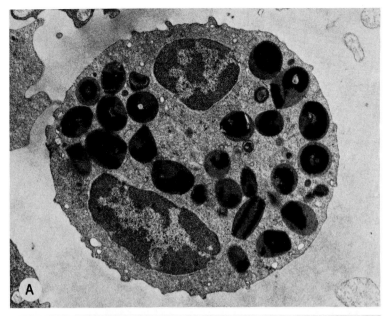

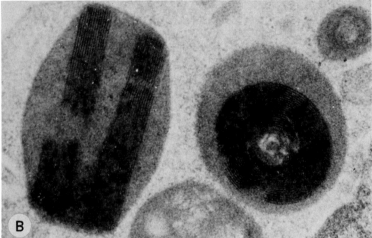

Fig. 14–3. *A*, Feline eosinophil with characteristic crystalloid granules and some "microgranules" (×11,200). *B*, Periodicity of lamellae in the crystalloid region of the granule is clearly visible at higher magnification (×50,000). (From Jain, N.C.: Schalm's Veterinary Hematology. 4th Ed. Philadelphia, Lea & Febiger, 1986, p. 734.)

appear to have consistently crystalloid (cat and guinea pig) or partially crystalloid (dog) granules, whereas others (cow and horse) have only homogeneous granules (Figs. 14–2, 14–3, and 14–4). The crystalloid granules have an electron-dense core in the form of a myelin figure surrounded by an electron-lucent matrix. Fowl, quail, and duck eosinophils contain crystalline and vacuolated granules (Maxwell, 1987). Small profiles of smooth endoplasmic reticulum, known as specific microgranules, are found in the mature eosinophils of many species, including the dog, cat, and horse (Figs. 14–2 and 14–3). These structures are visible only on electron microscopy.

Biochemical Constituents

Various substances, including lysosomal enzymes, have been found in the specific granules of eosinophils.

Cationic proteins, zinc, and phospholipase C are present in the granule core, peroxidase, acid phosphatase, and hydrolytic lysosomal enzymes are found in the granule matrix, and alkaline phosphatase and a nonspecific esterase are localized in the cytoplasm. Acid phosphatase, in association with arylsulfatase B, is also found in some smaller granules (0.1 to 0.5 μm). Specific cellular locations of histaminase, plasminogen and plasminogen activator, Hageman factor, kinin-producing activity and kininase, and thromboplastic activity remain uncertain. The eosinophil peroxidase differs from that in neutrophils with regard to antigenic, genetic, and physical characteristics. Feline eosinophils are devoid of peroxidase. The functional significance of various eosinophil constituents is outlined in Table 14–2.

The characteristic staining of eosinophil granules is attributed to their content of arginine-rich, highly cationic (basic) proteins. Several cationic proteins have

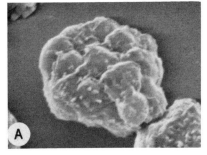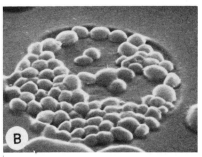

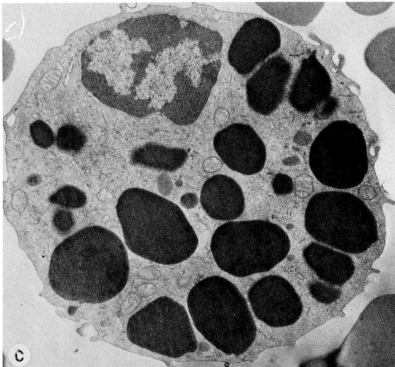

Fig. 14–4. Equine eosinophils. *A*, Scanning electron photomicrograph of a globular cell depicting some microvilli and granule contours (×4,400). *B*, Scanning electron photomicrograph showing distinctly dispersed granules in a cell flattened from smear making. The nucleus (region devoid of granules) and cell membrane have collapsed (×3,000). *C*, Transmission electron photomicrograph depicting characteristic large, round, homogeneous granules. Some mitochondria and rare profiles of rough endoplasmic reticulum are also present in the cytoplasm. A few microvillus-like projections are present on the cell surface (×10,000). (From Jain, N.C.: Schalm's Veterinary Hematology. 4th Ed. Philadelphia, Lea & Febiger, 1986, p. 735.)

been identified (Hamann et al., 1991); the principal ones are designated major basic protein (MBP) and eosinophil cationic protein (ECP). These proteins are rich in arginine and have molecular weights ranging from 12,000 in the guinea pig and 16,000 in the bovine to 21,000 in humans. Their concentrations in sputum and plasma can be measured by radioimmunoassay. Increased levels have been found in eosinophilic human patients and during acute infection and inflammation, probably because of the destruction of eosinophils in the blood or at inflammatory sites. ECPs have little bactericidal or phlogistic properties, but they are highly cytotoxic and tumoricidal in vitro and can activate the coagulation, kinin, and fibrinolytic systems.

Charcot-Leyden crystals found in lesions with massive eosinophilic infiltration consist of lysophospholipase derived from the plasma membrane of the cells. These are eosinophilic, bipyramidal crystals found in intracellular or extracellular locations where massive disintegration of eosinophils occurs—for example, in the bronchial or nasal mucus of human patients with

allergic asthma. Basophils also contain Charcot-Leyden protein (See Chapter 15).

FUNCTIONS

Although the functions of the eosinophils have yet to be fully defined, it is becoming apparent that eosinophils are important in controlling infection by metazoan parasites (Capron, 1991; Thorne and Mazza, 1991). It has been demonstrated that eosinophils participate in the regulation of allergic and acute inflammatory responses and may induce tissue damage (Kay, 1991; Weller, 1991; Williams et al., 1990). Eosinophils may also participate in coagulation and fibrinolysis through the activation of factor XII and plasminogen, respectively. The regulatory functions of several eosinophil components are summarized in Table 14–2. Species differences are found in biochemical responses of eosinophils to various stimuli (Sun et al., 1992).

The cytokines GM-CSF, IL-3, and IL-5 are impor-

Substance or Action	Functional Role
Cationic proteins (MBP, ECP)*	Responsible for characteristic staining of eosinophil granules; neutralize heparin; kill parasites; cytotoxic; promote coagulation and fibrinolysis, inhibit fibrin polymerization
Eosinophil-derived neurotoxin	Damages myelinated neurons in experimental animals
Hageman Factor	Activates coagulation sequence
Histaminase	Inactivates histamine
Kininase	Regulates kinin production and destruction activity
Lysosomal enzymes	Exert proteolytic action
Lysophospholipase	Destroys lysophospholipids
Oxygen products	Cytotoxic; kill parasites
Peroxidase	Some parasiticidal, antibacterial, and cytotoxic activities; inhibits SRS-A activity
Phagocytosis	Eosinophils engulf bacteria, immune complexes, mast cell granules, and inert particles
Phospholipase C	Degrades platelet-activating factor from mast cells
Plasminogen activator; plasminogen	Activate fibrinolysis
Prostaglandins (PGE$_1$, PGE$_2$)	Inhibit resynthesis of histamine and degranulation, increasing the level of cAMP in mast cells
Zinc	Inhibits release of histamine, serotonin, and platelet-activating factor from mast cells

* MBP, major basic protein; ECP, eosinophil cationic protein.

tant modulators of eosinophilia and eosinophil functions. Eosinophils from asthmatic individuals have increased metabolic activities (Bruijnzeel et al., 1992) and show increased propensity to release granule proteins (Carlson et al., 1991). Eosinophils from allergic individuals exhibit a markedly increased chemotactic response toward platelet activating factor (PAF) compared to eosinophils from normal persons (Warringa et al., 1992). Normal eosinophils incubated with minute amounts of GM-CSF, IL-3, and IL-5 mimic such an enhanced chemotactic response to PAF. Eosinophils incubated with these cytokines and IL-1 exhibit selective increases in phagocytic and microbicidal activities, enhanced capacity to release LTC4, reduced density, prolonged survival in tissue culture, and increased degranulation releasing arylsulfatase and beta-glucuronidase (Fabin et al., 1992; Tai et al., 1991; Weller, 1992). Therefore, release of various cytokines may be an important in vivo priming mechanism for eosinophil functions, particularly in allergic and asthmatic patients. PAF can also prime eosinophils for subsequent activation by receptor stimulated factors such as FMLP (Zoratti et al., 1992) and stimulate much greater superoxide anion production in eosinophils than in neutrophils (Zoratti et al., 1991). Primed eosinophils may cause increased tissue damage or enhance the host defense function. Furthermore, eo-

sinophils have been shown to produce some IL-3 and GM-CSF and may influence granulopoiesis (Kita et al., 1991).

Phagocytosis and Bactericidal Activity

It has been shown that eosinophils can phagocytize foreign particles, including bacteria, and undergo degranulation (Fig. 14–5). The major source of energy in eosinophils, as in neutrophils, is anaerobic glycolysis. Their NADPH oxidase activity is three to six times greater than in neutrophils, so the oxidative burst and hydrogen peroxide (H_2O_2) production are increased. Despite these phagocytosis-associated events, eosinophils have significantly lower phagocytic and bactericidal properties than neutrophils (Jain, 1986).

Eosinophils have surface receptors for IgG, IgE, IgM, IgA, IL-2, IL-5 complement components including C3b, leukotriene B4, histamine, and glucocorticoids. Individual variations may occur in the expression of surface receptors, and increased complement and IgG receptors per cell may be found during eosinophilias of diverse causes. ECF-A, histamine, and arachidonic acid metabolites can enhance the expression of IgG and C3b receptors. Interferon-gamma enhances expression of FcRI, FcRII, and FcRIII receptors on eosinophils, IL-1 induces expression of VLA-4 alpha (very late activation antigen-4 alpha) receptors, IL-3 upregulates the FcRII receptors, and PAF increases expression of CR3 receptors (Bochner et al., 1991; Hartnell et al., 1992; Zoratti et al., 1992). Leukocyte adhesion glycoproteins LFA-1 alpha (CD11a), CR3-alpha (CD11b), p150, 95-alpha (CD11c) and the common beta chain (CD18) are found on eosinophils, as on neutrophils (Hartnell et al., 1990). The expression of CD18 molecule is reduced on low-density eosinophils from hypereosinophilic patients.

Eosinophil peroxidase forms a complex with H_2O_2 and a halide (preferably iodide) and this complex has some bactericidal action, but it is more important for damaging parasites. A similar action has also been proposed for the other oxygen metabolites (superoxide anion, hydroxyl radical) produced following the metabolic activation of eosinophils. Eosinophil cationic proteins, in contrast to those of neutrophils, have weak or no bactericidal or inflammatory properties. Normal and leukemic human eosinophils have been found to contain lysozyme (Moscinski et al., 1992). Eosinophils lack lactoferrin, and phagocytin, both of which participate in bacterial killing in neutrophils. Thus, eosinophils seem to be functionally limited to provide host resistance to bacterial infection.

Parasiticidal Activity

The antibody-mediated killing of metazoan parasites by eosinophils has been demonstrated in several experimental studies with parasites such as Schistosoma

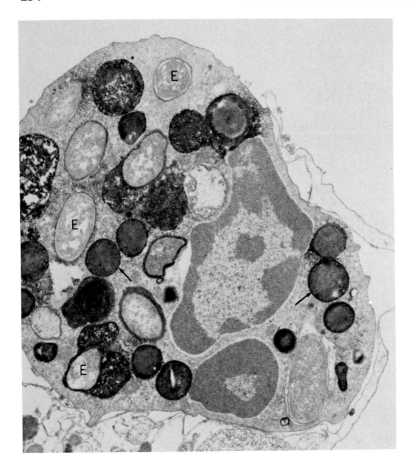

Fig. 14–5. Bovine eosinophil with intracellular *Escherichia coli* organisms *(E)* and intact peroxidase-positive eosinophil granules *(arrows).* Degranulation and accumulation of variable amounts of eosinophil granular material are evident in phagocytic vacuoles around some organisms (peroxidase stain; ×14,700). (From Jain, N.C.: Schalm's Veterinary Hematology. 4th Ed. Philadelphia, Lea & Febiger, 1986, p. 744.)

mansoni and Trichinella spiralis. The parasiticidal action is greater in the presence of antibody and/or complement. The killing process is mediated primarily by MBP, peroxidase-H_2O_2-halide complex, and oxygen metabolites, and is augmented by lysophospholipase present in the plasma membrane and by hydrolytic lysosomal enzymes. Neutrophils may also attach to the antibody- and complement-coated parasites, but they are less effective in inflicting damage than eosinophils. Eosinopenia in experimental animals increases their susceptibility to parasitic infection.

The current concept of the parasiticidal action of eosinophils through interactions with mast cells and lymphocytes is summarized in Figure 14–6 (also see Chap. 15). Parasitic infection may stimulate both humoral and cellular immune responses. Specific IgG antibodies so produced may bind to the parasite, fix complement, initiate an inflammatory reaction, and probably inflict some damage to the parasite. Specific IgE antibodies can bind to tissue mast cells and cause the degranulation and release of bioactive substances such as histamine, ECF-A, and platelet-activating factor (PAF). Special lymphokines (IL-3, IL-5, Eo-CSF and Eo-GSF) produced from T lymphocytes activated by parasitic antigens can stimulate eosinophil production and release. This may be reflected as blood eosinophilia. The eosinophil influx from the bone marrow to blood is also influenced by elevated circulating levels of histamine arising from mast cell de-

granulation in tissues. Tissue eosinophilia ensues in response to chemoattractants such as histamine, ECF-A, and activated complement components (C5a and C567) generated at the site of parasitic infection. When in tissues, eosinophils interact with the parasite through their surface receptors for IgG and complement. They become activated and undergo what is termed a "frustrated phagocytosis" that is, they exocytose granules or release granule contents to the exterior without actually phagocytosing the target. This also happens with neutrophils when the target cannot be internalized because it is too big, or for some other reason. Degranulation may also be augmented by interaction with IgE and parasitic antigen because the eosinophils also have receptors for IgE. The products of the eosinophil granules then begin to destroy the parasite and dampen the influence of mast cell factors. Enzyme release from eosinophils is dependent on calcium and GTP binding proteins (Cromwell et al., 1991) and is enhanced by IL-1-beta (Basker and Pincus, 1992).

Regulation of Allergic and Inflammatory Responses

A regulatory role for eosinophils in allergic response has been suggested by the following observations: (1) eosinophils can phagocytize immune complexes and mast cell granules; (2) prostaglandins (PGE_1 and PGE_2)

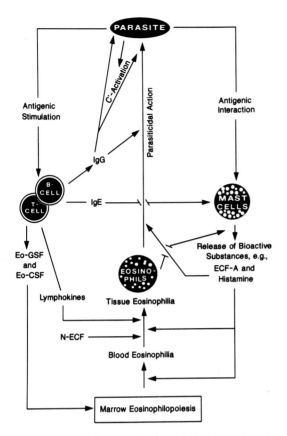

Fig. 14–6. Parasiticidal action of eosinophils by interaction with mast cells and lymphocytes. Parasitic antigens stimulate the lymphoid system. Stimulated T-lymphocytes produce eosinophil colony-stimulating factor (EO-CSF) and eosinophil growth-stimulating factor (EO-GSF), which promote bone marrow eosinophilopoiesis. IgE antibody, produced by certain subsets of stimulated B lymphocytes, coats tissue mast cells. Interaction of parasitic antigen with specific IgE-coated mast cells induces release of bioactive substances, such as eosinophil chemotactic factor of anaphylaxis (ECF-A) and histamine, from the mast cells. These substances are highly chemotactic for eosinophils and thus promote blood and tissue eosinophilia. Lymphokines from stimulated T lymphocytes and neutrophil-derived eosinophil chemotactic factor (N-ECF) also stimulate migration of eosinophils into tissues. Activation and degranulation of eosinophils are associated with parasiticidal action through eosinophil cationic proteins, including major basic protein, the eosinophil peroxidase-hydrogen peroxide-halide complex, and phospholipases. Eosinophil attachment and killing of parasite is high in the presence of IgG antibody and complement (C), intermediate in the presence of C alone, and low when only IgG is present. C activation can be initiated indirectly by parasitic antigen or directly by IgG antibody. ECF-A and histamine increase expression of C receptors on eosinophils and also accelerate C-dependent parasiticidal action of eosinophils. Eosinophils also regulate release of bioactive substances from mast cells; the eosinophil peroxidase-hydrogen peroxide-halide complex promotes such a release, whereas eosinophil prostaglandins E_1, E_2, and zinc are inhibitory. (From Jain, N.C.: Schalm's Veterinary Hematology. 4th Ed. Philadelphia, Lea & Febiger, 1986, p. 745.)

and zinc from eosinophils inhibit the mast cell release of histamine, serotonin, and PAF; (3) eosinophils contain factors that inhibit the replenishment of histamine in mast cells; (4) eosinophil histaminase inactivates free histamine; (5) eosinophil peroxidase inactivates the slow-reacting substance of anaphylaxis (SRS-A) of mast cell origin; and (6) eosinophil phospholipase C inactivates PAF released from mast cells. Leuko-

trienes C_4 (LTC$_4$), D_4 (LTD$_4$) and E_4 comprise the SRS-A. The SRS-A is probably inactivated by hypochlorous acid generated after eosinophil peroxidase-H_2O_2-halide complex formation, and not through the hydrolytic action of arylsulfatase, as had been suggested previously (see Fig. 15–2 for a depiction of some of these interactions).

A regulatory role in acute inflammation has been inferred from these antihistaminic and anti-inflammatory properties of eosinophils. In addition, eosinophil granules contain substances that inhibit the edema-inducing properties of serotonin and bradykinin.

Tissue Injury

Eosinophil is a potent inflammatory cell that takes active part in almost all types of inflammatory processes. Its activity is mediated by the secretion of four well characterized cytotoxic proteins, viz., ECP, MBP, peroxidase, and eosinophil protein X or eosinophil derived neutrotoxin (Venge, 1990). In addition, lipid mediators such as leukotriene C4 and PAF and oxygen metabolites have cytotoxic effects. Various proteins released from eosinophil granules in patients with significant and persistent eosinophilias may induce the various types of tissue damage (cutaneous, respiratory, neurologic, gastrointestinal, and cardiac lesions) seen in such patients (Nutman et al, 1988b, 1989a, 1989b). The measurement of the eosinophil proteins in various body fluids has provided evidence for the active participation of eosinophils in a number of diseases such as asthma, ulcerative colitis, rheumatoid arthritis, and psoriasis. Eosinophils are more toxic than neutrophils in antibody-mediated destruction of target cells as shown by the release of [51]Chromium from cultured tumor cells and lysis of chicken erythrocytes in vitro (Roberts et al., 1991). Both MBP and the peroxidase-H_2O_2-halide complex exhibit cytotoxic properties in vitro. Other cationic proteins, lysosomal hydrolases, and superoxide anions from stimulated eosinophils could augment tissue damage. Eosinophil cationic proteins and the eosinophil-derived neurotoxin can induce neuropathologic damage in rodents. Eosinophils can synthesize leukotrienes such as LTC$_4$ and LTD$_4$, which can induce smooth muscle contraction and bronchospasm.

The eosinophilia-myalgia syndrome in humans has been associated with ingestion of L-tryptophan-containing preparations leading to eosinophil activation and release of MBP and other toxic proteins into the extracellular space (Varga et al., 1992). Eosinophils are capable of both adhering to and releasing mitogens for fibroblasts, thus they may play a role in the development of fibrosis in disorders where they have been shown to be present (Noguchi et al., 1992; Shock et al., 1991). Eosinophils are susceptible to HIV-1 infection in vitro and may be an important reservoir for the virus in vivo (Freedman et al., 1991).

Interleukin-4 stimulates eosinophil and basophil

adhesion to endothelium by promoting endothelial cell expression of VCAM-1, which binds to eosinophil and basophil VLA-4 (Schleimer et al., 1992). Thus, local release of IL-4 in allergic diseases may partly explain the tissue infiltration of eosinophils and basophils observed in these situations.

EOSINOPHILIAS AND EOSINOPENIAS

Eosinophils constitute only a small part of the differential leukocyte count in health, yet their numbers are sufficient to reflect significant changes in pathophysiology under certain conditions. A diurnal variation in eosinophil number has been demonstrated in humans, with the highest count at midnight and the lowest at noon. This is inversely related to variations in the endogenous corticosteroid level. Eosinophilia may occur in some dogs in estrus, probably as a result of histamine release from mast cell degranulation during estrus.

Eosinophilias

A persistent eosinophilia generally reflects a chronic disease process, whereas an eosinopenia usually develops in acute diseases and may be a normal finding. Chronic eosinophilia is common to diseases of tissues and organs containing a high concentration of mast cells (e.g., the skin, lungs, gastrointestinal tract, and uterus). As mentioned above, eosinophilia is usually encountered in pathologic states associated with an interaction among specific antigen, IgE antibody, and mast cells or basophils. Thus, eosinophilia is not an expression of a single disease entity, such as parasitism or an allergic response, but is an occurrence to be anticipated in a wide variety of chronic diseases involving the continuous degranulation of mast cells (Table 14–1).

Eosinophils are found in increased numbers in blood and sputum of asthmatic persons, usually in relation to the severity of asthma (Busse and Sedgwick, 1992). Eosinophil toxic products have been incriminated as a cause of asthma. Eosinophilia seen in some cases of adult T-cell leukemia/lymphoma in humans may be caused by secretion of some lymphokines by the lymphoma cells (Murata et al., 1992b).

Peripheral blood eosinophilia may result from the following: (1) increased production; (2) increased release from bone marrow reserve; (3) preferential redistribution of cells from the marginal pool; and (4) prolonged intravascular survival. Eosinophilia in most situations, as in parasitism, is probably the result of the first two mechanisms. Eosinophilia in response to parasitism occurs only when a sensitivity to the protein of the parasite has developed and parasitic products are released in the body to trigger these responses. A transient eosinophilia may occur from the third mechanism in association with neutrophilia and lymphocytosis during the endogenous release of epinephrine

under physiologic stress. The effect is probably the result of the mobilization of eosinophils from the spleen, because it is not seen in splenectomized rats and guinea pigs. The fourth mechanism may be a major contributory factor in certain hypereosinophilic patients.

The term "pulmonary infiltrates with eosinophilia" (PIE) is applied to a clinical syndrome of pulmonary infiltrates (observed on radiologic examination) accompanied by blood eosinophilia. It has been observed in dogs and cats. Its causes include nonspecific allergic bronchitis, hypersensitivity to exogenous protein, heartworm disease, parasitic larval migration, and certain chronic infections. In most humans with PIE, serum IgE levels are increased and treatment with corticosteroids is beneficial.

Hypereosinophilic syndrome (HES) refers to a heterogeneous group of diseases characterized by persistent eosinophilia of undefined cause and by the eosinophilic infiltration of tissues, resulting in organ system dysfunction. A spectrum of HES, consisting of eosinophilic enteritis, disseminated eosinophilic infiltration of various organs and tissues, and eosinophilic leukemia, occurs in cats. Eosinophilic leukemia occurs also in the dog, and is suspected when the blood shows a prolonged, persistent, marked eosinophilia, with or without a left shift, and the bone marrow is dominated by a disordered differentiation and maturation of eosinophils. Other causes of eosinophilias should be eliminated before a definitive diagnosis of eosinophilic leukemia is made.

Eosinopenias

The eosinophil count may normally be zero in some animals; hence, eosinopenia is of limited significance. Animals with circulating eosinophils, however, characteristically develop eosinopenia after stress, the endogenous release or administration of corticosteroids, and acute infection.

Eosinopenia of acute physical and emotional stress is attributed to elevated levels of catecholamines, such as epinephrine, and adrenocorticosteroids. Epinephrine injection in laboratory animals initially (within 1 hour) induces a mild eosinophilia followed by an eosinopenia by 4 hours. The former response is related to the mobilization of eosinophils from the spleen, because it has not been seen in splenectomized rats and guinea pigs. The eosinopenic response is considered a β-adrenergic effect.

The mechanism of corticosteroid-induced eosinopenia remains to be established unequivocally. Various mechanisms have been proposed, including decreased marrow release, intravascular lysis, reversible sequestration in organs rich in the mononuclear phagocyte system, and increased migration in tissues. These effects are probably mediated through the corticosteroid-induced neutralization of circulating histamine, reduction in histamine release from mast cells, and increased release of undefined lymphokines as a result of lympholysis.

Eosinopenia characteristically accompanies acute infection and inflammatory reaction. It is attributed partly to the release of corticosteroids and catecholamines under such conditions, and is partly a consequence of infection and inflammation. The precise mechanisms remain to be established.

REFERENCES

Baskar, P. and Pincus, S.H.: Selective regulation of eosinophil degranulation by interleukin 1 beta. Proc. Soc. Exp. Biol. Med, 199:249, 1992.

Baumann, M.A., Paul, C.C. and Grace, M.J.: Effects of interleukin-5 on acute myeloid leukemias. Am. J. Hematol., 39:269, 1992.

Bochner, B.S., Luscinskas, F.W., Gimbrone, M.A. Jr., et al.: Adhesion of human basophils, eosinophils, and neutrophils to interleukin 1-activated human vascular endothelial cells: contributions of endothelial cell adhesion molecules. J. Exp. Med., 173:1553, 1991.

Bruijnzeel, P.L., Rihs, S., Virchow, J.C. Jr., et al.: Early activation or "priming" of eosinophils in asthma. Schweiz. Med. Wochenschr., 122:298, 1992.

Busse, W.W. and Sedgwick, J.B.: Eosinophils in asthma. Ann. Allergy, 68:286, 1992.

Capron, M.: Eosinophils and parasites. Ann. Parasitol. Hum. Comp., 66 Suppl 1:41, 1991.

Carlson, M., Hakansson, L., Peterson, C., et al.: Secretion of granule proteins from eosinophils and neutrophils is increased in asthma. J. Allergy Clin. Immunol., 87:27, 1991.

Cromwell, O., Bennett, J.P., Hide, I., et al.: Mechanisms of granule enzyme secretion from permeabilized guinea pig eosinophils. Dependence on Ca2+ and guanine nucleotides. J. Immunol., 147:1905, 1991.

Dvorak, A.M., Saito, H., Estrella, P., et al.: Ultrastructure of eosinophils and basophils stimulated to develop in human cord blood mononuclear cell cultures containing recombinant human interleukin-5 or interleukin-3. Lab. Invest., 61:116, 1989.

Fabian, I., Kletter, Y., Mor, S., et al.: Activation of human eosinophil and neutrophil functions by haematopoietic growth factors: comparisons of IL-1, IL-3, IL-5 and GM-CSF. Br. J. Haematol., 80:137, 1992.

Faccioli, L.H., Nourshargh, S., Moqbel, R., et al.: The accumulation of 111In-eosinophils induced by inflammatory mediators, in vivo. Immunology, 73:222, 1991.

Freedman, A.R., Gibson, F.M., Fleming, S.C., et al.: Human immunodeficiency virus infection of eosinophils in human bone marrow cultures. J. Exp. Med., 174:1661, 1991.

Hamann, K.J., Barker, R.L., Ten, R.M., et al.: The molecular biology of eosinophil granule proteins. Int. Arch. Allergy App. Immunol., 94:202, 1991.

Hartnell, A., Kay, A.B. and Wardlaw, A.J.: IFN-gamma induces expression of Fc gamma RIII (CD16) on human eosinophils. J. Immunol., 148:1471, 1992.

Hartnell, A., Moqbel, R., Walsh, G.M., et al.: Fc gamma and CD11/CD18 receptor expression on normal density and low density human eosinophils. Immunology, 69:264, 1990.

Jain, N.C.: Schalm's Veterinary Hematology. 4th ed. Philadelphia, Lea & Febiger, 1986, pp. 731–755.

Kay, A.B.: Biological properties of eosinophils. Clin. Exp. Allergy, 21 Suppl., 3:23, 1991.

Kita, H., Ohnishi, T., Okubo, Y., et al.: Granulocyte/macrophage colony-stimulating factor and interleukin 3 release from human peripheral blood eosinophils and neutrophils. J. Exp. Med., 174:745, 1991.

Maxwell, M.H.: The avian eosinophil—a review. World Poultry Sci. J., 43:190, 1987.

Moscinski, L.C., Kasnic, G. Jr. and Saker, A. Jr.: The significance of an elevated serum lysozyme value in acute myelogenous leukemia with eosinophilia. Am. J. Clin. Pathol., 97:195, 1992.

Murata, Y., Takaki, S., Migita, M., et al.: Molecular cloning and expression of the human interleukin 5 receptor. J. Exp. Med., 175:341, 1992a.

Murata, K., Yamada, Y., Kamihira, S., et al.: Frequency of eosinophilia in adult T-cell leukemia/lymphoma. Cancer, 69:966, 1992b.

Noguchi, H., Kephart, G.M., Colby, T.V., et al.: Tissue eosinophilia and eosinophil degranulation in syndromes associated with fibrosis. Am. J. Pathol., 140:521, 1992.

Nutman, T.B., Cohen, S.G. and Ottesen, E.A.: The eosinophil, eosinophilia, and eosinophil-related disorders. I. Structure and development. Allergy Proc., 9:629, 1988a.

Nutman, T.B., Cohen, S.G. and Ottesen, E.A.: The eosinophil, eosinophilia, and eosinophil-related disorders. II. Eosinophil infiltration and function. Allergy Proc., 9:641, 1988b.

Nutman, T.B., Ottesen, E.A. and Cohen, S.G.: The eosinophil, eosinophilia, and eosinophil-related disorders. III. Clinical assessments and eosinophil related disorders. Allergy Proc., 10:33, 1989a.

Nutman, T.B., Ottesen, E.A. and Cohen, S.G.: The eosinophil, eosinophilia, and eosinophil-related disorders. IV. Eosinophil related disorders (continued). Allergy Proc., 10:47, 1989b.

Roberts, R.L., Ank, B.J. and Stiehm, E.R.: Human eosinophils are more toxic than neutrophils in antibody-independent kiling. J. Allergy Clin. Immunol., 87:1105, 1991.

Schleimer, R.P., Sterbinsky, S.A., Kaiser, J., et al.: IL-4 induces adherence of human eosinophils and basophils but not neutrophils to endothelium. Association with expression of VCAM-1. J. Immunol., 148:1086, 1992.

Shock, A., Rabe, K.F., Dent, G., et al.: Eosinophils adhere to and stimulate replication of lung fibroblasts 'in vitro'. Clin. Exp. Immunol., 86:185, 1991.

Sorice, F. and De Simone, C.: Human eosinophil heterogeneity. Ric. Clin. Lab., 16:429, 1986.

Sun, F.F., Crittenden, N.J., Czuk, C.I., et al.: Biochemical and functional differences between eosinophils from animal species and man. J. Leukoc. Biol., 50:140, 1991.

Tai, P.C., Sun, L. and Spry, C.J.: Effects of IL-5, granulocyte/macrophage colony-stimulating factor (GM-CSF) and IL-3 on survival of human blood eosinophils in vitro. Clin. Exp. Immunol., 85:312, 1991.

Thorne, K.J., and Mazza, G.: Eosinophilia, activated eosinophils and human schistosomiasis. J. Cell. Sci., 98:265, 1991.

Tompkins, M.B., Novotney, C., Grindem, C.B., et al.: Human recombinant interleukin-2 induces maturation and activation signals for feline eosinophils in vivo. J. Leuk. Biol., 48:531, 1990.

Varga, J., Uitto, J. and Jimenez, S.A.: The cause and pathogenesis of the eosinophilia-myalgia syndrome. Ann. Intern. Med., 116:140, 1992.

Venge, P.: The human eosinophil in inflammation. Agents Actions, 29:122, 1990.

Warringa, R.A. Mengelers, H.J., Kuijper, P.H., et al.: In vivo priming of platelet-activating factor-induced eosinophil chemotaxis in allergic asthmatic individuals. Blood, 79:1836, 1992.

Weller, P.F.: The immunobiology of eosinophils. N. Engl. J. Med, 324:1110, 1991.

Weller, P.F.: Cytokine regulation of eosinophil function. Clin. Immunol. Immunopathol., 62:S55, 1992.

Williams, W.J., Beutler, E., Erslev, A.J., et al.: Hematology. 4th ed. New York, McGraw-Hill, 1990.

Zoratti, E.M., Sedgwick, J.B., Bates, M.E., et al.: Platelet-activating factor primes human eosinophil generation of superoxide. Am. J. Resp. Cell. Mol. Biol., 6:100, 1992.

Zoratti, E.M., Sedgwick, J.B., Vrtis, R.R., et al.: The effect of platelet-activating factor on the generation of superoxide anion in human eosinophils and neutrophils. J. Allergy Clin. Immunol., 88:749, 1991.

Chapter 15

The Basophils and Mast Cells

Basophils have not been investigated as extensively as other cells because of their rarity in blood and bone marrow. Consequently, little is known about their production, function, and response to disease. Basophils are frequently equated with tissue mast cells because of certain morphologic and functional similarities, so relative aspects are presented in this chapter. Mast cells may exhibit morphologic, biochemical and/or functional heterogeneity in different species. Functionally, the basophil is probably not an end-stage cell; it can resynthesize its granules, and might be able to undergo blast transformation under appropriate conditions. Details of mast cell and basophil development and functions can be found in recent reviews (Church et al., 1991; Galli, 1990; Kaplan et al., 1991; Melman, 1987; Miller and Schwartz, 1989; Stevens and Austen, 1989).

PRODUCTION AND DISTRIBUTION

Basophils are rare in blood, whereas mast cells are widely distributed in the connective tissue and are found in close association with blood vessels. The distribution of mast cells within the tissues and organs of the body varies among different species. An inverse relationship however exists between the numbers of basophils in blood and mast cells in tissues of many species; for example, the cat has few basophils in blood but many mast cells in tissues, whereas the reverse occurs in the rabbit.

It is generally believed that basophils are produced in the bone marrow, following a pattern similar to that of other granulocytes, whereas mast cells are produced from undifferentiated mesenchymal cells in the connective tissue. Mast cell production in the bone marrow probably also involves pluripotent hematopoietic stem cells. Early progenitor cells of both cell types have not been delineated morphologically. Basophil-specific myeloblasts and promyelocytes develop from the com-

mitted progenitor cells (CFU-Bas) and give rise to morphologically identifiable basophils (see Figs. 4–6 and 13–1).

Basophil production is antigen-specific and is regulated by "basophilopoietins" produced by activated T lymphocytes. In particular, interleukin-5, interleukin-3 and GM-CSF regulate basophil and mast cell production, differentiation, and maturation (Denburg et al., 1991; Ebisawa et al., 1989). Also, interleukin-4 and some uncharacterized microenvironmental (stromal) factors have similar effects of mast cells. Human bone marrow CD34+ pluripotent progenitor cells cultured in the presence of both human recombinant interleukin-3 and human recombinant hematopoietic stem cell factor give rise to cultures containing increased numbers of basophils and mast cells (Kirshenbaum et al., 1992).

CELL MORPHOLOGY AND GRANULE STRUCTURE

Basophils and mast cells have certain morphologic and biochemical features in common, so controversy continues regarding their separate origin and identity (Table 15–1). In Wright-stained film, typical basophil has intense reddish-violet granules that invariably fill the cytoplasm and mask the segmented nucleus. The number, size, and stainability of granules vary among species. For example, canine basophils have larger and fewer granules than bovine and equine basophils and feline basophil granules usually stain dull orange-gray against a grayish background, in contrast to the typical reddish-violet staining in other species (Plates VII–5, VII–6, and VII–7). The mast cell is large and has a round nucleus and many deeply stained violet granules that fill the cell and may mask the nucleus (Plate XII–4 and XXIV–6).

The characteristic metachromasia of basophils and mast cells can be ascribed to their granule content of sulfated glycosaminoglycans (mucopolysaccharides),

Table 15–1. Comparison of Features of Basophils and Mast Cells

Criterion	Basophils	Mast Cells
Location	Normally in blood and bone marrow; enter tissues during allergic and inflammatory processes	Normally in perivascular connective tissues; occasionally in bone marrow; rare in blood (abnormal)
Origin	Bone marrow; committed stem cell defined (CFU-Bas)	Undifferentiated mesenchymal connective tissue cell; in bone marrow, pluripotential hematopoietic stem cell
Mitotic potential	Absent (?)	Present
Morphology in Wright-stained films	Small, round cell; bi- or trilobed nucleus; large, less numerous, loosely packed, intense reddish-violet granules often masking the nucleus; species variation in granule size and staining	Relatively large, round to ovoid or stellate cell; round or oval nucleus; large, numerus, darkly stained granules densely packing the cytoplasm, with some eccentric distribution and covering the nucleus
Surface morphology	Many short villi and some smooth folds; "uropod" in motile cells	Prominent microvilli and long, villous processes
Granule ultrastructure	Immature granules, homogeneous; mature granules, homogeneous, coarsely or finely particulate, fibrillar, or reticulated	In most species, homogeneous; in humans, characteristic scrolls, whorls, gratings, or lattices
Granule composition and cytochemistry		
Histamine	Relatively low	Relatively high
Serotonin	Present in rats and mice	Present in rats and mice
Dopamine	?	Present in ruminants
Heparin	Variable amounts	Relatively more; species variations
Other proteoglycans	Variable amounts	Variable amounts
Alkaline phosphatase	Present or absent	Present
Acid phosphatase	Absent	Present
Acid hydrolases	Absent	Present
Peroxidase	Present in humans and rabbits	Present
Degranulation process	Slow	Fast
Generation of arachidonate metabolites	Small quantities of SRS-A and TxB_2	Comparatively larger amounts
Life span in tissues	Few days	Weeks to months

particularly heparin or chondroitin sulfate and dermatan sulfate, depending on the species. The absence of metachromatic staining of mature feline basophils perhaps indicates lack of these substances. Immature feline basophils, (myelocyte, metamyelocyte, and band forms) however, do contain metachromatic granules. These immature cells exhibit two types of large granules—darkly stained, reddish-purple granules and lightly stained, orange-gray granules common to mature basophils in this species (Plates V–2, XII–4, and XII–5). The former granule type probably corresponds to primary granules and the latter to secondary granules similar to those in neutrophil precursors. Basophil precursors in other species lack metachromatic granules and early immature cells have few such granules.

On electron microscopy, immature basophil granules appear homogeneous, whereas mature granules may present an array of dense particles, fibrils, or lamellae, or a honeycomb pattern, depending on the species and granule maturity. In comparison, mast cell granules in most species are homogeneous but, in humans, they show characteristic scrolls, whorls, gratings, and lattices. Morphology of basophil granules of some species resembles that of the mast cell granules rather than the basophil granules of other species; for example, guinea pig basophil and mouse mast cells granules are homogeneous (Eguchi, 1991). The granules in canine basophils vary markedly in size; large, moderately dense granules are found scattered among the numerous, small, light granules that fill the cell (Fig. 15–1). Granule formation occurs in the Golgi complex. Small granules coalesce to form large ones and their contents condense with granule maturation. The two important subcellular organelles in human mast cells include secretory granules, containing preformed mediators of inflammation, and lipid bodies, that contain large amounts of arachidonic acid (Dvorak, 1989).

BIOCHEMICAL CONSTITUENTS AND THEIR BIOLOGIC PROPERTIES

Basophils and mast cells contain various preformed substances of biologic importance, and can synthesize several equally important substances on immunologic and nonimmunologic stimulation (Table 15–2). The granule composition, however, may vary within and among species. The granules are particularly rich in histamine, heparin and, in some species, serotonin. Antigenically stimulated cells synthesize important factors such as platelet-activating factor (PAF), slow-reacting substance of anaphylaxis (SRS-A), and thromboxane A_2 (TxA_2). Leukotrienes C_4, D_4, and E_4 comprise the SRS-A. The mast cells contain a factor called

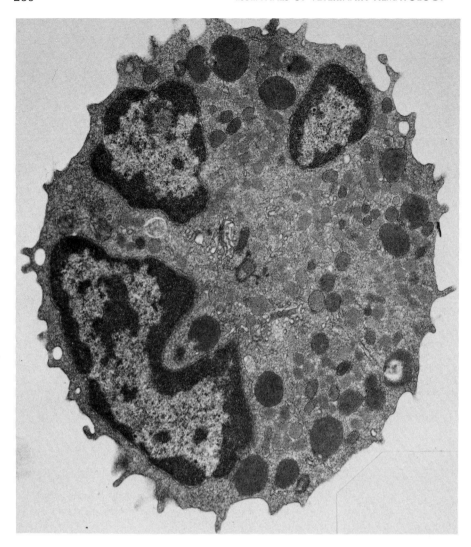

Fig. 15–1. Canine basophil containing numerous small to large, round granules of variable electron density. The central area of the cytoplasm contains profiles of the Golgi apparatus and centrioles. Some surface microvilli are also present (× 25,000). (From Jain, N.C.: Schalm's Veterinary Hematology. 4th Ed. Philadelphia, Lea & Febiger, 1986, p. 759.)

the eosinophilic chemotactic factor of anaphylaxis, (ECF-A) and basophils synthesize it on stimulation. The presence of these substances and their biologic properties are the basis of the pathophysiologic roles of basophils and mast cells in the induction of inflammation, anticoagulation, coagulation, fibrinolysis, and lipid metabolism (Jain, 1986; Williams et al., 1990).

Mast cells produce a broad panel of multifunctional cytokines by which they can influence many physiologic, immunologic, and pathologic processes (Galli et al., 1991; Gordon et al., 1990; Seder et al., 1991). These cytokines include interleukins-3, -4, -5, and -6 and GM-CSF. Interleukin-3 and GM-CSF produced by mast cells activated by IgE receptor cross-linking and other mechanisms can influence renewal of mast cells, and interleukin-4 can induce B cells to synthesize IgE (Heusser et al., 1991). Interferon-γ negatively regulates the IgE synthesis induced by interleukin-4; these two lymphokines may be produced by the same or different helper T cell clones (Romagnani et al., 1989). See Tables 17–3 and 17–4 for functions of various cytokines including interleukins.

It has been reported that human blood basophils comprise two populations having different densities and that these populations vary in their functional responses to various secretogouges and anti-allergic agents (Morita et al., 1989). Human basophils have been found to form Charcot-Lyden crystals (CLC) and to contain quantities of CLC protein comparable to that in eosinophils (Dvorak and Ackerman, 1989). The CLC is uniquely associated with the main, large, particle-filled granule population of human basophils.

Basophils and mast cells show some differences in cytochemical reactions of their granules. The basophil granules stain metachromatically with acid, but not neutral toluidine blue, are negative for chloroacetate esterase, and do not contain human mast cell tryptase. Mast cell granules stain with acid and neutral toluidine blue, are positive for chloroacetate esterase, and contain a mast cell specific tryptase (Bressler et al., 1990).

Feline and bovine basophils show alkaline phosphatase activity in their cytoplasm but not in granules. Feline basophil granules have a strong chloroacetate esterase activity (Plate X-10), but lack nonspecific esterase and peroxidase activities. Equine basophils are also peroxidase negative. Omega-exonuclease, a

Table 15–2. Various Substances Elaborated by Mast Cells and Basophils and Their Functions

Substance	Preformed	Newly Formed	Functions
Histamine	+	–	Smooth muscle contraction; increased vascular permeability; increased prostaglandin release; chemotactic and chemokinetic stimulation (H1 receptor) and inhibition (H2 receptors) of neutrophils and eosinophils; increased cAMP (H2 receptor); increased cGMP (H1 receptor); stimulation of suppressor T-lymphocytes
Slow-reacting substance of anaphylaxis (SRS-A: LTC_4, D_4, and E_4)	–	+	Smooth muscle contraction; increased vascular permeability; increased prostaglandin synthesis; synergistic with histamine and PGE
Serotonin	+	–	Smooth muscle contraction; increased vascular permeability
Platelet-activating factor	–	+	Platelet aggregation, sequestration, and release reaction; inflammatory mediator
Arachidonic acid metabolites	–	+	Various functions (e.g., smooth muscle contraction or relaxation, chemotactic for neutrophils and eosinophils, increase cAMP and cGMP)
Eosinophil chemotactic factor of anaphylaxis (ECF-A)	+ (mast cells)	+ (basophils)	Chemotactic activation and deactivation of neutrophils and eosinophils
ECF-oligopeptides	+	–	Same as ECF-A
Neutrophil chemotactic factor (NCF)	+	–	Chemotactic activation and deactivation of neutrophils
Lipid chemotactic factors	–	+	Chemotactic for neutrophils and eosinophils; Chemotactic deactivation of neutrophils
Proteoglycans	∣	–	
Heparin			Anticoagulation after interaction with antithrombin III; inhibition of activation of complement
Chondroitin sulfate			Platelet factor 4 interaction; granule binding of mediators
Dermatan sulfate			?
Basophil kallikrein-like activities (BK-A)	+	–	
Hageman factor cleaving protease			Activates Hageman factor
Kinin cleaving protease			Generates kinin from kininogen
Chymase			Proteolysis; mast cell degranulation
Arylsulfatases A, B	+	–	Hydrolysis of SRA-S
Plasminogen activator (in plasma membrane)	+	–	Activates plasminogen
Elastase	+	–	Capable of inducing severe lung injury
IL-3, IL-4, IL-5, IL-6, GM-CSF	–	+ (mast cells)	Produced by activated mast cells; see Tables 17–3 and 17–4 for function.

marker for human basophils, is present in the cytoplasm of basophils of the dog, cat, rhesus monkey, and gibbon, but not in basophils of the horse, cattle, goat, pig, and alpaca (Jain and Kono, 1991).

INTERRELATIONSHIP OF BASOPHILS AND EOSINOPHILS

Several observations indicate an interrelationship between basophils and eosinophils (see Table 14–2). Histamine and the ECF-A elaborated by basophils are chemotactic for eosinophils. The release of these factors in tissues causes the local accumulation of eosinophils. In some conditions, an increase in basophil and eosinophil numbers in the blood may occur simultaneously; similarly, eosinophils often infiltrate tissues rich in mast cells. Important regulatory interactions of eosinophil and mast cell products are shown in Figure 15–2.

Experimental studies have shown that mast cells are responsible for the mediator release in acute allergic inflammatory reaction, while eosinophils and basophils are involved in the mediator release that occurs during the late phase of inflammatory reactions (Lichtenstein and Bochner, 1991). Prednisone inhibits the influx of eosinophils and basophils and associated appearance of inflammatory mediators, thereby modifying the late phase inflammatory response associated with an allergic reaction (Charlesworth et al., 1991). Cyclosporin A strongly inhibits histamine and leukotriene release from human basophils (Ezeamuzie and Assem, 1990).

BIOLOGIC PROPERTIES AND FUNCTIONS

The biologic functions of basophils are thought to be similar to those of mast cells because of similarities in their biochemical constituents (see above). In addition, they respond instantaneously to substances in their environment through interactions with surface receptors. Basophils and mast cells express a unique immunologic surface marker profile including binding sites for a variety of immunomodulating ligands and

MAST CELL - EOSINOPHIL INTERACTIONS

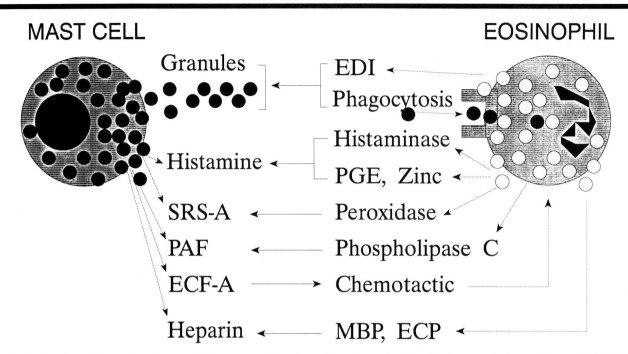

Fig. 15–2. Regulatory interactions of eosinophil and mast cell products. Histamine and eosinophil chemotactic factor of anaphylaxis (ECF-A) released from mast cells in tissue attract eosinophils. Mast cell degranulation is controlled by eosinophil-derived inhibitors (EDIs) consisting of PGE$_1$ and PGE$_4$ and through phagocytosis of exocytosed granules. Various mediators released from mast cells in the milieu are inactivated by eosinophil components: histamine by histaminase, PGEs, and zinc; slow-reacting substance of anaphylaxis (SRS-A) by hypochlorous acid generated from the action of eosinophil peroxidase-hydrogen peroxide-halide complex; platelet-activating factor (PAF) by phospholipase C in eosinophil membrane; and heparin by major basic protein (MBP) and eosinophil cationic protein (ECP). See table 14–2 for additional information.

adhesion molecules (Valent et al., 1990b). Basophils and mast cells have surface receptors for IgE, IgG, β-adrenergic catecholamines, prostaglandins, histamine, and cholera enterotoxin. The Fc gamma receptors present on human basophils are exclusively of the Fc gamma RII (CDw32) subtype; Fc gamma RI (CD64) is absent (Anselmino et al., 1989). Human basophils have receptors for various lymphokines such as interleukin-1, interleukin-2, interleukin-3, interleukin-4, and interleukin-5, GM-CSF, and C3a (Bischoff et al., 1990a, 1990b; Lopez et al., 1990; Massey et al., 1989; Stockinger et al., 1990; Valent et al., 1990a). Basophils are sluggishly motile, but respond chemotactically to bacterial products, complement components C5a and C567, kallikrein, a monocyte chemotactic and activating factor (MCAF), and certain undefined lymphokines (Alam et al., 1992; Williams et al., 1990). MCAF induces histamine release from human basophils (Kuna et al., 1992).

The most important function of mast cells and basophils is the elicitation of an immediate hypersensitivity reaction through the secretion of their stored vasoactive mediators and the elaboration of some potent mediators on stimulation. Both cells exhibit mediator release followed by degranulation on interaction of appropriate antigens (pollens, dust, dandruff) with specific, cell-bound IgE. IgE molecules

bind reversibly through the Fc region and the amount of basophil-bound IgE may vary with plasma IgE levels. In vitro IgE-mediated release of histamine by basophils can be used as a screening test to evaluate immediate hypersensitivity responses in horses (Magro et al., 1988). Many physical, chemical, and mechanical stimuli can also induce the degranulation of mast cells and basophils. Respiratory viruses can cause nonimmunologic release of histamine from human basophils (Sanche-Legrand and Smith, 1989). Neuraminidase on the surface of influenza A virus was found to potentiate the effect of the virus on basophil histamine release (Clementsen et al., 1988). Basophils also degranulate in blood in response to postprandial lipemia. A unique property of basophils and mast cells that is now recognized is that they can resynthesize granules following degranulation.

Basophils from normal and allergic individuals vary in their sensitivity for mediator release, and basophils from allergic persons may develop a reversible or irreversible desensitization to an agonist. Basophils from approximately 20% of normal humans seem to be unresponsive (nonreleasers), in terms of both histamine and leukotriene release, to an IgE cross-linking stimulus, such as anti-IgE antibody (Nguyen et al., 1990). Nonreleasing basophils probably have a defect in early signal transduction, possibly involving the influx of Ca^{++}. Basophils from allergic patients, such as those with asthma and atopic dermatitis, are more sensitive to histamine-releasing factors than are basophils from normal persons (Alam et al., 1990; Sainte-Laudy and Henocq, 1990). Basophils from approximately 50% of AIDs patients are sensitive to cytokine-induced histamine release that is mediated by a cell-bound IgE (Pedersen et al., 1991). In patients with food hypersensitivity, exposure to the relevant antigens produces a cytokine (histamine-releasing factor) that interacts with IgE bound to the surface of basophils, causing them to release histamine (Sampson et al., 1989).

Several interleukins, GM-CSF, PAF, and TNF, variably influence the mediator release from basophils (Alam et al., 1989; Bischoff et al., 1990a, 1990b; Dahinden et al., 1989; Haak-Frendscho et al., 1988; Lopez et al., 1990; Massey et al., 1989). Interleukin-1 augments IgE-dependent release of histamine from human basophils. Interleukin-3 primes basophils for mediator release by interleukin-8, formerly termed neutrophil-activating peptide, NAP-1 (Dahinden et al., 1989). GM-CSF renders basophils capable of responding to C3a. Interleukin-3 also promotes basophil adhesion to endothelium by increasing cell surface expression of CD11b/CD18 antigens on basophils (Bochner et al., 1990). Interleukin-3 therapy in human patients with cancer causes basophilia, eosinophilia, and in vivo histamine release (Merget et al., 1990). Interleukin-5 primes basophils for enhanced histamine release and leukotriene-C4 generation in response to various basophil agonists such as C5a, C3a, and IL-8. Interleukin-8 both promotes and inhibits histamine and leukotriene release from human basophils exposed to interleukin-3; release induced by C5a, anti-IgE, and FMLP is not inhibited (Bischoff et al., 1991; Kuna et al., 1991). PAF can induce a release of inflammatory mediators (histamine and leukotriene C4) from human basophils primed by interleukin-3, GM-CSF, and interleukin-5 and this response is decreased in the absence of neutrophils (Brunner et al., 1991; Columbo et al., 1990). A recently cloned cytokine, MCAF, is a potent secretogogue for basophils (Alam et al., 1992).

The receptor-mediated secretion and degranulation processes involve signal transduction mechanisms (see Fig. 13–5). Stimuli such as anti-IgE antibody and FMLP activate protein kinase C and an increase in intracellular free calcium, but substantial degranulation can occur in the absence of any increase in intracellular calcium (Warner and MacGlashan, 1990). A protein-kinase-C-independent pathway may also be involved in release of inflammatory mediators from basophils (Knol et al., 1990). Histamine and leukotriene C4 release from human basophils is inhibited by many pharmacologic agents such as some arachidonic analogues, activators of adenylate cyclase, and inhibitors of phospholipase A_2, phosphodiesterase, and protein kinase C (Morita et al., 1988; Warner et al., 1988).

The degranulation process has been studied using the electron microscope (Jain, 1986; Dvorak et al., 1991). Initially, granules become stripped of their membranes and granular substances, rather than whole granules, are then released to the exterior through the formation of a single pore (guinea pig basophils) or multiple pores (human basophils and rat mast cells) in the plasma membrane. During this phase, membranes from the granules fuse with the plasma membrane to form an invaginated degranulation sac (or sacs). Next, both the intact and membrane-stripped granules are extruded through the pore(s) formed in the plasma membrane (Fig. 15–3). Granule exocytosis may begin within minutes and continues for hours.

The degranulation of mast cells and basophils immediately initiates an acute inflammatory reaction, whereas continuous slow degranulation contributes to the delayed phase of an inflammatory reaction. The increase in capillary permeability can be attributed to the release of histamine, serotonin, and PAF, whereas leukocyte infiltration is promoted by the neutrophil chemotactic factor of anaphylaxis (NCF-A) and ECF-A. The PAF causes platelet aggregation and the release reaction, and is considered to have several times more phlogistic activity than histamine. Histamine release at sites of inflammation may suppress local immune responses as histamine was found to cause a dose dependent inhibition of blastogenesis of canine peripheral blood lymphocytes to phytohemagglutinin-P (Daniel et al., 1990).

Basophil and mast cell products may regulate local and systemic coagulation and fibronolysis. Heparin released in the blood binds to antithrombin to effect the anticoagulation of circulating blood and also of blood escaping in body cavities. The serosal linings of body cavities contain many mast cells. Thus, chronic bleeding into the chest or abdominal cavity is not followed by blood clotting. This is a protective mechanism referable to the heparin in mast cells. The clotting of blood in body cavities would lead to the formation of extensive adhesions.

The extent of the procoagulant and fibrinolytic activities of basophils and mast cells remains unknown. Activation of the Hageman factor by the PAF and a bradykinin-like activity promotes coagulation and fibrinolysis is activated by the action of plasminogen activator, leading to the formation of plasmin.

Heparin released from degranulated basophils during postprandial lipemia promotes the release of lipoprotein lipase from endothelial cells of the vessel wall. Lipoprotein lipase causes the clearing of chylomicra and facilitates the metabolism of triglycerides.

BASOPHIL NUMBERS IN BLOOD

Basophils are rare in blood and bone marrow. The normal range in various species is 0 to 300/μl of blood. They are found more frequently in ruminants and horses than in dogs and cats. Rabbits generally have as many as 10 to 15% basophils in blood. Basopenia seen in normal animals is of little significance, but basophilia is considered significant. Basophilia may be seen in various conditions (see Table 14–1), but usually

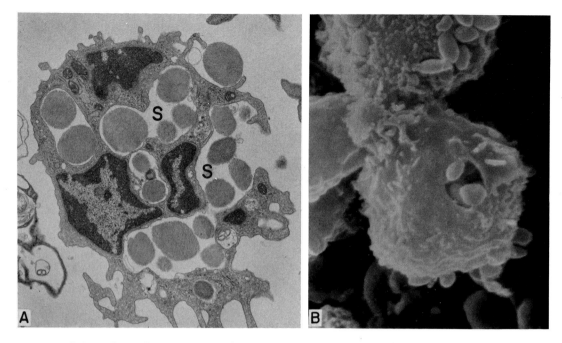

Fig. 15–3. In vitro anaphylactic degranulation of guinea pig basophils. *A,* Transmission electron photomicrograph (× 9,000). *B,* Scanning electron photomicrograph (× 10,000). (From Dvorak, A.M., et al.: Surface membrane alterations in Guinea pig basophils undergoing anaphylactic degranulation: A scanning electron microscopy study. Lab. Invest., 45:58, 1981.)

its mechanism remains unknown. Sometimes basophilia and eosinophilia may occur concurrently, perhaps reflecting a functional interaction of the two cell types. Basophilia is common in conditions associated with IgE production and the release of lymphokines, as in allergic dermatitis, eczema, and delayed hypersensitivity reaction. A slight basophilia occurs frequently in humans with chronic myelogenous leukemia and sometimes in acute myelogenous leukemia. Although glucocorticoids induce basopenia in different species, some dogs with Cushing's syndrome may have a small number of basophils in their blood.

Mast cells are normally absent in blood and are rare in the bone marrow. A rare mast cell may be found in a severely stressed animal or an animal in shock. Mastocytosis may occur in some dogs with a malignant mast cell tumor. Mastocytosis or mastocytemia may also occur in dogs with parvovirus infection or may have other, nonspecific causes.

A diagnosis of mast cell leukemia in human patients is made when greater than 10% atypical mast cells are found in blood (Torrey et al., 1990).

REFERENCES

Alam, R., Forsythe, P.A., Rankin, J.A., et al.: Sensitivity of basophils to histamine releasing factor(s) of various origin: dependency of allergic phenotype of the donor and surface-bound IgE. Allergy Clin. Immunol., 86:73, 1990.

Alam, R., Lett-Brown, M.A., Forsythe, P.A., et al.: Monocyte chemotactic and activating factor is a potent histamine-releasing factor for basophils. J. Clin. Invest., 89:723, 1992.

Alam, R., Welter, J.B., Forsythe, P.A., et al.: Comparative effect of recombinant IL-1, -2, -3, -4, and -6, IFN-gamma, granulocyte-macrophage-colony-stimulating factor, tumor necrosis factor-

alpha, and histamine-releasing factors on the secretion of histamine from basophils. J. Immunol., 142:3431, 1989.

Anselmino, L.M., Perussia, B. and Thomas, L.L.: Human basophils selectively express the Fc gamma RII (CDw32) subtype of IgG receptor. J. Allergy Clin. Immunol., 84:907, 1989.

Bischoff, S.C., Baggiolini, M., De Weck, A.L., et al.: Interleukin 8-inhibitor and inducer of histamine and leukotriene release in human basophils. Biochem. Biophys. Res. Commun., 179:628, 1991.

Bischoff, S.C., Brunner, T., De Weck, A.L., et al.: Interleukin 5 modifies histamine release and leukotriene generation by human basophils in response to diverse agonists. J. Exp. Med, 172:1577, 1990a.

Bischoff, S.C., De Weck, A.L. and Dahinden, C.A.: Interleukin 3 and granulocyte/macrophage-colony-stimulating factor render human basophils responsive to low concentrations of complement component C3a. Proc. Natl. Acad. Sci. USA, 87:6813, 1990b.

Bochner, B.S., McKelvey, A.A., Sterbinsky, S.A., et al.: IL-3 augments adhesiveness for endothelium and CD11b expression in human basophils but not neutrophils. J. Immunol., 145:1832, 1990.

Bressler, R.B., Friedman, M.M., Kirshenbaum, A.S., et al.: Sequential appearance of basophils and mast cells from human bone marrow in long-term suspension culture. Int. Arch. Allergy Appl. Immunol., 91:403, 1990.

Brunner, T., De Weck, A.L. and Dahinden, C.A.: Platelet-activating factor induces mediator release by human basophils primed with IL-3, granulocyte-macrophage colony-stimulating factor, or IL-5. J. Immunol., 147:237, 1991.

Charlesworth, E.N., Kagey-Sobotka, A., Schleimer, R.P., et al.: Prednisone inhibits the appearance of inflammatory mediators and the influx of eosinophils and basophils associated with the cutaneous late-phase response to allergen. J. Immunol., 146:671, 1991.

Church, M.K., el-Lati, S., and Okayama, Y.: Biological properties of human skin mast cells. Clin. Exp. Allergy, 21 Suppl 3:1, 1991.

Clementsen, P., Jensen, C.B., Jarlov, J.O., et al.: Virus enhances histamine release from human basophils. Agents Actions, 23:165, 1988.

Columbo, M., Casolaro, V., Warner, J.A., et al.: The mechanism of mediator release from human basophils induced by platelet-activating factor. J. Immunol., 145:3855, 1990.

Dahinden, C.A., Kurimoto, Y., De Weck, A.L., et al.: The neutrophil-activating peptide NAF/NAP-1 induces histamine and leukotriene release by interleukin 3-primed basophils. J. Exp. Med., 170:1787, 1989.

Daniel, S.L., Ogilvie, G.K. and Felsburg, P.J.: Modulation of canine lymphocyte blastogenesis via histamine. Vet. Immunol. Immunopathol., 24:69, 1990.

Denburg, J.A., Silver, J.E. and Abrams, J.S.: Interleukin-5 is a human basophilopoietin: induction of histamine content and basophilic differentiation of HL-60 cells and of peripheral blood basophil-eosinophil progenitors. Blood, 77:1462, 1991.

Dvorak, A.M.: Human mast cells. Adv. Anat. Embryol. Cell. Biol., 114:1, 1989.

Dvorak, A.M. and Ackerman, S.J.: Ultrastructural localization of the Charcot-Leyden crystal protein (lysophospholipase) to granules and intragranular crystals in mature human basophils. Lab. Invest., 60:557, 1989.

Dvorak, A.M., Warner, J.A., Kissell, S., et al.: F-met peptide-induced degranulation of human basophils. Lab. Invest., 64:234, 1991.

Ebisawa, M., Saito, H., Reason, D.C., et al.: Effects of human recombinant interleukin 5 and 3 on the differentiation of cord blood-derived eosinophils and basophils. Arerugi, 38:442, 1989.

Eguchi, M.: Comparative electron microscopy of basophils and mast cells, in vivo and in vitro. Electron Microsc. Rev., 4:293, 1991.

Ezeamuzie, C.I. and Assem, E.S.: Anti-allergic properties of cyclosporin A: inhibition of mediator release from human basophils and rat basophilic leukemia cells (RBL-2H3). Immunopharmacology, 20:31, 1990.

Galli, S.J.: New insights into "the riddle of the mast cells": microenvironmental regulation of mast cell development and phenotypic heterogeneity. Lab. Invest., 62:5, 1990.

Galli, S.J., Gordon, J.R. and Wershil, B.K.: Cytokine productions by mast cells and basophils. Curr. Opin. Immunol., 3:865, 1991.

Gordon, J.R., Burd, P.R. and Galli, S.J.: Mast cells as a source of multifunctional cytokines. Immunol. Today, 11:458, 1990.

Haak-Frendscho, M., Dinarello, C. and Kaplan, A.P.: Recombinant human interleukin-1 beta causes histamine release from human basophils. J. Allergy Clin. Immunol., 82:218, 1988.

Heusser, C.H., Bews, J., Brinkmann, V., et al.: New concepts of IgE regulation. Int. Arch. Allergy Appl. Immunol., 94:87, 1991.

Jain, N.C.: Schalm's Veterinary Hematology. 4th ed. Philadelphia, Lea & Febiger, 1986, pp. 756–767.

Jain, N.C. and Kono, C.S.: Omega-exonuclease activity in basophils of certain animal species. Comp Haematol Int, 1:166, 1991.

Kaplan, A.P., Reddigari, S., Baeza, M., et al.: Histamine releasing factors and cytokine-dependent activation of basophils and mast cells. Adv. Immunol., 50:237, 1991.

Kirshenbaum, A.S., Goff, J.P., Kessler, S.W., et al.: Effect of IL-3 and stem cell factor on the appearance on human basophils and mast cells from CD34+ pluripotent progenitor cells. J. Immunol., 148:772, 1992.

Knol, E.F., Koenderman, L., Mul, E., et al.: Differential mechanisms in the stimulus-secretion coupling in human basophils: evidence for a protein-kinase-C-dependent and a protein-kinase-C-independent route. Agents Actions, 30:49, 1990.

Kuna, P., Reddigari, S.R., Kornfeld, D., et al.: IL-8 inhibits histamine release from human basophils induced by histamine-releasing factors, connective tissue activating peptide III, and IL-3. J. Immunol., 147:1920, 1991.

Kuna, P., Reddigari, S.R., Rucinski, D., et al.: Monocyte chemotactic and activating factor is a potent histamine-releasing factor for human basophils. J. Exp. Med., 175:489, 1992.

Lichtenstein, L.M. and Bochner, B.S.,: The role of basophils in asthma. Ann. N.Y. Acad. Sci, 629:48, 1991.

Lopez, A.F., Eglinton, J.M., Lyons, A.B., et al.: Human interleukin-3 inhibits the binding of granulocyte-macrophage colony-stimulating factor and interleukin-5 to basophils and strongly enhances their functional activity. J. Cell. Physiol., 145:69, 1990.

Magro, A.M., Rudofsky, U.H., Schrader, W.P., et al.: Characterisation of IgE-mediated histamine release from equine basophils in vitro, Equine Vet. J., 20:352, 1988.

Massey, W.A., Randall, T.C., Kagey-Sobotka, A., et al.: Recombinant human IL-1 alpha and -1 beta potentiate IgE-mediated histamine release from human basophils. J. Immunol., 143:1875, 1989.

Melman, S.A.: Mast cells and their mediators. Emphasis on their role in type I immediate hypersensitivity in canines. Int. J. Dermatol., 26:335, 1987.

Merget, R.D., Maurer, A.B., Koch, U., et al.: Histamine release from basophils after in vivo application of recombinant human interleukin-3 in man. Int. Arch. Allergy Appl. Immunol., 92:366, 1990.

Miller, J. and Schwartz, L.B.: Heterogeneity of human mast cells. Prog. Clin. Biol. Res., 297:115, 1989.

Morita, Y., Asakawa, M., Hirai, K., et al.: Functional differences of human basophils with different densities. Int. Arch. Allergy Appl. Immunol., 88:332, 1989.

Morita, Y., Takaishi, T., Honda, Z., et al.: Role of protein kinase C in histamine release from human basophils. Allergy, 43:100, 1988.

Nguyen, K.L., Gillis, S. and MacGlashan, D.W. Jr.: A comparative study of releasing and nonreleasing human basophils: nonreleasing basophils lack of early component of the signal transduction pathway that follows IgE cross-linking. J. Allergy Clin. Immunol., 85:1020, 1990.

Pedersen, M., Permin, H., Bindslev-Jensen, C., et al.: Cytokine-induced histamine release from basophils of AIDS patients. Interaction between cytokines and specific IgE antibodies. Allergy, 46:129, 1991.

Romagnani, S., Maggi, E., Del Prete, G., et al.: Role of interleukins in induction and regulation of human IgE. Clin. Exp. Rheumatol., 7 Suppl 3:S117, 1989.

Sainte-Laudy, J. and Henocq, E.: Reactivity of human basophils to anti-IgE and protein A in atopic dermatitis. Agents Actions, 30:250, 1990.

Sampson, H.A., Broadbent, K.R. and Bernhisel-Broadbent, J.: Spontaneous release of histamine from basophils and histamine-releasing factor in patients with atopic dermatitis and food hypersensitivity [see comments]. N. Engl. J. Med., 321:228, 1989.

Sanchez-Legrand, F. and Smith, T.F.: Interaction of paramyxoviruses with human basophils and their effect on histamine release. J. Allergy Clin. Immunol., 84:538, 1989.

Seder, R.A., Paul, W.E., Ben-Sasson, S.Z., et al.: Production of interleukin-4 and other cytokines following stimulation of mast cell lines and in vivo mast cells/basophils. Int. Arch. Allergy Appl. Immunol., 94:137, 1991.

Stevens, R.L. and Austen, K.F.: Recent advances in the cellular and molecular biology of mast cells. Immunol. Today, 10:381, 1989.

Stockinger, H., Valent, P., Majdic, O., et al.: Human blood basophils synthesize interleukin-2 binding sites. Blood, 75:1820, 1990.

Torrey, E., Simpson, K., Wilbur, S., et al.: Malignant mastocytosis with circulating mast cells. Am. J. Hematol., 34:283, 1990.

Valent, P., Besemer, J., Kishi, K., et al.: Human basophils express interleukin-4 receptors. Blood, 76:1734, 1990a.

Valent, P., Majdic, O., Maurer, D., et al.: Further characterization of surface membrane structures expressed on human basophils and mast cells. Int. Arch. Allergy Appl. Immunol., 91:198, 1990b.

Warner, J.A. and MacGlashan, D.W. Jr: Signal transduction events in human basophils. A comparative study of the role of protein kinase C in basophils activated by anti-IgE antibody and formyl-methionyl-leucyl-phenylalanine. J. Immunol., 145:1897, 1990.

Warner, J.A., MacGlashan, D.W. Jr., Peters, S.P., et al.: The pharmacologic modulation of mediator release from human basophils. J. Allergy Clin. Immunol., 82:432, 1988.

Williams, W.J., Buetler, E., Erslev, A.J., et al.: Hematology. 4th ed. New York, McGraw-Hill, 1990.

The Monocytes and Macrophages

The monocytes are derived from hematopoietic stem cells in the bone marrow and, shortly after entering the circulation, they randomly migrate into various tissues and body cavities and become macrophages. Considerable heterogeneity exists in the morphologic, metabolic, and functional features among macrophages from different sites, among macrophages from the same sites, and between macrophages from normal animals and animals manipulated to yield "activated" macrophages (Jain, 1986; Winkler, 1988; Williams et al., 1990). Similarly, monocyte heterogeneity, in the form of less mature and more mature monocytes, may also exist, analogous to that of neutrophils (band and segmented neutrophils).

The blood monocytes, the promonocytes and their precursors in the bone marrow, and the tissue macrophages comprise the mononuclear phagocyte system (MPS). Members of the MPS include histiocytes in connective tissue, fixed and free macrophages in the lymph nodes, spleen, and bone marrow, serosal macrophages in the pleural and peritoneal cavities, Kupffer cells of the liver, alveolar macrophages, osteoclasts, Langerhans cells in the epidermis, intraglomerular mesangial macrophages in the kidneys, and microglial cells in the nervous system. The MPS replaces the reticuloendothelial system, which also included other cells capable of phagocytosis, such as the reticular cells of the spleen and lymph nodes and the endothelial cells of the lymph and blood sinuses. These cell types are excluded from the MPS, because they are not derived from monocytes. Current concepts of monocyte and macrophage production and biology have been summarized (Henry and Moore, 1991; Johnston, 1988; Metcalf, 1991; Nielsen, 1990; Papadimitriou and Ashman, 1989; Stein and Keshav, 1992; van Furth, 1989; van Kessel and Verhoef, 1990).

PRODUCTION AND KINETICS

Monocytes

The monocyte is a descendant of a bipotential progenitor cell, the colony-forming unit–granulocyte-monocyte (CFU-GM), committed to produce both neutrophils and monocytes (Fig. 16–1). This progenitor cell originates from the pluripotential stem cell (PPSC). The differentiation of PPSC and CFU-GM is influenced by the hematopoietic inductive microenvironment in the bone marrow and several cytokines (Metcalf, 1991). Interleukin-3 and granulocyte-monocyte colony-stimulating factor (GM-CSF) regulate the entire process of monocytopoiesis, from the PPSC to the monocyte stage. The differentiation of the CFU-GM into the CFU-M and the proliferation of monocyte precursors (monoblast and promonocyte) to monocytes, however, is influenced by a monocyte-specific colony-stimulating factor (M-CSF). This CSF is a glycoprotein with a molecular weight of 45,000 to 70,000 and is produced by various cells, including activated monocytes, macrophages, T lymphocytes, and endothelial cells. A factor increasing monocytosis (FIM) synthesized and secreted by macrophages stimulates monocyte production by its effect on the mitotic activity of monoblasts and promonocytes in the bone marrow (Sluiter et al., 1990). Prostaglandin E_2 (PGE_2) produced by macrophages inhibits monocyte production, whereas lactoferrin stimulates monocytopoiesis through its inhibitory effect on PGE_2 production. Factors regulating the release of monocytes in blood remain poorly defined (see Chap. 4 for additional comments).

A single intravenous injection of M-CSF in rats induced a dose-dependent monocytosis, neutrophilia,

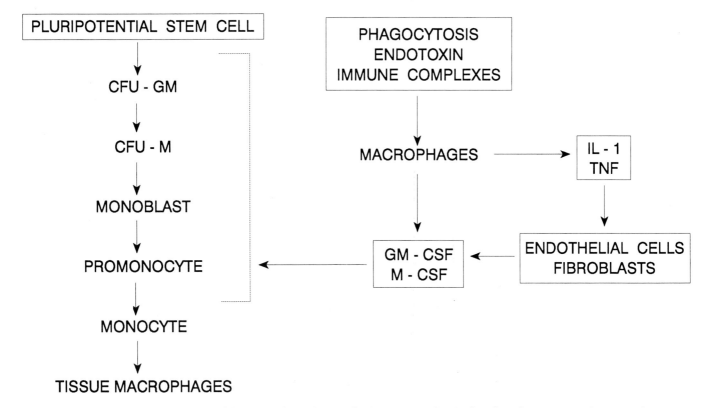

Fig. 16–1. Development of monocytes and factors regulating their production. Nonspecific stimuli such as phagocytosis, endotoxin, and immune complexes activate macrophages to elaborate cytokines such as interleukin 1 (IL-1), tumor necrosis factor (TNF), and granulocyte-monocyte colony and monocyte colony-stimulating factors (GM-CSF, M-CSF). IL-1 and TNF in turn stimulate endothelial cells and fibroblasts to produce more GM-CSF and M-CSF. GM-CSF and M-CSF, along with IL-3, regulate monocyte production at all levels—that is, from the differentiation of the pluripotential stem cell into the committed stem cell CFU-GM through the formation of a mature monocyte.

and lymphopenia (Ulich et al., 1990). The monocytosis peaked at 28 to 32 hours, with a seven- to eight-fold increase in the number of circulating monocytes and promonocytes, and it was preceded by a transient monocytopenia at 15 minutes postinoculation. The monocytosis resulted from marrow monocyte precursor proliferation, maturation, and release. Similarly, a single intravenous injection of recombinant human interleukin-3 in rats induced a neutrophilia and monocytosis by 4 to 6 hours postinoculation, peaking at 8 hours and then subsiding to normalcy by 12 to 24 hours (Ulich et al., 1989). The neutrophilia resulted from release of cells from the marrow reserve rather than from demargination of cells in the microvasculature. Myeloid and erythroid hyperplasias were evident at 8 hours. A combination of interleukin-3 and interleukin-6 induced synergistic changes in the peripheral blood and bone marrow monocyte populations.

The monoblast divides once and the promonocyte once or twice, but the monocyte usually does not divide in the bone marrow. In bone marrow aspirates stained with Wright stain monocytes may occasionally be found but promonocytes and monoblasts are rare, except in cases of acute myelomonocytic and monocytic leukemia.

Kinetic studies of radioisotope-labelled blood monocytes in humans have provided some information about their production, release, and circulation. The mean time of production and release of monocytes from bone marrow to blood is about 50 to 60 hours. No bone marrow reserve of monocytes is present, unlike that for neutrophils. Thus, newly formed monocytes are delivered to the circulation as soon as they are produced; the minimum emergence time in blood is about 6 hours. Monocytes are distributed in the vascular system between the circulating and marginal pools in a ratio of 1:3.5. Their mean half-life of survival in blood is estimated as 8.4 hours (range 4.5–10 hours) using $DF^{32}P$ (di-isopropyl fluorophosphate) and 71 hours (range, 36 to 104 hours) using ^3H-TdR (tritiated thymidine) as a label for newly formed monocytes. The latter data are considered to be fairly accurate. Monocytes normally leave blood randomly to enter tissues. Kinetic studies of inflammatory conditions have revealed that a monocytosis observed in blood during disease states actually reflects increased bone marrow production and release, rather than a shift of monocytes from the intravascular marginal pool.

Species differences may exist in monocyte kinetics, as indicated by studies of some other species. For example, about two to three times more monocytes are present in the bone marrow of the mouse than in its blood. The intravascular half-life is about 1 day in mice and 2 days in rats. The mean monocyte production time in calves is about 36 hours and the circulatory half-life is about 21 hours. The bone marrow of healthy calves contains monoblasts, promonocytes, and monocytes in a ratio of 1:2.31:4.96, and these proportions change little during infection. Thus, monocytosis of chronic infection or inflammatory response in cattle may result from an overall increase in monocytopoiesis, as in humans, rather than from the increased release of marrow monocytes.

Macrophages

Tissue macrophages originate from monocytes, but are far more numerous than circulating monocytes; a ratio of 50:1 has been found in humans. Such a high tissue distribution of macrophages might be related to their long life span, several weeks to years (van Furth, 1989).

The migration of monocytes into tissues may increase during inflammatory response, but may be reduced in animals on corticosteroids and other immunosuppressive drugs. Non-steroidal anti-inflammatory drugs, such as indomethacin, phenylbutazone, oxyphenylbutazone, and flunixin, have been found to inhibit movement of equine monocytes and neutrophils in vitro (Dawson et al., 1987). The monocytes migrate into tissues through interendothelial regions of the venular wall, but factors regulating their migration remain to be clearly defined. An increased demand for macrophages may be met, at least in part, by the local proliferation of macrophages rather than by blood monocytes.

Tissue macrophages are classified as fixed or free. Fixed macrophages are found in most tissues, such as in the splenic sinusoids, liver (Kupffer cells), bone marrow (reticulum cells), lymph nodes, and lamina propria of the gastrointestinal tract. Free macrophages are found primarily in the pleural, peritoneal, and synovial cavities, alveolar spaces, and inflammatory sites. Free macrophages may move from one tissue to the other; in contrast, monocytes, once in tissues, do not re-enter the blood. For example, free macrophages from the peritoneal cavity may migrate through the draining lymphatics into other organs, such as the spleen. Macrophages can be cultured in vitro from bovine bone marrow (Pontzer and Russell, 1989) and swine peripheral blood (Genovesi et al., 1989).

MORPHOLOGY AND COMPOSITION

Monocytes and Their Precursors

The first morphologically recognizable cell of the series is the monoblast, whereas the PPSC, CFU-GM, and CFU-M remain morphologically unidentifiable. The monoblast resembles a myeloblast but has a slightly convoluted, round nucleus, with a wavy or indented outline (Plates VIII–1, VIII-2, and XXVI-2 to XXVI-4). The nuclear chromatin may be finely stippled or lacy, one or more distinct or indistinct nucleoli may be present, and the cytoplasm may be scanty or fairly abundant and moderately blue. The next stage, the

promonocyte, has a more convoluted nucleus, which tends to become increasingly dented or elongated with maturation. The nuclear chromatin at this stage may be lacier or remain stippled, but the nucleoli disappear and the cytoplasm becomes slightly more abundant, and may contain some vacuoles (Plates VIII-3 and XXVI-3).

The monocyte is characterized by an ameboid nucleus that can assume any form. A typical monocyte nucleus may be fat, irregularly contoured, folded, horseshoe shape, or slightly lobed, with a coiled appearance (Plates VII-2, VII-4, and VII-10). Some canine monocytes may have nuclei resembling those of young neutrophils—bands, metamyelocytes, or myelocytes (Plate VIII). The nuclear chromatin is lacy or reticular and may exhibit some areas of condensation. The cytoplasm is relatively abundant, stains slightly blue, and has a ground glass or foamy appearance. Some large vacuoles are found in a typical monocyte and occasionally it may contain some indistinct reddish-purple (azurophilic) granules (Plate VIII-7).

Prominent surface folds or ridges can be seen on scanning electron microscopy of monocytes, which may appear as microvillus-like projections or blebs on transmission electron microscopy (Fig. 16–2). Extensive membrane ruffling is considered of functional significance. Monocytes contain fewer and small lysosomal granules than neutrophils. The granules originate from the Golgi apparatus and appear to be primary granules. The granules give a positive reaction for acid phosphatase and arylsulfatase, but may be either peroxidase-positive or peroxidase-negative. The cytoplasmic basophilia of monocytes is attributed to the scattered cisternae of the rough endoplasmic reticulum and to diffuse clusters of polyribosomes. A distinguishing feature of promonocytes and monocytes is the presence of some bundles of microfilaments near the nucleus.

Cytochemical staining reveals slight peroxidase activity in some monocytes, but no alkaline phosphatase activity. Monocytes characteristically show diffuse nonspecific esterase (NSE) activity in the cytoplasm, a feature highly useful for distinguishing monocytes from neutrophils (Plates X-8 and X-9). This enzyme activity can be inhibited by sodium fluoride, in contrast to the coarsely granular, fluoride-resistant NSE activity seen in some lymphocytes. Sometimes, monocytic cells may show localized globular NSE activity that can be inhibited by sodium fluoride (Plate XXVI-6).

Macrophages

The transformation from monocyte to macrophage is accompanied by many morphologic and biochemical changes. A macrophage is usually larger than a monocyte because of its more abundant cytoplasm. The nuclear chromatin appears more open. The cytoplasm stains more blue or red and contains many more vacuoles. Macrophages show an increase in cytoplasmic organelles, but the number and content of lysosomes

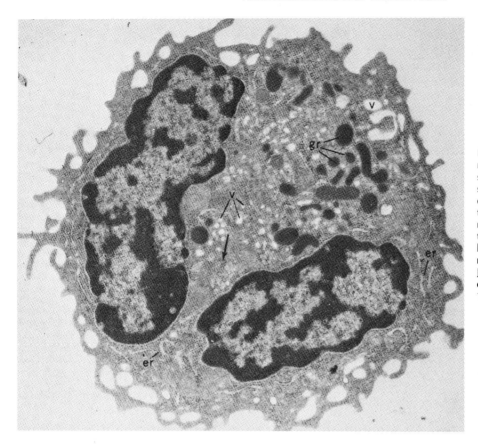

Fig. 16–2. Canine monocyte having many lysosomal granules (gr), several small to large vesicles (v), abundant ribosomes *(arrow)*, and prominent rough endoplasmic reticulum (er), especially along the cell periphery. This cell also presents many microvillus-like projections along the cellular outline. The nucleus appears bilobed and shows heavy areas of chromatin condensation (×17,500). (From Jain, N.C.: Schalm's Veterinary Hematology. 4th Ed. Philadelphia, Lea & Febiger, 1986, p. 773.)

may vary with the stage of cellular maturation, location, and activity of the cell (Figs. 16–3 and 16–4). Macrophages are metabolically and functionally more active than monocytes. For example, they show increases in protein content, glucose utilization, lactate production, pinocytotic and phagocytic activities, and enzyme synthesis.

Macrophages at different stages of maturation and at different sites may have varied but distinct morphologic features and different metabolic and functional characteristics. For example, peritoneal macrophages derive energy from anaerobic glycolysis, but alveolar macrophages do so largely from oxidative metabolism. The principal source of energy in monocytes and most tissue macrophages, however, is anaerobic glycolysis.

Macrophages are generally peroxidase-negative but some may be peroxidase-positive, depending on their stage of differentiation and environmental conditions. Epithelioid cells and multinucleated giant cells, which also originate from monocytes, are peroxidase-negative. A strong NSE activity that can be inhibited by sodium fluoride is seen in bone marrow macrophages.

Surface Receptors of Monocytes and Macrophages

Human monocytes and macrophages have surface receptors for IgG, IgM, IgA, IgE, C3b, C3bi, C3d, tumor necrosis factor (TNF), glucocorticoids, and some other hormones, such as insulin. Species variation has been found in the receptor expression. Monocyte subpopulations in humans may differ in the expression of IgG (FcRI) receptors; they may be FcRI-positive or negative. Bovine and canine cells were found to have IgG and C3 receptors, but not IgM receptors. Receptors for the chemoattractant N-formyl-methionyl-leucyl-phenylalanine (FMLP) are present on the surface of equine monocytes, but not on neutrophils (Sedgwick et al., 1987). The receptor activity may become altered in vitro and in vivo during disease—for example, surface receptors increase during macrophage activation.

Several antigens have been identified on the surface of monocytes; some are specific to monocytes and some are shared also by neutrophils and platelets. Monoclonal antibodies to monocyte-specific antigens have been developed to characterize human monocytes and to obtain a definitive diagnosis of acute monocytic and myelomonocytic leukemias. Similar observations on monoclonal antibodies that react with monocytes of animal species are being described (Haig et al., 1991; Saalmuller and Reddehase, 1988; Whitehurst et al., 1991). Some leukocyte adhesion molecules (Mac-1 or CD11b/CD18) are also present on the monocytes. Monocytes and macrophages carry Ia and CD4 antigens. The former is necessary to recognize the appropriate lymphocytes for antigen presentation and to

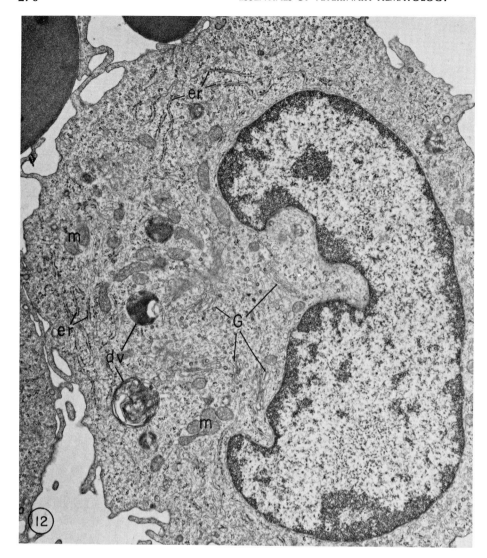

Fig. 16–3. Rabbit macrophage taken from a 96-hour peritoneal exudate. Numerous digestive vacuoles (dv) varying in size and content are present, but no secretory granules are evident. The Golgi complex (G) is large and contains numerous vesicles, many of which are coated. Rough endoplasmic reticulum (er) is moderately abundant, and mitochondria (m) are numerous (×12,000). (From Bainton, D.F.: The cell of inflammation: A general view. *In* Handbook of Inflammation, Vol. 2. Edited by L.E. et al., New York, Elsevier-North Holland, 1980, p.1.)

initiate an immune response. The effect of the latter on mononuclear phagocytes is not known. Ia (immune activation) molecules are now recognized as class II major histocompatibility complex (MHC) glycoproteins (HLA-DR antigen). The expression of MHC class II molecules on macrophages may be reduced in bacterial infections (e.g., Staphylococcus aureus) which can diminish interleukin-1 production and macrophage-T cell interaction (Politis et al., 1992). The CD4 molecule on the T lymphocytes is involved in the induction of T-lymphocyte helper functions and T-cell proliferative responses to antigen stimulation. CD4 molecules on T-lymphocytes act as adhesion molecules and bind to class II MHC molecules on macrophages. They are also an important part of the receptor for the human immunodeficiency virus (HIV). Tissue macrophages may serve as a reservoir of HIV, and CD4-positive T cells carry much of the viral burden in the blood and ultimately are depleted by infection with HIV (Kalter et al., 1991). Similarly, the macro-

phage is a major target of simian immunodeficiency virus infection in the bone marrow (Kitagawa et al., 1991).

FUNCTIONS

Monocytes and macrophages are important in the body's defense against microbial infections and are also important under physiologic conditions. Because monocytes are normally a source of free and fixed macrophages of the MPS, various functions of the MPS can be indirectly assigned to monocytes (Table 16–1).

Phagocytosis and Microbicidal Activity

Because they are highly phagocytic, cells of the MPS engulf and destroy pathogens that cannot be effectively

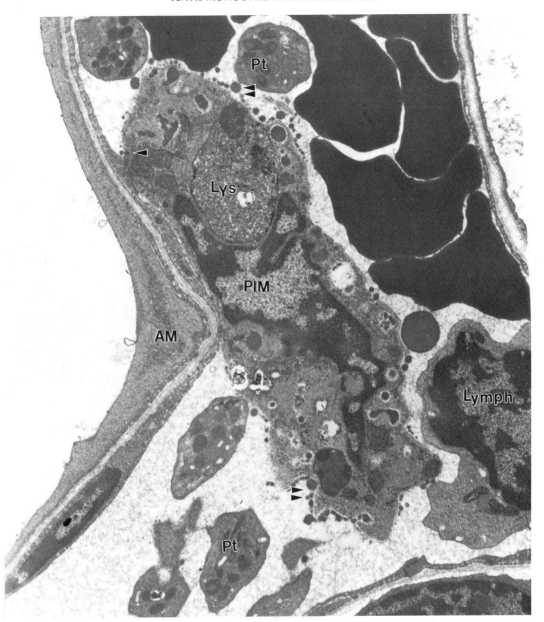

Fig. 16.4. Transmission electron photomicrograph of an equine alveolar capillary depicting a pulmonary intravascular macrophage (PIM) with its globular surface coat *(double arrows)*. The surface coat is comprised of a chain of electron-dense globules of different sizes. Some of these globules seem to undergo internalization at the coated pits *(single arrow)* and can be found as endocytic structures. The lymphocyte (Lymph) and platelets (Pt) present in the vicinity lack surface globules that are characteristic of PIM. An alveolar macrophage (AM) is present in the surfactant layer (uranyl acetate and lead citrate stain; ×15,000). (Courtesy of Dr. Onkar S. Atwal, Department of Biomedical Sciences, Ontario Veterinary College, University of Guelph, Ontario, Canada.) See Atwal et al., 1989, for comparative morphology of PIMS in ruminants.

controlled by neutrophils, especially intracellular organisms and those causing a granulomatous inflammatory response (e.g., fungi, protozoa, viruses, the tubercle bacillus, and Listeria and Brucella species). Differences in macrophage function may contribute to increased resistance to some infectious diseases in animals. For example, mammary gland macrophages from cows resistant to Brucella abortus produced significantly higher oxidative burst activity and had greater bacteriostatic activity than did macrophages from susceptible cows (Harmon et al., 1989). Intramammary macrophages may be most important in

defense of the mammary gland during the early nonlactating period, primarily because of their comparatively greater phagocytic activity for Staphylococcus aureus and Escherichia coli during that period (Fox et al., 1988).

Macrophages from different locations vary in the expression of surface glycoproteins or adhesion molecules (see Fig. 13–6). Various surface glycoproteins are important in monocyte adhesion, chemotaxis, and migration into inflammatory sites. Expression of adhesion molecules on monocytes (Mac-1 and p150,95) is augmented several fold by chemoattractants (Springer

Table 16–1. Functions of the Mononuclear Phagocyte Systems (MPS)

Transformation of monocytes into effector cells of the MPS (i.e., fixed and free macrophages in various tissues)

Phagocytosis and microbicidal action, principally against intracellular bacteria, viruses, fungi, and protozoa

Regulation of the immune response in both the afferent and efferent limbs of the immune response

Scavenger role: phagocytic removal of tissue debris, effete cells, antibody-coated cells, and other foreign material

Secretion of monokines, lysosomal enzymes, and other substances (see Table 16–2)

Cytotoxic effect against tumor cells and red cells

Regulation of hematopoiesis: control of granulopoiesis, monocytopoiesis, lymphopoiesis, and erythropoiesis

Other regulatory roles; in inflammation, tissue repair, and remodeling of embryonic tissues and bones

Coagulation and fibrinolysis: generation of several clotting factors and a plasminogen activator

and Anderson, 1986), and exudate macrophages in the peritoneal cavity show increased expression of adhesion molecules compared to resident macrophages (Rabinowitz and Gordon, 1989).

Phagocytosis is promoted by specific opsonins, such as IgG and nonspecific opsonins, such as C3b, C3bi, and fibronectin, The opsonized organisms are recognized by the phagocyte through its appropriate surface receptors. This receptor-mediated endocytosis and postphagocytic events are analogous to those in neutrophils. Regardless of the opsonization, killing of a rough strain of Pasteurella multocida by bovine alveolar macrophages was much higher than that of the smooth strain (Ashfaq and Campbell, 1986). Both microfilaments and microtubules are important for attachment and ingestion of opsonized particles, but different signal transducing mechanisms for phagocytosis may be triggered by the binding of particles to different surface adhesion or receptor molecules (Newman et al., 1990).

The ingested organisms reside in membrane-bound phagocytic vacuoles and are usually destroyed by cellular microbicidal actions. The mechanisms of bacterial killing by monocytes and macrophages have been less clearly defined, but are thought to be similar to those of neutrophils involving both oxygen-dependent and oxygen-independent mechanisms (Jain, 1986). Oxygen metabolites, peroxidase, lysozyme, a specific basic protein (monocytin), and proteolytic enzymes may be involved. Phagocytically stimulated macrophages undergo oxidative respiratory burst and produce increased amounts of oxygen metabolites (such as superoxide anions) as compared to unstimulated macrophages (Dyer et al., 1989). As described for the neutrophil (see Chapter 13), activation of protein kinase C and increase in intracellular Ca^{++} lead to activation of NADPH oxidase and subsequent conversion of oxygen to superoxide anions (Shepherd, 1986). Interferons produced by the mononuclear phagocytes aid in protection against viral infection. Monocyte cationic proteins possess fungicidal activity. Inorganic nitrogen oxides produced by activated macrophages

have been implicated in the microbicidal activity against Leishmania and Schistosoma species and Mycobacterium avium (Denis, 1991).

The phagocytic ingestion of an organism may not necessarily result in its death (Jain, 1986). An organism (e.g., Toxoplasma species) may resist destruction by hydrogen peroxide (H_2O_2) through the protection afforded by its catalase and glutathione peroxidase, which detoxify H_2O_2 to water. In other cases, the organism may inhibit phagolysosome formation through the release of certain substances (sulfolipids by Mycobacterium tuberculosis) or may armor itself with a protective chemical (polysaccharide by Leishmania donovanii) to ward off the destructive action of lysosomal substances. Leishmanial organisms are intracellular parasites of macrophages and may occasionally appear in circulating monocytes and neutrophils. Infected dogs show hyperproteinemia or hypoproteinemia, regenerative or nonregenerative anemia, WBC counts in the normal to leukopenic range, lymphopenia, and/or thrombocytopenia.

The MPS is thought to be immature at birth, probably because it requires antigenic exposure for full expression of functional activity. Macrophages have been linked to the natural resistance of cats to viral infection. Macrophages from kittens are five times more susceptible to feline leukemia virus (FeLV) infection than those from adult cats, and the temporary suppression of macrophage function in cats markedly increases their susceptibility to viral infection. Corticosteroids are known to depress the functional competence of the MPS. In addition, acquired and genetic defects of MPS function are associated with an increased incidence of infections. A classic example is chronic granulomatous disease of children in which monocytes, in addition to neutrophils, show genetic defects in host resistance (see Chap. 13). Studies on genetically selected obese and lean swine indicate that genetically transferred factors are of primary importance in alveolar phagocytic responses. Cells from obese pigs were significantly more effective at Fc (gamma)-mediated phagocytosis of opsonized sheep erythrocytes than those from lean pigs, and linolenic acid enhanced this phagocytic activity (Caruso and Jeska, 1990).

Regulation of the Immune Response

Macrophages are assigned a crucial role in most immune responses. They are involved in both phases of the immune response—in the afferent limb (induction of immunity to an antigen) and in the efferent limb (expression of cellular immunity). In the afferent limb of the immune response, they pick up and process the antigen before it is made available to lymphocytes to trigger an antibody response or cellular immunity. The antigen-binding property of macrophages is associated with their surface Ia antigens. It is believed that monocytes process the antigen in a highly immunogenic form. The antigen is then made available to lymphocytes by mechanisms that are still not clearly defined, but secretion of the antigen bound to a soluble macrophage product (RNA) or cell-to-cell interaction may be involved. Macrophages secrete interleukin-1, which stimulates T lymphocytes to elaborate various lymphokines, (Table 17–4) which recruit specific clones of T and B cells to participate in the efferent limb of the immune response (Dinarello, 1992). Interleukin-1 (MW 17,000 to 19,000) has been purified from bovine monocytes (Lederer and Czuprynski, 1989) and equine osteoarthritic joint effusions (Morris et al., 1990a). Human and murine macrophages stimulated with galactose oxidase have been found to secrete a novel monokine other than interleukin-1. This monokine, termed macrophage-derived blastogenic factor (MW 29,000 to 35,000), stimulates resting T cells to produce interferon-gamma and proliferate (Antonelli et al., 1988).

In the efferent limb of the immune response, augmented phagocytosis, destruction of antibody-coated pathogens, or cytotoxicity is effected by "activated" or "armed" macrophages (Jain, 1986; Shinomiya et al., 1989). Soluble factors secreted from activated macrophages may augment or suppress the immune response. Macrophage activation occurs nonspecifically through various substances or conditions such as endotoxin, immune complexes, complement components, and disease states. Endotoxin-induced priming of macrophages causes a significant increase in HLA-DR and C3bi receptor (CR3) expression which is associated with an increase in intracellular Ca^{++} mobilization (McLeish et al., 1989). Macrophage activation can occur under the influence of lymphokines secreted by activated T cells (e.g., macrophage-activating factor or other lymphokines) or may be independent of T-cell participation. Cytokines such as α-interferon, TNF, interleukin-3, and GM-CSF can activate macrophages.

Activated macrophages are metabolically more active, and manifest enhanced functional activities of a broader, less discriminatory type. Thus, the resulting enhanced host defense is nonspecific. In comparison, armed macrophages are produced in response to a specific activating agent, probably through the action of a "specific macrophage-arming factor" produced by sensitized T cells. These macrophages are actively cytotoxic against a specific target, such as tumor cells. Purified human monocytes activated in vitro by interferon-gamma have been infused into humans as a potential treatment for certain types of cancer (Stevenson et al., 1988).

Rhodococcus equi is a facultative intracellular organism infecting alveolar macrophages of foals. It usually persists and multiplies within the phagosome, apparently by inhibiting phagosome-lysosome fusion by an unknown mechanism (Zink et al., 1987). Opsonization of R. equi with antibody against its capsular components is associated with increased phagosome-lysosome fusion and significantly enhanced killing. Macrophages from uninfected foals incubated in the presence of lymphocyte factors (derived by in vitro incubation of sensitized lymphocytes with R. equi

surface antigen) showed a 50% increase in killing of R. equi. In comparison, sensitized macrophages (from foals experimentally exposed to R. equi) incubated with lymphocyte factors had a greater than 100% increase in killing capacity (Hietala and Ardans, 1987). Opsonized Rhodococcus equi and zymosan particles can activate the respiratory burst of resident alveolar macrophages from adult horses (Brumbaugh et al., 1990).

Scavenger Role

A scavenger role for macrophages has been suggested from observations that they remove tissue debris from areas of tissue destruction and ingest cellular remnants, effete cells, antibody-coated cells, and other foreign material. Some examples are the phagocytic destruction of the ejected nuclei of metarubricytes in bone marrow, the removal of Howell-Jolly bodies from circulating red cells in the spleen, and phagocytosis of antibody-coated red cells by the MPS in immune-mediated hemolytic anemia. Macrophages recognize the material to be phagocytosed through their surface receptors. An early event in the destruction of red cells by macrophages is modification of band 3 protein in senescent or damaged red cell membrane, followed by deposition of anti-band 3 antibodies and activation of complement (C3 fragment). The band 3-antiband 3-C3b complex is recognized by monocytes through their C3b receptors (CR1) and phagocytosis ensues (Bussolino et al., 1989). Oxidative damage to the red cells, as by phenylhydrazine, exposes galactosyl residues on the red cell membrane, which are then recognized by lectin-like receptors on the macrophages (Horn et al., 1990).

The phagocytosed material is normally degraded and the debris exocytosed. In certain circumstances, however, the debris may accumulate in the macrophages as a result of a defective disposal process because of genetic defects of the enzymes involved, cellular overload, or other reasons. Such cells become prominent in tissues because of their intracellular contents. Some examples follow.

Gaucher cells are highly vacuolated macrophages that contain glucocerebroside in the form of tubular or fibrillar elements because of a deficiency of β-glucosidase or β-glucocerebrosidase, which catalyzes the hydrolysis of glucocerebroside. These cells are seen in the bone marrow, spleen, and liver in Gaucher disease. The principal source of cerebroside may be the membranes of the effete leukocytes and red cells. In Niemann-Pick disease types A and B, sphingomyelin accumulates in macrophages because of a deficiency of the catabolic enzyme sphingomyelinase. These macrophages characteristically appear foamy or vacuolated but do not show fibrils, as seen in Gaucher cells. The vacuoles are lipid-filled lysosomes. Sea blue histiocyte syndrome is a non-neurological form of Niemann-Pick disease. Macrophages accumulate cellular debris (sphingomyelin and ceroid) because of a deficiency of sphingomyelinase and consequently, they appear granular blue in Wright stained marrow films. Large, reddish-purple granules known as Alder-Reilly bodies are found in neutrophils, macrophages, and sometimes in lymphocytes in patients with mucopolysaccharidosis developing from an abnormality of mucopolysaccharide catabolism resulting from an enzyme deficiency (see Chap. 13).

Secretory Role and Related Functions

A secretory role of macrophages involves the production of many soluble substances, collectively referred to as monokines (Table 16–2). Although secretion of these substances occurs normally, increased production follows nonspecific stimulation of the MPS by various agents, such as bacteria, endotoxin, cytokines, mitogens, and ionophores. Agents known to increase the intracellular level of cyclic AMP inhibit secretory activity, whereas those increasing the intracellular level of cyclic GMP promote secretion.

Stimulation of macrophage secretory activity may be selective, e.g., endotoxin causes augmented release of chemoattractants for neutrophils, superoxide, interleukin-1, and TNF, but does not affect the production of macrophage-derived growth factor activity for fi-

Table 16–2. Secretory Products of the Mononuclear Phagocyte System

Complement components
  C1 through C9, factors B and D, properdin
Antimicrobial or cytotoxic substances
  Interferons, a listericidal factor, oxygen metabolites (superoxide anion, hydroxyl radical, H_2O_2, and singlet oxygen), other cytotoxic factor(s)
Products of arachidonic acid metabolism
  Mostly PGE_2 and some PGI_2, $PGF_{2\alpha}$, thromboxane A_2, leukotrienes C_4 and D_4
Lysosomal enzymes
  Acid hydrolases (e.g., proteinases, esterases, lipases, sulfatases, ribonucleases, and cathepsins), neutral proteinases (e.g., collagenase, elastase, and plasminogen activator), arginase, and lysozyme
Factors modulating functions of other cells including interleukins
  Factors enhancing growth of committed erythroid stem cells; colony-stimulating factors enhancing granulopoiesis; lymphocyte-activating factors for T and B cells; lymphocyte differentiation factors for T and B cells; lymphocyte proliferation inhibitor; mononuclear cell factor; angiogenic factor inducing microvascular proliferation; fibroblast cell proliferation factor; factor enhancing collagen synthesis by fibroblasts; fibronectin as a chemotactic factor for monocytes, promoting phagocytosis, and with other activities; chemotactic factors for neutrophils and eosinophils; platelet-activating factor
Procoagulant and fibrinolytic factors
  Vitamin K-dependent clotting factors X, IX, VII, and prothrombin, factor V, and tissue thromboplastin-like activity; plasminogen activator
Binding proteins
  Transferrin, ferritin, transcobalamin II
Other factors
  Endogenous pyrogen, haptoglobin, leukotriens, α_2-macroglobulin (a plasma proteinase inhibitor), growth factor promoting wound healing, plasmin inhibitor, tumor necrosis factor, macrophage inflammatory proteins 1 and 2

broblasts (Christman et al., 1988, 1989; Morris et al., 1990b). Monocyte subpopulations, which vary in expression of Fc receptor for human IgG, differ in secretion of monokines, e.g., both FcRI-positive and FcRI-negative monocytes secrete similar amounts of TNF and interleukin-6, but the latter cells have significantly enhanced ability to secrete interleukin-1 (Pryjma et al., 1992). Sustained subacute endotoxemia in sheep was found to cause a monocytosis and increased superoxide production by monocytes, particularly in non-survivors (Polla et al., 1991). Release of TNF from endotoxin-stimulated human monocytes requires the presence of endogenous retinoids. Removal of endogenous serum retinoids by delipidization inhibited TNF release, but not intracellular accumulation of TNF mRNA or protein (Turpin et al., 1990).

Various monokines exhibit diverse biologic activities, such as roles in host defense, the inflammatory process, regulation of activities of other cells, regulation of hematopoiesis, cytotoxic and antitumor activities, and coagulation and fibrinolysis. Some functions may be speculative, and some require confirming evidence. Most of these functions, however, depend on the secretory activity of macrophages (see above). Some examples follow.

Plasminogen activator cleaves plasminogen to produce plasmin, which can lyse fibrin and dissolve clots at sites of inflammation. This effect, however, may be controlled by plasmin inhibitors and α_2-macroglobulin secreted by macrophages. A plasminogen activator is produced by bovine blood monocytes and milk macrophages, particularly from mastitic quarters (Politis et al., 1991). Equine monocytes and macrophages express a tissue thromboplastin-like procoagulant activity that is augmented by platelets and endotoxin (Henry and Moor, 1988; Grunig et al., 1991). This procoagulant activity of mononuclear cells may be important in coagulopathies associated with endotoxemia in horses (Henry and Moore, 1991). Monocytes can reversibly bind heparin and this interaction decreases the expression of tissue factor on the cell surface, thus hampering the cellular procoagulant potential (Abbate et al., 1990).

Lysosomal collagenase, elastase, and acid hydrolases can degrade tissue components and activate complement and kinin systems, thereby potentiating the inflammatory response. Various oxygen metabolites produced by activated macrophages can cause cell damage and have cytotoxic effects on tumor cells, and virus-infected cells (van Kessel and Verhoef, 1990). Cytolytic mechanisms may differ depending on the type of target cells as well as the source of mononuclear phagocytes (Chung and Kim, 1988). A high molecular weight tumoricidal activity secreted by activated murine bone-marrow derived macrophages has been recently characterized (Schwamberger et al., 1991). "Macrophage inflammatory proteins 1 and 2" are macrophage-derived mediators of vascular changes in inflammation (Sherry et al., 1988; Wolpe et al., 1989).

TNF has been implicated as an important mediator of inflammatory processes and has clinical relevance in chronic infectious diseases. Chronic administration of recombinant bovine TNF to cattle produced clinical and pathologic changes similar to those observed in some chronic parasitic and viral infections (Bielefeldt et al., 1989). TNF production from bovine alveolar macrophages in vitro is increased significantly after stimulation by bovine respiratory viruses and bacterial endotoxins (Bienhoff et al., 1992) and from equine alveolar cells treated with bacterial lipopolysaccharide (MacKay et al., 1991). TNF has been found to be directly cytotoxic to schistosomula of Schistosoma mansoni (James et al., 1990). TNF, alone or in combination with interleukin-2, is associated with killing of Mycobacterium avium by macrophages (Bermudez and Young, 1988). TNF seems to be intimately associated with peroxidase-induced macrophage-mediated cytotoxicity, which indicates a possible role for peroxidases as immunomodulator (Lefkowitz et al., 1989).

Interleukin-1 and TNF cause fever through their effects on the temperature-regulating center of the hypothalamus. Interleukin-1 has been implicated in the induction and augmentation of the pathologic processes involved in arthritis and articular cartilage destruction in humans and possibly horses (Morris et al., 1990a) and in endotoxin-induced lung injury in dogs (Tabor et al., 1988). Intravenous administration of endotoxin (30 or 1000 ng/kg) induces increased production of TNF and interleukin-6, peaking at 2 hours and 3 to 4 hours postinoculation, respectively (MacKay and Lester, 1992; Morris et al, 1992). Interleukin-6 acts synergistically with interleukin-1 and TNF to promote synthesis of acute phase proteins (see Fig. 21–5). Interleukin-1 production can be modulated, e.g., chemical antagonists of arachidonic acid metabolism can inhibit its production (Newton, 1990). Interleukin-4 has been found to inhibit the secretion of interleukin-1-beta and TNF-alpha by activated monocytes almost 100%. The secretion of interleukin-6 is reduced by 70 to 80%, while secretion of interleukin-1-alpha, which is mainly cell associated, is not inhibited (te Velde et al., 1990).

Colony-stimulating factors (GM-CSF, G-CSF, and M-CSF) are important regulators of hematopoiesis, particularly granulocyte and monocyte production in the bone marrow.

Some monokines (interleukin-1 and TNF) may play a role in the pathogenesis of anemia associated with chronic inflammatory or malignant diseases. In vitro production of erythropoietin is inhibited by interleukin-1 and TNF-alpha, but not by interleukin-6, transforming growth factor beta 2, and interferon-gamma (Jelkmann et al., 1992). Furthermore, interleukin-1 blocked erythropoietin formation in isolated serumfree perfused rat kidneys. Chronic exposure of nude mice to TNF in vivo preferentially inhibited erythropoiesis (Johnson et al., 1989).

MONOCYTE NUMBERS IN BLOOD AND TISSUES

The number of monocytes in blood is usually less than 1500/μl in the dog and cat and less than 1000/μl in the horse, cow, sheep, and goat. Monocytosis generally indicates a chronic inflammatory response. Monocytes respond to elevations in blood corticosteroid concentrations, but species differences are seen with regard to the type of response—for example, monocytosis invariably occurs in the dog but is inconsistent in the cow, horse, and cat. In contrast, monocytopenia occurs in humans and laboratory animals. Steroid-induced monocytopenia can be attributed to an increased shift of cells into the marginal pool, inhibition of marrow release, or decreased production, but the mechanisms of monocytosis remain unknown. In species not consistently responding with monocytosis, monocytopenia may develop in the initial stages of stress but, after the acute phase of the disease is over, it is followed by monocytosis.

Monocytosis characteristically occurs in subacute and chronic inflammatory conditions. Monocytosis in humans is strongly correlated with proportionate increases in the total blood monocyte pool and monocyte turnover rate, a moderate change in the ratio of the circulating to the marginal pool of monocytes, and a slight increase in intravascular life. Monocyte production in the bone marrow increases and is associated with an accelerated release of mature and sometimes immature monocytes into the blood. The presence of many immature monocytic cells in the blood or a persistent, marked monocytosis may suggest acute or chronic monocytic leukemia, which can be confirmed by bone marrow examination and the elimination of other causes. Common hematologic findings in cats infected with feline immunodeficiency virus include anemia, neutropenia, lymphopenia, and monocytosis (Hopper et al., 1989).

Monocytes accumulate in areas of inflammation and tissue destruction in response to appropriate chemotactic factors. Lipid or lipid-rich bacterial substances, such as products from the tubercle bacillus and lipopolysaccharides of gram-negative bacteria, complement components C3a and C5a, and soluble substances from T lymphocytes (certain lymphokines), neutrophils, and tumor cells are some chemotactic factors for monocytes. Surface receptors on neutrophils and monocytes, similar to lymphocyte homing receptors, are regulated by chemotactic factors and appear to be involved in homing of these cells to inflamed tissues (Jutila et al., 1989). This process is aided by increased endothelial cell adhesiveness for leukocytes through expression of adhesion molecules. Under appropriate circumstances, monocytes in tissues transform to macrophages, epithelioid cells, and giant cells, all of which are important cellular components of chronic inflammation. Some tissue macrophages may also originate locally.

In some situations, transformation of monocytes to macrophages may occur in the circulation. "Reactive" or "toxic" monocytes have been found in the blood of dogs with severe bacterial infections, septicemia, and acute bacterial endocarditis. These cells may appear as macrophages with a convoluted or indented nucleus and highly vacuolated, pale blue, more abundant cytoplasm, with or without fine pinkish azurophilic granules (Plate VIII-10). Such cells have been found in humans with severe bacterial infections.

REFERENCES

Abbate, R., Gori, A.M., Modesti, P.A., et al.: Heparin, monocytes, and procoagulant activity. Haemostasis, 20 Suppl 1:98, 1990.

Antonelli, G., Dianzani, F., Van Damme, J., et al.: A macrophage-derived factor different from interleukin 1 and able to induce interferon-gamma and lymphoproliferation in resting T lymphocytes. Cell. Immunol., 113:376, 1988.

Ashfaq, M.K. and Campbell, S.G.: The influence of opsonins on the bactericidal effect of bovine alveolar macrophages against Pasteurella multocida. Cornell Vet., 76:213, 1986.

Atwal, O.S., Minhas, K.J., Frenczy, B.G., et al.: Morphology of pulmonary intravascular macrophages (PIMs) in ruminants: Ultrastructural and cytochemical behavior of dense surface coat. Am. J. Anat., 186:285, 1989.

Bermudez, L.E. and Young, L.S.: Tumor necrosis factor, alone or in combination with IL-2, but not IFN-gamma, is associatd with macrophage killing of Mycobacterium avium complex. J. Immunol., 140:3006, 1988.

Bielefeldt Ohmann, H., Campos, M., Snider, M., et al.: Effect of chronic administration of recombinant bovine tumor necrosis factor to cattle. Vet. Pathol., 26:462, 1989.

Bienhoff, S.E., Allen, G.K. and Berg, J.N.: Release of tumor necrosis factor-alpha from bovine alveolar macrophages stimulated with bovine respiratory viruses and bacterial endotoxins. Vet. Immunol. Immunopathol., 30:341, 1992.

Brumbaugh, G.W., Davis, L.E., Thurmon, J.C., et al.: Influence of Rhodococcus equi on the respiratory burst of resident alveolar macrophages from adult horses. Am. J. Vet. Res., 51:766, 1990.

Bussolino, F., Fischer, E., Turrini, F., et al.: Platelet-activating factor enhances complement-dependent phagocytosis of diamide-treated erythrocytes by human monocytes through activation of protein kinase C and phosphorylation of complement receptor type one (CR1). J. Biol. Chem., 264:21711, 1989.

Caruso, J.P. and Jeska, E.L.: Phagocytic functions of pulmonary alveolar macrophages in genetically selected lean and obese swine and the effects of exogenous linolenic acid upon cell function. Vet. Immunol. Immunopathol., 24:27, 1990.

Christman, J.W., Petras, S.F., Hacker, M., et al.: Alveolar macrophage function is selectively altered after endotoxemia in rats. Infect. Immunol., 56:1254, 1988.

Christman, J.W., Petras, S.F., Vacek, P.M., et al.: Rat alveolar macrophage production of chemoattractants for neutrophils: response to Escherichia coli endotoxin. Infect. Immunol., 57:810, 1989.

Chung, T. and Kim, Y.B.: Two distinct cytolytic mechanisms of macrophages and monocytes activated by phorbol myristate acetate. J. Leuk. Biol., 44:329, 1988.

Dawson, J., Lees, P. and Sedgwick, A.D.: Actions of non-steroidal anti-inflammatory drugs on equine leucocyte movement in vitro. J. Vet. Pharmacol. Ther., 10:150, 1987.

Denis, M.: Tumor necrosis factor and granulocyte macrophage-colony stimulating factor stimulate human macrophages to restrict growth of virulent Mycobacterium avium and to kill avirulent M. avium: Killing effector mechanism depends on the generation of reactive nitrogen intermediates. J. Leuk. Biol., 49:380, 1991.

Dinarello, C.A.: The biology of interleukin-1. Chem. Immunol., 51:1, 1992.

Dyer, R.M., Erney, S., Spencer, P., et al.: Oxidative metabolism of the bovine alveolar macrophage. Am. J. Vet. Res., 50:448, 1989.

Fox, L.K., McDonald, J.S., Hillers, J.K., et al.: Function of phagocytes obtained from lacteal secretions of lactating and nonlactating cows. Am. J. Vet. Res., 49:678,1988.

Genovesi, E.V., Knudsen, R.C., Gerstner, D.J., et al.: In vitro induction of swine peripheral blood monocyte proliferation by the fibroblast-derived murine hematopoietic growth factor CSF-1. Vet. Immunol. Immunopathol., 23:223, 1989.

Grunig, G., Hulliger, C., Winder, C., et al.: Spontaneous and lipopolysaccharide-induced expression of procoagulant activity by equine lung macrophages in comparison with blood monocytes and blood neutrophils. Vet. Immunol. Immunopathol., 29:295, 1991.

Haig, D.M., Thomson, J. and Dawson, A.: Reactivity of the workshop monoclonal antibodies with ovine bone marrow cells and bone marrow-derived monocyte/macrophage and mast cell lines. Vet. Immunol. Immunopathol., 27:135, 1991.

Harmon, B.G., Adams, L.G., Templeton, J.W., et al.: Macrophage function in mammary glands of Brucella abortus-infected cows and cows that resisted infection after inoculation of Brucella abortus. Am. J. Vet. Res., 50:459, 1989.

Henry, M.M. and Moore, J.N.: Endotoxin-induced procoagulant activity in equine peripheral blood monocytes. Circ. Shock., 26:297, 1988.

Henry, M.M. and Moore, J.N.: Clinical relevance of monocyte procoagulant activity in horses with colic. J. Am. Vet. Med. Assoc., 198:843, 1991.

Hietala, SK. and Ardans, A.A.: Interaction of Rhodococcus equi with phagocytic cells from R. equi-exposed and non-exposed foals. Vet. Microbiol., 14:307, 1987.

Hopper, C.D., Sparkes, A.H., Gruffydd-Jones, T.J., et al.: Clinical and laboratory findings in cats infected with feline immunodeficiency virus. Vet. Rec., 125:341, 1989.

Horn, S., Gopas, J. and Bashan, N.: A lectin-like receptor on murine macrophage is involved in the recognition and phagocytosis of human red cells oxidized by phenylhydrazine. Biochem. Pharmacol., 39:775, 1990.

Jain, N.C.: Schalm's Veterinary Hematology. 4th ed. Philadelphia, Lea & Febiger, 1986, pp. 768–789.

James, S.L., Glaven, J., Goldenberg, S., et al.: Tumour necrosis factor (TNF) as a mediator of macrophage helminthotoxic activity. Parasite Immunol., 12:1, 1990.

Jelkmann, W., Pagel, H., Wolff, M., et al.: Monokines inhibiting erythropoietin production in human hepatoma cultures and in isolated perfused rat kidneys. Life Sci., 50:301, 1992.

Johnson, R.A., Waddelow, T.A., Caro, J., et al.: Chronic exposure to tumor necrosis factor in vivo preferentially inhibits erythropoiesis in nude mice. Blood, 74:130, 1989.

Johnston, R.B. Jr.: Current concepts: immunology. Monocytes and macrophages. N. Engl. J. Med., 318:747, 1988.

Jutila, M.A., Berg, E.L., Kishimoto, T.K., et al.: Inflammation-induced endothelial cell adhesion to lymphocytes, neutrophils, and monocytes. Role of homing receptors and other adhesion molecules. Transplantation, 48:727, 1989.

Kalter, D.C., Gendelman, H.E. and Meltzer, M.S.: Monocytes, dendritic cells, and Langerhans cells in human immunodeficiency virus infection. Dermatol. Clin., 9:415, 1991.

Kitagawa, M., Lackner, A.A., Martfeld, D.J., et al.: Simian immunodeficiency virus infection of macaque bone marrow macrophages correlates with disease progression in vivo. Am. J. Pathol., 138:921, 1991.

Lederer, J.A. and Czuprynski, C.J.: Production and purification of bovine monocyte-derived interleukin 1. Vet. Immunol. Immunopathol., 23:201, 1989.

Lefkowitz, D.L., Mone, J., Mills, K., et al.: Peroxidases enhance macrophage-mediated cytotoxicity via induction of tumor necrosis factor. Proc. Soc. Exp. Biol. Med., 190:144, 1989.

MacKay, R.J., King, R.R., Dankert, J.R., et al.: Cytotoxic tumor necrosis factor activity produced by equine alveolar macrophages: preliminary characterization. Vet. Immunol. Immunopathol., 29:15, 1991.

MacKay, R.J. and Lester, G.D.: Induction of the acute-phase cytokine, hepatocyte-stimulating factor/interleukin 6, in the circulation of horses treated with endotoxin. Am. J. Vet. Res., 53:1285, 1992.

McLeish, K.R., Dean, W.L., Wellhausen, S.R., et al.: Role of intracellular calcium in priming of human peripheral blood monocytes by bacterial lipopolysaccharide. Inflammation, 13:681, 1989.

Metcalf, D.: Control of granulocytes and macrophages: molecular, cellular, and clinical aspects. Science, 254:529, 1991.

Morris, E.A., McDonald, B.S., Webb, A.C., et al.: Identification of interleukin-1 in equine osteoarthritic joint effusions. Am. J. Vet. Res., 51:59, 1990a.

Morris, D.D., Moore, J.N., Fischer, K., et al.: Endotoxin-induced tumor necrosis factor activity production by equine peritoneal macrophages. Circ. Shock., 30:229, 1990b.

Morris, D.D., Moore, J.N., Crowe, N., et al.: Effect of experimentally induced endotoxemia on serum interleukin-6 in horses. Am. J. Vet. Res., 53:753, 1992.

Newman, S.L., Bucher, C., Rhodes, J., et al.: Phagocytosis of Histoplasma capsulatum yeasts and microconidia by human cultured macrophages and alveolar macrophages. Cellular cytoskeleton requirement for attachment and ingestion. J. Clin. Invest., 85:223, 1990.

Newton, R.C.: The production of human interleukin-1 beta by blood monocytes. Prog. Clin. Biol. Res., 349:217, 1990.

Nielsen, H.: Chemotaxis of human blood monocytes. Methodological and clinical aspects. Dan. Med. Bull., 37:406, 1990.

Papadimitriou, J.M. and Ashman, R.B.: Macrophages: current views on their differentiation, structure, and function. Ultrastruct. Pathol., 13:343, 1989.

Politis, I., Zhao, X., McBride, B.W., et al.: Function of bovine mammary macrophages as antigen-presenting cells. Vet. Immunol. Immunopathol., 30:399, 1992.

Politis, I., Zhao, X., McBride, B.W., et al.: Plasminogen activator production by bovine milk macrophages and blood monocytes. Am. J. Vet. Res., 52:1208, 1991.

Polla, B.S., Clerc, J., Pittet, J.F., et al.: Superoxide production by peripheral blood monocytes during sustained endotoxaemia in sheep. Clin. Sci., 81:815, 1991.

Pontzer, C.H. and Russell, S.W.: Culture of macrophages from bovine bone marrow. Vet. Immunol. Immunopathol., 21:351, 1989.

Pryjma, J., Mytar, B., Loppnow, H., et al.: FcR+ and FcR− monocytes differentially secrete monokines during pokeweed mitogen-induced T-cell-monocyte interactions. Immunology, 75:355, 1992.

Rabinowitz, S. and Gordon, S.: Differential expression of membrane sialoglycoproteins in exudate and resident mouse peritoneal macrophages. J. Cell. Sci., 93:623, 1989.

Saalmuller, A. and Reddehase, M.J.: Immune system of swine: dissection of mononuclear leucocyte subpopulations by means of two-colour cytofluorometric analysis. Res. Vet. Sci., 45:311, 1988.

Schwamberger, G., Flesch, I. and Ferber, E.: Tumoricidal effector molecules of murine macrophages. Pathobiology, 59:248, 1991.

Sedgwick, A.D., Dawson, J. and Lees, P.: Influence of chemotactic agents on the locomotion of equine polymorphonuclear and mononuclear leucocytes. Res. Vet. Sci., 43:55, 1987.

Shepherd, V.L.: The role of the respiratory burst of phagocytes in host defense. Semin. Respir. Infect., 1:99, 1986.

Sherry, B., Tekamp-Olson, P., Gallegos, C., et al.: Resolution of the two components of macrophage inflammatory protein 1, and cloning and characterization of one of those components, macrophage inflammatory protein 1 beta. J. Exp. Med., 168:2251, 1988.

Shinomiya, H., Shinomiya, M., Stevenson, G.W., et al.: Activated killer monocytes: preclinical model systems. Immunol. Ser., 48:101, 1989.

Sluiter, W., Nibbering, P.H., van Furth, R., et al.: Increased activity of FIM in serum of mice during a Mycobacterium bovis (BCG) infection. Immunology, 70:327, 1990.

Springer, T.A. and Anderson, D.C.: The importance of the Mac-1, LFA-1 glycoprotein family in monocyte and granulocyte adherence, chemotaxis, and migration into inflammatory sites: insights from an experiment of nature. Ciba Found. Symp., 118:102, 1986.

Stein, M. and Keshav, S.: The versatility of macrophages. Clin. Exp. Allergy, 22:19, 1992.

Stevenson, H.C., Lacerna, L.V., Jr. and Sugarbaker, P.H.: Ex vivo activation of killer monocytes (AKM) and their application to the treatment of human cancer [published erratum appears in J Clin Apheresis 1989;5(1):59]. J. Clin. Apheresis, 4:118, 1988.

Tabor, D.R., Burchett, S.K. and Jacobs, R.F.: Enhanced production of monokines by canine alveolar macrophages in response to endotoxin-induced shock. Proc. Soc. Exp. Biol. Med., 187:408, 1988.

te Velde, A.A., Huijbens, R.J.F., Heije, K., et al.: Interleukin-4 (IL-4) inhibits secretion of IL-1beta, tumor necrosis factor alpha, and IL-6 by human monocytes. Blood, 76:1392, 1990.

Turpin, J., Mehta, K., Blick, M., et al.: Effect of retinoid on the release and gene expression of tumor necrosis factor-alpha in human peripheral blood monocytes. J. Leuk. Biol., 48:444, 1990.

Ulich, T.R., del Castillo, J., Busser, K., et al.: Acute in vivo effects of IL-3 alone and in combination with IL-6 on the blood cells of the circulation and bone marrow. Am. J. Pathol., 135:663, 1989.

Ulich, T.R., del Castillo, J., Watson, L.R., et al.: In vivo hematologic effects of recombinant human macrophage colony-stimulating factor. Blood, 75:846, 1990.

van Furth, R.: Origin and turnover of monocytes and macrophages. Curr. Top. Pathol., 79:125, 1989.

van Kessel, K.P. and Verhoef, J.: A view to a kill: cytotoxic mechanisms of human polymorphonuclear leukocytes compared with monocytes and natural killer cells. Pathobiology, 58:249, 1990.

Whitehurst, C.E., Hill, R.J., Day, N.K., et al.: Phenotypic markers for the feline monocyte: rosette formation with human erythrocytes and a monoclonal antibody which binds myeloid cells. Proc. Soc. Exp. Biol. Med., 197:317, 1991.

Williams, W.J., Beutler, E., Erslev, A.J., et al.: Hematology. 4th ed. New York, McGraw-Hill, 1990, Chaps. 93, 98.

Winkler, G.C.: Pulmonary intravascular macrophages in domestic animal species: Review of structural and functional properties. Am. J. Anat., 181:217, 1988.

Wolpe, S.D., Sherry, B., Juers, D., et al.: Identification and characterization of macrophage inflammatory protein 2. Proc. Natl. Acad. Sci. USA, 86:612, 1989.

Zink, M.C., Yager, J.A., Prescott, J.F., et al.: Electron microscopic investigation of intracellular events after ingestion of Rhodococcus equi by foal alveolar macrophages. Vet. Microbiol., 14:295, 1987.

The Lymphocytes and Plasma Cells

Lymphocytes represent a heterogeneous group of cells, both morphologically and functionally. They are pivotal in the initiation and execution of the immune response. Acquired and hereditary disorders of the immune response are being increasingly recognized in humans and animals, which has prompted in-depth studies of lymphocyte pathophysiology. New techniques have been developed to recognize lymphocyte subpopulations (Wilson, 1991). Molecular mechanisms of immune response in health and disease are being elucidated. Plasma cells are the descendants of lymphocytes involved in the humoral antibody response.

LYMPHOCYTES

Lymphocytes can be categorized in several ways. Based on the cell size, they are grouped as small, medium, or large, or simply as small (6 to 9 μm) or large (9 to 15 μm) lymphocytes. In consideration of their life span, they can be designated as short-lived or long-lived lymphocytes. On the basis of functional differences in immune response, they are referred to as B (bursa-dependent), T (thymus-dependent), and non-T, non-B or null cells. In most species, 80 to 95% of the peripheral blood lymphocytes are classified as T and B cells.

Morphology and Composition

The nucleus in the lymphocyte has coarsely clumped chromatin and is generally round, but may be oval or slighted indented. A nucleolus is not seen in Wright-stained blood films from various species, except for an occasional cell in cattle. Lymphocytes from normal animals, however, may show nucleoli using special staining methods or an electron microscope (Fig. 17–1). The amount of cytoplasm is usually scanty in small lymphocytes but may be more generous, particularly in large lymphocytes. A few small azurophilic granules can be seen in the cytoplasm of an occasional lymphocyte. Cells with large azurophilic granules (1 to 2 μm) are known as large granular lymphocytes, and usually include natural killer cells and a component of non-MHC (major histocompatibility complex) restricted cytotoxic T cells.

Cytoplasmic color is related to the amount of free ribosomes, polyribosomes, and/or rough endoplasmic reticulum (RER), and varies with the activity of the lymphocyte (Figs. 17–1, 17–2, and 17–3). Highly active cells that synthesize more protein or immunoglobulins have dark blue cytoplasm, compared to the pale cytoplasm of functionally inactive cells. The RER is most developed in plasma cells and less so in immunocytes (compare Figs. 17–3 and 17–7). Scanning electron microscopy reveals a smooth or villous surface, unrelated to the functional identity of the lymphocytes.

The cell size, degree of cytoplasmic basophilia and, to a certain extent, the nuclear chromatin pattern are thought to indicate relative cell age or maturity. The larger cell size, basophilic cytoplasm, and smooth chromatin are characteristics of relatively immature lymphocytes. The presence of one or more prominent nucleoli or nucleolar rings characterizes the cell as a lymphoblast. The proportion of small and large lymphocytes in blood may change during disease.

The exposure of lymphocytes to various mitogens (plant lectins, bacterial products, and enzymes) stimulates small lymphocytes to undergo complex morphologic and biochemical changes that lead to blastogenesis (formation of blast cells). Similar processes are probably involved in the antigenic stimulation of T and B cells and in the formation of plasmacytic cells.

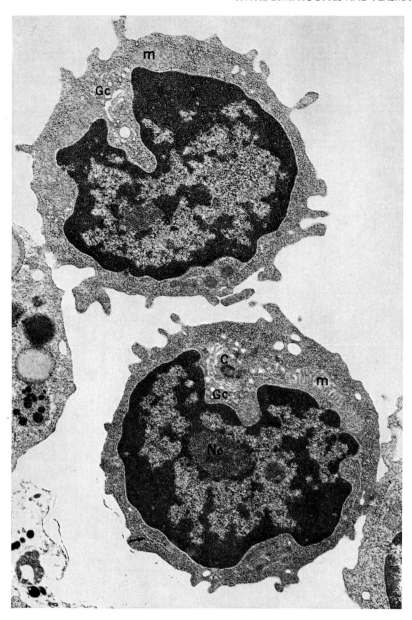

Fig. 17–1. Two canine lymphocytes from blood. The cytoplasm of both lymphocytes contains numerous ribosomes (dense particles), some indistinct mitochondria (m), and an inconspicuous inactive area of the Golgi complex (Gc) represented by smooth, small, round vesicles or elongated tubules. The nuclei appear irregular in outline and contain areas of chromatin condensation, principally along the nuclear membrane. The lower lymphocyte also has a centriole (C) a few profiles of rough endoplasmic reticulum in the cytoplasm along the periphery (arrow), and a distinct nucleolus (No) with areas of chromatin condensation along the margin. A few cytoplasmic projections are also present on these cells (×19,000). (From Jain, N.C.: Schalm's Veterinary Hematology. 4th Ed. Philadelphia, Lea & Febiger, 1986, p. 793.)

Early biochemical events are similar in B and T cells stimulated through receptor-ligand interaction or any other mechanism (see Fig. 13–5).

Lymphocytes do not stain for peroxidase and other usual myeloid cytochemical markers, such as Sudan black B and chloroacetate esterase. Alkaline phosphatase activity, like that present in the neutrophils of most species, is usually absent. Some T lymphocytes may show a nonspecific esterase (NSE) activity that is not inhibited by sodium fluoride, compared to a sodium fluoride-inhibitable NSE activity in monocytes. NSE-positive lymphocytes reveal localized, coarse, cytoplasmic granules or a single or multiple globular reaction, whereas monocytes usually show a diffuse cytoplasmic staining (Plate X-9). Lymphocytes contain many other lysosomal acid hydrolytic enzymes (e.g., acid phosphatase and β-glucuronidase) and enzymes for purine and pyrimidine synthesis. A genetic defi-

ciency of two enzymes of purine metabolism, adenosine deaminase and purine nucleoside phosphorylase, is associated with genetic defects in the development and function of the lymphoid system in humans. Inherited lysosomal storage diseases, such as fucosidosis, mannosidosis, mucopolysaccharidosis, and gangliosidosis are characterized by cytoplasmic vacuolation of lymphocytes (Plates IX–7, IX–8) and abnormal lysosomal granulation of leukocytes (Plates XIII-1 to 4) in blood (Alroy et al., 1989a, 1989b, 1992; Cantz and Ulrich-Bott, 1990; Keller and Lamarre, 1992).

Production

Lymphocytes are produced in the bone marrow, in the lymphoid organs, which include the thymus, lymph nodes, and spleen, and in gut-associated lymphoid

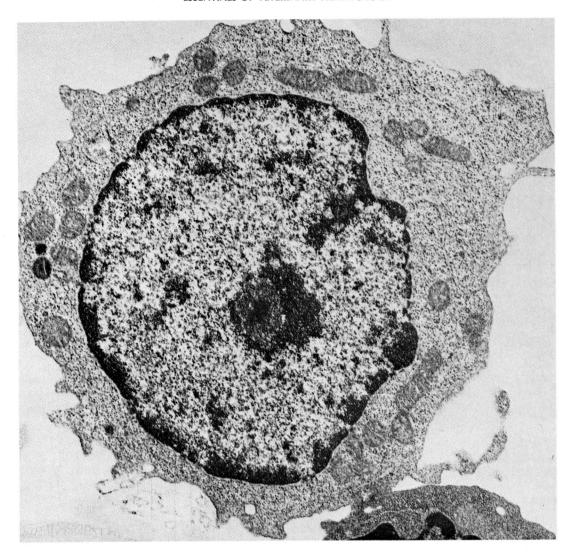

Fig. 17–2. Lymphocyte with a moderate amount of cytoplasm and a vesicular nucleus with a nucleolus. Nuclear pores and some chromatin condensation are evident along the nuclear membrane. The cytoplasm is rich in free ribosomes, has some profiles of rough endoplasmic reticulum and scattered mitochondria, and has a few dense granular structures, (×26,000). (From Jain, N.C.: Schalm's Veterinary Hematology. 4th Ed. Philadelphia, Lea & Febiger, 1986, p. 794.)

tissues (GALT), which include Peyer's patches, the tonsils, and the appendix. Quantitative studies have shown that the bone marrow is the body's largest lymphopoietic organ (Williams et al., 1990). Except for supplying lymphoid precursors to seed the peripheral lymphoid organs, however, lymphopoiesis in the bone marrow and thymus is largely ineffective in that most of the cells die in situ, with a turnover time of 2 to 4 days.

During intrauterine life, undifferentiated pluripotential stem cells (PPSCs) originate first from the yolk sac and later from the fetal liver, spleen, and bone marrow. In adult life, these cells continue to develop in the bone marrow. The PPSCs initially differentiate into committed lymphoid stem cells under the influence of an appropriate microenvironment and some undefined stimuli. These lymphoid progenitors from the bone marrow continually seed the primary or central lymphoid organs—the bursa of Fabricius in

birds or its mammalian equivalent (perhaps the bone marrow) and the thymus (Fig. 17–4). At these sites, at least two functionally and phenotypically different populations of lymphocytic precursors develop. These cells then migrate to the secondary or peripheral lymphoid organs (e.g., lymph nodes and spleen), where they become preferentially located and give rise to immunocompetent subsets of T or B lymphocytes in response to appropriate antigenic stimuli.

Three stages of T lymphocyte development were characterized in horses by six monoclonal antibodies that reacted with T lymphocytes at different stages of maturation (Wyatt et al., 1988). Monoclonal antibodies EqT12 and EqT13 identified cells with the functional characteristics of prothymocytes, EqT6 and EqT7 identified resident cortical thymocytes, and EqT2 and EqT3 identified a subpopulation of mature T lymphocytes and all mature T lymphocytes, respectively. In horses with inherited severe combined immuno-

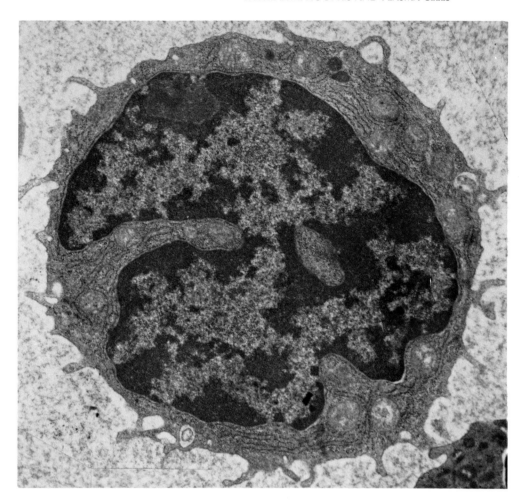

Fig. 17–3. Lymphocyte with a small amount of cytoplasm, rich in rough endoplasmic reticulum, and with an indented nucleus with condensed chromatin. This cell would appear blue in Wright-stained blood film and may be referred to as an "immunocyte." Some mitochondria and surface microvilli are also evident (×25,000). (From Jain, N.C.: Schalm's Veterinary Hematology. 4th Ed. Philadelphia, Lea & Febiger, 1986, p. 795.)

DEVELOPMENT OF LYMPHOCYTES

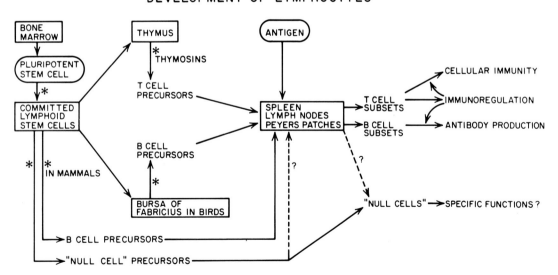

*Local Microenvironment

Fig. 17–4. Sequential development of lymphocytes and their functional differentiation at various primary and secondary sites of lymphopoiesis. See text for details. (From Jain, N.C.: Schalm's Veterinary Hematology. 4th Ed. Philadelphia, Lea & Febiger, 1986, p. 799.)

deficiency, both prothymocytes and mature thymocytes are present but cortical thymocytes are virtually absent. The production of mature B and T lymphocytes is inhibited because of the genetic defect, but the development of large granular lymphocytes with cytotoxic activity is not affected (Perryman et al., 1988). In normal foals, T lymphocytes appeared as early as the 75th day of fetal development.

Factors controlling the migration and specific development of various lymphocytes at different locations are largely unknown. Lymphoid differentiation toward a T-cell lineage in the thymus occurs primarily in the cortex and is influenced by such factors as the thymic microenvironment, thymic hormones, and soluble substances produced by cells of the thymic medulla and by macrophages. Thymic hormones also influence T-cell production in secondary lymphoid organs. The differentiation of pre-T cells and T-cell precursors in the thymus and of pre-B cells and B-cell precursors in the bone marrow are antigen-independent. In comparison, B-cell production in the bone marrow, spleen, and lymph nodes is primarily antigen-dependent and is promoted by γ-interferon. Thus, it is understandable why thymectomized and germ-free animals develop lymphopenia and have impaired immune responses. Interferon-γ may also amplify the immune response of T cells to tissue-associated antigens (Fuller et al., 1992) and augments expression of class I and class II MHC antigens on the surface of lymphocytes (Walrand et al., 1989). T cell development in thymus is influenced by IL-1, IL-2, IL-4, IL-6, and IL-7 and in secondary lymphoid organs by IL-1, IL-2, IL-4, IL-7, and IL-9. B cell development in primary lymphoid organs is influenced by IL-1 through IL-7 and in secondary lymphoid organs by IL-1 through IL-6.

Lymphocytes, as supplied to the blood, are produced primarily in the lymph nodes and, to a limited extent, in other lymphoid tissues. All lymph nodes, however, are not active at a given time; some are resting. The development of mature lymphocytes occurs in a stepwise manner (Fig. 17–5). The recognition of various sequential stages is based primarily on cell surface properties and functional criteria. Lymphoblasts, prolymphocytes, and lymphocytes can be identified morphologically, but their B- or T-cell lineage cannot be determined morphologically. The lymphocyte generation time is estimated to be 6 to 8 hours and, in some cases, may even be less than 2 hours. The number of mitoses involved seems to vary with the cell type (six

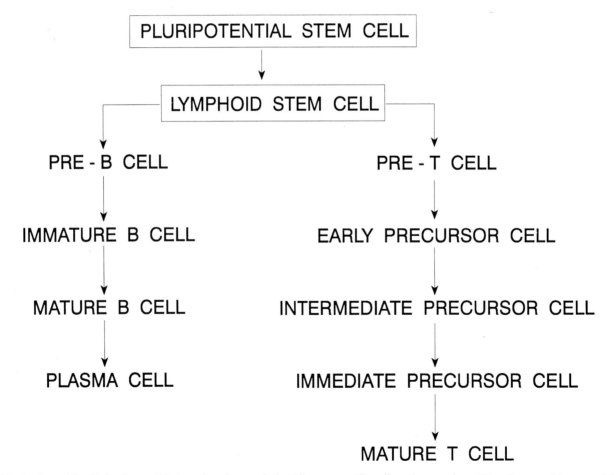

Fig. 17–5. B- and T-cell developmental stages based on analysis of lineage specific cell markers, such as CD antigens and immunoglobulin receptors.

Table 17–1.   Criteria for Characterization of Lymphocyte Subpopulations in Various Species

B Cells	T Cells
Specific surface antigens	Specific surface antigens
Ia antigens	Brain-associated antigens
Surface immunoglobulin (sIg)	Reaction with antithymocyte serum
Cytoplasmic Ig (in pre-B cells)	Subsets with Fc receptors for various immunoglobulins
Receptors for Fc portion of various immunoglobulins	Spontaneous E rosettes with erythrocytes of heterologous species
Erythrocyte-antibody rosettes	Stimulation by phytomitogens: phytohemagglutinin (PHA), con-
Receptors for C3: erythrocyte-antibody-complement rosettes (C3b and C3d)	canavalin A, PWM, wax bean, and bovine serum albumin
Receptors for Epstein-Barr virus	Receptors for Helix pometia antigen, peanut agglutinin, and C-reactive protein
Stimulation by pokeweed mitogen (PWM), antiglobulin serum, dextran, protein A, trypsin, lipopolysaccharides, insoluble PHA, concanavalin A	Receptors for measles virus
Adherence to nylon wool	Positive staining for Tdt in precursor cells and acid phosphatase, β-glucuronidase, and α-naphthyl acetate esterase in mature T cells
Positive staining for terminal deoxyribonucleotidase (Tdt) in pre-B cells and 5′-nucleotidase in mature B cells.	

to eight for T cells and two to three for B cells). Lymphopoiesis is generally stimulated by antigenic exposure and depressed by corticosteroids, sex hormones, and malnutrition.

Surface Markers and Subpopulations

The subpopulations of lymphocytes and their subsets can be defined by various functional, cell surface, and enzymatic markers (Table 17–1). B lymphocytes are generally characterized by the presence of surface immunoglobulins and by the formation of rosettes with antibody-coated or antibody-complement–coated erythrocytes (Table 17–1). In comparison, T lymphocytes form spontaneous rosettes with erythrocytes of suitable heterologous species (usually sheep erythrocytes) and are stimulated by certain phytomitogens to undergo blastogenesis in vitro (e.g., phytohemagglutinin [PHA] and concanavalin A). T-helper and T-suppressor cells from feline blood rosette with guinea pig and gerbil erythrocytes, respectively (Gengozian et al., 1991). Removal of cells rosetting with gerbil erythrocytes resulted in a 2-3 fold increase in immunoglobulin synthesis in cultured lymphocytes, while depletion of cells rosetting with guinea pig erythrocytes yielded a much reduced response.

The immunoglobulin receptors and immunoglobulins on the surface of B lymphocytes are unique. Immunoglobulin expression varies with the stage of B-cell differentiation. Immature B cells express cytoplasmic IgM, but mature cells express surface IgM, IgG, and IgD antibody bound to specific Fc receptors on their surface membrane. These Ig molecules are involved in cell activation and antigen processing during the immune response. Surface receptors for Ig are not found on plasma cells.

Lymphocytes also have cell surface adhesion molecules, known as lymphocyte function-associated antigens (LFAs). The major surface adhesion molecules include LFA1, LFA2 (CD2), and LFA3 (see Fig. 13–6). Adhesion molecules, "homing receptors" present on lymphocytes, and "addressins" present on endothelial cells in lymphoid and other tissues appear to be important in lymphocyte recirculation (Abernethy and Hay, 1992; Chin et al., 1991; Salmi and Jalkanene, 1991; Stoolman, 1989). Adhesion molecules are required for proper T-cell function and the immune response. They are involved in the interactions of lymphocytes with the antigen-presenting cells (usually macrophages) and in T-cell–mediated cytolysis of target cells. Monoclonal antibodies to these antigens block T-cell functions, such as cytotoxic T-cell–mediated killing of target cells and the T-cell proliferative response to lectins and antigens.

Subsets of B and T cells can be differentiated further by detecting various specific cell membrane antigens. Many clusters of differentiation antigens (CD units) have been defined on lymphocytes by using monoclonal antibodies to human leukocytes (Williams et al., 1990). Some common antigens found on human B lymphocytes and their precursors include CD9, CD10, CD19, CD20, CD21, CD22, CD24, CD37, CD38, and CD39, and those present on T lymphocytes include CD2, CD3, CD4, CD7, and CD8. CD antigens may be acquired or lost during the differentiation, maturation, and activation of lymphocytes, and many of the antigens can also be found in varying degrees on other leukocytes and body cells. For example, committed progenitors and pre-B cells express CD9, CD10, and CD38, whereas immature and mature B lymphocytes express CD21, CD37, and CD39. CD19 and CD24 are considered pan B-cell markers, and CD3 and CD7 are pan T-cell markers. CD4 is expressed not only on helper T cells, but also on monocytes, CD45 is a panleukocyte marker and its two isoforms, CD45RA and CD45RO, have been hypothesized to identify "naive" and "memory" T cells, respectively (Clement, 1992). Many of these and other leukocyte antigenic markers are being used to classify leukemias and lymphomas in humans (Stewart, 1992). Monoclonal antibodies are being increasingly used to characterize lymphocyte subpopulations in animal blood and lymphoid tissues (Alders and Shelton, 1990; Djilali et al., 1991; Hein et al., 1991; Lunn et al., 1991; Naessens, 1991; Roy et al., 1988; Wyatt et al., 1988).

Functionally, some of these surface antigens on lymphocytes have been found to be important in the immune response involving antigen recognition (e.g., CD3 antigen on T cells), cell activation, and cell proliferation. They are also useful in the identification of lymphocyte types and cell maturity, based on their distribution on the developing lymphocytes. T-helper cells express CD4 but not CD8, whereas T-suppressor cells express CD8 but not CD4. In normal humans, CD4 antigen is found on about two-thirds and CD8 on about one-fourth of T cells in blood. The distribution of CD4 and CD8 subpopulations in feline blood is similar to that in humans (Tompkins et al., 1990a). Canine helper and suppressor T cells can be distinguished using mouse monoclonal antibodies (Hotzl et al., 1991). CD4 and CD8 antigens facilitate antigen recognition by binding to the glycoproteins of the MHC II and MHC I, respectively. They may also enhance the antigen responsiveness of appropriate T cells. CD4 antigen also serves as the receptor for the human immunodeficiency virus (HIV). The receptor for antigen recognition on most T cells consists of an α-β heterodimer associated with the CD3 molecule. A receptor-ligand interaction on the T cell causes the degradation of phosphatidylinositol and activation of protein kinase C, increases intracellular free calcium, and ultimately results in the activation and proliferation of T cells (Kay, 1991). A similar signal transduction mechanism seems to be involved in MHC class-II-mediated B cell activation (Charron et al., 1991).

The application of such immunophenotyping methods in humans has provided new insights regarding the characterization of leukemias, lymphomas, immune-mediated diseases, and immunodeficiency syndromes. This has become possible because of the availability of many unique monoclonal antibodies and of the use of flow cytometry to characterize lymphoid and myeloid populations routinely in clinical settings. Blast cells that cannot be precisely identified by morphologic and cytochemical staining criteria can be characterized by their antigenic diversity in this way. Similar studies in animals are being conducted, but these have been hampered by the limited availability of specific monoclonal antibodies.

Subtypes in Blood and Tissues

The total population of B and T cells in the blood of most animal species is about 80 to 95%, with about 70% T cells and 20% B cells, and the remaining probably comprise the null cells, although wide variations have been reported among and within species. Among lymphoid tissues, T cells predominate in the thymus, lymph nodes, and thoracic duct lymph, and B cells predominate in the bone marrow and spleen. In blood and various tissues, most T cells are generally long-lived, most B cells are short-lived, and memory T and B cells are long-lived. The average life span of long-lived human lymphocytes is estimated to be 4.3 years and about 1% may live for at least 20 years. The short-lived lymphocytes survive for a few hours to 5 days.

The number of T and B lymphocytes in the blood and lymphoid tissues varies with the age and the health of an individual. For example, B cells are few during fetal life and steadily increase after birth until adult values are attained, and again decline during old age. About twice as many T cells (30.6 ± 4.7%) are found in the peripheral blood of 1- to 2-year-old calves than in 2- to 3-month-old calves (16.5 ± 3.2%; Sulochana et al., 1985). Leukemic cows and cows with persistent lymphocytosis have increased numbers of B cells compared to normal cows. B lymphocytes are low or absent in agammaglobulinemic animals. In addition to quantitative changes, the disease state may also affect the functional properties of lymphocytes. For example, the mitogenic properties of T cells may be transiently reduced during bacterial, viral, mycotic, and parasitic infections, autoimmune diseases, and lymphoid and nonlymphoid malignancies.

Hemal lymph nodes may play a specialized role in the immune system because they display germinal centers and a unique distribution of lymphocyte subsets (Thorp et al., 1991). It has been shown that marked differences are found in the percentage and distribution of lymphocyte subsets in sheep hemal lymph nodes compared to those in mesenteric lymph nodes and blood. A greater number of T19 (gamma/delta)+ lymphocytes and fewer CD8+ lymphocytes are present in hemal nodes than in mesenteric lymph nodes and a higher percentage of CD4+ lymphocytes occurs in hemal and mesenteric lymph nodes than in blood. T19+ cells are found throughout hemal nodes except the lymphoid follicles. The leukocyte common antigen, CD45, is expressed on 80% of the hemal node lymphocytes.

Recirculation

In contrast to granulocytes, about 70% of the peripheral blood lymphocytes that go into tissues re-enter the vascular system to recirculate (Fig. 17–6). Recirculation has been observed during fetal life, as early as 96 days of gestation in sheep. This property of lymphocytes has made the estimation of lymphocyte life span difficult and somewhat inaccurate.

The recirculating population consists primarily of T lymphocytes; B lymphocytes, except for memory cells, are considered noncirculating. Various lymphocytes recirculate at different rates and follow different pathways. T lymphocytes generally take longer to recirculate (24 to 48 hours) as compared to B cells (15 to 18 hours) and recirculating cells spend relatively much more time in the homing (specific) lymphoid organs than in the blood. Circulation through the thymus, spleen, and bone marrow is by way of the hematogenous route, whereas re-entry of lymphocytes from the lymph nodes is largely through the lymph except in the pig, in which it is hematogenous because of the inverted architecture of the lymph node. Lymphocytes

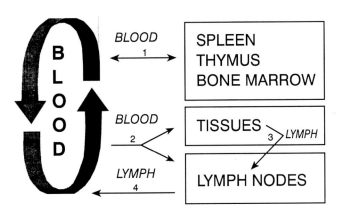

Fig. 17–6. Recirculation of lymphocytes through peripheral blood *(left)*, spleen, bone marrow, lymphoid organs, and other body tissues. Recirculation is either through blood (1) or primarily involves migration successively through blood (2), afferent lymph (3), and efferent lymph (4).

enter various tissues primarily at the region of postcapillary venules, which peculiarly have cuboidal or cylindric endothelial cells and are known as high endothelial venules (HEV). Lymphocyte and endothelial surface contact at these sites involves interactions between cell surface adhesion molecules and homing receptors on lymphocytes and appropriate ligands on the HEV that contribute to an organ-specific homing mechanism. For example, Peyer's patches contain mainly B cells and some CD4-positive T cells, whereas lymph nodes predominantly contain T cells, including CD8-positive T cells. The path of migration is between the endothelial cells and interendothelial migration takes 10 to 20 minutes in most species.

The recirculation phenomenon is of prime biologic importance because it provides a mechanism for the

generalized distribution of lymphoid cells concerned with a systemic immune response. As a result, a great number of lymphocytes can be exposed to an antigen deposited locally in the tissue. Antigenically primed cells can then be relocated elsewhere in the body to propagate and mount a vigorous immune response. It is also important for immune surveillance, whereby harmful or undesirable clones of cells are destroyed by special cytotoxic lymphocytes. A therapeutic advantage of the recirculation phenomenon is targeting tumor cells using labelled lymphocytes to deliver radiation or antibodies preferentially to affected tissues.

The mechanisms involved in lymphocyte recirculation and its regulation are not definitively known but cell membrane properties, including surface adhesion molecules, seem to be important (Abernethy and Hay, 1992; Chin et al., 1991; Salmi and Jalkanene, 1991; Stoolman, 1989). Lymphocyte recognition and binding to endothelial cells in lymphoid organs and other body tissues is controlled by several homing molecules present on their surface (Table 17–2). Cytokines secreted at sites of inflammation increase the expression of ICAM-1, VCAM-1, and ELAM-1 and facilitate the migration of lymphocytes and other leukocytes to sites of inflammation. The expression of homing receptors on lymphocytes may decrease with age of the animal (Walcheck et al., 1992). For example, virtually 100% blood lymphocytes from young bovine calves (less than 1 month old) expressed LECAM-1 (equivalent to human MEL-14) compared to 17–67% lymphocytes in older animals (greater than 1 year old).

Recirculation can be altered by the exposure of lymphocytes to enzymes (neuraminidase and trypsin), viruses (influenza and New Castle disease viruses), and heparin. Variations in the blood and bone marrow distribution of lymphoid cells in lymphomas might be

Table 17–2.   Homing Receptors of Lymphocytes Involved in Recirculation through Various Lymphoid Organs and Tissues*

Lymphocyte Receptors	Ligand	Location of Ligands	Comments
LFA-1 (CD11a/CD18)	ICAM1 and 2	Endothelial cells in most organs	Belongs to integrin family; is a two-chain protein, non-organ specific, and important in antigen recognition by T cells and in cytotoxic T cell mediated cytotoxicity; more abundant on memory T cells than on naive T cells
MEL-14	MECA-79	HEV in lymph nodes	Organ specific; may function as a lectin, binds to carbohydrate moieties of lymph node HEV cells; more abundant on naive T cells than on memory T cells
CD44	MECA-79 MECA-367	HEV in peripheral lymph nodes HEV in mucosal lymphoid tissues such as Peyer's patches and mesenteric lymph nodes	Expression is increased on memory T cells; present also on many epithelial cells, neural, and connective tissue cells; also acts as a receptor for matrix component (e.g., hyaluronate); murine MECA-367 and MECA-79 antigens have been termed "addressins"
VLA-4 α-chain (CDw49d/β-chain CD29)	VCAM-1	HEV in Peyer's patches	Belongs to integrin family, expression is increased on memory T cells, fibronectin also serves as a ligand

* HEV, high endothelial venule; LFA, lymphocyte function associated antigen; ICAM, intercellular adhesion molecule; MEL-14, an antigen recognized by MEL-14 antibody in mice; CD, cluster designation for "cluster of differentiation" antigen; VLA, very late activation antigen; MECA-367 and MECA-79 antigens recognized by respective monoclonal antibodies; VCAM, vascular cell adhesion molecules; other adhesion molecules referred to in the text include ELAM, endothelial leukocyte adhesion molecule, and LECAM, leukocyte endothelial cell adhesion molecule.
Source: Abbas et al., 1991; Abernethy and Hay, 1992; Springer, 1990.

a manifestation of disturbed recirculation of leukemic cells, probably because of altered surface properties. General anesthesia of sheep with ketamine and xylazine was found to produce a marked depression in lymphocyte traffic through primary peripheral lymph nodes that correlated with elevated PGE2 levels and diminished lymphocyte output into efferent lymph (Moore et al., 1988).

Numbers in Blood

The number of lymphocytes in blood varies with age and adrenal cortical activity. Young animals have higher lymphocyte counts than adults and lymphopenia occurs following an increase in the circulatory concentration of corticosteroids. The number of lymphocytes in blood may be influenced by the rates of production, recirculation, and utilization or destruction of lymphocytes. Hence the existence of a lymphopenia or a lymphocytosis does not necessarily signify an altered lymphopoiesis. Abnormalities of B- and T-cell functions that result in a defective immune response are discussed in Chapter 21.

LYMPHOPENIA

Corticosteroid-induced lymphopenia is attributed to lympholysis in blood and lymphoid tissues, increased shift of lymphocytes from blood to other body compartments, or both. T cells in blood and tissues are most sensitive to the lympholytic effect. Lymphocytes have high-affinity receptors for corticosteroids in their cytoplasm. After ligand-receptor interaction in the cytoplasm, the ligand-receptor complexes bind to specific DNA sequences and induce the synthesis of mRNA, which in turn triggers the synthesis of proteins that inhibit intracellular glucose transport and lipid synthesis. In addition, an endonuclease may become activated, causing DNA fragmentation. Glucocorticoids also markedly inhibit the synthesis of IL-1 by macrophages and IL-2 by activated T cells, thereby thwarting an immune response (an immunosuppressive effect).

Lymphopenia from decreased lymphopoiesis occurs after thymectomy, irradiation, and chemotherapy. A similar mechanism is involved in the lymphopenia associated with combined immune deficiency in foals and in uremic dogs with end-stage kidney disease. Lymphopenia seen in acute viral infections may be the result of increased destruction and/or increased sequestration of lymphocytes in lymphoid or other tissues because of altered surface properties. Lymphopenia may occur in some cases of acute lymphocytic leukemia and lymphoma, and is probably associated with the decreased release of lymphocytes in blood. Lymphopenia associated with protein-losing enteropathy results from the loss of lymphocytes in the lymph drained from the body. Zinc deficiency may cause lymphopenia and abnormal lymphocyte functions, but the mechanisms involved are unknown.

Lymphopenia observed in various diseases may be associated with a proportionate or disproportionate decrease or increase in the numbers of B and T cells or their subsets. For example, sheep and cattle experimentally infected with bluetongue virus develop a lymphocytopenia one week after infection (Ellis et al., 1990). The lymphopenia is associated with an increase in the CD4:CD8 ratio (greater than 3) because of a greater decrease in absolute numbers of circulating CD8+ lymphocytes compared to CD4+ lymphocytes. Bluetongue-infected cattle, however, develop a lymphopenia without a significant change in the CD4:CD8 ratio. Sheep infected with tick-borne fever develop a lymphopenia six days after experimental infection, with recovery by 13 to 16 days of infection. This transient lymphopenia was associated with a significant reduction in both B and T (CD4+, CD5+, and CD8+) lymphocytes and an increase in null cells (Woldehiwet, 1991). Development of lymphocytic leukemia and lymphoma in sheep inoculated with bovine leukemia virus (BLV) is characterized by an increase in the number of circulating B cells and a decrease in the CD4:CD8 ratio from a much greater increase in CD8+ cells than in CD4+ cells in blood, lymph nodes, and spleen (Dimmock et al., 1990). Lymphocytotic cattle infected with BLV show increased numbers of B, T helper, and T suppressor cells, while aleukemic BLV infected cattle have reduced numbers of B and T helper cells compared to noninfected healthy cattle (Taylor et al., 1992). T helper immunosuppression is observed in cats with FeLV (feline leukemia virus)-induced lymphoproliferative diseases as well as with FeLV-associated acquired immune deficiency syndrome-like diseases (Pardi et al., 1991; Tompkins et al., 1989a) and in FIV (feline immunodeficiency virus) infected cats (Bishop et al., 1992). FIV infected cats, like humans with HIV infection, have a reduced number of CD4+ cells and an inverted CD4:CD8 ratio (Barlough et al., 1991; Novotney et al., 1990). Cattle infected with bovine virus diarrhea develop a transient leukopenia and a decrease in the absolute numbers of B and T lymphocytes (Bolin et al., 1985).

Lymphocyte functions in various species may also be altered under physiologic and pathologic conditions. Calves with lethal trait A46, a genetic disorder affecting zinc absorption, have normal numbers of functional subpopulations at birth, but numbers of both T and B cells are reduced following development of zinc deficiency by 3 weeks of age (Perryman et al., 1989). In pregnant cows, the number of lymphocytes is decreased during the week before calving, being lowest on the day before calving and is associated with diminished in vitro stimulation with phytohemagglutinin, concanavalin A, and pokeweed mitogen (Saad et al., 1989). Lymphocyte blastogenesis is significantly reduced in heat-stressed pregnant sheep in pre- and post-parturient period; the immunosuppressive effect seems to be partly mediated by an unidentified serum factor (Niwano et al., 1990). Lymphocytes from sheep given dietary selenium supplementation may show increased or decreased mitogen response depending on the amount given (Larsen et al., 1988). Lymphopenia caused by endotoxemia in sheep is associated with a reduction in numbers of T and B lymphocytes in blood and lung lymph (Duke et al., 1990).

LYMPHOCYTOSIS

Lymphocytosis may be physiologic, reactive, or proliferative (Jain, 1986). A transient physiologic lymphocytosis is seen with a marked release of epinephrine because of physical or emotional stress. It usually occurs in association with neutrophilia. A "rapidly accessible pool" of lymphocytes, analogous to the marginal pool of neutrophils, exists in the body. Its size in calves, sheep, and dogs has been estimated to be about seven to ten times that of the lymphocytes in circulating blood. Cells from this pool can be mobilized easily and can cause physiologic lymphocytosis—for example, after excitation and physical exercise, particularly in young animals. The exact anatomic location of this pool is unknown.

Reactive lymphocytosis often occurs because of chronic infections, and proliferative lymphocytosis results from the malignant proliferation of lymphocytes as in lymphoma and acute and chronic lymphocytic leukemias (Thurmond et al., 1990). Both types of lymphocytosis are persistent, but the former usually abates with recovery from disease. An immune response leading to antibody formation is often not reflected as lymphocytosis in the blood, although some morphologic evidence (e.g., increased basophilia) may be found occasionally, particularly in those with chronic, marked antigenic stimulation. Thus, reactive lymphocytosis is generally accompanied by atypical, highly basophilic lymphocytes or immunocytes in the blood. Lymphocytosis and immature lymphocytes in blood are not consistently found in lymphoid malignancies; only about 25% of dogs with lymphoma show such abnormalities. Persistent lymphocytosis may be seen in chronic viremias associated with FeLV, bovine leukemia virus (BLV), and bovine immunodeficiency virus infections.

Functions

Lymphocytes constitute the immunologic armor of the body. They are important for the production of humoral antibodies and for conferring cellular immunity, and are responsible for antibody diversity. The immune response is age-dependent, with younger and older individuals being less competent. Aberrations of one or both types of the immune response occur in humans and animals and may manifest as an increased or decreased response (e.g., multiple myeloma, immune deficiency syndromes, immune-mediated hemolytic anemia, immune-mediated thrombocytopenia).

HUMORAL IMMUNITY

Antibody synthesis occurs in B lymphocytes predominantly in the lymph nodes, to a lesser extent in the spleen and bone marrow, and to a variable extent locally in various tissues, including Peyer's patches. Antibody formation generally requires the participation of macrophages, B cells, and T cells. Macrophages initially bind the antigen through their surface receptors and process it so that it becomes highly immunogenic. This antigen is then presented to participating virgin T-helper cells and B cells. Through their surface immunoglobulins, T cells recognize the carrier portion and B cells recognize the hapten portion of the foreign antigen. Cell-to-cell interaction similarly involves the recognition of surface Ia antigens. These interactions initiate the clonal proliferation of both T and B cells. Lymphokines from antigen-stimulated T cells promote lymphopoiesis, which is further regulated by factors from T-suppressor cells and stimulatory (interleukin-1, also known as lymphocyte-activating factor) and inhibitory (prostaglandins E) substances from macrophages. The antigen-specific "primed" progeny of lymphocytes recognize the same antigen on subsequent presentation and undergo a similar secondary but heightened proliferation. Some of the progeny become memory cells but most express the specific immune response, humoral or cellular, depending mainly on the type of antigen.

The antigenic activation of B cells for the immune response may also occur independently of T-cell participation. T-cell–independent antigens are usually high-molecular-weight polymers. They directly cross-link cell surface receptors on B cells and activate them. The transformation of B cells into antibody-producing immunocytes or plasma cells is the basis of humoral antibody response. The initial antibody formed is IgM, but, with a continued immune response, it switches to IgG. Clonal amplification results in the production of increasing amounts of antibody. Memory cells may survive for decades.

CELLULAR IMMUNITY

Cellular immunity is expressed primarily by T lymphocytes and to some extent also by the null cells. In this respect, the T cells are responsible for immune regulation, a delayed type of hypersensitivity, homograft rejection, graft-versus-host reaction, cytotoxicity, and the production of many lymphokines with diverse biologic activities. Different subpopulations of T lymphocytes may be involved in different functions.

IMMUNE REGULATION

It involves the participation of T-helper and T-suppressor cells in antibody synthesis (see above). Disturbances of this function of T cells have been associated with the development of many autoimmune diseases, including immune-mediated hemolytic anemia and immune-mediated thrombocytopenia.

CYTOTOXIC ACTIVITY

Cytotoxic activity mediated by lymphocytes involves the expression of the following: (1) cytotoxic T-cell activity, which is antigen-dependent; (2) killer (K) cell activity, which is antibody-dependent; and (3) natural killer (NK) cell activity, which is antibody–independent. The various cytotoxic effector cells show distinct differences in origin, phenotype, morphology, and target cell specificity, but all of them destroy the target cells by a contact-dependent, non-phagocytic process (Groscurth, 1989). Cytotoxic T cells are characterized by typical lysosomal granules and expression of a unique profile of surface antigens. They recognize specific antigens which are presented in association with class I MHC molecules. K cells and most NK cells are considered subpopulations of null cells, although they have Fc receptors for IgG and form low-affinity rosettes at 4°C with sheep erythrocytes (Williams et al., 1990). Because their cytotoxic potential can be activated by lymphokines such as IL-2, they form an important component of the lymphokine activated killer (LAK) cell population exploited for cancer therapy. Interferons can also regulate NK cell function. K cells can be found in normal animals. NK cells in humans and rats have been morphologically identified as large, granular lymphocytes (cells containing prominent azurophilic granules). Human NK cells mostly express CD16, and a minor population expresses CD3 molecules. NK cells kill the appropriate targets without antibody participation and do not require MHC mol-

ecules to recognize the target cells. LAK cells are heterogeneous in the expression of surface antigens and selection of target cells. They contain peculiar intranuclear inclusion bodies which are believed to develop from prolonged stimulation by IL-2 (Groscurth, 1989).

A unique CD45R+ granular subpopulation of lymphocytes, equivalent to NK cells of mice and humans, was found in the sheep uterus and considered to have an important role in local immunity (Lee et al., 1988). Large granular lymphocyte with NK activity have been isolated from cattle vaccinated against foot and mouth disease (Amadori et al., 1992).

The mechanism of killing is largely unknown, but may involve degranulation of the large granular lymphocytes after attachment to target cells and subsequent enzymatic (protease and/or phospholipase) or cytotoxin-induced membrane damage and colloidal osmotic lysis (Tompkins et al., 1989b; Williams et al., 1990). A pore-forming proteolytic enzyme, perforin, has been identified in the granules of cytotoxic T cells. Fragmentin, a 32-kD granule protein was found to induce DNA fragmentation and apoptosis (Shi et al., 1992).

The cytotoxic activity of T lymphocytes is being manipulated for cancer therapy (Melief, 1992; Rosenberg, 1992; Whiteside et al., 1992). Cytokines are being

Table 17–3. Lymphokines Secreted by Lymphocytes and Possible Biologic Functions

Lymphokine*	MW	Source	Biologic Role
MIF	23,000–65,000	T4 cells B cells	Inhibits migration of monocytes and macrophages, increases their phagocytic and oxidative activities; a similar factor acting on neutrophils is called leukocyte inhibition factor (LIF)
MAF	30,000	T and B cells	Induces morphologic and metabolic changes in macrophages for enhanced functional activities such as protein synthesis, lysosome formation, pinocytosis, phagocytosis, and bactericidal and tumoricidal capacities
LMF	30,000–40,000	T and B cells	Promotes blastogenesis of lymphocytes, particularly B cells
Lymphotoxin (LT)	35,000–150,000	T cells and some B cells	Destroys a wide variety of cells in tissue culture; may function in allograft rejection and tumor immunity
Interferons	20,000–160,000	B and T cells	B cells produce α- and β-interferons, and T cells produce γ-interferon; antiviral, inhibit tumor growth, regulate cellular and humoral immune responses and macrophage functions, may cause lymphopenia during viral infections. Interferon γ augments expression of class I and class II MHC antigens on lymphocytes.
TNF-β	25,000	T cells, activated macrophages	Activated macrophages produce TNF-α and activated T cells produce TNF-β. TNF-β exerts cytotoxic (antitumor and antiviral) activity and systemic toxicity; stimulates production of inflammatory cytokines (IL-1, IL-6, IL-8, multiple CSFs, interferon-γ, and TGF-β).
TGF-β	28,000	T cells, activated macrophages, and many other cells	Switches B cells to produce IgA; a negative regulator of immune response as it inhibits T cell proliferation induced by mitogens, maturation of cytotoxic T cells, macrophage activation, and cytokine-mediated effects on neutrophils and endothelial cells; promotes angiogenesis; causes synthesis of cellular matrix proteins (collagen) and cellular receptors for matrix proteins
CSFs			See Table 4-3
ILs			See Table 17-4

* MIF, macrophage migration inhibition factor; MAF, macrophage-activating facor; LMF, lymphocyte mitogenic factor; TNF, tumor necrosis factor; CSFs, colony-stimulating factors; ILs, interleukins; TGF, transforming growth factor.

utilized to increase the functional competence of cytotoxic T cells and act as antitumor agents (Patel and Collins, 1992; Lotze, 1992; Rees, 1992; Wu et al., 1992). Five T-cell growth factors have now been recognized (IL-2, IL-4, IL-5, IL-7, and IL-10) and four of these (except IL-10) have been shown to induce LAK cell activity from sensitive precursors. In animal models, complete destruction of tumors can be achieved by transfusing tumor specific T cells, combined with IL-2. The most active cells are CD8+ cytotoxic T lymphocytes, which recognize peptides of 8-10 amino acid length, bound to the antigen presenting groove of MHC class I molecules. In the case of virus-induced tumors these peptides are derived from viral antigens. Potentially immunogenic human tumors include melanoma and renal cell carcinoma in addition to virus-associated cancers, Burkitt's lymphoma and cervical carcinoma (Melief and Kast, 1991). Although the exact mechanism of IL-2 based immunotherapy in cancer remains unclear, it has been hypothesized that both IL-2 activated lymphocytes and their secretory products such as interferon-γ or tumor necrosis factor-β may contribute to the lysis of tumor cells in vivo (Atzpodien and Kirchner, 1990). Thus, efforts are underway toward enhancing both the activation state and the specificity of IL-2 induced killer cells in humans. Retransfusion of tumor-derived activated lymphocytes has been shown to mediate the regression of metastatic neoplasms in up to 50% of patients receiving systemic IL-2. Attempts are also being made to develop a low-dose IL-2 therapeutic regimen as high dose therapy is associated with con-

Table 17–4.   Characteristics of Interleukins

Interleukin	MW	Source	Biologic Role
IL-1	17,500	Monocytes, macrophages, endothelial cells, other cells	Enhances T- and B-cell activation, synthesis of IL-2 and chemotoxis; triggers synthesis of IL-6; acts as endogenous pyrogen and early hematopoietic growth factor; induces production of PGE_2, acute phase proteins, neutral proteases, and collagenase; activates NK cells and other macrophages; has antiviral activity; may promote chemotaxis and extravasation of neutrophils; releases histamine from basophils
IL-2 (T-cell growth factor)	15,000–20,000	Activated T cells	Promotes proliferation of T and B cells, lymphokine secretion, and production of cytotoxic T cells, causes eosinophilia and bone marrow eosinophil hyperplasia in cats
IL-3	14,000–30,000	Activated T and B-cells, macrophages, other cells	Acts as multipotential hematopoietic growth factor and mast cell growth factor, causes neutrophilia and monocytosis, enhances histamine release from basophils
IL-4	15,000–19,000	Activated T cells	Promotes growth of and activates B and T cells; promotes B_j cells to switch to IgE synthesis and induces Fc épsilon RII receptors on B cells
IL-5	45,000	T cells, mast cells	Induces B-cell, T-cell, and eosinophil differentiation
IL-6	26,000	Monocytes, macrophages, fibroblasts, many other cell types such as megakaryocytes	B-cell differentiation factor (causes B cells to become plasma cells); enhances T-cell activation and cytotoxicity; induces production of acute phase proteins, has CSF activity; causes neutrophilia and monocytosis
IL-7	25,000	Bone marrow stromal cells	Induces differentiation of human and murine pre-B cells and T cells; stimulates development of cytolytic T lymphocytes and lymphokine-activated killer cells from CD8+ cells
IL-8	8,500	Monocytes, macrophages, T cells, fibroblasts, endothelial cells, many other cells	Potent neutrophil chemoattractant; exerts proinflammatory activities (e.g., neutrophil degranulation and adherence to endothelial cells); has anti-inflammatory effects (neutrophil emigration into tissues)
IL-9	32,000–39,000	T cells	Acts as an erythroid colony stimulating factor, a T cell growth factor, and as stimulating factor for mast cells
IL-10	~18,700	T cells (T-$_{H2}$ cells) B cells	Inhibits cytokine synthesis (acts as an anticytokine) by T helper-1 cells in the presence of macrophages
IL-11	~23,000	Bone marrow stromal cells	Promotes proliferation of T-dependent Ig-producing B cells and committed macrophage progenitors; acts synergistically with IL-3 or directly to stimulate megakaryocytopoiesis
IL-12	35,000–40,000 (heterodimer)	B cells	Acts synergistically with IL-2 as a growth factor for activated T cells (CD4+ and CD8+ subsets) and NK cells

Source: Balkwill, 1991; Druez et al., 1990; Mosmann and Moore, 1991; Podlaski et al., 1992; Shaw, 1991; Teramura et al., 1992.

siderable systemic toxicity. Recombinant cytokine therapy is being initiated to treat tumors also in animals (Moore et al., 1991).

IMMUNE SURVEILLANCE

This role is assigned to NK cells, in that they mediate natural resistance to tumors and certain bacterial and viral infections. Hence, modification of this function may be expected to result in disease. NK activity seems to be poorly developed during fetal life and at birth.

SECRETION OF LYMPHOKINES

It is generally a property of stimulated T lymphocytes, but resting or nonstimulated T lymphocytes may also express this activity. Some B lymphocytes can also produce lymphokines to a limited extent, but these

lymphokines have not been characterized. Exposure to an antigen or a nonspecific stimulus is usually required to activate lymphocytes for lymphokine production. Many lymphokines have been described; most are glycoproteins. Lymphokines are generally identified by their functional activities, so some may be the same molecules with overlapping properties. These diverse properties include inhibitory, toxic, stimulatory and inflammatory activities. Commonly known lymphokines include various hematopoietic growth factors (colony stimulating factors) and interleukins (Tables 17–3 and 17–4).

Cytokine therapy is a recent molecular advance in the treatment of cancer, infectious diseases, hematopoietic disorders, and immunodeficiency syndromes. Selected references are presented to obtain further details on immunobiology of various cytokines includ-

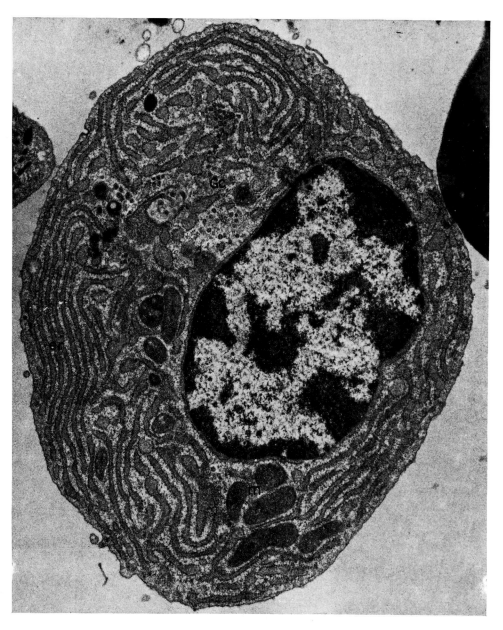

Fig. 17–7. Plasma cell from canine bone marrow. This cell characteristically displays patchy areas of chromatin condensation, in the form of a cartwheel, in the round eccentric nucleus and numerous elongated cisternae of endoplasmic reticulum (er) that almost fill the cytoplasm. Some mitochondria (m) are distributed among the cisternae of the rough endoplasmic reticulum. In the upper cytoplasmic portion, near the nucleus, remnants of the Golgi complex (Gc) cut transversely and, represented as small, round saccules, seem to be present. This area appears as a clear zone in the plasma cells in bone marrow smears stained with a Romanowsky stain (see Plate XI-4). The rough endoplasmic reticulum contains flocculent proteinaceous material representing immunoglobulin molecules (×18,000). (From Jain, N.C.: Schalm's Veterinary Hematology. 4th Ed. Philadelphia, Lea & Febiger, 1986, p. 813.)

ing hematopoietic growth factors and interleukins in humans and animals (Balkwill, 1991; Bardy et al., 1991; Bauer and Olson, 1988; Blecha, 1990; Burgess, 1990; Dower et al., 1992; Dreuz et al., 1990; Elmslie et al., 1991; Gasson, 1991; Gimbrone, 1989; Goodwin and Namen, 1991; Matsushima et al., 1992; Moore, 1991; Mosmann and Moore, 1991; Nagata, 1990; Neta et al., 1992; Podlaski et al., 1992; Riegel et al., 1992; Spooner et al., 1992; Teramura, 1992; Thomsen et al., 1991; Tompkins et al., 1990b; van Damme, 1991).

In vivo administration of recombinant IL-2 in humans causes anemia, thrombocytopenia, and eosinophilia (Lafreniere et al., 1990). In mice, IL-2 causes a dose-dependent increase in total leukocyte count, which is associated with increases in numbers of monocytes and granulocytes, but not lymphocytes. Simultaneously, CFU-GM proliferation is also increased in the bone marrow. Administration of recombinant IL-6 in monkeys causes a dose-dependent increase in platelet count, anemia, neutrophilia, monocytosis, and elevations in serum C-reactive protein and α-1 acid glycoprotein (Asano et al., 1990). The increase in platelet counts is associated with a marked increase in megakaryocyte size.

Interferons are produced by B and T cells in response to viral or bacterial infection or stimulation by chemical agents (Table 17–2). They exert antiviral, antitumor, and immunomodulatory effects. The antiviral activity of interferons is ascribed to induction of two enzymes, 2′,5′-oligoadenylate synthetase (2′,5′-OAS) and protein kinase. Activation of an RNAse by 2′,5′-oligoadenylates, synthesized through the action of 2′,5′-OAS, degrades mRNA and rRNA and thus inhibits virus production. Decreased OAS activity in macrophages has been related to loss of the antiviral state. Recombinant bovine interferon-α can induce an increase in 2′,5′-OAS activity in alveolar macrophages and blood mononuclear cells (Holland et al., 1991).

PLASMA CELLS

Plasma cells are recognized by their characteristic morphologic features, which include a small, usually eccentric nucleus with clumped chromatin, often in the form of a cartwheel, an abundant, highly basophilic cytoplasm, and a small clear area in the cytoplasm near the nucleus (Plate XI-4). A nucleolus may be seen in the plasmablast. The basophilia is attributed to a complex rough endoplasmic reticulum (RER) that occupies most of the cytoplasm and the clear area is represented by the Golgi apparatus (Fig. 17–7). The well-known pyroninophilia of the plasma cells is the result of their elaborate RER, which is rich in RNA (Plate X-12). Plasma cells lack peroxidase and NSE, but are strongly positive for β-glucuronidase.

Morphologic abnormalities are found in plasma cells, infrequently during an immune response and frequently in multiple myelomas and other pathologic conditions associated with plasmacytosis. A plasma cell engorged with antibody protein in its cytoplasm in the form of pinkish or bluish globules (Russell bodies) is occasionally seen in the bone marrow or lymph node aspirate, but rarely in the blood (Plate XI-5; Fig. 17–8). It is called a Mott cell. Plasma cells with reddish peripheral cytoplasmic staining, flame cells, have been found in IgA myeloma (Plates XIII-7, XIII-8, and XIII-9). Multinucleated plasma cells are seen occasionally during a vigorous immune response or gammopathy.

Plasma cells are derived from B lymphocytes in response to antigenic stimulation, proliferation, and maturation. Their developmental stages include plasmablast, transitional (immature) plasma cells, and terminally differentiated mature plasma cells. The entire process takes about 4 to 5 days and includes the participation of IL-4, IL-5, and IL-6 released from activated T-helper cells. Plasma cells can be found in any tissue, but are most numerous in tissues engaged in antibody formation. They are common in the medullary cords and germinal centers of lymph nodes, in the splenic white pulp and perivascular sheaths, and in connective tissue. Small numbers are found in the bone marrow. Plasmablasts and transitional (immature) plasma cells, along with mature plasma cells, are

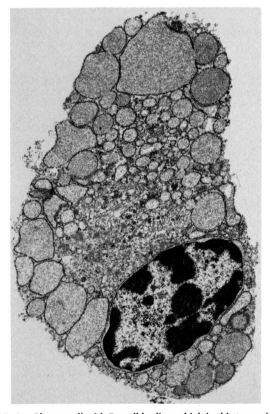

Fig. 17–8. Plasma cell with Russell bodies, which in this transmission electron photomicrograph appear as dilated vesicular structures (endoplasmic reticulum) containing amorphous material (immunoglobulin molecules). The eccentrically placed nucleus shows the characteristic cartwheel pattern of condensed chromatin. Although the cell membrane appears discontinuous or lost, cellular integrity is remarkably intact (× 22,000). (From Jain, N.C.: Schalm's Veterinary Hematology. 4th Ed. Philadelphia, Lea & Febiger, 1986, p. 814.)

often seen in antigen-stimulated lymphoid tissues, primarily the lymph nodes, spleen, and bone marrow. Plasma cells are extremely rare in blood, even in multiple myeloma. Circulating plasmacytoid cells, referred to as immunocytes, may be found in the blood during chronic antigenic stimulation (Fig. 17–3).

Plasma cells are concerned with the synthesis, storage, and secretion of immunoglobulins. Normally, one type of plasma cell or B cell synthesizes one type of antibody. The production of immunoglobulin is rapid, about 1 to 2 minutes, and its appearance outside the cell takes about 15 minutes. Abnormalities in the synthesis and secretion of immunoglobulins have been found in humans and animals. Particular examples include multiple myeloma and immunodeficiency syndromes (see Chap. 21). Malignant plasma cells secrete a lymphotoxin that stimulates osteoclasts to resorb bone, thus producing lytic lesions characteristic of those of multiple myeloma.

REFERENCES

Abbas, A.K., Lichtman, A.H. and Pober, J.S.: Cellular and molecular immunology. Philadelphia, W.B. Saunders Company, 1991, pp. 32, 151, 157–159.

Abernethy, N.J. and Hay, J.B.: The recirculation of lymphocytes from blood to lymph: physiological considerations and molecular mechanisms. Lymphology, 25:1, 1992.

Alders, R.G. and Shelton, J.N.: Lymphocyte subpopulations in lymph and blood draining from the uterus and ovary in sheep. J. Reprod. Immunol., 17:27, 1990.

Alroy, J., Freden, G.O., Goyal, V., et al.: Morphology of leukocytes from cats affected with alpha-mannosidosis and mucopolysaccharidosis VI (MPS VI). Vet. Pathol., 26:294, 1989a.

Alroy, J., Orgad, U., DeGasperi, R., et al.: Canine GM1-gangliosidosis. A clinical, morphologic, histochemical, and biochemical comparison of two different models. Am. J. Pathol., 140:675, 1992.

Alroy, J., Warren, C.D., Raghavan, S.S., et al.: Animal models for lysosomal storage diseases: their past and future contribution. Hum. Pathol., 20:823, 1989b.

Amadori, M., Archetti, I.L., Verardi, R., et al.: Isolation of mononuclear cytotoxic cells from cattle vaccinated against foot-and-mouth disease. Arch. Virol., 122:293, 1992.

Asano, S., Okano, A., Ozawa, K., et al.: In vivo effects of recombinant human interleukin-6 in primates: stimulated production of platelets. Blood, 75:1602, 1990.

Atzpodien, J. and Kirchner, H.: Cancer, cytokines, and cytotoxic cells: interleukin-2 in the immunotherapy of human neoplasms. Klin. Wochenschr., 68:1, 1990.

Balkwill, F.R.: Cytokines. A practical approach. Oxford, Oxford University Press, 1991.

Bardy, P.G., Lopez, A.F., Shannon, M.F., et al.: Future prospects of therapy with haematopoietic growth factors. In: Thomson, A.W. (eds), The cytokine handbook, San Diego, Academic Press, p. 325, 1991.

Barlough, J.E., Ackley, C.D., George, J.W., et al.: Acquired immune dysfunction in cats with experimentally induced feline immunodeficiency virus infection: comparison of short-term and long-term infections. J. Acquir. Immune. Defic. Syndr., 4:219, 1991.

Bauer, R.M. and Olsen, R.G.: Parameters of production and partial characterization of feline interleukin 2. Vet Immunol. Immunopathol., 19:173, 1988.

Bishop, S.A., Williams, N.A., Gruffydd-Jones, T.J., et al.: Impaired T-cell priming and proliferation in cats infected with feline immunodeficiency virus. AIDS, 6:287, 1992.

Blecha, F.: In vivo use of interleukins in domestic food animals. Adv. Vet. Sci. Comp. Med., 35:231, 1990.

Bolin, S.R., McClurkin, A.W. and Coria, M.F.: Effects of bovine viral diarrhea virus on the percentages and absolute numbers of circulating B and T lymphocytes in cattle. Am. J. Vet. Res., 46:884, 1985.

Burgess, A.W.: Granulocyte-macrophage colony stimulating factor. In: Sporn, M.B. Roberts, A.B. (eds), Peptide growth factors and their receptors I, Springer-Verlag, p. 723, 1990.

Cantz, M. and Ulrich-Bott, B.: Disorders of glycoprotein degradation. J. Inherit. Metab. Dis., 13:523, 1990.

Charron, D., Brick-Ghannam, S., Ramirez, R., et al.: HLA class-II-mediated B-lymphocyte activation: signal transduction and physiologic consequences. Res. Immunol., 142:467, 1991.

Chin, Y.H., Sackstein, R. and Cai, J.P.: Lymphocyte-homing receptors and preferential migration pathways. Proc. Soc. Exp. Biol. Med., 196:374, 1991.

Clement, L.T.: Isoforms of the CD45 common leukocyte antigen family: markers for human T-cell differentiation. J. Clin. Immunol., 12:1, 1992.

Dimmock, C.K., Ward, W.H. and Trueman, K.F.: Lymphocyte subpopulations in sheep with lymphosarcoma resulting from experimental infection with bovine leukaemia virus. Immunol. Cell Biol., 68:45, 1990.

Djilali, S., Dacosta, B., Kessler, J.L., et al.: Preparation and characterization of a monoclonal antibody against bovine CD5 lymphocyte surface antigen. Comp. Immunol. Microbiol. Infect. Dis., 14:257, 1991.

Dower, S.K., Sims, J.E., Cerretti, D.P., et al.: The interleukin-1 system: receptors, ligands and signals. Chem. Immunol., 51:33, 1992.

Dreuz, C., Coulie, P., Uyttenhove, C., et al.: Functional and biochemical characterization of mouse P40/IL-9 receptors. J. Immunol., 145:2494, 1990.

Duke, S.S., Guerry-Force, M.L., Forbes, J.T., et al.: Acute endotoxin-induced lymphocyte subset sequestration in sheep lungs. Lab. Invest., 62:355, 1990.

Ellis, J.A., Luedke, A.J., Davis, W.C., et al.: T lymphocyte subset alterations following bluetongue virus infection in sheep and cattle. Vet. Immunol. Immunopathol., 24:49, 1990.

Elmslie, R.E., Dow, S.W. and Ogilvie, G.K.: Interleukins: biological properties and therapeutic potential. J. Vet. Intern. Med., 5:283, 1991.

Fuller, L., Fernandez, J., Zheng, S., et al.: Immunochemical and biochemical characterization of purified canine interferon-gamma. Production of a monoclonal antibody, affinity purification, and its effect on mixed lymphocyte culture and mixed lymphocyte kidney culture reactions. Transplantation, 53:195, 1992.

Gasson, J.C.: Molecular physiology of granulocyte-macrophage colony-stimulating factor. Blood, 77:1131, 1991.

Gengozian, N., Hill, R.J., Good, R.A., et al.: Two populations of guinea pig erythrocyte-rosetting cells in the cat: evidence for their T-helper function in mitogen-induced synthesis of Ig and interleukin-2. Cell. Immunol., 133:1, 1991.

Gimbrone, M.A. Jr., Obin, M.S., Brock, A.F., et al.: Endothelial interleukin-8: A novel inhibitor of leukocyte-endothelial interactions. Science, 246:1601, 1989.

Goodwin, R.G. and Namen, A.E.: Interleukin-7. In: Thomson, A.W. (eds), The Cytokine Handbook. San Diego, Academic Press, 1991, p. 191.

Groscurth, P.: Cytotoxic effector cells of the immune system. Anat. Embryol. (Berl), 180:109, 1989.

Hein, W.R., Dudler, L., Beya, M.F., et al.: Epitopes of the T19 lymphocyte surface antigen are extensively conserved in ruminants. Vet. Immunol. Immunopathol., 27:173, 1991.

Holland, S.P., Fulton, R.W., Short, E.C., et al.: In vitro and in vivo 2′,5′-oligoadenylate synthetase activity induced by recombinant DNA-derived bovine interferon αI1 in bovine alveolar macrophages and blood mononuclear cells. Am. J. Vet. Res., 52:1779, 1991.

Hotzl, C., Kolb, H.J., Holler, E., et al.: Functional characterization of canine lymphocyte subsets. Ann. Hematol., 63:49, 1991.

Jain, N.C.: Schalm's Veterinary Hematology. 4th ed. Philadelphia, Lea & Febiger, 1986, pp. 790–820.

Kay, J.E.: Mechanisms of T lymphocyte activation. Immunol. Lett., 29:51, 1991.

Keller, C.B. and Lamarre, J.: Inherited lysosomal storage disease in an English Springer Spaniel. J. Am. Vet. Med. Assoc., 200:194, 1992.

Lafreniere, R., Houwen, B., Rankin, C., et al.: In vivo administration of recombinant interleukin-2 induces granulocyte-macrophage colony formation in a murine system. J. Biol. Response Mod., 9:420, 1990.

Larsen, H.J., Overnes, G. and Moksnes, K.: Effect of selenium on sheep lymphocyte responses to mitogens. Res. Vet. Sci., 45:11, 1988.

Lee, C.S., Gogolin-Ewens, K. and Brandon, M.R.: Identification of a unique lymphocyte subpopulation in the sheep uterus. Immunology, 63:157, 1988.

Lotze, M.T.: T-cell growth factors and the treatment of patients with cancer. Clin. Immunol. Immunopathol., 62:S47, 1992.

Lunn, D.P., Holmes, M.A. and Duffus, W.P.: Three monoclonal antibodies identifying antigens on all equine T lymphocytes, and two mutually exclusive T-lymphocyte subsets. Immunology, 74:251, 1991.

Matsushima, K., Baldwin, E.T. and Mukaida, N.: Interleukin-8 and MCAF: novel leukocyte recruitment and activating cytokines. Chem. Immunol., 51:236, 1992.

Melief, C.J.: Tumor eradication by adoptive transfer of cytotoxic T lymphocytes. Adv. Cancer Res., 58:143, 1992.

Melief, C.J. and Kast, W.M.: Cytotoxic T lymphocyte therapy of cancer and tumor escape mechanisms. Semin. Cancer Biol., 2:347, 1991.

Moore, A.S., Theilen, G.H., Newell, A.D., et al.: Preclinical study of sequential tumor necrosis factor and interleukin 2 in the treatment of spontaneous canine neoplasms. Cancer Res., 51:233, 1991.

Moore, M.A.S.: The clinical use of colony stimulating factors. Annu. Rev. Immunol., 9:159, 1991.

Moore, T.C., Spruck, C.H. and LeDuc, L.E.: Depression of lymphocyte traffic in sheep by anaesthesia and associated changes in efferent-lymph PGE2 and antibody levels. Immunology, 63:139, 1988.

Mosmann, T.R. and Moore, K.W.: The role of IL-10 in crossregulation of T_H1 and T_H2 responses. Immunol. Today, 12:A49, 1991.

Naessens, J.: Characterization of lymphocyte populations in African buffalo (Syncerus caffer) and waterbuck (Kobus defassa) with workshop monoclonal antibodies. Vet. Immunol. Immunopathol., 27:153, 1991.

Nagata, S.: Granulocyte colony-stimulating factor. In: Sporn, M.B. Roberts, A.B. (eds), Peptide Growth Factors and Their Receptors I. New York, Springer-Verlag, 1990, p. 697.

Neta, R., Sayers, T.J. and Oppenheim, J.J.: Relationship of TNF to interleukins. Immunol. Ser., 56:499, 1992.

Niwano, Y., Becker, B.A., Mitra, R., et al.: Suppressed peripheral blood lymphocyte blastogenesis in pre- and postpartal sheep by chronic heat-stress, and suppressive property of heat-stressed sheep serum on lymphocytes. Dev. Comp. Immunol., 14:139, 1990.

Novotney, C., English, R.V., Housman, J., et al.: Lymphocyte population changes in cats naturally infected with feline immunodeficiency virus. AIDS, 4:1213, 1990.

Pardi, D., Hoover, E.A., Quackenbush, S.L., et al.: Selective impairment of humoral immunity in feline leukemia virus-induced immunodeficiency. Vet. Immunol. Immunopathol., 28:183, 1991.

Patel, P.M. and Collins, M.K.: Cytokine modulation of cell growth and role in tumour therapy. Eur. J. Cancer, 28:298, 1992.

Perryman, L.E., Leach, D.R., Davis, W.C., et al.: Lymphocyte alterations in zinc-deficient calves with lethal trait A46. Vet. Immunol. Immunopathol., 21:239, 1989.

Perryman, L.E., Wyatt, C.R., Magnuson, N.S., et al.: T lymphocyte development and maturation in horses. Anim. Genet., 19:343, 1988.

Podlaski, F.J., Nanduri, V.B., Hulmes, J.D., et al.: Molecular characterization of interleukin 12. Arch. Biochem. Biophys., 294:230, 1992.

Rees, R.C.: Cytokines as biological response modifiers. J. Clin. Pathol., 45:93, 1992.

Riegel, J.S., Corthesy, B., Flanagan, W.M., et al.: Regulation of the interleukin-2 gene. Chem. Immunol., 51:266, 1992.

Rosenberg, S.A.: Karnofsky Memorial Lecture. The immunotherapy and gene therapy of cancer. J. Clin. Oncol., 10:180, 1992.

Roy, C. and Izaguirre, C.A.: Origin of T lymphocyte colony-forming cells in cell populations depleted of sheep erythrocyte rosette forming cells. Clin. Exp. Immunol., 73:46, 1988.

Saad, A.M., Concha, C. and Astrom, G.: Alterations in neutrophil phagocytosis and lymphocyte blastogenesis in dairy cows around parturition. Zentralbl. Veterinarmed. [B], 36:337, 1989.

Salmi, M. and Jalkanen, S.: Regulation of lymphocyte traffic to mucosa-associated tissues. Gastroenterol. Clin. North Am., 20:495, 1991.

Shaw, A.R.: Molecular biology of cytokines: An introduction. In: Thomson, A. (eds), The Cytokine Handbook. San Diego, Academic Press, 1991.

Shi, L., Kraut, R.P., Aebersold, R., et al.: A natural killer cell granule protein that induces DNA fragmentation and apoptosis. J. Exp. Med., 175:553, 1992.

Spooner, C.E., Markowitz, N.P. and Saravolatz, L.D.: The role of tumor necrosis factor in sepsis. Clin. Immunol. Immunopathol., 62:S11, 1992.

Springer, T.A.: Adhesion receptors of the immune system. Nature, 346:425, 1990.

Stewart, C.C.: Clinical applications of flow cytometry. Immunologic methods for measuring cell membrane and cytoplasmic antigens. Cancer, 69:1543, 1992.

Stoolman, L.M.: Adhesion molecules controlling lymphocyte migration. Cell, 56:907, 1989.

Sulochana, S., James, P.D., Pillai, R.M., et al.: Lymphocyte subpopulations in the peripheral blood of normal and tumor bearing cattle. Ind. J. Ani. Health, 24:117, 1985.

Taylor, B.C., Stott, J.L., Thurmond, M.A., et al.: Alteration in lymphocyte subpopulations in bovine leukosis virus-infected cattle. Vet. Immunol. Immunopathol., 31:35, 1992.

Teramura, M., Kobayashi, S., Hoshino, S., et al.: Interleukin-11 enhances human megakaryocytopoiesis in vitro. Blood, 79:327, 1992.

Thomsen, M.K., Larsen, C.G., Thomsen, H.K., et al.: Recombinant human interleukin-8 is a potent activator of canine neutrophil aggregation, migration, and leukotriene B4 biosynthesis. J. Invest. Dermatol., 96:260, 1991.

Thorp, B.H., Seneque, S., Staute, K., et al.: Characterization and distribution of lymphocyte subsets in sheep hemal nodes. Dev. Comp. Immunol., 15:393, 1991.

Thurmond, M.C., Carter, R.L., Picanso, J.P., et al.: Upper-normal prediction limits of lymphocyte counts for cattle not infected with bovine leukemia virus. Am. J. Vet. Res., 51:466, 1990.

Tompkins, M.B., Gebhard, D.H., Bingham, H.R., et al.: Characterization of monoclonal antibodies to feline T lymphocytes and their use in the analysis of lymphocyte tissue distribution in the cat. Vet. Immunol. Immunopathol., 26:305, 1990a.

Tompkins, M.B., Novotney, C., Grindem, C.B., et al.: Human recombinant interleukin-2 induces maturation and activation signals for feline eosinophils in vivo. J. Leuk. Biol., 48:531, 1990b.

Tompkins, M.B., Ogilvie, G.K., Gast, A.M., et al.: Interleukin-2 suppression in cats naturally infected with feline leukemia virus. J. Biol. Response Mod., 8:86, 1989a.

Tompkins, M.B., Pang, V.F., Michaely, P.A., et al.: Feline cytotoxic large granular lymphocytes induced by recombinant human IL-2. J. Immunol., 143:749, 1989b.

van Damme, J.: Interleukin-8 and related molecules. In: Thomson, A.W. (eds), The Cytokine Handbook. San Diego, Academic Press, 1991, p. 201.

Walcheck, B., White, M., Kurk, S., et al.: Characterization of the bovine peripheral lymph node homing receptor: a lectin cell adhesion molecule (LECAM). Eur. J. Immunol., 22:469, 1992.

Walrand, F., Picard, F., McCullough, K., et al.: Recombinant bovine interferon-gamma enhances expression of class I and class II bovine lymphocyte antigens. Vet. Immunol. Immunopathol., 22:379, 1989.

Whiteside, T.L., Jost, L.M., and Herberman, R.B.: Tumor-infiltrating lymphocytes. Potential and limitations to their use for cancer therapy. Crit. Rev. Oncol. Hematol., 12:25, 1992.

Williams, W.J., Beutler, E., Erslev, A.J., et al.: Hematology. 4th ed. New York, McGraw-Hill, 1990.

Wilson, C.B.: The ontogeny of T lymphocyte maturation and function. J. Pediatr., 118:S4, 1991.

Woldehiwet, Z.: Lymphocyte subpopulations in peripheral blood of sheep experimentally infected with tick-borne fever. Res. Vet. Sci., 51:40, 1991.

Wu, H.K., Hirai, H., Inamori, K., et al.: Anti-tumor effects of interleukin-4 and interleukin-5 against mouse B cell lymphoma and possible mechanisms of their action. Jpn. J. Cancer Res., 83:200, 1992.

Wyatt, C.R., Davis, W.C., McGuire, T.C., et al.: T lymphocyte development in horses. I. Characterization of monoclonal antibodies identifying three stages of T lymphocyte differentiation. Vet. Immunol. Immunopathol., 18:3, 1988.

Interpretation of Leukocyte Parameters

A systematic approach to the evaluation of hematologic data is necessary to make the most of information obtained from the laboratory analysis of blood samples from animal patients. Proper interpretation requires knowledge of the factors that can influence hematologic values. Information about sample size and site of blood collection, laboratory procedures used and their advantages and disadvantages, reference (normal) values, normal cell morphology, species-specific characteristics, and physiologic variations are necessary for recognizing hematologic abnormalities. The functional significance of various blood components and their response to disease, singly or together, are essential for determining the clinical significance of various abnormalities. A thorough history and clinical examination of the patient complements the laboratory findings to diagnose the disease.

Total and differential leukocyte counts, which comprise the leukogram, are valuable hematologic aids in the evaluation of the host's response to microbial infection, and in the diagnosis of leukemias and other diseases. In evaluating a leukogram, it is necessary to know not only the total and differential leukocyte counts, but to recognize that morphologic changes in leukocytes are pertinent, and that ancillary information about other blood components should be obtained. The total plasma protein and fibrinogen concentrations, red cell parameters (PCV, hemoglobin, and RBC count), and nucleated erythrocyte and reticulocyte counts indirectly assist in interpretating the leukogram. Bone marrow findings may have a direct or indirect bearing. Functional defects of leukocytes cannot be detected from the leukogram findings alone.

The art of hemogram interpretation can be mastered with practice and by following a methodical approach that encompasses general and more specific criteria when analyzing laboratory data (Jain, 1986). The discussion here is concerned with the interpretation of leukocyte values. A computer-generated flow chart has been developed to systematize leukogram interpretation (Fig. 18–1). The checklist includes common and unusual abnormal findings so that a more inclusive interpretive approach of leukocytic responses to disease can be developed. A similar approach to the interpretation of erythrocyte parameters is discussed in Chapter 8. Additional information can be found in other veterinary clinical pathology texts (Duncan and Prasse, 1986; Jain, 1986; Meyer et al., 1992; Willard et al., 1989).

TOTAL LEUKOCYTE COUNT

The total leukocyte count varies with the animal species and is influenced by age. It is high at birth and diminishes gradually to attain adult values at 2 to 12 months of age. The total leukocyte count is evaluated for increases (leukocytosis) or decreases (leukopenia) in cell numbers beyond the reference range and to determine the various leukocyte types that cause such changes (Tables 18–1 through 18–5). The suffixes -*cytosis* and -*philia* denote an increase in the leukocyte count, whereas -*penia* indicates a decrease compared to the reference values. Leukocytosis is much more common than leukopenia and is not as serious a prognostic sign as a leukopenia. Leukocytosis may be physiologic, reactive, or proliferative (autonomous).

A change in the total leukocyte count may involve abnormalities of production, release, intravascular distribution, life span, and tissue egress of various leukocytes. For example, circulating neutrophils are in a dynamic equilibrium with neutrophils in the marginal

INTERPRETATION OF LEUKOCYTE PARAMETERS

WBC COUNT
- ☐ Normal
- ☐ Increased
- ☐ Decreased

FIBRINOGEN
- ☐ Normal
- ☐ Increased
- ☐ Decreased

NucRBC
- ☐ Present
- ☐ Absent

RETICULOCYTES
- ☐ Normal
- ☐ Increased
- ☐ Decreased

+ ANEMIA −
- ☐ Blood loss
- ☐ Depression
- ☐ Hemolytic

NEUTROPHILS

COUNT (/µl)
- ☐ Normal
- ☐ Increased
- ☐ Decreased

LEFT SHIFT
1+, 2+, 3+, 4+
- ☐ Regenerative
- ☐ Degenerative
- ☐ Leukemoid
- ☐ Leukoerythr-
  oblastic

MORPHOLOGY
Toxic Changes
- ☐ Vacuolation
- ☐ Basophilia
- ☐ Döhle Bodies
- ☐ Azurophilic granules
- ☐ Polyploidy
- ☐ Bizarre giant forms
- ☐ Leukergy
- ☐ Other

Other Abnormalities
- ☐ Hypersegmentation
- ☐ Pelger Huët Anomaly
- ☐ Chédiak Higashi Syndrome
- ☐ Mucopolysaccharidosis
- ☐ Intracellular objects
- ☐ Other

LYMPHOCYTES

COUNT (/µl)
- ☐ Normal
- ☐ Increased
- ☐ Decreased

TYPE
- ☐ N:L ratio
- ☐ Immature
  - ☐ Prolymph
  - ☐ Lymphblst
- ☐ Immunocytes
- ☐ Atypical/
  Reactive
- ☐ Other

MONOCYTES

COUNT (/µl)
- ☐ Normal
- ☐ Increased
- ☐ Decreased

MORPHOLOGY
- ☐ Normal
- ☐ Activated
- ☐ Immature
- ☐ Macrophages
- ☐ Phagocytic
- ☐ Other

EOSINOPHILS

COUNT (/µl)
- ☐ Normal
- ☐ Increased
- ☐ Decreased

MORPHOLOGY
- ☐ Large grn
- ☐ Vacuolated
- ☐ Other

BASOPHILS

COUNT (/µl)
- ☐ Normal
- ☐ Increased

MORPHOLOGY
- ☐ Normal
- ☐ Immature
- ☐ Other

BONE MARROW MYELOPOIESIS
- ☐ Not done
- ☐ Normal
- ☐ Increased
- ☐ Decreased
- ☐ Left shifted
- ☐ Right shifted
- ☐ M:E ratio
- ☐ Other

CYTOCHEMISTRY IMMUNOPHENOTYPING
- ☐ Myeloid markers
- ☐ Monocytic markers
- ☐ Lymphoid markers

INTERPRETATION
- ☐ Normal
- ☐ Age-related
- ☐ Corticosteroid effect
- ☐ Epinephrine effect
- ☐ Acute inflammation/infection
- ☐ Chronic inflammation/infection
- ☐ Chronic active inflammation
- ☐ Endotoxemia/Septicemia
- ☐ Viral/Rickettsial infection
- ☐ Immune-mediated
- ☐ Parasitic/Allergic
- ☐ Other

- ☐ LEUKOPENIA
  - ☐ Decreased production
  - ☐ Increased destruction
  - ☐ Increased sequestration

- ☐ LEUKOCYTOSIS
  - ☐ Physiologic
  - ☐ Reactive

- ☐ LEUKEMIA
  - ☐ Lymphoid (Acute/Chronic)
  - ☐ Myeloid (Acute/Chronic)
  - ☐ Monocytic (Acute/Chronic)
  - ☐ Myelomonocytic (Acute/Chronic)

Fig. 18–1. Interpretation of leukocyte parameters.

Table 18-1. Causes of Neutrophilia and Neutropenia

Neutrophilia
  Physiologic
    Epinephrine release
    Corticosteroids, endogenous or exogenous
  Reactive
    Established local or systemic infections: bacterial, rickettsial, viral, fungal, parasitic
    Tissue-necrosis
    Immune-mediated diseases: inflammatory (e.g., rheumatoid arthritis) or noninflammatory (e.g., autoimmune hemolytic anemia)
    Tumors
    Estrogen toxicity (early stage)
  Proliferative or autonomous
    Myeloid leukemias, acute or chronic
Neutropenia
  Decreased survival
    Acute bacterial infections
    Septicemia
    Toxemia
    Anaphylaxis
    Hypersplenism
  Decreased production
    Acute infections: bacterial, viral, rickettsial
    Drug toxicity, e.g. estrogen
    Radiation
    Myeloid or lymphoid leukemia
    Canine cyclic hematopoiesis
    Myelophthisis
  Increased ineffective granulopoiesis
    Feline leukemia virus infection
    Myelophthisis
    Acute myeloid or lymphoid leukemia

Table 18-2. Causes of Lymphocytosis and Lymphopenia

Lymphocytosis
  Physiologic
  Chronic suppurative inflammation
  Persistent lymphocytosis in cattle
  Lymphocytosis in young pigs
  Lymphoma
  Lymphocytic leukemia
Lymphopenia
  Corticosteroids
  Viral infection
  Septicemia
  Endotoxemia
  Lymphoma
  Lymphocytic leukemia
  Immunosuppressive drugs
  Radiation
  Immunodeficiency syndromes
  Loss of lymph

Table 18-3. Causes of Monocytosis and Monocytopenia

Monocytosis
  Corticosteroids in dogs
  Chronic infection or inflammation
  Monocytic and myelomonocytic leukemias
  Granulomatous diseases
Monocytopenia
  Acute infection or inflammation
  Corticosteroids (in some species)

Table 18-4. Causes of Eosinophilia and Eosinopenia

Eosinophilia
  Parasitism
  Allergic conditions (IgE-mediated)
  Diseases of certain body tissues or organs rich in mast cells: skin, lungs, uterus, intestine
  Eosinophilic leukemia
  Undefined causes
Eosinopenia
  Epinephrine (β-adrenergic effect)
  Corticosteroids
  Acute infection

Table 18-5. Causes of Basophilia and Basopenia

Basophilia
  Generally in association with eosinophilia
  Basophilic leukemia
Basopenia: not seen

pool (capillary beds) and in the bone marrow reserve. An immediate functional demand of neutrophils is met first by mobilization of cells from the marginal and circulating pools, then from the bone marrow reserve, and finally by increased granulopoiesis and accelerated release. The latter is often reflected in the blood as a left shift. Thus, the size of the marginal and circulating pools, the size of the marrow reserve, and the proliferative capability of the bone marrow are important determinants of the leukocyte response to disease. Generalized causes of increases and decreases in numbers of different leukocytes are presented in Tables 18-1 through 18-5. (See Chapters 13 to 17 for additional information on the responses of various types of leukocytes to disease.) Mast cells are usually present in tissues. They may be found in the blood of about 10% of dogs with mastocytoma or transiently in dogs experiencing severe stress from trauma and/or acute inflammation.

Leukocytosis

PHYSIOLOGIC LEUKOCYTOSIS

Physiologic leukocytosis may occur as an epinephrine response, in which the marginal pools of neutrophils and/or lymphocytes are mobilized into the general circulation, raising the total leukocyte count and absolute neutrophil and/or lymphocyte numbers. Thus, a transient neutrophilia or lymphocytosis, or both, may manifest. It is common in young animals and is generally triggered by emotional and physical disturbances. Rarely, monocyte and eosinophil numbers may also increase (see Chap. 13).

Corticosteroid-induced or "stress" leukocytosis may occur in health or disease, so it may be physiologic or pathologic. Such a response must be distinguished from the epinephrine response. Glucocorticosteroids released endogenously or administered therapeutically cause predictable hematologic changes. They typically produce leukocytosis caused by neutrophilia, usually without a left shift, and also induce lymphopenia and eosinopenia. In addition, monocytosis is characteristic of the dog. Monocytosis occurs inconsistently in the cat, cow, and horse. Monocytopenia is typically seen in humans and laboratory animals. Neutrophilia occurs mainly from the mobilization of segmented (mature) neutrophils from the bone marrow reserve and from the decreased diapedesis of cells into the tissues. In addition, it may partly be the result of a shift of marginal pool cells into the circulation. Lymphopenia occurs mainly from lympholysis of steroid-sensitive T lymphocytes in the blood and lymphoid tissue, or from the margination and sequestration of lymphocytes in extravascular sites. Eosinopenia occurs largely as a result of diminished inflow of cells from the bone marrow because of interference with the chemotactic effect of histamine on eosinophils. The cause of monocytosis remains unknown. The basophil response to corticosteroids is similar to that of eosinophils but is usually not recognized, because basophils are normally rare in blood.

In this context, it is important to note that lymphopenia and eosinopenia are the only consistent changes characteristic of the leukogram in hypercorticism (Cushing's syndrome) in dogs (Table 18–6). In a study of 117 cases of canine Cushing's syndrome, 80% of patients had eosinopenia and lymphopenia, whereas leukocytosis was seen in only 24% of cases (Ling et al., 1979). Conversely, in the absence of glucocorticoid action, the total and differential leukocyte patterns characteristic of the "stress phenomenon" would not be expected. Thus, normal eosinophil counts and normal or elevated lymphocyte numbers in sick dogs should suggest the inclusion of hypoadrenocorticism (Addison's disease) in the differential diagnosis. Formerly, adrenocortical function was indirectly assessed by using the Thorn test, which is based on the premise that, in the presence of a functioning adrenal cortex, an intramuscular injection of ACTH should cause a reduction in lymphocytes and eosinophils and an increase in neutrophils and monocytes. Use of the Thorn test has been supplanted by the direct measurement of plasma cortisol and ACTH levels, which provides a highly accurate assessment of endocrine functions.

REACTIVE LEUKOCYTOSIS

Reactive leukocytosis occurs in response to disease. Certain diseases may induce a specific response, but usually a general pattern of leukocyte response is evident, regardless of disease. A reactive leukocytosis may occur with or without a left shift. The degree of leukocytosis varies with the species and is usually relative to the neutrophil:lymphocyte (N:L) ratio. Animals with a high N:L ratio (dogs and cats) mount a much greater response than animals with a low N:L ratio (horses and cows). In fact, in cattle, reversal of the N:L ratio may be the only indication of a mild inflammatory response. Reversal of the N:L ratio has also been observed in racehorses with "poor performance" syndrome (Fogarty and Leadon, 1987).

Often, a corticosteroid-induced response and, less commonly, an epinephrine-induced response may occur simultaneously with a reactive leukocytosis.

Table 18–6. Hemograms in Canine Hyperadrenocorticism (Cushing's Syndrome)

Parameter	Dog Number								
	1	2	3	4	5	6	7	8	9
Breed	Corgi	Beagle	Boxer	Chihuahua	Poodle	Terrier	Dachshund	Dachshund	Dachshund
Sex	F	M	F	M	XF	XF	M	F	F
Age (yr)	1	6	7	8	10	10	12	6	11
RBC ($\times 10^6/\mu$l)	7.24	4.82	7.39	7.32	4.67	8.00	6.18	8.07	8.19
Hb (g/dl)	17.7	12.7	16.3	18.5	12.1	18.8	15.2	15.3	18.5
PCV (%)	50	37	51	58	36	53	44	44	57
MCV (fl)	69.0	76.7	69.0	79.2	77.0	66.2	71.1	54.5	69.5
MCHC (%)	35.0	34.3	35.9	31.8	33.6	35.4	34.5	34.7	32.4
Plasma proteins (g/dl)	6.8	7.2	7.5	7.8	6.9	6.8	6.5	7.3	9.1
Fibrinogen (g/dl)	0.2	0.5	0.4	0.3	0.7	0.5	0.3	0.4	0.4
Icterus index (units)	2	2	2	2	2	2	2	2	2
ESR (corrected)	1+	39+	2+	0	42+	1+	6+	6+	5+
Nucleated RBC/100 WBC	0	0	0	1	2	0	0	0	0
WBC/μl	11,000	32,300	13,400	12,100	20,550	12,100	7,000	16,400	12,650
Band neutrophil	0	807	201	181	1,332	544	805	1,394	0
Mature neutrophil	9,625	28,585	11,189	10,588	17,015	11,011	4,550	13,038	10,626
Lymphocyte	715	1,292	1,072	666	512	242	490	492	1,075
Monocyte	660	1,615	871	484	1,435	302	1,120	1,394	948
Eosinophil	0	0	67	121	205	0	35	82	0
Basophil	0	0	0	60	0	0	0	0	0
Leukocytes (%)									
Band neutrophil	0	2.5	1.5	1.5	6.5	4.5	11.5	8.5	0
Mature neutrophil	87.5	88.5	83.5	87.5	83.0	91.0	65.0	79.5	84.0
Lymphocyte	6.5	4.0	8.0	5.5	2.5	2.0	7.0	3.0	8.5
Monocyte	6.0	5.0	6.5	4.0	7.0	2.5	16.0	8.5	7.5
Eosinophil	0.0	0.0	0.5	1.0	1.0	0.0	0.5	0.5	0.0
Basophil	0.0	0.0	0.0	0.5	0.0	0.0	0.0	0.0	0.0

Thus, a reactive leukocytosis resulting from disease must be distinguished from a physiologic leukocytosis caused by the endogenous release of corticosteroids or epinephrine. A leukocytosis is considered reactive when one or more of the following are seen concurrently: (1) neutrophilia with a left shift; (2) hyperfibrinogenemia; (3) monocytosis in a species other than the dog; (4) a positive corrected erythrocyte sedimentation rate (ESR); and (5) the absence of a frank lymphopenia or eosinopenia. In the dog, monocytosis should accompany one or more of the other four criteria, or its value (absolute monocyte count) must be greater than twice normal.

PROLIFERATIVE LEUKOCYTOSIS

Proliferative or autonomous leukocytosis results from a neoplastic change in the hematopoietic stem cells. More common forms of leukemia include lymphocytic, myelogenous, myelomonocytic, and monocytic leukemias. Eosinophilic and basophilic leukemias are rare. It should be noted, however, that blood cell cancer does not always manifest as leukocytosis. Sometimes, in leukemias, the leukocyte counts may be normal or even leukopenic, and the cell population in the bone marrow may be abnormal, with little or no evidence of abnormality in the peripheral blood.

Leukopenia

Leukopenias develop mainly from neutropenia and lymphopenia in most animals (Tables 18–1 and 18–2). Neutropenia, however, is the primary cause of leukopenia in animals with an N:L ratio greater than 1, and lymphopenia is a concomitant finding in animals with an N:L ratio less than 1. Neutropenia is more common in bacterial infections, and lymphopenia is common in viral infections. Severe bacterial and viral infections, though, may cause leukopenia associated with both neutropenia and lymphopenia and may also reduce the number of other leukocyte types. Salmonellosis in the horse and coliform mastitis are classic examples of the former, and feline panleukopenia viral infection is an example of the latter. Leukopenia may be seen in some cases of lymphoma and myeloproliferative disorders and is common in myelodysplastic syndrome, particularly in cats. Eosinopenia generally results because of a corticosteroid effect, but it may also occur as a result of the disease. The return of lymphocytes and eosinophils in blood, as determined from sequential hemograms, indicates convalescence, and is generally a good prognostic sign.

Cats infected with panleukopenia virus develop leukopenia from neutropenia and lymphopenia by 2 to 4 days because of depressed myelopoiesis. Anemia and thrombocytopenia manifest in more protracted cases from marked inhibition of erythropoiesis and megakaryocytopoiesis. Similarly, dogs infected with parvovirus develop marked leukopenia from neutropenia and lymphopenia. During convalescence granulopoiesis becomes re-established, and blood at this time may show a marked degenerative left shift (Table 18–7). Initially, the neutrophils released to blood are giant forms, with bizarre nuclear patterns (Plates XV–8, XV–9, and XV–10). Such leukocyte patterns characteristic of the early convalescence of panleukopenic cats must be distinguished from a similar pattern seen in other diseases that seriously depress granulopoiesis (e.g., chronic myelogenous leukemia, Table 18–8, and myelophthisis from lymphoma). Gradually, neutrophil morphology improves, so that by the fourth or fifth day a normal neutrophil morphology is attained. Surviving cats show dramatic changes in the leukogram— from a degenerative left shift to that of a regenerative left shift within a few days.

Leukopenia is believed to occur during the early stage of distemper and is followed by leukocytosis because of secondary bacterial infection. A marked lymphopenia is a consistent feature of distemper (Table 18–9). It is an expression of the widespread atrophy and necrosis of lymphoid tissue produced by

Table 18–7. Rapidly Changing Total and Differential Leukocyte Counts During Convalescence From Panleukopenia in the Cat

	Time Since Admission to Clinic					
	Day 5		Day 6		Day 8	
Parameter	No.	%	No.	%	No.	%
PCV (%)		28		28		31
WBC/µl	1,100	(Corrected)	6,900		36,100	
Blasts	44	4.0	0	0.0	0	0.0
Progranulocytes	11	1.0	69	1.0	0	0.0
Myelocytes	440	40.0	897	13.0	541	1.5
Metamyelocytes	55	5.0	1,518	22.0	2,166	6.0
Bands	22	2.0	2,001	29.0	9,205	25.5
Neutrophils	22	2.0	1,311	19.0	18,411	51.0
Lymphocytes	484	44.0	897	13.0	5,415	15.0
Monocytes	0	0.0	0	0.0	0	0.0
Eosinophils	22	2.0	69	1.0	361	1.0
Basophils	0	0.0	138	2.0	0	0.0
Nucleated RBC/100 WBC	8		0		0	

Table 18–8.   Leukocyte Response to Disease in the Dog

Parameter	Case 1: Pyometra With Regenerative Left Shift	Case 2: Pyometra With Degenerative Left Shift	Case 3: Leukemoid Reaction in Chronic Peritonitis	Case 4: Chronic Myelomonocytic Leukemia
RBC ($\times 10^6/\mu$l)	6.10	6.70	3.90	1.21
Hemoglobin (g/dl)	13.2	13.9	8.6	2.7
PCV (%)	41.0	44.0	25.0	9.0
MCV (fl)	67.0	65.7	64.1	74.4
MCHC (%)	32.2	31.6	34.4	30.0
MCH (pg)	21.6	20.7	22.1	22.3
ESR (mm/hr)	33 +	25 +	33 +	15 +
Reticulocytes (%)	—	—	1.0	0
nRBC/100 WBC	—	0.5	0	Rare
Anisocytosis	Slight	Slight	Slight	Marked
Polychromasia	Slight	—	Slight	Slight
Leptocytosis	—	—	Moderate	—
Icterus index (units)	10	5	2	2
Plasma proteins (g/dl)	8.3	7.5	6.9	—
WBC/μl	59,500	33,200	104,000	116,000
Myeloblasts	0	0	Rare	3,712
Promyelocyte	0	0	Rare	2,784
Myelocytes	298	0	1,040	2,784
Metamyelocytes	7,438	1,826	23,400	1,160
Bands	17,850	11,122	36,920	812
Neutrophils	23,800*	12,118†	38,480‡	53,940
Lymphocytes	3,272	2,324	1,560	22,852**
Monocytes	5,950	4,482	2,600	26,216
Eosinophils	892	0	0	464
Basophils	0	0	0	0
Unclassified cells	—	332	0	1,276
Degenerated cells	—	996	0	0
Platelets/μl	—	—	—	Abnormal
M:E ratio	—	—	—	36.1:1

* Large with basophilic, foamy cytoplasm.
† Slightly basophilic cytoplasm. Atypical left shift.
‡ Cytoplasmia basophilia and polyploid nuclei in some cells.
** May be in error.

the virus. Both T and B lymphocytes are depleted, and cellular and humoral immunity are suppressed in surviving animals. In convalescent dogs, blood lymphocyte numbers remain at low levels for a considerable period. Erythrocyte parameters are near the low-normal range. Although the total plasma concentration may also be within the normal range for the age of the animals, dogs may present with hypoproteinemia or hyperproteinemia. The fibrinogen concentration is also usually normal. The erythrocyte sedimentation rate may be negative or positive.

An important finding is the rare occurrence of distemper inclusions in immature erythrocytes and leukocytes in the blood and, infrequently, in the bone marrow of dogs with distemper (Figs. 18–2 and 18–3; Plates XIV–7 and XVII–9). On electron microscopy,

Table 18–9.   Hemograms in Canine Distemper Grouped on the Basis of Total Leukocyte Count

No. of Dogs	Hemogram Class	RBC ($\times 10^6/\mu$l)	Hb (g/dl)	PCV (%)	Plasma* Proteins (g/dl)	Plasma* Fibrinogen (g/dl)	WBC/μl	Band Neutrophils	Neutrophils	Lymphocytes	Monocytes	Eosinophils	Basophils
8	Leukopenia												
	Range	4.12–7.50	8.6–18.0	26–50	6.0–8.3 (6)	0.4–0.6 (5)	1,300–5,500	0–690	720–4,977	27–360	120–1,240	0–55	0–27
	Mean ± 1 SD	5.61 ± 1.31	12.0 ± 2.8	36 ± 8	6.9 ± 0.8	0.5 ± 0.1	3,863 ± 1,586	237 ± 249	2,858 ± 1,533	227 ± 118	513 ± 334	9 ± 18	3 ± 9
20	Low normal												
	Range	3.08–8.25	6.7–18.1	23–54	5.3–7.6 (10)	0.1–0.8 (9)	6,000–9,500	0–1,974	998–8,052	44–1,653	484–7,315	0–585	0–88
	Mean ± 1 SD	5.48 ± 1.33	12.1 ± 3.0	37 ± 8	6.6 ± 0.9	0.4 ± 0.2	8,185 ± 1,206	349 ± 504	5,737 ± 1,705	582 ± 423	1,384 ± 1,464	99 ± 171	7 ± 21
21	High normal												
	Range	3.74–9.30	7.1–19.6	23–58	4.5–9.4 (15)	0.2–0.6 (11)	9,900–15,300	0–2,632	6,720–12,852	54–994	288–2,550	0–610	0
	Mean ± 1 SD	5.87 ± 1.5	13.1 ± 3.5	40 ± 10	6.6 ± 1.2	0.4 ± 0.1	11,980 ± 1,512	400 ± 600	9,880 ± 1,463	441 ± 249	1,145 ± 552	98 ± 161	0
15	Leukocytosis												
	Range	3.50–6.70	7.5–16.9	25–49	4.9–8.8 (11)	0.2–0.8 (10)	18,000–53,000	0–10,822	8,640–42,480	0–2,976	481–9,824	0–1,800	0–343
	Mean ± 1 SD	5.61 ± 0.9	13.1 ± 2.2	40 ± 6	6.8 ± 1.0	0.6 ± 0.2	30,620 ± 10,663	1,922 ± 3,032	24,593 ± 9,270	577 ± 734	2,845 ± 2,310	221 ± 496	35 ± 94
64	All classes												
	Range	3.08–9.3	6.7–19.6	23–58	4.5–9.4 (42)	0.1–0.8 (35)	1,300–53,000	0–10,822	720–42,480	0–2,976	120–9,824	0–1,800	0–343
	Mean ± 1 SD	5.67 ± 1.3	12.7 ± 3.1	38 ± 8	6.7 ± 1.0	0.5 ± 0.2	14,148 ± 10,846	720 ± 1,676	11,153 ± 9,086	490 ± 467	1,539 ± 1,620	116 ± 282	11 ± 50

* Number in parentheses represents number of samples when less than the total for the group.

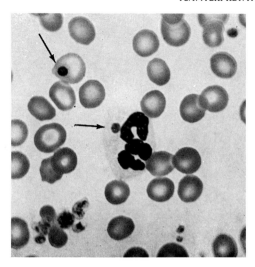

Fig. 18–2. Viral inclusions in an erythrocyte and neutrophil (× 2320). (From Jain, N.C.: Schalm's Veterinary Hematology. 4th Ed. Philadelphia, Lea & Febiger, 1986, p. 1131.)

these inclusions appear to be aggregates of filamentous viral structures (nucleocapsid tubules) compatible with distemper virus (Fig. 18–4). The inclusions are not seen throughout the course of the disease but only during certain periods, and then only occasionally. Usually hardening of the foot pads is also described. In experimental cases of distemper, the inclusions were more frequent in lymphocytes than in neutrophils, and more leukocytes were found to contain inclusions by electron microscopy than by light microscopy.

In dogs infected with canine infectious hepatitis, the leukogram typically shows leukopenia to low-normal WBC counts; the WBC counts for 11 dogs were 1800 to 9500/μl, with a mean value of 5900. Lymphocytes

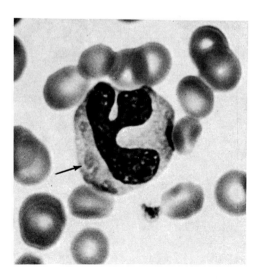

Fig. 18–3. Viral inclusions in a monocyte (× 3870). (From Jain, N.C.: Schalm's Veterinary Hematology. 4th Ed. Philadelphia, Lea & Febiger, 1986, p. 1131.)

decrease more than neutrophils and monocytes remain within the normal ranges. Distinction between activated lymphocytes and monocytes often becomes difficult, however, because of morphologic abnormalities such as dark-staining cytoplasm, irregular nuclear outline, and the presence of small, distinct, azurophilic granules in the cytoplasm. These lymphoid/monocytoid cells occur early in the course of the disease and are replaced by normal lymphocytes and monocytes as convalescence begins. Other important manifestations of the disease are marked thrombocytopenia and disseminated intravascular coagulation. Anemia is not common, but mild to severe nonresponsive anemia normoblastemia without reticulocytosis, and normoproteinemia have been seen in experimentally infected dogs. The icterus index remains within the normal range.

Additional Considerations

Fibrinogen is an acute phase protein. In acute inflammation from various causes, the fibrinogen concentration may become elevated within 3 to 5 days and remain high for days or weeks as the disease becomes chronic. Generally, the fibrinogen response follows the initial leukocytic response, but it persists longer than the leukocyte response. In cows, fibrinogen is an important parameter to evaluate because it may be the only indication of an active inflammatory response. In diseases in which excessive fibrinogen deposition occurs in tissues, the fibrinogen concentration in blood may not be elevated beyond reference values.

A plasma protein to fibrinogen (PP:F) ratio is calculated to determine whether the increase in the fibrinogen concentration is real (because of inflammation or disease) or results from hemoconcentration caused by dehydration. In general, the former is associated with an increase in the fibrinogen level only, and the latter causes increases in both components. In most species, a ratio lower than 10 is considered significant for disease-induced hyperfibrinogenemia and a value between 10 and 15 is considered equivocal.

Nucleated erythrocytes (nRBCs) may be found in blood (normoblastemia) in various conditions, but occur more frequently in association with reticulocytosis in response to anemia (acute blood loss or hemolytic anemia). They are also commonly found in dogs with lead poisoning, in cats and dogs with a myeloproliferative disorder (MPD), and in animals with acute stress and shock, endotoxemia, and septicemia. Normoblastemia in these conditions is unaccompanied by reticulocytosis. The total leukocyte count should be corrected for the presence of nRBCs in blood, because *all* nucleated cells are counted when a total leukocyte count is made using manual or automated methods.

Anemias and the associated erythropoietic response may influence the total and differential leukocyte counts. An intense erythropoietic response to acute blood loss or hemolytic anemia, as evidenced by in-

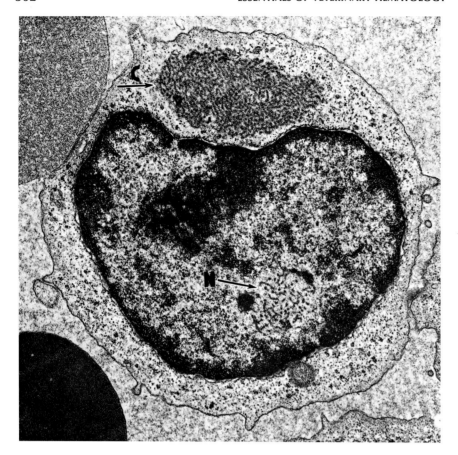

Fig. 18–4. Filamentous viral structures, compatible with canine distemper virus, are present in the nucleus (N) and cytoplasm (C) of a lymphocyte (× 16,500). (From Jain, N.C.: Schalm's Veterinary Hematology. 4th Ed. Philadelphia, Lea & Febiger, 1986, p. 1132.)

creased reticulocytosis in the blood and bone marrow, may be accompanied by leukocytosis and neutrophilia with a left shift. This is probably the result of the generalized stimulation of hematopoietic stem cells in the bone marrow from cytokines produced in response to disease. Conversely, chronic inflammatory conditions suppress erythropoiesis, resulting in a mild, nonresponsive anemia. Prominent reactive leukocytosis, neutrophilia, and monocytosis are common findings in such conditions.

DIFFERENTIAL LEUKOCYTE COUNTS

Quantitative and qualitative changes may occur in various leukocytes (Tables 18–1 through 18–5). Some understanding of the response to disease, disease associations, and pathophysiologic mechanisms of leukocyte abnormalities is essential to evaluate numeric and morphologic changes in leukocytes. Absolute counts rather than percentages of various leukocytes should be used for the interpretation of a leukogram. A total leukocyte count corrected for nRBCs, when present, should be used to calculate the absolute leukocyte count for each cell type, as discussed above. In patients presenting with borderline hematologic abnormalities, sequential hemograms should be obtained to follow patterns of changes in hematologic values, rather than relying on a single observation.

Left Shifts

The peripheral blood normally contains only a small number of immature neutrophils. In most species, these consist of fewer than 300 band cells/μl of blood. The increased release of immature neutrophils from the bone marrow into the blood occurs when the functional demand for neutrophils in tissues increases or in cases of acute and chronic myelogenous or myelomonocytic leukemias. The presence of above-normal numbers of immature neutrophils in blood constitutes a shift to the left. A left shift may be graded 1+ to 4+, depending on the types of myeloid cells found: 1+ (slight), bands only; 2+ (moderate), metamyelocytes; 3+ (marked), myelocytes and promyelocytes; 4+ (extreme), myeloblasts. *The extent of the left shift indicates severity of the disease, whereas the magnitude of the cell count reflects the ability of the bone marrow to meet the demand.* The left shift in reactive leukocytosis is usually pyramidal and complete, whereas in leukemias it is generally nonpyramidal and disordered, and may be hiatal.

In regenerative left shift, the total leukocyte count is slightly to markedly elevated because of neutrophilia and the number of immature neutrophils is usually below that of mature (segmented) neutrophils. It indicates a good host response, and occurs when the bone marrow has had sufficient time (usually 3 to 5 days) to respond to the increasing neutrophil demands in tissues. The bone marrow usually shows myeloid hyperplasia, with normal to increased maturation to segmented neutrophils.

In degenerative left shift, the total leukocyte count varies from being below normal to occasionally slightly elevated. The main feature is the presence of immature neutrophils in excess of mature neutrophils. A degenerative left shift indicates that the bone marrow, at the moment, has a depleted reserve of mature neutrophils and is consequently releasing excessive numbers of immature cells instead of mature neutrophils. It also indicates that the bone marrow either has had insufficient time to respond or cannot meet the overwhelming demand. In most species, it is an unfavorable prognostic sign that requires vigorous therapeutic management. A degenerative left shift in cattle is common, however, during the initial stages of acute to peracute inflammatory or infectious disease. This probably occurs because of a limited supply of mature neutrophils in the bone marrow reserve in this species, so that the supply is rapidly exhausted. Species differences in the regenerative capability of the bone marrow might also be involved. A degenerative left shift in cattle is not considered as serious a prognostic sign as in other species, unless it has persisted for several days.

Occasionally, a leukogram may show an intermediate left shift pattern in that a moderate to marked neutrophilia with immature neutrophils exceeding mature ones or a neutropenia with mature neutrophils predominating the immature cells may be present. These transitional patterns of left shift should be interpreted in light of sequential changes in the leukograms or clinical status of the patient, because they might indicate recovery or worsening of the disease.

Leukemoid Reaction

A leukemoid reaction is generally a reactive leukocytosis consisting of an unusual elevation in the total leukocyte count, or absolute count of a leukocyte type or a marked to extreme left shift suggestive of leukemia. A leukemoid reaction involving neutrophils is generally similar to a regenerative left shift and, infrequently, a severe degenerative left shift may give that indication. Occasionally, a leukemoid blood picture may involve other leukocytes, such as lymphocytes or eosinophils. Additional laboratory findings and clinical evaluation of the patient, however, reveal that the disease is not a leukemia. A physiologic leukocytosis may sometimes mimic a leukemoid reaction. Examples of leukemoid reactions include the following: (1) an extreme regenerative left shift seen in pyometra and chronic active peritonitis in the dog (Table 18–8); (2) a marked lymphocytosis in chronic suppurative conditions (e.g., traumatic reticulitis), a persistent lymphocytosis associated with bovine leukemia virus infection in cattle, or lymphocytosis in kittens, foals, and puppies; (3) salmon disease in dogs, in which aberrant and immature lymphoid and monocytoid cells are present in the blood (Plate XI–6); and (4) extreme eosinophilia from non-neoplastic causes. A leukemoid reaction involving neutrophilic lineage was found to occur as a paraneoplastic syndrome in two dogs with renal carcinoma and adenocarcinoma; the WBC counts in these dogs were 256,000 and 136,800/µl, respectively (Lappin and Latimer, 1988; Madewell et al., 1990).

Leukoerythroblastic Reaction

The presence of nRBCs in association with a left shift characterizes a leukoerythroblastic reaction (LER), which is a nonspecific finding. It may be seen in cases with neutropenia or neutrophilia from various causes. Diseases associated with LER include hematopoietic and nonhematopoietic malignancies, autoimmune hemolytic anemia, autoimmune thrombocytopenia, trauma, myelophthisis, endotoxemia, septicemia, and certain systemic diseases. Generally, LER is attributed to abnormalities of bone marrow architecture that promote the inappropriate release of immature erythroid cells into the blood along with granulocytes. If anemia is a concomitant finding, the designation "leukoerythroblastic anemia," can be used.

MORPHOLOGIC CHANGES IN LEUKOCYTES

Various morphologic abnormalities, acquired and hereditary, may be found in neutrophils and, less commonly, in other leukocytes (Table 13–7).

Bacterial toxins, toxic products of metabolism, and products of tissue necrosis may affect leukocytes in the blood and bone marrow. The toxic influences of these substances are noticed chiefly in neutrophil morphology; these changes include basophilia of cytoplasm resulting from the retention of cytoplasmic ribonucleic acid (Plate VIII–11), cytoplasmic vacuolation and foaminess from restricted cytolysis by digestive enzymes released intracellularly from lysosomal granules (Plate VIII–12), Döhle bodies as remnants of RER (Plates IX–2 and XII–6), azurophilic granules from the retention of acid mucopolysaccharides in the primary granules generally lost after the promyelocyte stage (Plates XI–12 and XV–12), and polyploidy and bizarre giant forms resulting from reduced mitosis or early maturation (Plates IX–4, XV–8, XV–9, and XV–10). The first two types of changes are the most common morphologic abnormalities in leukocytes. Döhle bodies are common in cats and horses, and giant bizarre neutrophils are frequently seen in cats during the early stage of recovery from toxic granulopoiesis. Azurophilic granules are more frequent in cattle, sheep, and horses than in dogs and cats. Leukergy is the nonspecific clumping of neutrophils, occasionally seen in the blood of horses with acute inflammatory disease (Plate XII–7).

Artifactual morphologic changes, such as slight vacuolation of cytoplasm, uneven distribution of cytoplasmic granules, irregular cell membrane, and pyknosis, may occur in canine neutrophils as storage artifacts in EDTA-anticoagulated blood (Gossett and Carakostas, 1984). Such morphologic artifacts are not seen in smears prepared within 1 hour of blood collection. These mild morphologic changes, however, should be distinguished from toxic changes in neutrophils associated with infectious and inflammatory diseases. Compared to normal leukocytes, leukemic cells are more prone to such artifacts.

Hypersegmentation (five or more lobes) of neutrophil nuclei may result from the aging of blood in vitro but, more commonly, it indicates the increased intravascular sojourn of cells as a corticosteroid effect. Increased numbers of hypersegmented neutrophils in the blood is referred to as a right shift. Hypersegmentation occurs in humans with macrocytic normochromic anemia caused by vitamin B_{12} and folate deficiency. It may occur in certain poodles with red cell macrocytosis simulating vitamin B_{12}-folate deficiency. Rarely, it may be an idiopathic finding (Plate XI–7).

Hyposegmentation of neutrophil nuclei occurs less commonly. It is of hereditary occurrence in dogs and cats with Pelger-Hüet anomaly and is detected as an incidental finding (Plate IX–5). An occasional Pelger-Hüet cell may be found in the blood of any species as an acquired abnormality (Plate IX–6). The functional competence of Pelger-Hüet cells may be slightly reduced, but the host's defense is not compromised.

Chédiak-Higashi syndrome is an inherited anomaly in which the formation of lysosomal granules is aberrant. It occurs in several species, including cats, cattle, Aleutian mink, and humans. Neutrophils, eosinophils, and monocytes have unusually large granules (Plates IX–10, IX–11, IX–12). Such neutrophils are phagocytically active, but their bacterial killing ability is reduced because of defective degranulation. In mucopolysaccharidosis, neutrophils, lymphocytes, and monocytes may show a few large, azurophilic granules (Plates XIII–1 to XIII–4). An occasional granule has a prominent halo around it. This granulation is not a toxic effect, but is a manifestation of the genetic absence of enzymes involved in the catabolism of acid mucopolysaccharides. The disease has been reported in dogs and cats (for a discussion of other neutrophil anomalies, see Chap. 13).

Intracellular inclusions or organisms may be found in leukocytes in the blood and/or bone marrow in certain diseases. Examples include the following: (1) distemper inclusions in lymphocytes, monocytes, and neutrophils (Plate XIV–7; Figs. 18–2, 18–3); (2) Ehrlichia equi morulae in neutrophils and, rarely, in eosinophils of horses and dogs (Plates XIV–1, XIV–2, and XIV–3); (3) Ehrlichia canis morulae in lymphocytes, neutrophils, and monocytes of dogs (Plates XIII–5, XIII–6, and XIV–4); (4) phagocytized platelets, erythrocytes, and bacteria in neutrophils and monocytes (Plates XIV–10 and XV–6 and Fig. 6–1D); (5) Leishmania, Histoplasma, and Toxoplasma organisms in bone marrow macrophages (Plates XIV–8 and XIV–

9); (6) Chlamydia in a neutrophil (Plate XIV–5); and (7) sideroleukocytes in the blood in equine infectious anemia or idiopathic anemia (Plate XIV–11). Gamonts of Hepatozoon canis may be found in the cytoplasm of occasional neutrophils in Giemsa-stained blood films, but are best observed after staining with a modified naphthol ASD-chloroacetate esterase method (Mercer and Craig, 1988). Leukopenia associated with lymphopenia and neutropenia are characteristic of toxoplasmosis in the cat and may be accompanied by Döhle bodies as a toxic change in the neutrophils.

Lymphocyte morphology should be carefully examined for cytoplasmic and nuclear changes. Immunocytes are small to medium-sized cells with deep blue cytoplasm. They are B lymphocytes engaged in antibody synthesis, and are occasionally found in the blood in diseases associated with prolonged antigenic stimulation of the immune system. Plasma cells are extremely rare in blood, even in animals with multiple myeloma. Atypical or reactive lymphocytes are abnormal cells other than immature lymphocytes. They may be found in leukemic and nonleukemic conditions and sometimes may be storage artifacts in anticoagulated blood. Large, bizarre lymphocytes with lobed or irregular nuclei (Reider's cells) are atypical lymphocytes and monocytoid lymphocytes in salmon disease in dogs are reactive lymphocytes. Atypical lymphoid-monocytoid cells with dark-staining cytoplasm, with or without azurophilic granules, are found in dogs during early periods of infection with infectious canine hepatitis. Immature lymphocytes include lymphoblasts and prolymphocytes. A lymphoblast has a round nucleus with fine or coarse well-dispersed chromatin, one or more distinct or indistinct nucleoli, and a high nucleus: cytoplasm ratio (Plates XIX–1 and XIX–2). A prolymphocyte resembles a lymphoblast except that it lacks nucleoli (Plate XIX–4). Immature lymphocytes are diagnostic of acute lymphocytic leukemia or lymphoma, although an occasional lymphoblast is found in the blood of normal cattle. Prominent cytoplasmic vacuoles occur in many lymphocytes in lysosomal storage diseases like gangliosidosis, fucosidosis, and mannosidosis (Plates IX–7 and IX–8) and prominent coarse azurophilic granules are found in some lymphocytes besides monocytes and neutrophils in mucopolysaccharidosis (Plates XIII–1 and XIII–2).

Immature monocytes, promonocytes and monoblasts, are found in the blood and bone marrow in acute and chronic monocytic and myelomonocytic leukemias (Plates XXVI–2 to XXVI–4). Monoblasts and promonocytes have round, cauliflower-like nuclei with a characteristic convoluted nuclear membrane and stippled or stringy chromatin. Nucleoli are present in monoblasts but not in promonocytes, which have more abundant cytoplasm than monoblasts. Sometimes, seemingly immature monocytes, not necessarily promonocytes or monoblasts, are found in dogs with chronic inflammatory conditions. These cells have large ameboid nuclei, but the nuclear chromatin is finely stippled or stringy and the cytoplasm is more basophilic than usual for a monocyte.

The activation or transformation of monocytes to macrophages occurs in tissues but, rarely, may occur in the circulation. Activated monocytes in blood resemble macrophages in that they have abundant, vacuolated cytoplasm, with or without fine, pinkish granules. Such cells may be found in the blood in certain conditions, such as subacute bacterial endocarditis in the dog (Plate VIII–10).

Morphologic abnormalities are rare in eosinophils and basophils. Eosinophil granules in the dog are normally small and uniformly stained, and an occasional granule may be partially vacuolated. In rare cases of eosinophilia, eosinophil granules as large as erythrocytes may be found (Plate XII–2) and granule vacuolation may be slightly more exaggerated (Plate IX–9). Rarely, a mature eosinophil may also contain a few small, dark reddish-purple, "toxic" granules. Basophils in the cat usually have small, round, light pink or orange granules compared to the deep magenta granules typical of other species (compare Plates VII–5, VII–6, and VII–7). Sometimes, basophils with a few to many reddish-purple granules may be found in the blood of cats with basophilia (Plate XII–5). The bone marrow of cats contains developing basophils (myelocytes and metamyelocytes) with large, deep purple and light pink or orange granules as a species characteristic (Plates V–2 and XII–4). The significance of these findings is unknown.

BONE MARROW EVALUATION

A bone marrow examination is necessary to evaluate changes in blood cells properly, particularly cytopenias. Whenever possible, the bone marrow examination should be performed simultaneously with the blood examination. Changes in the rates of myelopoiesis and erythropoiesis influence the myeloid:erythroid (M:E) ratio. The M:E ratio varies with the species, but is generally greater than unity. An M:E ratio greater than the reference value may result from increased granulopoiesis or decreased erythropoiesis. Conversely, an M:E ratio less than the reference value may be the result of decreased granulopoiesis or increased erythropoiesis. Therefore, the neutrophil and reticulocyte numbers in blood must be obtained to determine how changes in respective bone marrow hematopoietic activities are reflected in blood. Generally, increased effective myelopoiesis results in neutrophilia, whereas decreased myelopoiesis is reflected as neutropenia. In right-shifted granulopoiesis, mature and band neutrophils combined are more numerous, whereas in left-shifted marrow these cells are less numerous compared to all cells, from metamyelocytes through myeloblasts. The myeloid maturation index is high in the former and low in the latter. Left-shifted marrow is common in patients with neutropenias, but right-shifted marrow is found in those with neutrophilias resulting from established inflammatory conditions or infections. Toxic changes in cell morphology may also be present in bone marrow myeloid cells.

Bone marrow findings vary in leukemias. Increased numbers of lymphocytes may be seen in bone marrow in a small percentage of cases of lymphocytic leukemia in dogs and cats. Lymphocytes are more common in lymphocytic leukemia in calves than in adult cattle. Acute myeloid leukemias are characterized by highly left-shifted granulopoiesis. The blast cell population in these cases is usually greater than 30%. In comparison, granulopoiesis in chronic leukemias is intensified but appears to be irregularly right-shifted, and the blast cell population is above normal but less than 30%. Monocytes and their precursors are rarely identified in normal bone marrow, but are increased in acute and chronic monocytic and myelomonocytic leukemias. Increased numbers of monocytes may also be seen in some chronic inflammatory conditions, such as pyometra (Table 18–8).

Increased numbers of eosinophils and basophils are occasionally found in the bone marrow but their significance, other than a heightened granulopoiesis from some undetermined cause, remains unknown. The bone marrow of cows usually contains more eosinophils than that in other species; this probably reflects the higher blood eosinophil count in this species.

CYTOCHEMICAL PROFILE OF LEUKEMIC LEUKOCYTES

Cytochemical analyses can be performed to determine cell lineage in acute leukemias in the dog and cat (Jain, 1989; Jain et al., 1991). The cytochemical staining of blood and bone marrow smears is essential to differentiate the blast cells found in acute myeloid leukemias from those found in acute lymphocytic leukemias. Acute myeloid leukemias can be subclassified into acute myelogenous, myelomonocytic, and monocytic leukemias. Suitable cytochemical markers of neutrophils include positive reactions with peroxidase (Plates X–4 and X–6), Sudan black B (Plate X–7), and chloroacetate esterase (Plates X–8 and X–9). Nonspecific esterase (NSE) is a commonly used marker for monocytes (Plates X–8 and X–9). Lymphocytes do not react for these enzymes except for some NSE activity, which can be distinguished from that in monocytes by its staining pattern and resistance to fluoride inhibition. Monocytes usually show a slight to strong diffuse cytoplasmic NSE activity that can be inhibited by sodium fluoride, but lymphocytes when positive reveal a coarsely globular localized cytoplasmic activity that is resistant to fluoride inhibition. Neutrophils of the dog and cat normally lack alkaline phosphatase (ALP) activity (Plates X–2 and X–3). In these species, increased numbers of ALP-positive cells are usually found in acute myeloid leukemias (Plate XXV–6), increased numbers of NSE-positive cells are seen in acute monocytic leukemia, and both ALP-positive and NSE-positive cells occur in acute myelomonocytic leukemia (Plates XXVI–5 and XXVI–6). Peroxidase activity and sudanophilia manifest in unison and usually characterize the neutrophilic component in acute myeloid leukemias that present equivocal morphologic features.

A major limitation of the application of cytochemical staining in the identification of cell lineage in leukemias is that the diagnosis of acute lymphocytic leukemia is by a negative cytochemical profile (Plate XIX–6). Highly undifferentiated myeloid and monocytic stem cells may also stain negative or poorly with routinely used methods. In such cases, it is important to consider the combined results of various cytochemical reactions, as a cytochemical profile, rather than individual results, to arrive at a conclusion. Additional cytochemical markers, electron microscopy, and the ultrastructural demonstration of peroxidase may be useful in some cases to determine cell lineage. More importantly, the immunophenotyping of leukemic cells by the use of lineage-specific monoclonal antibodies is now in vogue for the classification of acute leukemias in humans. This diagnostic approach to the classification of acute leukemias in animals is forthcoming, although it is now limited by the availability of lineage- and species-specific monoclonal antibodies.

SUMMARY

The proper interpretation of a leukogram requires several considerations, such as the age and clinical evaluation of the patient, total and differential leukocyte counts, leukocyte morphology, N:L ratio, bone marrow cytology, and certain ancillary hemogram findings. Age-related changes include high lymphocyte counts in young animals and a slight increase in the N:L ratio with age. Physiologic leukocytosis resulting from the effects of epinephrine is reflected in neutrophilia and/or lymphocytosis, exclusively because of increases in mature cells. It is common in young animals, but may also occur in adults. Corticosteroids, released endogenously in diseased animals or administered exogenously, induce predictable changes in leukocyte counts. Corticosteroid effects in a leukogram typically manifest as leukocytosis, neutrophilia, lymphopenia, and eosinopenia. In addition, monocytosis is characteristic of the dog, but is infrequent in other species. Thus, convalescence is heralded by the return of lymphocytes and eosinophils to the blood.

An acute inflammatory response or bacterial infection is associated with slight to moderate neutrophilia, with or without a left shift, whereas monocytosis generally indicates the chronic nature of the disease process. A marked, persistent neutrophilia may be seen in chronic suppurative conditions, such as abscess formation. Neutrophilia with a variable left shift may also occur in various noninfectious conditions, such as a postoperative state and responsive anemias. A chronic active inflammatory process is characterized by monocytosis, neutrophilia with or without a left shift, and ancillary hematologic changes, such as a positive erythrocyte sedimentation rate and hyperfibrinogenemia. Severe endotoxemia and septicemia initially produce a neutropenia or degenerative left shift, which later transforms into a neutrophilia or regenerative left shift as the condition improves. Uncomplicated viral and rickettsial infections are usually associated with leukopenia, neutropenia, and lymphopenia. Eosinophilia is common in conditions associated with the continuous degranulation of mast cells, as in certain parasitic infections and allergic (IgE-mediated) conditions. Immune-mediated neutropenia is rare in humans; it remains to be defined in veterinary medicine. Mast cells may be found in the blood of dogs with mastocytoma or transiently in those with severely stressful conditions.

Morphologic changes in leukocytes are commonly the result of the deleterious effects of exogenous or endogenous toxic substances, and rarely are caused by hereditary diseases. Viral inclusions, rickettsial morulae, bacteria, and protozoa may sometimes be found in circulating leukocytes during systemic infections. Acute or chronic myeloid and lymphoid leukemias can be diagnosed cytologically based on leukocyte counts, cell morphology, and the cytochemical profile. Immunophenotyping, however, may be necessary to diagnose cytologically equivocal cases of acute leukemias.

REFERENCES

Duncan, J.R. and Prasse K.W.: Veterinary laboratory medicine. 2nd ed. Ames, Iowa State University Press, 1986, pp. 31–60.
Fogarty, U. and Leadon, D.: Poor performance syndrome: A review of the literature and some data on the haematological and blood biochemical changes in two groups of thoroughbred racehorses performing below expectation. Irish Vet. J., 41:203, 1987.
Gossett, K.A. and Carakostas, M.C.: Effect of EDTA on morphology of neutrophils of healthy dogs with inflammation. Vet. Clin. Pathol., 13:22, 1984.
Jain, N.C.: Schalm's Veterinary Hematology. 4th ed. Philadelphia, Lea & Febiger, 1986, pp. 821–837.
Jain, N.C.: Cytochemistry of canine and feline leukocytes and leukemias. In: Kirk, R. (eds), Current Veterinary Therapy X—Small Animal Practice. Philadelphia, W.B. Saunders Co., 1989, p. 465.
Jain, N.C., Blue, J.T., Grindem, C.B., et al.: A report of the animal leukemia study group: Proposed criteria for classification of acute myeloid leukemia in dogs and cats. Vet. Clin. Pathol., 20: 63, 1991.
Lappin, M.R. and Latimer, K.S.: Hematuria and extreme neutrophilic leukocytosis in a dog with renal tubular carcinoma. J. Am. Vet. Med. Assoc., 192:1289, 1988.
Ling, G.V., Stabenfeldt, G.H., Comer, K.M., et al.: Canine hyperadrenocorticism: Pretreatment clinical and laboratory evaluation of 117 cases. J. Am. Vet. Med. Assoc., 174:1211, 1979.
Madewell, B.R., Wilson, D.W., Hornof, W.J., et al.: Leukemoid blood response and bone marrow infarcts in a dog with renal tubular adenocarcinoma. J. Am. Vet. Med. Assoc., 197:1623, 1990.
Mercer, S.H. and Craig, T.M.: Comparison of various staining procedures in the identification of Hepatozoon canis gamonts. Vet. Clin. Path., 17:63, 1988.
Meyer, D.T., Coles, E.H. and Rich, L.J.: Veterinary Laboratory Medicine Interpretation and Diagnosis. Philadelphia, W.B. Saunders Co., 1992, pp. 27–42.
Willard, M.D., Tvedten, H., and Turnwald, G.H.: Small Animal Clinical Diagnosis by Laboratory Methods. Philadelphia, W.B. Saunders Co., 1989, pp. 57–85.

The Leukemias: General Aspects

Neoplastic processes involving hematopoietic cells can be grouped broadly as myeloproliferative and lymphoproliferative disorders. A myeloproliferative disorder (MPD) is a disorder of the hematopoietic stem cells concerned with the production of the granulocytic, monocytic, erythrocytic, and megakaryocytic series, whereas a lymphoproliferative disorder (LPD) is restricted to the cells of the lymphoid series (Table 19-1).

Leukemia is a neoplastic disease involving one or more cell types of the hematopoietic tissues. Typically, the total leukocyte (WBC) count is extremely elevated or above normal and abnormal or primitive cells are present in the blood, which permit the diagnosis to be made. The neoplastic proliferation of hematopoietic cells, however, is not always associated with leukocytosis, and the neoplastic blood cells may not be observed in blood films. In fact, in some instances, leukopenia may exist, as is common in lymphoma. The diagnosis of leukemia becomes challenging when a leukopenia is present, when the neoplastic cells are either absent (aleukemic leukemia) or present in such a low number (subleukemic leukemia) as to defy diagnosis, or when an extreme leukocytosis occurs mainly because of increases in more differentiated cells (leukemoid reaction). The diagnosis in such cases might require the examination of buffy coat smears for abnormal cells, several sequential blood examinations, and cytologic examination of other hematopoietic tissues such as the bone marrow, lymph nodes, and spleen. Sometimes, hematologic abnormalities of an undefined nature may precede the development of a recognizable leukemia; the condition is then referred to in retrospect as a myelodysplastic syndrome (MDS), preleukemia, or smoldering leukemia (Bennett, 1986).

The leukemias may further be categorized as acute or chronic based on cellular maturity, apparent onset, and clinical course. Acute leukemias are characterized by the presence of predominantly immature (blast) cells in the blood and/or hematopoietic tissues and a relatively shorter clinical course. The clinical course of the disease may, however, change with therapy. In

Table 19–1. Classification of Hematopoietic Neoplasms

Myeloproliferative disorders
  Acute myeloid leukemia
    AUL: Acute undifferentiated leukemia
    M0: Minimally differentiated myeloblastic leukemia
    M1: Myeloblastic leukemia without differentiation
    M2: Myeloblastic leukemia with differentiation
    M3: Promyelocytic leukemia
    M4: Myelomonocytic leukemia
    M5: Monocytic leukemia
    M6: Erythroleukemia (M6-Er, M6 with erythroid predominance)
    M7: Megakaryocytic leukemia
  Chronic myeloid leukemia
    Chronic myelogenous leukemia
    Chronic eosinophilic leukemia
    Chronic basophilic leukemia
    Chronic monocytic leukemia
    Chronic myelomonocytic leukemia
  Myelodysplastic syndromes
    Refractory anemia
    Refractory anemia with excess blasts
    Refractory anemia with excess blasts "in transformation"
    Erythremic myelosis (acute or chronic; MDS-Er, MDS with erythroid predominance)
  Others
    Polycythemia vera
    Essential (primary) thrombocythemia
    Mast cell leukemia
    Histiocytic medullary reticulosis (malignant histiocytosis)
Lymphoproliferative disorders
  Lymphocytic
    Lymphoma
    Acute lymphoblastic leukemia
    Acute prolymphocytic leukemia
    Chronic lymphocytic leukemia
    "Histiocytic lymphoma" or "reticulum cell sarcoma"
    Hodgkin's or Hodgkin's-like disease
    Burkitt's lymphoma
  Plasmocytic
    Multiple myeloma
    Waldenström's macroglobulinemia

Table 19–2.   Cytologic and Cytochemical Features of Blood and Bone Marrow Cells in Leukemia*

Characteristic	Lymphocytic†	Granulocytic†	Monocytic†
Cell size	Usually small	Usually large	Usually large
Nuclear shape	Round to oval, smooth contour, rare clefting or slight indentation	Round to oval, smooth contour	Irregular, smooth or clefted contour; nuclear folds may be present
Nuclear chromatin	Fine to coarsely granular (gravel-like) or clumped	Finely stippled (sand-like)	Finely stippled or reticular (linearly fibrillar)
Nucleoli	One or more; distinct or inconspicuous	One or more; distinct or inconspicuous	One or more; distinct or inconspicuous
Amount of cytoplasm	Scant to moderately abundant	Moderately abundant	Moderately abundant
Nuclear: cytoplasmic ratio	High	Low to high	Low to high
Cytoplasmic basophilia	Slight to marked	Moderate	Moderate
Cytoplasm	Smooth, featureless, rarely vacuolated	Ground glass-like; no vacuoles unless toxic	Grayish blue, foamy or vacuolated
Azurophilic granules	Generally absent; rarely, few and large	Many, small but distinct	Usually absent; sometimes fine and indistinct
Specific granules	−	+	−
Cytochemical markers			
Peroxidase	−	+, usually strong	+, usually weak
Alkaline phosphatase	−	+, some cells	−
Lipase	−	−	+
Nonspecific esterase	−	−	+
Cell rafts	−	+	+
Proliferative cell line	Recognizable lymphocytic	Maturation toward neutrophilic series	Maturation toward monocytic cells

* Cell morphology varies with the patient and with time in the same patient. All cytologic criteria do not manifest in every case; mixed leukemias are sometimes encountered.

† −, absent; +, present.

humans, the presence of more than 30% blast cells in the bone marrow is considered sufficient for the diagnosis of acute myeloid leukemia (AML) and this is also true for the dog and cat. Blast cells are found in the blood of almost all dogs and cats with AML, but only about one-third have more than 30% circulating blast cells. Chronic leukemias are characterized by the predominance of mature leukocytes in the blood and bone marrow and a relatively longer clinical course. Similarly, a chronic MPD, such as essential thrombocythemia or polycythemia vera, show an overabundance of circulating platelets and mature red cells, respectively.

A number of cytomorphologic features have been found helpful in distinguishing among lymphocytic, myelogenous, and monocytic cell lines in leukemic patients (Table 19-2). Although acute lymphocytic leukemias (ALL) and AML with some lineage specific differentiation can usually be distinguished, acute leukemias comprised essentially of blast cells with little differentiation in regard to typical cell types are often difficult to classify. In such cases, cytochemical staining, electron microscopy, cytogenetic analysis and, more recently, immunophenotyping have been found useful. Chronic lymphocytic leukemias (CLL) and chronic myelogenous leukemias (CML) can be readily distinguished based on their distinctive cell morphology.

INCIDENCE AND CAUSES OF LEUKEMIA

The incidence of leukemia varies with the type of leukemia, the species involved, and the geographic location (Jain, 1986; Williams et al., 1990). Although leukemia can occur at any age, myeloid leukemias are common in young animals. A study published in 1983 reported the annual incidence for all leukemias per 100,000 cats or dogs as 224.3 and 30.5, respectively (Schneider, 1983). Cats had 6.1 times more lymphoma and 15.7 times more MPD than dogs. In the cat, a bimodal age pattern was seen for all leukemias and for lymphoma alone, and a single early peak was seen for MPD. In the dog, all age-specific patterns increased with age and peaked later in life. Neutered female cats and neutered male dogs were at the lowest risk. Neutering decreased the risk of leukemia in the female cat by approximately 50%, but not in the dog. The age and sex preferences resembled those in humans. The overall incidence of ALL and AML in humans is about equal, but the former is more common in childhood and the latter is prevalent in adults. The incidence increases with age and is slightly higher in males than in females (1.3:1). A recent study showed that dogs less than 6 months in age were 3.3 times more likely to have a hematopoietic neoplasm than dogs over 6 months of age (Keller and Madewell, 1992). Age, sex, and breed patterns and the influence of other factors, such as season, however, might not be apparent.

The causes of leukemia are being extensively investigated and still remain elusive. Although the molecular mechanisms associated with the neoplastic transformation of the cell are unknown, cellular abnormalities leading to leukemia may develop as a result of certain viral infections, exposure to certain chemicals or physical agents, genomic alterations, defective immune surveillance, or undefined causes. One or more of these factors may act in concert in the development of leukemia. Benzene, alkylating agents, and radiation are documented leukemogenic agents.

A viral cause of leukemia was first postulated by Ellermann and Bang, in 1908, who reported the transmission of avian leukemia to two of five chickens given cell-free material. More recently, leukemias and lymphomas of seemingly viral origin have been reported to occur in a wide variety of species, such as chickens, rodents, cats, cattle, sheep, and nonhuman primates. In addition, human T-cell leukemia-lymphoma virus (HTLV-I) has been found to have a causative association with adult T-cell leukemias in humans from southern Japan and the Caribbean (Williams et al., 1990). Genetic or vertical transmission has also been demonstrated in studies on leukemia in mice. The avian and murine leukemogenic viruses can cause different forms of leukemia and tumors, depending to some extent on the dose, route of infection, and genetic make-up of the host. Leukemogenic viruses may be present in some mice throughout life without producing leukemia. A high incidence of leukemia could be induced in these virus-infected mice, however, by exposure to x-irradiation. Such observations are consistent with the "multihit theory" of oncogenesis, which states that cancer development requires at least two steps. Retrovirus is an example of the first step; excessive radiation is an example of the second step.

The viral induction of tumorigenesis has been attributed to particular gene sequences carried by the virus, termed "viral oncogenes" (Williams et al., 1990). Similar genes are found in normal uninfected vertebrate cells and these are referred to as cellular oncogenes or proto-oncogenes. Proto-oncogenes have been found to give rise to corresponding viral oncogenes during the course of viral infection of a cell—for example, c-src gives rise to v-src and c-mic to v-mic. Proto-oncogenes regulate the proliferation and differentiation of normal cells and are potentially tumorigenic. They are classified according to their location or biologic activity of their protein products, such as growth factors and their cell surface receptors. The activation of proto-oncogenes through mutation, gene amplification, gene rearrangement, or retroviral infection has been implicated in the pathogenesis of hematopoietic malignancies in humans. For example, in humans, the N-ras gene has been demonstrated in AML and MDS, c-myc in B-cell lymphomas, B-cell ALL, and T-cell ALL, and c-abl gene in CML. FeLV induced diseases may be caused by an activation of cellular proto-oncogenes, particularly *myc* gene, or by viral mutation of FeLV-A (Jarrett, 1991).

Viruses are classified by ultrastructural examination as A, B, and C types and by their nucleic acid content as RNA or DNA viruses. The avian, murine, and feline leukemia viruses are C-type RNA viruses and are further classified as oncornaviruses. Although most RNA viruses are retroviruses (contain RNA-dependent DNA polymerase—reverse transcriptase), only a few are oncogenic. Reverse transcriptase activity and par-

ticles of retroviral density have been found in short-term cultures of lymphoid tissue from sheep and dogs with lymphocytic leukemia or lymphoma. A few DNA viruses have been associated with tumor formation (e.g., Epstein-Barr virus with Burkitt's lymphoma in humans, Marek's disease virus with Marek's lymphoma of T cells in chickens, and Herpes sylvilagus with lymphoma in cottontail rabbits).

CLONAL ORIGIN OF LEUKEMIAS

Current concepts of hematopoietic differentiation are summarized in Figure 4-6. In human studies, it has been shown that most hematopoietic neoplasms have a clonal origin. For example, chromosomal analyses and the determination of glucose-6-phosphate dehydrogenase (G-6-PD) isoenzymes have shown that CML originates from the multipotential myeloid stem cell; thus, such abnormalities are expressed not only in mature neutrophils, but also in the erythroid and megakaryocytic series. In comparison, AML originates primarily at the committed myeloid stem cell level and ALL from committed lymphoid stem cells.

Although most hematopoietic neoplasms, being clonal in origin, are often characterized by the predominance of a single cell line, the disease sometimes appears to involve two cell lines, but rarely more (Fig. 19-1). Rarely, leukemic clones of lymphoid and myeloid cells may proliferate in the same patient, thereby indicating a neoplastic involvement of the pluripotential stem cell or its uncommitted progeny. It has also been recognized that hematopoietic malignancies are progressive. Thus, the disease involving a single cell line may progress or change to involve other cell lines—for example, AML may evolve into acute myelomonocytic leukemia (AMMoL). Myelodysplastic syndromes involving the clonal proliferation of hematopoietic stem cells slowly progress into a mixed or well-defined leukemia (e.g., erythremic myelosis transforms into erythroleukemia and in turn into myelogenous leukemia). In some cases, transformations may occur within the same cell line, so that different patterns of cellular differentiation become apparent (e.g., the "blast crisis" of CML in humans). Such changes may occur rapidly within weeks or slowly over a period of months or years. Progressions or conversions are more common in an MPD than in an LPD. Rarely, hybrid or mixed leukemias may occur (Catovsky et al., 1991; Ruiz-Arguelles et al., 1988; Sun et al., 1991). Mixed leukemias can be biphenotypic (e.g., having blast cells with markers for two cell lines, such as both lymphoid and myeloid markers) or bilineal (e.g., having blast cells of two separate cell lines, such as some blast cells with lymphoid features and others with myeloid features). Such leukemias probably arise from neoplastic transformation of multipotent hematopoietic stem cells.

The mechanisms associated with the clonal expansion of leukemic stem cells have not been delineated. An interplay among the hematopoietic inductive mi-

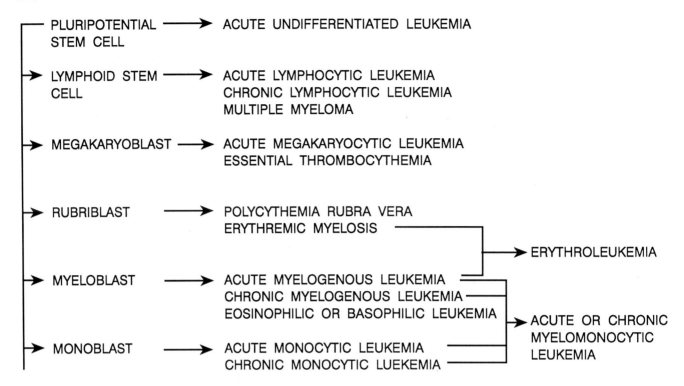

Fig. 19–1. Neoplasms of blood cells.

croenvironment, hematopoietic growth factors, surface receptors for growth factors, and transduction process is suspected. The activation of cellular oncogenes in leukemic cells that code for cell surface receptors or signal transduction may also be involved. Similarly, the exact mechanisms of pancytopenia associated with MPD or MDS remain unknown. In such cases, anemia, thrombocytopenia, and neutropenia may result from the inability of normal stem cells to undergo lineage-specific proliferation, differentiation, and maturation. These abnormalities may result from a deficiency of hematopoietic growth stimulators or increased production of growth inhibitors. The simplistic explanation that they result from overcrowding of the marrow by leukemic cells (myelophthisis) is untenable. The pathogenesis of neoplasia-associated thrombocytopenia may also involve immune-mediated megakaryocyte or platelet destruction, platelet consumption from disseminated intravascular coagulation (DIC) or bleeding tumors, and the sequestration of platelets in vascular beds (spleen) or vascular tumors (Helfand, 1988).

CLASSIFICATION OF HEMATOPOIETIC MALIGNANCIES

An accurate diagnosis of leukemia is essential for proper therapeutic management. The FAB (French-American-British) classification of leukemias groups acute leukemias into myeloid and nonmyeloid or lymphoid leukemias based primarily on their cell morphology and cytochemical reactivity for peroxidase

and nonspecific esterase (Bennett et al., 1985a, 1985b, 1989, 1991; Cheson et al., 1990). Acute myelogenous leukemias are subclassified into eight categories (M0, M1, M2, M3, M4, M5a and M5b, M6, and M7) and acute lymphoid leukemias into three categories (L1, L2, and L3) according to the direction and degree of cellular differentiation. FAB criteria have been adapted for the classification of AML in dogs and cats, and their features are summarized in Table 19-3 (Jain et al., 1991). Myelogenous leukemias (acute or chronic) may present a spectrum from a pure myelogenous leukemia to a pure monocytic leukemia, with the intermediate form being a mixture of the two (myelomonocytic leukemia). Pure acute monoblastic leukemia is rare in humans and animals in comparison to pure AML. Although cytochemical staining is helpful in distinguishing most subtypes of AML, electron microscopy and immunophenotyping are needed to define minimally differentiated forms of AML (M0) and acute undifferentiated leukemia (AUL).

The lymphoproliferative malignancies are classified in various ways using a multitude of criteria. A traditional approach has simply been to designate the tumor-forming disease as a lymphoma, malignant lymphoma, or lymphosarcoma. Formerly, lymphosarcoma was preferred to describe lymphoid tumors of animals, whereas lymphoma was commonly used for humans. The current trend in veterinary medicine, however, is to use lymphoma. The disease in the blood and/or bone marrow is called ALL or CLL. A patient with lymphoma might not have an overt leukemia, though, and conversely, a patient with ALL or CLL might not show tumor masses in tissues or organs. The FAB

Table 19–3. FAB Criteria for Classification of Acute Myeloid Leukemias in Humans*

Type	Characteristic Findings in Blood and Bone Marrow
AUL	Blast cells nonreactive for usual myeloid or lymphoid cytochemical markers or antibodies
M0	Blast cells show restricted myeloid differentiation on electron microscopy (PO+ granules) and/or by immunophenotyping
M1	Blast cells >90% of NEC, differentiated granulocytes or monocytes <10%, PO+ or SB+ blast cells >3%
M2	Myeloblasts >30 to <90% of NEC, differentiated granulocytes >10%, monocytic cells <20%, NSE+ cells <20% of NEC
M3	Not yet reported in dogs and cats; human cases have blast cells >30% of NEC; predominantly hypergranular, hypogranular, or microgranular abnormal promyelocytes with folded, reniform, or bilobed nuclei; bundles (faggots) of Auer rods in myeloid cells
M4	Myeloblast and monoblasts >30%, differentiated granulocytes >20%, monocytic cells >20%, NSE+ cells >20% of NEC
M5	Monocytic cells >80% of NEC, most are NSE+; granulocytes <20%; M5a has >80% monoblasts and promonocytes, M5b has <80% monoblasts and promonocytes, with prominent differentiation to monocytes
M6	Bone marrow erythroid cells >50%; myeloblasts and monoblasts <30% of ANC, but >30% of NEC in bone marrow
M6-Er	Bone marrow erythroid cells >50%; M6 with erythroid predominance considered when rubriblasts plus myeloblasts and monoblasts comprise >30% of ANC in bone marrow
M7	Megakaryoblasts >30% of NEC, increased megakaryocytes in bone marrow; abnormal megakaryoblasts may be present in blood; blasts are positive for platelet glycoprotein IIb-IIIa, show focal fluoride-sensitive NAE positivity, are negative for PO, SB, NBE; myelofibrosis or increased amount of reticulin seen in histologic sections of bone marrow from human cases
MDS	Bone marrow erythroid cells <50%; blast cells <30% of ANC; usually normocellular to hypercellular and sometimes hypocellular marrow, and single, bilineal, or trilineal dyshematopoiesis; blood shows refractory anemia
MDS-Er	Bone marrow erythroid cells >50%; MDS with erythroid predominance considered when myeloblasts and monoblasts combined are <30% of NEC, or blast cell count including rubriblasts is <30% of ANC

From Jain, N.C., Blue, J.T., Grindem, C.B., et al.: A report of the leukemia study group: Proposed criteria for classification of acute myeloid leukemias in dogs and cats. Vet. Clin. Pathol., 20:63, 1991.
* With some modifications for dogs and cats.

criteria for the morphologic classification of ALL in humans remain to be adapted for the dog and the cat.

The anatomic categorization of lymphoid neoplasms is based on the major locations of tumor masses or neoplastic cells in various organs or tissues (e.g., thymic, alimentary, multicentric, cutaneous, or leukemic form). The histologic classification of lymphoma involves determining the microscopic distribution of neoplastic cells—diffuse and nodular or their variants—and the cell types involved—poorly differentiated, well differentiated, and "histiocytic" lymphoma. The current trend is to characterize various lymphoid malignancies by their immunologic cell surface markers—B, T, pre-B, pre-T, mixed (both B and T), and non-B, non-T cell types or their subtypes. The usefulness of these various classifications in the prognosis and therapy of lymphoid malignancies is a subject of much interest that is currently being investigated. Lymphomas involving lymphocytes with abundant cytoplasm and many azurophilic granules, called large granular lymphocytes, have been observed in humans and in the dog (Plate XXI-5), cat (Plate XXI-6), horse, and Fischer rats (Franks et al., 1986; Grindem et al., 1989; Wellman et al., 1989). Functionally, large granular lymphocytes have natural killer (NK) and antibody-dependent cell-mediated cytotoxic (ADCC) activities.

Leukemic leukocytes exhibit morphologic and kinetic, biochemical, and functional abnormalities. Leukemic blast cells may sometimes reveal nuclear and cytoplasmic features unlike those of normal blast cells. Various cell features may be abnormal, including DNA, RNA, and protein syntheses, enzyme activities, kinetic behavior, distribution in blood vasculature, rates of egress and ingress, recirculation, surface antigens and properties, and functional characteristics.

These features can aid in the clinical and laboratory diagnoses of leukemias but can also impose difficulty in establishing a correct diagnosis.

CLINICAL AND LABORATORY ABNORMALITIES OF HEMATOPOIETIC MALIGNANCIES

The clinical manifestations of hematopoietic malignancies are generally related to the quantitative and qualitative abnormalities of the blood cells. These aspects are reviewed here; details can be found under specific types of leukemias (Chapter 20). Nonspecific clinical signs include weight loss, anorexia, depression, and fever. Weakness, pale mucous membranes, and other signs of anemia are seen in most patients. The anemia is usually nonregenerative. Recurrent infections, fever of unknown origin, and delayed wound healing are common in patients with compromised immune competence resulting from severe leukopenia, functional defects of circulating neutrophils, or deficiency of protective antibodies. Enlargement of the superficial and internal lymph nodes, spleen, liver, and kidneys may be detected in LPDs and in MPDs. Rare cases of chronic myeloid leukemia may develop discrete tumors of leukemic granulocytes, known as chloromas or granulocytic sarcomas, in various body tissues. An infrequent finding is the accumulation of leukemic cells in the anterior chamber of the eyes (hypopyon). The radiologic examination of long bones and vertebrae can reveal characteristic punched-out osteolytic lesions in patients with multiple myeloma. Such bones are prone to fracture.

Petechial and ecchymotic hemorrhages in the mucous membranes, epistaxis, hematuria, bleeding into the gut and, rarely, hyphema may occur in severely thrombocytopenic patients. These signs may also be apparent when platelets are functionally defective, as in essential thrombocythemia. Microvascular thrombosis and DIC have been reported in human AML, particularly in acute promyelocytic leukemia and, less often, in other forms of AML. The release of a procoagulant, probably from the lysosomal granules of leukemic cells, is believed to initiate these coagulopathies (Falanga et al., 1988).

Excessive leukocytes in patients with acute or chronic leukemias may impede blood flow because of leukocyte clumps and thrombi in many organs including the lungs, brain, eyes, and ears. The local release of toxic products from the leukocytes may cause endothelial damage and hemorrhage. Abnormalities such as stupor, coma, retinal enlargement, papilledema, acute respiratory distress, and severe neurologic deficits have been detected in human patients with hyperleukocytic leukemias.

Serum chemistries may reveal spurious hypoglycemia in cases of leukemia with marked leukocytosis and hyperkalemia caused by the release of platelet potassium in essential thrombocythemia. Hypercalcemia is a characteristic finding in some cases of lymphoma and lymphocytic leukemia. Hyperproteinemia and monoclonal gammopathy are unique to multiple myeloma, although they may also occur in some cases of lymphoma. These abnormalities result in the hyperviscosity of blood and associated clinical signs. The icterus index, total bilirubin, and conjugated bilirubin values may be elevated when hepatic function is compromised because of neoplastic infiltration.

CLASSIFICATION OF ACUTE MYELOID LEUKEMIA

Acute myeloid leukemias and myelodysplastic syndromes in humans are classified according to FAB criteria, based primarily on the number and morphology of blast cells in Romanowsky-stained blood and bone marrow films. These criteria can be used to classify AML in dogs and cats, and perhaps in other animal species (Table 19-3 and Fig. 19-2). The consistent use of these criteria can help enhance the understanding of the clinical, pathobiologic, and therapeutic aspects of these diseases in animals, as has been the

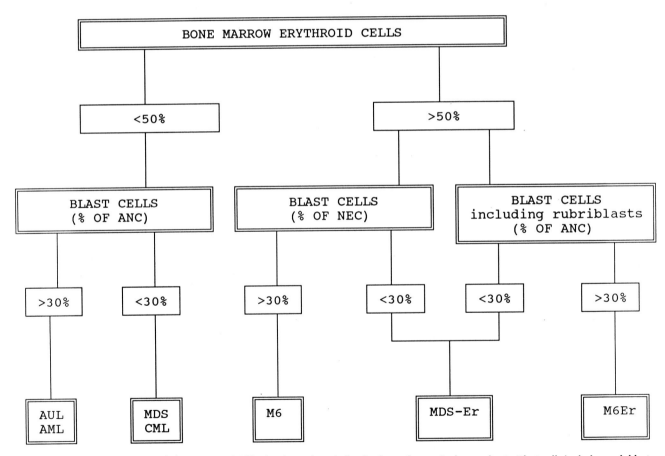

Fig. 19-2.   Schematic to classification of acute myeloid leukemias and myelodysplastic syndromes in dogs and cats. Blast cells include myeloblasts, monoblasts, and megakaryoblasts. ANC, all nucleated cells in bone marrow excluding lymphocytes, plasma cells, macrophages, and mast cells; NEC, nonerythroid cells in bone marrow; AUL, acute undifferentiated leukemia; AML, acute myeloid leukemias M1 to M5 and M7; CML, chronic myeloid leukemias including chronic myelogenous, chronic myelomonocytic, and chronic monocytic leukemias; MDS, myelodysplastic syndrome; MDS-Er, myelodysplastic syndrome with erythroid predominance; M6, erythroleukemia; M6Er, erythroleukemia with erythroid predominance. (From Jain, N.C., et al.: A report of the animal leukemia study group: Proposed criteria for classification of acute myeloid leukemias in dogs and cats. Vet. Clin. Pathol., 20:63, 1991.)

case in humans. Note that the cytomorphologic diagnosis of AML and MDS requires bone marrow examination, blood examination alone is usually not diagnostic (Bennett et al., 1985a, 1985b, 1986, 1991; Cheson et al., 1990; Jain et al., 1991).

Ideally, blood, bone marrow aspirates, and bone marrow core biopsies should be collected simultaneously for the diagnosis of AML and MDS. Wright- or Wright-Giemsa–stained blood and bone marrow films are examined to determine blast cell number and morphology. A 200-cell differential leukocyte count is performed on blood films. Similarly, 200 cells (or more, if needed) are differentiated in bone marrow films to determine the percentages of blast cells and various maturative stages of the myeloid and erythroid series and to calculate a myeloid:erythroid (M:E) ratio. Blast cells include myeloblasts (types I and II), monoblasts, and megakaryoblasts. Blast cell percentages are calculated in relation to all nucleated cells (ANC) and to nonerythroid cells (NEC) in the bone marrow. Lymphocytes, macrophages, mast cells, and plasma cells are excluded when calculating ANC, and erythroid cells are excluded for NEC counts.

When the erythroid component is less than 50%, the presence of more than 30% blast cells in the bone marrow indicates AML or AUL (Fig. 19-2). When the marrow blast cell number is less than 30%, MDS, CML, or even a leukemoid response may be suspected. In comparison, when the erythroid component is greater than 50%, M6 is diagnosed with a blast cell count of more than 30% NEC, whereas M6-Er (see Table 19-1) is considered if the addition of rubriblasts increases the blast cell count to more than 30% ANC. MDS-Er is considered with a blast cell count of less than 30% NEC or when the blast count inclusive of rubriblasts is less than 30% ANC. Additional criteria are used to distinguish AUL and various subtypes of AML (Table 19-3). A bone marrow core biopsy is needed to determine the overall marrow cellularity, to define myelofibrosis (Plate XXII-6), and to identify rare cases of hypocellular AML, as described in humans. Core "imprints" may be used for light microscopy in case of a dry marrow tap. Typical Auer rods, common in immature myeloid cells in AML in humans and relied on heavily to distinguish a leukemic from a leukemoid reaction and AML from ALL (Jain et al., 1987), have not been found in dogs and cats with AML. Auer-rod like granules, however, were seen in a cat with AML-M2 (Jain et al., 1991).

The identity of blast cells should be ascertained using appropriate cytochemical markers of neutrophilic, monocytic, and megakaryocytic differentiation (Facklam and Kociba, 1985, 1986; Grindem et al., 1985, 1986; Jain 1986; Jain et al., 1981). Peroxidase (PO), Sudan black B (SB), and chloroacetate esterase (CAE) are generally considered neutrophil markers, whereas nonspecific esterase (NSE) is a monocytic marker and acetylcholine esterase (ACE) is a specific marker for megakaryocytes. Unfortunately, these methods identify lymphoblasts only by their negativity. In cases in which the usual cytomorphologic and cytochemical markers fail to identify the blast cell type, electron microscopy may be used to delineate lineage-specific ultrastructural features and ultrastructural myeloperoxidase in cytoplasmic organelles, including positive primary granules in myeloblasts, and to demonstrate platelet PO in megakaryoblasts (Breton-Gorius et al., 1984; Lee et al., 1987; Madewell et al., 1991; Polli et al., 1989). Immunophenotyping with lineage-specific antibodies to cytoplasmic and surface determinants of blood cells is being used to establish the identity of human leukemic cells (Bassan et al., 1989; Loffler, 1990; Matutes et al., 1988; Parwaresch et al., 1991; Stewart, 1992). Such reagents and procedures are being developed for general use in veterinary medicine. Their use as diagnostic reagents may be necessary in some but not in all cases of acute leukemias. The clinical relevance of cytomorphologic, cytochemical, and immunophenotypic characterizations of AML in dogs and cats remains to be determined. Cytogenetic and molecular analyses may also be important in the diagnosis of leukemias in animals, as in humans (Castro et al., 1988; Cuneo et al., 1990; Grindem and Buoen, 1986, 1989). The artificial, subjective grouping of a leukemia may change with the progression of disease, and cognizance of the biologic characteristics of a leukemia is more important for the development of a rational therapy than its mere classification.

Canine and Feline Bone Marrow Cells

Myeloblast Type I. This large cell has a round to oval nucleus, finely stippled or smooth nuclear chromatin, one or more distinct or indistinct nucleoli, a small amount of moderately blue cytoplasm, and no azurophilic granules (Plates XXIV-2, XXV-1). Usually, the nucleus is centrally located and the nuclear outline is regular and smooth. The nucleus may, however, sometimes be slightly off center and the nuclear outline may (rarely) be slightly irregular (Plate V-3). The nuclear:cytoplasmic (N:C) ratio is high (more than 1.5) and the cell diameter is about 1.5 to 3 times that of the red cell. The cell morphology is often distorted in hypercellular smears. A clear area representing the Golgi apparatus may be seen infrequently in the cytoplasm. The cytoplasm may have a ground glass appearance. Infrequently, a few small cytoplasmic vacuoles may occur, but this does not necessarily indicate monocytic transformation.

Myeloblast Type II. This cell has features similar to those of a type I myeloblast, but it also has some (less than 15) tiny azurophilic granules scattered in the cytoplasm (Plate VI-1). The nucleus is usually centrally located, but may be eccentrically placed.

Promyelocyte. This cell has smooth or slightly stippled nuclear chromatin, with or without a nucleolus or nucleolar ring, and many distinct azurophilic granules well dispersed in a slightly to moderately blue abundant cytoplasm (Plate XXIV-2). The nucleus may be centrally located or eccentrically placed. Prominent nucleoli may be present, even in cells with heavy cytoplasmic granulation (Plate V-4). A clear Golgi zone, surrounded or sprinkled by azurophilic granules, may be apparent in some promyelocytes.

Monoblast. This large cell has a round, slightly to moderately irregular or folded nucleus, a stippled or finely reticular nuclear chromatin, one or more prominent nucleoli, and a moderate amount of basophilic agranular cytoplasm (Plates VIII-1 and VIII-2). A clear area representing the Golgi zone may be prominent in the cytoplasm, particularly near the site of nuclear indentation. The N:C ratio may be similar to or lower than that in the myeloblast.

Promonocyte. This large cell has a cerebriform nucleus with prominent nuclear folds, stippled or lacy chromatin, and no distinct nucleoli (Plate VIII-3). Compared to monoblasts, the cytoplasm may be more abundant and less basophilic, with a ground glass appearance. Fine azurophilic granules are rare; therefore, the cytoplasm is generally nongranular. Cytoplasmic vacuoles may be present.

Lymphoblast. This small to large cell has a round to oval nucleus, finely stippled to slightly coarse nuclear chromatin, one or more distinct or indistinct nucleoli, and a small to moderate amount of pale blue, featureless cytoplasm without azurophilic granules (Plate XIX-1). Rarely, the nuclear outline may appear slightly indented or irregular and the cytoplasm may contain few vacuoles (Plate XIX-5). The N:C ratio is usually higher than in a typical myeloblast and the cytoplasm does not have a granular appearance. It is distinguished from the myeloblast by its coarser nuclear chromatin, small amount of cytoplasm, and negative staining for neutrophilic markers such as PO, SB, and CAE (Plate XIX-6).

Rubriblast. This large cell has a round nucleus, finely stippled or smooth nuclear chromatin, one or more distinct nucleoli, and a moderate amount of deep blue cytoplasm devoid of azurophilic granules (Plates IV-1 and IV-5). The N:C ratio is high. The prorubricyte has cytoplasmic features similar to those of a rubriblast, but the nuclear chromatin shows minimal condensation and nucleoli or nucleolar rings are absent (Plate IV-2).

Dysplastic Changes. These changes are developmental morphologic abnormalities in bone marrow cells. Dysmyelopoiesis is indicated by polyploid or hypersegmented neutrophil nuclei, giant cell size (particularly metamyelocytes and bands), abundance of azurophilic granules or hypogranular cytoplasm, and Pelger-Huët cell morphology. Multiple nuclei, nuclear fragmentation, megaloblastic appearance (Plate XV-4), excessive cytoplasm relative to the nucleus, and an abnormal distribution of siderosomes (Plate XV-5) constitute dyserythropoiesis. Abnormal rubriblasts (neoplastic or dysplastic) have enlarged nucleoli, eccentric nuclei, and more abundant deep blue cytoplasm. Some abnormal blast cells with characteristics mimicking erythroid features may have broad pseudopods (Plate XV-3) or a few coarse, reddish-purple cytoplasmic granules that stain PO-negative or SB-negative. The definitive identity of such cells remains to be established. Dysmegakaryocytopoiesis is indicated by decreased numbers of megakaryocytes, megakaryocytes with a nonlobed, large nucleus or multiple small nuclei, and dwarf megakaryocytes or micromegakaryocytes in the blood and bone marrow.

Subtypes of Acute Myeloid Leukemia and Other Myeloid Disorders

Acute Undifferentiated Leukemia (AUL). Included in this category are cases with a predominance of blast cells with eccentric nuclei and pseudopodia (Plates XV-3 and XXII-5). These cases were formerly described by the now obsolete term "reticuloendotheliosis." Blast cell leukemias with uncertain lineage or lymphoid morphology and strong ALP activity may be placed in this category until additional evidence for lineage specificity has been obtained. Also included here are cases in which the bone marrow has almost 100% blast cells that cannot be classified properly by the usual morphologic and cytochemical criteria. The myeloid identity of blast cells in such cases should be defined by electron microscopy, ultrastructural cytochemistry, and/or immunophenotyping, as done for AUL and M0 in humans, and they should then be recategorized.

Myeloblastic Leukemia Without Maturation (M1). The predominant cell in the bone marrow is the type I myeloblast, whereas type II myeloblasts are rare. Both types of blast cells comprise more than 90% of the ANC (Plate XX-1). Differentiated granulocytes are less than 10% of the NEC, and often include promyelocytes through segmented neutrophils and eosinophils. Rarely, megaloblastic erythroid cells and mitotic figures are present.

Myeloblastic Leukemia With Maturation (M2). Myeloblasts constitute more than 30% to less than 90% of the ANC, with a variable proportion of type II blasts. Differentiated granulocytes are more than 10% of the NEC, with a predominance of promyelocytes or a disproportionate number of promyelocytes through segmented neutrophils and occasional eosinophils (Plate XX-2). Promyelocytes have many more azurophilic granules than type II myeloblasts. The granules are usually uniformly distributed in the bluish cytoplasm but sometimes may be concentrated in one area, particularly near the Golgi region. The amount of cytoplasm is generally more than that in a myeloblast, but may be similar. The monocytic component is less than 20% of the NEC. Delicate, Auer rod-like granules are extremely rare.

Promyelocytic Leukemia (M3). This type has not been reported so far in dogs and cats. In human M3 cases, promyelocytes show irregular, reniform, folded, or bilobed nuclei and hypergranular, hypogranular, or microgranular cytoplasm. Bundles (faggots) of Auer rods are common in abnormal blast cells and promyelocytes.

Myelomonocytic Leukemia (M4). This AML subtype is recognized by the presence of prominent granulocytic and monocytic cell lines. Myeloblasts and monoblasts together constitute more than 30% of the ANC and differentiated granulocytes and monocytes each comprise more than 20% of the NEC (Plates XX-3 and -4). More neutrophilic differentiation may be seen in this subtype than in M2.

Monocytic Leukemia (M5).   The predominant population is monocytic, as determined by characteristic nuclear morphology and confirmed by cytochemical staining for NSE. Monoblasts and promonocytes constitute more than 80% of the NEC in M5a, whereas M5b has more than 30% to less than 80% monoblasts and promonocytes, with prominent differentiation to monocytes (Plates XX-5 and -6). The blast cells of M5a may have more prominent clear areas of the Golgi zone in the cytoplasm that the blast cells in M5b. The granulocytic component is less than 20%. Occasional dyserythropoiesis is present in the form of megaloblastic erythroid cells.

Erythroleukemia (M6 and M6-Er).   The erythroid component in M6 is characteristically more than 50% and the myeloblasts and monoblasts combined are less than 30% of the ANC. M6 is recognized when at least one of the following criteria is met: myeloblasts and monoblasts are more than 30% of the NEC, or a blast cell count that includes rubriblasts is more than 30% of the ANC (Plate XXI-1). An M6-Er designation may be used to define the latter situation when rubriblasts predominate in the erythroid component (Plate XXIII-3). M6 disorders generally exhibit a significant amount of granulocytic differentiation, and may progress to AML-M2 (Plate XXIII-4).

Megakaryoblastic Leukemia (M7).   Megakaryocytic leukemia is rare in dogs and cats. Megakaryocytes can be differentiated in dogs and cats by a positive ACE reaction. In addition, α granules and the formation of demarcation membrane systems may be observed on transmission electron microscopy. A diagnosis of MDS with megakaryocyte predominance or essential thrombocythemia is considered when the megakaryoblast count is less than 30%.

Megakaryoblastic leukemia, according to FAB criteria, is diagnosed when the bone marrow aspirate contains more than 30% of the NEC as megakaryoblasts. Megakaryoblasts are also detected in the peripheral blood. Megakaryocytes in the blood and bone marrow vary in size but are often small (micromegakaryocytes) (Plates XXI-1 and -2). They are identified by the platelet PO reaction on electron microscopy or by a positive reaction for platelet glycoproteins IIb-IIIa by immunologic methods. Myelofibrosis and increased reticulum in core biopsies are prominent in most patients with M7 and sometimes increased numbers of mature megakaryocytes are found.

Myelodysplastic Syndrome (MDS and MDS-Er).   Features include less than 30% blast cells of ANC or NEC, whether the erythroid component is greater or less than 50%. The bone marrow is usually normocellular to hypercellular, but may be hypocellular. Dysplastic changes are prominent and involve one or more of the erythroid, myeloid, and megakaryocytic cell lines.

Peripheral blood often shows pancytopenia, with or without a left shift. Typically, MDS is recognized when blast cells are less than 30% of the ANC in a bone marrow with less than 50% erythroid cells. The designation MDS-Er may be used to indicate erythroid predominance when the erythroid component is more than 50% and the myeloblasts and monoblasts combined are less than 30% of the NEC or ANC, inclusive of rubriblasts (Fig. 19-2). Erythremic myelosis may be classified as M6-Er or MDS-Er because the erythroid component is more than 50% of the ANC and the blast cell count, including rubriblasts, may be more or less than 30% of the ANC, respectively (Plates XXII-4, XXII-6, and XXIII-2). Cats with MDS do not show extramedullary leukemic infiltrates unlike cats with AML (Blue et al., 1988).

Chronic Myeloid Leukemias.   CML, chronic monocytic leukemia (CMoL), and chronic myelomonocytic leukemia (CMMoL) may be classified under MDS because the blast cell counts in these leukemias are less than 30% of the ANC and the erythroid component is less than 50%. Although CMoL is considered an MDS under the FAB system, CML and CMMoL are distinct entities. These leukemias can be distinguished from classic MDS by the absence of prominent dysplastic changes in the bone marrow and by the presence of a marked leukocytosis in the blood. The latter is often accompanied by a disorderly left shift in CML and by absolute monocytosis in CMoL and CMMoL. Some dysplastic granulocytes and megakaryocytes are found in CMMoL in humans.

CHEMOTHERAPY OF HEMATOPOIETIC MALIGNANCIES

Lymphoma, lymphoid leukemias, myeloid leukemias, and other hematopoietic neoplastic diseases remain essentially incurable by currently available methods. The primary aim of cancer chemotherapy in such patients, therefore, is to control the disease process and prolong the life of the patient. The treatment of hematopoietic malignancies generally involves chemotherapy, immunotherapy, radiation, and marrow transplantation (Wiernik, 1991; Wiernik and Dutcher, 1992). The purpose of various treatments is to destroy leukemic clones of cells and allow the propagation of normal hematopoietic cells. Hematopoietic growth factors have been used in conjunction with intensive radiation and chemotherapy to promote the repopulation of normal hematopoietic stem cells (Galvani, 1991; Testa and Dexter, 1990). Similarly, erythropoietin administration has been tried in MDS in humans (Verhoef et al., 1992). Prolonged survival without therapy is rare.

Many drugs are used for the treatment of neoplasms, including hematopoietic malignancies, in human and veterinary medicine (Table 19-4). These drugs are broadly categorized as cycle-dependent drugs, which selectively kill cells in mitotic and DNA synthetic phases, and noncycle-dependent agents, which kill cells

Table 19–4. Some Drugs Used for Chemotherapy of Canine and Feline Hematopoietic Neoplasms

Drug	Indications*	Dose†
Busulfan (Myleran)	MPD	3–4 mg/m², orally, per day
Chlorambucil (Leukeran)	LPD	2 mg/m², orally, alternate days
Cyclophosphamide (Cytoxan)	LPD	50 mg/m², IV or orally, 3–4 days a week
Cytosine arabinoside (Cytosar)	LPD, MPD	100 mg/m², IV or SC, for 2–4 days
Doxorubicin (Adriamycin)	LPD	30 mg/m², IV, every 21 days
L-Asparaginase	LPD	10,000–40,000 units, SC or IP, once or twice weekly, 15 min after giving antihistamine
Melphalan (Alkeran)	Myeloma	1.5 mg/m², orally, per day, for 7–10 days every 2–3 weeks
6-Mercaptopurine	LPD, MPD	50 mg/m², orally, per day
Methotrexate	LPD, MPD	2.5 mg/m², orally, 2–3 times a week
Nitrogen mustard (Mustargen)	LPD	5 mg/m², orally or IV, per day or in divided dosage for 2–4 days
Prednisone	LPD	10–40 mg/m², orally, per day, for 7 days, then half the dose alternate days
Vinblastine (Velban)	LPD	2 mg/m², IV, once a week
Vincristine (Oncovin)	LPD	0.5 mg/m², IV, once a week

 * LPD, lymphoproliferative disorder; MPD, myeloproliferative disorder.
 † m², body surface area; IV, intravenous; SC, subcutaneous.

in all phases of the cell cycle. This distinction, however, is not absolute. Based on the hypothesis that the primary defect in leukemia is the lack of stem cell differentiation and maturation, drugs inducing cellular differentiation and maturation in vitro have also been used to treat leukemias; these drugs include cytosine arabinoside (ara-C) and *cis*-retinoic acid.

Antineoplastic agents are more effective when used in combination and other drugs should be substituted when the animal becomes refractory to the initial therapy or shows signs of toxicity. The reason for the relative success of combination therapy is that different drugs attack tumor cells at different stages of the cell cycle and by different mechanisms, perhaps thereby producing a synergistic action and a higher rate of tumoricidal effect with minimal toxicity. Unless every neoplastic cell is destroyed, relapses may occur after the discontinuation of therapy or a refractoriness to chemotherapeutic drugs eventually develops, and the disease again becomes progressive.

Whole body irradiation alone has been used to treat lymphoma in dogs, but prolonged periods of remission have been observed in such dogs treated with combination chemotherapy followed by total body irradiation and the transplantation of autologous bone marrow. Immunotherapy has been used to induce a systemic antitumor immune response by the patient. Immunotherapy with an autogenous vaccine (injection of chemically modified tumor cell extracts in Freund's complete adjuvant) has been found beneficial when given following cytoreductive chemotherapy.

Immunotherapy may be directed to destroy tumor cells or virus-infected cells by stimulating nonspecific or tumor-specific or virus-specific immune response (Weiss, 1988). Nonspecific stimuli induce macrophage activation, interferon-gamma production, and NK cell activity. Specific immunostimulation is aimed at destroying tumor- or virus-infected cells in particular. Purified staphylococcal protein A and interferon-gamma appear to be potential immunostimulants to treat FeLV-induced neoplastic and non-neoplastic diseases. Purified staphylococcal protein A induces formation of cytotoxic T lymphocytes and production of

interferon-gamma. Interferon-gamma in cats promotes NK cell-mediated lysis of FeLV-infected B cells, but not of T cells (Rojko and Olson, 1984). Low dose oral administration of interferon-gamma in FeLV-cats has been found to increase survival, but possible mechanisms remain undetermined (Weiss et al., 1991). Other nonspecific immunomodulators, such as acemannan (a complex carbohydrate) and killed Propionibacterium acnes, were found to cause clinical and hematologic improvements, enhance quality of life, and increase the survival rate of FeLV-infected cats (Sheets et al., 1991; Tizard 1991).

Various treatment programs involving single, sequential, and combination therapy have been developed for canine and feline patients. These programs are being constantly modified with experience to increase their therapeutic effectiveness and reduce side effects. The treatment of bovine and equine patients has generally not been attempted, primarily for economic reasons. A subunit recombinant vaccine, consisting of gp51 and gp30 antigens of bovine leukemia virus (BLV) expressed in vaccinia virus, may induce a protective immunity against BLV infection (Portetelle et al., 1990). See Chapter 20 for FeLV vaccine.

The general experience has been that prospective clinical staging of the disease has prognostic significance. Also, individual variations are noted in response to therapy, probably reflecting a varied nature of the disease process. The ideal canine candidate is one in which the diagnosis has been made in the early stage of the disease and in which the generalized spread of neoplastic cells to visceral organs has not occurred. Major organ involvement presents too large a mass of neoplastic tissue to be destroyed for best results. The initial drug doses should be large enough to produce rapid remissions; the dose should then be reduced to the level that maintains remission as long as possible. In a study of 147 lymphoma dogs treated with a combination of chemotherapy (vincristine, L-asparaginase, cyclophosphamide, and methotrexate), response to therapy and duration of the response were influenced by gender; females had a significantly prolonged remission and survival time (MacEwen et al., 1987). Cyclophosphamide, being a potent myelo-suppressive agent, may be substituted by cytosine arabinoside in neutropenic leukopenic animals (Helfand, 1987).

Normally functioning kidneys are important to successful cancer therapy because, with the regression of large tumor masses, nitrogenous wastes are released and must be excreted. A blood urea nitrogen level should be determined before and during treatment to monitor kidney function. Blood cytology should also be routinely monitored. A significant change in kidney function or evidence of developing thrombocytopenia, leukopenia, or anemia should call for an immediate reduction in dose or discontinuance of the cytotoxic drug(s).

The treatment of leukemia and lymphoma with cytotoxic drugs may produce signs of intoxication during the period of rapid regression of neoplastic tissue. Therefore, proper supportive care is essential to successful management. The principal sign is depression. Other chronic signs of drug toxicity are sepsis, bone marrow suppression, gastrointestinal irritation, hemorrhagic cystitis, and alopecia. Corticosteroids used in combination with cytotoxic drugs may largely prevent the depression of hematopoiesis through their stimulatory effect on the bone marrow. With a properly controlled drug regimen, severe anemia, leukopenia, or thrombocytopenia is not a common occurrence. In fact, platelet numbers in the blood have increased in some dogs during therapy with prednisolone combined with a cytotoxic drug. The appearance of Howell-Jolly bodies and/or nucleated erythrocytes in the peripheral blood during therapy has been conjectured to be an expression of suppression of the "pitting" function of the spleen, primarily by the action of the corticosteroids administered.

The value of splenectomy in canine lymphoma has been studied (Brooks et al., 1987). Splenectomy may rapidly reverse anemia and thrombocytopenia in lymphomatous dogs with massive splenomegaly. Splenectomized dogs treated with chemotherapy may go into remission and attain survival times comparable to those dogs given combination chemotherapy alone, but survival may be reduced in some dogs by complications of sepsis and DIC.

REFERENCES

Bassan, R., Rambaldi, A., Viero, P., et al.: Integrated use of morphology, cytochemistry, and immune marker analysis to identify acute leukaemia subtypes. Haematologica, 74:487, 1989.
Bennett, J.M., Catovsky, D., Daniel, M.T., et al.: Criteria for the diagnosis of acute leukemia of megakaryocyte lineage (M7). Ann. Intern. Med., 103:460, 1985a.
Bennett, J.M., Catovsky, D., Daniel, M.T., et al.: Proposed revised criteria for the classification of acute myeloid leukemia. Ann. Intern. Med., 103:620, 1985b.
Bennett, J.M., Catovsky, D., Daniel, M.T., et al.: Classification of the myelodysplastic syndromes. Clin. Haematol., 15:909, 1986.
Bennett, J.M., Catovsky, D., Daniel, M.T., et al.: Proposals for the classification of chronic (mature) B and T lymphoid leukaemias. French-American-British (FAB) Cooperative Group. J. Clin. Pathol., 42:567, 1989.

Bennett, J.M., Catovsky, D., Daniel, M.T., et al.: Proposal for the recognition of minimally differentiated acute myeloid leukaemia. Br. J. Haematol., 78:325, 1991.
Blue, J.T., French, T.W. and Kranz, J.S.: Non-lymphoid hematopoietic neoplasia in cats: a retrospective study of 60 cases. Cornell Vet., 78:21, 1988.
Breton-Gorius, J., van Haeke, D., Pryzwansky, K.B., et al.: Simultaneous detection of membrane markers with monoclonal antibodies and peroxidatic activities in leukaemia: ultrastructural analysis using a new method of fixation preserving the platelet peroxidase. Br. J. Haematol., 58:447, 1984.
Brooks, M.B., Matus, R.E., Leifer, C.E., et al.: Use of splenectomy in the management of lymphoma in dogs: 16 cases (1976–1985) J. Am. Vet. Med. Assoc., 191:1008, 1987.
Castro, N.H., Walter, J., dos Santos, R., et al.: Cytogenetic study of cattle affected by persistent lymphocytosis. Zentralbl Veterinarmed [A]., 35:380, 1988.
Catovsky, D., Matutes, E., Buccheri, V., et al.: A classification of acute leukaemia for the 1990s. Ann. Hematol., 62:16, 1991.
Cheson, B.D., Cassileth, P.A., Head, D.R., et al.: Report of the National Cancer Institute-sponsored workshop on definitions of diagnosis and response in acute myeloid leukemia. J. Clin. Oncol., 8:813, 1990.
Cuneo, A., Orshoven, A., Michaux, J.L., et al.: Morphologic, immunologic and cytogenetic studies in erythroleukemia: evidence for multilineage involvement and identification of two distinct cytogenetic-clinicopathologic types. Br J Haematol, 75:346, 1990.
Facklam, N.R. and Kociba, G.J.: Cytochemical characterization of leukemic cells from 20 dogs. Vet. Pathol., 22:363, 1985.
Facklam, N.R. and Kociba, G.J.: Cytochemical characterization of feline leukemic cells. Vet. Pathol., 23:155, 1986.
Falanga, A., Alessio, M.G., Donati, M.B., et al.: A new procoagulant in acute leukemia. Blood, 71:870, 1988.
Franks, P.T., Harvey, J.W., Mays, M.C., et al.: Feline large granular lymphoma. Vet. Pathol., 23:200, 1986.
Galvani, D.W.: The current status of myeloid growth factor therapy. J. R. Coll. Physicians. Lond., 25:213, 1991.
Grindem, C.B. and Buoen, L.C.: Cytogenetic analysis of leukaemic cells in the dog. A report of 10 cases and a review of the literature. J. Comp. Pathol., 96:623, 1986.
Grindem, C.B. and Buoen, L.C.: Cytogenetic analysis in nine leukaemic cats. J. Comp. Pathol., 101:21, 1989.
Grindem, C.B., Roberts, M.C., McEntee, M.F., et al.: Large granular lymphocyte tumor in a horse. Vet. Pathol., 26:86, 1989.
Grindem, C.B., Stevens, J.B. and Perman, V.: Cytochemical reactions in cells from leukemic cats. Vet. Clin. Pathol., 14:6, 1985.
Grindem, C.B., Stevens, J.B. and Perman, V.: Cytochemical reactions in cells from leukemic dogs. Vet. Pathol., 23:103, 1986.
Helfand, S.C.: Low-dose cytosine arabinoside-induced remission of lymphoblastic leukemia in a cat. J. Am. Vet. Med. Assoc., 191:707, 1987.
Helfand, S.C.: Platelets and neoplasias. Vet. Clin. North. Am.: Small Anim. Pract., 18:131, 1988.
Jain, N.C.: Schalm's Veterinary Hematology. 4th ed. Philadelphia, Lea & Febiger, 1986, pp. 838–908.
Jain, N.C., Blue, J.T., Grindem, C.B., et al.: A report of the animal leukemia study group: Proposed criteria for classification of acute myeloid leukemia in dogs and cats. Vet. Clin. Pathol., 20:63, 1991.
Jain, N.C., Cox, C. and Bennett, J.M.: Auer rods in the acute myeloid leukemias: frequency and methods of demonstration. Hematol. Oncol., 5:197, 1987.
Jain, N.C., Madewell, B.R., Weller, R.E., et al.: Clinico-pathological findings and cytochemical characterization of myelomonocytic leukemia in 5 dogs. J. Comp. Pathol., 91:17, 1981.
Jarrett, O.: Overview of feline leukemia virus research. J. Am. Vet. Med. Assoc., 199:1279, 1991.
Keller, E.T. and Madewell, B.R.: Locations and types of neoplasms in immature dogs: 69 cases (1964–1989). J. Am. Vet. Med. Assoc., 200:1530, 1992.
Lee, E.J., Pollak, A., Leavitt, R.D., et al.: Minimally differentiated acute nonlymphocytic leukemia: a distinct entity. Blood, 70:1400, 1987.
Loffler, H.: Morphology, immunology, cytochemistry, and cytoge-

netics and the classification of subtypes in AML. Haematol. Bluttransfus., 33:239, 1990.

MacEwen, E.G., Hayes, A.A., Matus, R.E., et al.: Evaluation of some prognostic factors for advanced multicentric lymphosarcoma in the dog: 147 cases (1978–1981). J. Am. Vet. Med. Assoc., 190:564, 1987.

Madewell, B.R., Jain, N.C., and Munn, R.J.: Unusual cytochemical reactivity in canine acute myeloblastic leukaemia. Comp. Haematol. Intl., 1:117, 1991.

Matutes, E., Pombo de Oliveira, M., Foroni, L., et al.: The role of ultrastructural cytochemistry and monoclonal antibodies in clarifying the nature of undifferentiated cells in acute leukemia. Br. J. Haematol., 69:205, 1988.

Parwaresch, M.R., Kreipe, H., Radzun, H.J., et al.: Lineage-specific receptors in the diagnosis of malignant lymphomas and myelomonocytic neoplasms. Curr. Top. Pathol., 83:495, 1991.

Polli, N., Lambertenghi-Deliliers, G., Schiro, R., et al.: Relevance of ultrastructural immunocytochemistry in the characterization of unclassifiable leukemias: correlation with phenotypic and genic studies. Haematologica. (Pavia), 74:129, 1989.

Portetelle, D., Burny, A., Desmettre, P., et al.: Development of a specific serological test and an efficient subunit vaccine to control bovine leukemia virus infection. Dev. Biol. Stand., 72:81, 1990.

Rojko, J.L. and Olsen, R.G.: The immunobiology of the feline leukemia virus. Vet. Immunol. Immunopathol., 6:107, 1984.

Ruiz-Arguelles, G.J., Lobato-Mendizabal, E. and Marin-Lopez, A.: The incidence of hybrid acute leukaemias. Leuk. Res., 12:707, 1988.

Schneider, R.: Comparison of age- and sex-specific incidence rate patterns of the leukemia complex in the cat and the dog. J. Nat. Cancer Inst., 70:971, 1983.

Sheets, M.A., Unger, B.A., Giggleman, G.F., Jr., et al.: Studies of the effect of acemannan on retrovirus infections: clinical stabilization of feline leukemia virus-infected cats. Mol. Biother., 3:41, 1991.

Stewart, C.C.: Clinical applications of flow cytometry. Immunologic methods for measuring cell membrane and cytoplasmic antigens. Cancer, 69:1543, 1992.

Sun, G.X., Wormsley, S., Sparkes, R.S., et al.: Where does transformation occur in acute leukemia? Leuk. Res., 15:1183, 1991.

Testa, N.G. and Dexter, T.M.: Haemopoietic growth factors and haematological malignancies. Baillieres. Clin. Endocrinol. Metab., 4:177, 1990.

Tizard, I.: Use of immunomodulators as an aid to clinical management of feline leukemia virus-infected cats. J. Am. Vet. Med. Assoc., 199:1482, 1991.

Verhoef, G.E., Zachee, P., Ferrant, A., et al.: Recombinant human erythropoietin for the treatment of anemia in the myelodysplastic syndromes: A clinical and erythrokinetic assessment. Ann. Hematol., 64:16, 1992.

Weiss, R.C.: Immunotherapy for feline leukemia, using staphylococcal protein A or heterologous interferons: immunopharmacologic actions and potential use. J. Am. Vet. Med. Assoc., 192:681, 1988.

Weiss, R.C., Cummins, J.M. and Richards, A.B.: Low-dose orally administered alpha interferon treatment for feline leukemia virus infection. J. Am. Vet. Med. Assoc., 199:1477, 1991.

Wellman, M.L., Couto, C.G., Starkey, R.J., et al.: Lymphocytosis of large granular lymphocytes in three dogs. Vet. Pathol., 26:158, 1989.

Wiernik, P.H.: New agents in the treatment of acute myeloid leukemia. Semin. Hematol., 28:95, 1991.

Wiernik, P.H. and Dutcher, J.P.: Clinical importance of anthracyclines in the treatment of acute myeloid leukemia. Leukemia, 6 Suppl 1:67, 1992.

Williams, W.J., Beutler, E., Erslev, A.J., et al.: Hematology. 4h ed. New York, McGraw-Hill, 1990.

The Leukemias

General aspects of hematopoietic neoplasms are discussed in Chapter 19. Table 19–1 provides a simplified classification of various myeloproliferative and lymphoproliferative disorders and Table 19–2 lists various distinguishing characteristics of acute myelogenous, acute lymphocytic, and acute monocytic leukemias. A brief description of various types of leukemias encountered in dogs, cats, cattle, horses, sheep, goats, and pigs is presented here; further details can be found elsewhere (Jain, 1986; Theilen and Madewell, 1987).

FELINE LEUKEMIAS

Hematopoietic neoplasms represent about one-third of all cat tumors and most are lymphoid. The demonstration of virus particles in transmissible lymphoma in neonatal kittens by Jarrett in 1964 was followed by extensive investigations of the nature of the virus,

incidence of natural infection, immune responses, and associated clinical diseases. The virus became known as the feline leukemia virus (FeLV), even though the incidence of leukemia is low in the presence of a high natural infection rate. Current information on various aspects of FeLV infection have been reviewed (Cotter, 1992; Hardy, 1991; Hoover and Mullins, 1991; Jarrett, 1991; Lutz, 1990; Rojko et al., 1988; Rojko and Kociba, 1991).

Feline Leukemia Virus

The FeLV is a C-type oncornavirus (retrovirus) similar to the avian and murine leukemia viruses. Virus particles budding from cell membranes can be demonstrated by electron microscopy (Fig. 20–1) of bone marrow and various other tissues and organs of the body. The FeLV has several structural proteins, all of which are immunogenic.

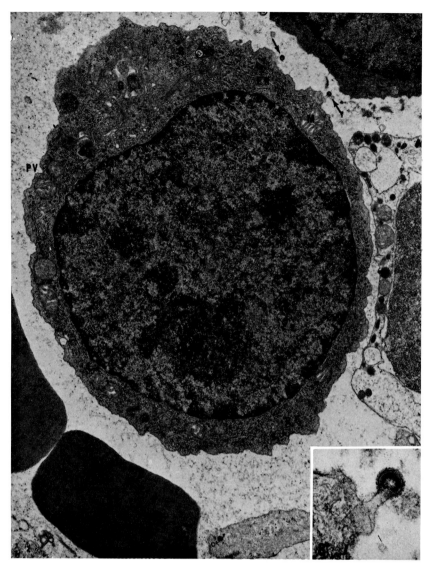

Fig. 20.–1. Electron photomicrograph of a prominent atypical cell from the bone marrow of a cat with a myeloproliferative disorder. Arrows indicate two virus particles budding from the cell membrane (×11,040). *Inset,* Higher magnification (×64,560) of one of the virus particles. Ultrastructure of the cell reveals pinocyotic vesicles (PV) along the cell membrane. The nucleus (N) is round and eccentrically located and presents a large nucleolus (Nu). A small amount of chromatin (C) is visible along the nuclear membrane. Numerous round mitochondria (M) and a well-developed Golgi apparatus (G) are evident. Free ribosomes and polysomes (R) are present in large numbers in the cytoplasm. The endoplasmic reticulum (ER) is limited to moderate numbers of long cisternae having numerous ribosomes along their surfaces. The cytoplasmic matrix is characteristically electron-dense, resembling that of a polychromatophilic rubricyte. (From Herz, A., et al.: C-type virus particles demonstrated in bone marrow cells of a cat with myeloproliferative disease Cal. Vet., 23:16, 1969.)

DIAGNOSIS

FeLV infection in cats can be demonstrated by virus isolation in tissue cultures and by immunodiagnostic tests, such as immunofluorescence and the enzyme-linked immunosorbent assay (ELISA), immunoblot (western blot), radioimmunoassay, and immunodiffusion test (Hardy, 1991; Hardy and Zuckerman, 1991). The most commonly used methods are immunofluorescence antibody (IFA) test and ELISA. A 27-kD group specific antigen, p27, is present in the viral core of FeLV. The antibody to this antigen has no protective significance, but it is of importance in IFA test. In the blood, this antigen occurs in leukocytes and platelets and in the bone marrow, it is also found in cells of the granulocytic, erythrocytic, and megakaryocytic series. Therefore, a positive IFA test on blood or bone marrow films indicates that the cat is viremic. The sensitivity and specificity of IFA test are over 98% (Hardy and Zuckerman, 1991). A positive IFA test does not, however, indicate the presence of leukemia or lymphoma.

An ELISA test has been developed to detect soluble viral antigens in serum, plasma, saliva, and tears (Hawkins, 1991). Either polyclonal or monoclonal antibodies are used in the direct ELISA test to detect viral antigen p27. Serum or plasma p27 ELISA test is very sensitive and specific. Results of the IFA and ELISA tests generally show an excellent concordance, their sensitivity and specificity exceeding 98%. General principles of various immunodiagnostic tests have been outlined (Hardy, 1991) and the sensitivity and specificity of several commercially available ELISA kits for detecting FeLV antigen (p27) in blood, tears, and saliva have been compared (Hawkins, 1991; Hawks et al., 1991; Lopez et al., 1989, 1990; Tonelli, 1991). False-positive ELISA test results have been associated with the presence of heterophil antibodies cat serum directed primarily against mouse immunoglobulins (Lopez and Jacobson, 1989).

Positive ELISA or IFA test results in cats without clinical signs of disease should be interpreted with caution, because a high proportion can be false-positive due to the low prevalence of FeLV infection in general cat population. On the other hand, a negative test is a good predictor of absence of FeLV infection because a false negative test occurs very rarely (Jacobson, 1991; Romatowski, 1989). About 10% of healthy cats that test positive by ELISA do not have infective virus in their blood (Jarrett, 1991).

An antigen distinct from the virus structure is produced on the membrane of altered host cells through the action of the virus. This antigen is called FOCMA (feline oncornavirus cell membrane antigen). Host cells are induced to produce FOCMA by both the FeLV and the feline sarcoma virus, FSV. This tumor-specific antigen has been found on the membranes of naturally occurring feline lymphoma, myelogenous leukemia, and multicentric fibrosarcoma cells. High FOCMA antibody titers commonly protect against tumor development and leukemia, and about 25 to 38% of cats exposed to FeLV may develop such titers of FOCMA antibodies. Cats infected with FeLV and exhibiting leukemia or lymphoma or cats with FeLV-associated disease commonly have low or undetectable FOCMA titers, whereas those exposed to FeLV but who remain healthy develop high FOCMA titers. A strong correlation was found between antibody levels against FeLV and FOCMA antigen in cats recovered from FeLV infection. Cats with FOCMA antibody titers had a higher prevalence of history of disease than cats without FOCMA antibody, and the prevalence of FOCMA antibody titer was identical in young and adult cats (Swenson et al., 1990).

DISEASES CAUSED BY OR ASSOCIATED WITH FeLV INFECTION

A host of neoplastic and non-neoplastic diseases are caused by or associated with the FeLV infection in cats; the latter group of diseases occurs much more frequently than the former group. These diseases include lymphoid and myeloid malignancies, immunodeficiency, secondary bacterial infections, regenerative and nonregenerative or aplastic anemias, thrombocytopenia, pancytopenia, panleukopenia-like syndrome, thymic atrophy, glomerulonephritis, abortion and fetal resorption, and neurologic syndrome.

In cats naturally infected with FeLV, a nonregenerative anemia is indicated by erythroid hypoplasia, reticulocytopenia, ferrokinetics suggestive of decreased erythropoiesis, and low numbers of BFU-E and CFU-E in spite of increased serum erythropoietin values (Wardrop et al., 1986). Cyclic hematopoiesis has been observed in association with FeLV infection in cats. Cyclic variations in neutrophil, monocyte, reticulocyte, and platelet counts, with a cycle of 8 to 12 days, were evident and could be corrected by treatment with prednisolone (Swenson et al., 1987).

A characteristic of FeLV infection is the development of immunosuppression, which places the cat in jeopardy of developing intercurrent infections and other associated diseases (Pardi et al., 1991; Reinacher, 1989). Various viral, bacterial, and parasitic diseases have been found in association with FeLV-induced immunosuppression. The pathogenesis of immunosuppression remains to be fully elucidated, although several mechanisms have been described. A viral envelope polypeptide (MW, 15,000), p15E, impairs normal lymhocyte functions in vitro and in vivo. Neutrophils of cats infected with FeLV have reduced respiratory burst activity, and chemotactic property is impaired particularly in young viremic cats (Kiehl et al., 1987). Immunosuppression of T helper cells is observed in cats with FeLV-induced lymphoproliferative diseases as well as with FeLV-associated acquired immune deficiency syndrome-like diseases (Pardi et al., 1991; Quackenbush et al., 1990; Tompkins et al., 1989a) and feline immunodeficiency virus (FIV) infected cats (Bishop et al., 1992). FIV-infected cats, like humans with HIV infection, have a reduced number of CD4+ cells and a normal number of CD8+ cells leading to an inverted CD4:CD8 ratio (Barlough et al., 1991; Novotney et al., 1990). In contrast, FeLV-infected cats have reduced numbers of both CD4+ and CD8+ cells, with a normal CD4:CD8 ratio (Tompkins et al., 1991). Thus, both groups of cats develop a T cell lymphopenia but by different mechanisms. Prolonged administration of diethylcarbamazine was found to prevent or delay the development of lymphopenia in two FeLV-infected cats (Kitchen et al., 1988).

The FeLV exists in three subgroups (A, B, and C) based on the presence of a type-specific envelope glycoprotein antigen, gp70. The antibody to gp70 is virus-neutralizing and a significant titer renders the cat immune to FeLV infection. All FeLV isolates are comprised of FeLV-A, and about half, in addition, contain FeLV-B, whereas only about 1% contain FeLV-C (Jarrett, 1991). Viruses of subgroup A usually infect only feline cells, whereas subgroup B and C viruses can grow in cells of several species. Subgroups A and AB were commonly present in cats with lymphoma and in FeLV-positive but clinically normal cats. Cats have age-related variations in their susceptibility to various subgroups of FeLV. In experimentally inoculated kittens, a macrocytic anemia, associated with active erythropoiesis in the bone marrow and extramedullary hematopoiesis in the spleen, occurred from infection with the subgroup A virus. Infection with the subgroup C virus resulted in a fatal aplastic or nonregenerative normocytic-normochromic anemia, and infection with the subgroup B virus was not accompanied by anemia. The anemia caused by FeLV-C infection results from marked inhibition of growth and/or differentiation of early erythroid progenitor cells (BFU-E) in the bone marrow. The erythroid inhibitory activity of FeLV-C has been localized in the N-terminus of the envelope surface glycoprotein, gp70 (Riedel et al., 1988).

Infection with the Kawakami-Theilen strain of FeLV caused a marked increase in the number of macrothrombocytes in association with thrombocytopenia (Boyce et al., 1986). The Rickard strain of FeLV (FeLV-R) causes thymic lymphoma composed of prothymocytes or immature cortical thymocytes (Rojko et al., 1989). A new FeLV isolate (FeLV-AB/GM-1) was found to induce acute myeloid leukemia in a high proportion of cats by 5 to 8 weeks of infection (Toth et al., 1986). It also induced myelodysplastic changes in in vitro assays for hematopoietic and stromal bone marrow cells (Testa et al., 1988). Cytologic and histologic studies suggested two stages in the development of leukemia. The first stage appeared to be equivalent to the syndrome of bone marrow dysplasia or preleukemia, which rapidly converted to leukemia. The WBC counts were low or normal, but the number of leukemic and abnormal cells increased in the peripheral blood as the disease progressed. Another new strain of FeLV (FeLV-FAIDS) was found to cause a severe immunodeficiency syndrome in kittens by destroying T cells (Mullins et al., 1989; Overbaugh et al., 1988).

Studies on the pathogenesis of FeLV-induced leukemia have shown that FeLV induced diseases may be caused by an activation of cellular proto-oncogenes, particularly *myc* gene, or by viral mutation of FeLV-A (Jarrett, 1991). For example, the generation of a recombinant virus, such as that involving FeLV-A and *myc* (FeLV-*myc*), appears to cause thymic lymphoma, while FeLV-C and FeLV-FAIDS may be variants of the prototype FeLV-A and cause anemia and immunodeficiency, respectively.

INCIDENCE AND SPREAD OF INFECTION

Healthy cats in a natural environment generally do not show persistent FeLV infection. Little evidence of viremia (0 to less than 1%) is found in stray cats, cats in single-cat households, and cats in multiple-cat households with no history of FeLV-related diseases. In contrast, cats in multiple-cat households with a history of lymphoma or exposure to FeLV show a higher level (about 30%) of persistent FeLV infection. Thus, natural infection with FeLV occurs commonly among cats in close contact, as in multiple-cat households or catteries.

In viremic cats, large quantities of the virus are present in saliva (in about 3 weeks of infection), but rarely in urine, feces, and milk or in fleas recovered from such cats. Healthy viremic cats excrete about 5- to 10-fold higher levels of virus than leukemic cats and are found at 10- to 20-fold higher rates than sick cats. Horizontal spread of the virus between cats, by contact with infected cats or their secretions and excretions, is the primary means of disease propagation. Infection spreads through the skin, oral, or respiratory routes, although the FeLV can survive in the cat's environment for only a few hours.

Pathogenetic studies have indicated that after initial host-virus interactions cats either become persistently infected and immunosuppressed, or develop a self-limiting infection and immunity and recover, or recover partially and develop a latent infection (Hayes et al., 1992; Hoover and Mullins, 1991). Subsequently, leukemogenesis or the induction of fatal, non-neoplastic, FeLV-related disease occurs in persistently infected cats. The induction period for development of lymphoma, leukemia, or an FeLV-related disease in naturally infected cats may vary from 3 to 41 months (mean 17.6). Seroepidemiologic studies have suggested the following: (1) about 30% of FeLV-exposed cats (category 1) do not mount an adequate immune response to FeLV and become persistently infected within the first 4 to 6 weeks (ELISA+, IFA+, and virus neutralizing antibody, VNAb-). (2) About 60% of cats (category 2) develop a self-limiting infection (regressive infection; ELISA-, IFA-, VNAb+). The risk of development of FeLV-related disease in these cats is rare. About 30 to 40% of cats in this category may harbor latent provirus. They rarely become progressively viremic (category 1) and develop FeLV-related diseases or develop a FeLV-negative lymphoma. (3) About 30 to 40% of cats in category 2 (category 3) become transiently viremic or antigenemic during the early period of FeLV exposure (ELISA+, IFA-/+, VNAb-). (4) About 5 to 10% of cats (category 4) show an atypical or sequestered infection (ELISA+, IFA-, VNAb+/-). These cats have localized FeLV infection in selected tissues (bone marrow, spleen, lymph nodes, and small intestine). They may show a low degree of or intermittent antigenemia or viremia and eventually progress to either category 1 or 2.

A significant association exists between FeLV seropositivity and FIV infection; FeLV-positive cats were nearly four times more likely to be seropositive for FIV than were FeLV-negative cats (Cohen et al., 1990).

The spread of FeLV among cats can be prevented by detecting viremic cats with use of the IFA test, followed by removal of such cats from the environment. The occurrence of lymphoproliferative and myeloproliferative disorders, as well as the many FeLV-associated diseases, can be prevented by eliminating FeLV from the environment of cats. In addition to testing and removing viremic cats, the vaccination of cats with an effective vaccine may reduce the spread of infection. Efforts are being made to develop a highly protective vaccine, such as those containing a recombinant FeLV envelope protein gp70 (Kensil et al., 1991; Marciani et al., 1991), a molecularly cloned inactivated virus, or a mixture of immunogenic synthetic viral peptides (Hoover et al., 1991), or immune-stimulating complexes (Weijer et al., 1989). Protocols of chemotherapy to prolong the survival of cats with lymphoma have been developed but treatment is usually not recommended because of the nature of the FeLV infection. Stage of disease significantly affects response to chemotherapy and both stage of disease and FeLV status influence survival (Mooney et al., 1989). Nonspecific immunomodulation can also be attempted (Tizard, 1991).

Lymphoproliferative Disorders

Lymphoma and lymphocytic leukemia may occur singly or in combination. The combined incidence of lymphoma and lymphocytic leukemia in cats is up to

200/100,000 annually and accounts for 80 to 90% of all feline hematopoietic neoplasms. Lymphoma is the most frequently occurring form. About 70% of cases of lymphoma are found in FeLV-positive cats and about 30% of cases occur in cats that are recognized as nonviremic or FeLV-negative. Serologic studies, however, have indicated that FeLV is also the cause of lymphoma in cats that are FeLV-negative. Most FeLV-negative lymphomatous cats are over 7 years of age, and most such cases involve alimentary or unclassified forms of the tumor. Two morphologically similar C-type viruses have been described in association with feline lymphoma; the first, FeLV, is the causative agent of lymphoma, and the second, feline C-type virus (RD-114), is an endogenous virus of the cat not known to cause disease.

ANATOMIC FORMS OF LYMPHOMA

Clinical manifestations of lymphoma are so varied that several somewhat distinct anatomic patterns have been recognized. These are designated as thymic or mediastinal, alimentary or abdominal, multicentric, and unclassified forms. The first two are generally limited to the neoplastic involvement of the viscera and their associated lymph nodes. The multicentric form generally includes enlargement of some or all peripheral lymph nodes, as well as variable involvement of the internal organs. In the rare unclassified form, lymphoma may be located in the skin, eye, central nervous system, or any other nonlymphoid tissue. The thymic and alimentary forms, considered together, occur most frequently, so that generalized superficial lymph node enlargement is not the most common finding in lymphoma of the cat, as is the case in the dog. Variations have been noted in the geographic distribution of various forms of lymphoma and FeLV-associated hematologic diseases.

Clinical signs applicable to all forms of lymphoma are depression, rapid wasting, fluctuating temperature elevations (with some cats remaining afebrile and others experiencing continuous pyrexia), vomiting and/or diarrhea, and progressive refractory anemia. Age and sex distributions reveal equal susceptibility of the sexes, with distribution throughout the entire life span of the cat. Cats as young as 6 months of age have had lymphoma, most commonly the thymic or mediastinal form. The thymic form is common in younger cats (mean age, 2.5 years), the multicentric form is common in relatively older cats (mean age, 4 years), and the alimentary form is common at a much higher age (mean age, 8 years). The average age of FeLV-infected cats with lymphoma is 3 years, whereas that of FeLV-negative cats with lymphoma is 7 years. No breed susceptibility has been reported.

Immunologic cell surface marker studies have shown that thymic lymphomas are composed of T cells, alimentary lymphomas are composed of B cells, and multicentric lymphomas either lack B- or T-cell surface markers or are composed of T cells. All histologic types of lymphoma—undifferentiated lymphocytic, poorly differentiated lymphocytic, well-differentiated lymphocytic, and "histiocytic" types—may occur in any of the various anatomic forms.

The thymic form is characterized by a rapidly developing space-occupying mass in the anterior ventral portion of the thorax. The mass may extend into the thoracic inlet, where it becomes palpable. Displacement of the trachea, esophagus, and regional lung lobes produces coughing, gagging, vomiting, and eventually dyspnea of varying degrees. A radiograph of the chest with the cat in the standing position reveals a fluid line and, after withdrawal of the fluid, the mass can be visualized radiographically. Similar clinical signs may be produced by pyothorax, chylothorax, diaphragmatic hernia, and chronic heart failure. In such cases, stained films of the centrifuged sediment of pleural effusions are generally diagnostic. Neutrophils and bacteria are present in large numbers in pyothorax. Chylothorax is characterized by a fluid that remains milky after centrifugation and contains small mature lymphocytes. The chest fluid of cats with thymic lymphoma usually has a high nucleated cell count (5,000 to 295,000/μl), with lymphoblasts or prolymphocytes predominating and mitotic figures often present.

The alimentary or abdominal form of lymphoma involves primarily the terminal ileum, mesenteric lymph nodes, liver, kidneys, and spleen. It is the most frequent form of lymphoma encountered in FeLV-negative cats. Depression, anorexia, and rapid weight loss are frequent accompanying signs. Palpation reveals a firm mass in the midabdomen or, when the kidneys are grossly involved, bilateral firm masses in the region of the kidneys.

The multicentric form includes peripheral lymphadenopathy and internal lymph node and organ involvement. The spleen may be enlarged several times, and the liver may present a distinctly lobular pattern or numerous small foci of tumor cell infiltrations. The mesenteric lymph nodes, kidneys, and mediastinal lymph nodes may be involved. Clinical signs are referable to the extent and degree of tissue and organ involvement.

HEMATOLOGY OF LYMPHOID MALIGNANCIES

Hematologic changes in lymphoid malignancies are not usually characteristic of a leukemia (Table 20–1). A mild to severe anemia may be seen in one-third to two-thirds of FeLV-positive lymphoma cats. Anemia is common in the thymic or multicentric form, but not in the alimentary form. Erythrocyte morphology is usually of a persistent, normocytic-normochromic, nonregenerative anemia. The total plasma protein concentration may be elevated from hemoconcentration, or sometimes may be reduced because of decreased synthesis or loss through the kidneys or intestinal tract. In general, plasma fibrinogen values are within the normal range. WBC counts vary from leukopenia (less than 5,500/μl) to leukocytosis (more than 19,500/μl) because of neutrophilia. Almost 50% of cats may show frank lymphopenia (less than 1,500 lymphocytes/μl). Only a small number of cats (approx-

Table 20-1.   Selected Hematologic Findings in Lymphoid Malignancies in the Cat

Parameter	Form of Disease		
	Thymic Lymphoma	Alimentary and Multicentric Lymphoma	Histiocytic Lymphoma
No. of cats	19	22	8
PCV (%)			
Range	9–46	4–39	20–37
Mean ± 1 SD	32.7 ± 8.3	23.5 ± 8.9	25.6 ± 6.8
No. cats tested	19	22	8
Plasma protein (g/dl)			
Range	6.9–8.8	6.1–8.2	4.8–10.0
Mean ± 1 SD	7.7 ± 0.7	7.3 ± 0.7	7.3 ± 1.8
No. cats tested	6	11	8
Fibrinogen (g/dl)			
Range	0.10–0.40	0.10–0.50	0.10–0.40
Mean ± 1 SD	0.26 ± 0.11	0.30 ± 0.15	0.24 ± 1.00
No. cats tested	5	11	7
Total WBC/μl			
Range	3,200–33,600	1,600–30,800	800–25,500
Mean ± 1 SD	15,605 ± 9,791	11,614 ± 8,149	11,468 ± 8,927
No. cats tested	18*	17†	8
Absolute lymphocyte count			
Range	56–6,200	500–9,009	240–2,719
Mean ± 1 SD	1,692 ± 1,441	2,935 ± 2,724	1,000 ± 757
No. cats tested	18*	17†	8

*One cat showed leukemia: WBC, 118,000; absolute lymphocytic count, 116,200.

† Five leukemic cats showed a WBC range of 65,000 to 693,000, with a mean of 210,000; six leukemic cats showed absolute lymphocyte counts ranging between 19,559 and 693,000, with a mean of 56,221 ± 43,576.

imately 10%) may show leukemic blood pictures, with WBC counts ranging from 65,000 to 693,000/μl and absolute lymphocyte counts ranging from 19,559 to 693,000/μl. Although neoplastic involvement of lymphocytic tissues with tumor formation may be present, the blood may be lymphocytopenic in as many as 50% of cats. Immunosuppression characteristic of FeLV infection may cause lymphocytopenia from thymic atrophy and the depletion of other lymphoid tissues. Lymphopenia may also result from the inability of neoplastic lymphocytes to enter the blood from lymphoid tissues because of alterations in their surface membrane properties.

Lymphoblasts and prolymphocytes are larger than normal mature lymphocytes (Figs. 20–2 and 20–3). Although a finely stippled chromatin pattern is the hallmark of immaturity, the chromatin may sometimes be coarsely granular (compare Plates XIX-1, XIX-3, and XIX-4). When a nucleolar ring or rings are present, the cell is identified as a lymphoblast. The cytoplasm of lymphoblasts and prolymphocytes is sparse and stains a deeper blue compared to that of the mature lymphocyte. Vacuoles may occasionally be present in the cytoplasm, and rarely in the nucleus (Plates XIX-5 and XIX-6). In histiocytic lymphoma, neoplastic cells tend to be larger than typical lymphoblasts and prolymphocytes, the cytoplasm tends to stain a darker blue, and many round, discrete vacuoles commonly appear in both the cytoplasm and nucleus (Figs. 20–4 and 20–5). Large reddish purple cytoplas-

mic granules characterize the lymphocytes found in blood of cats with large granular lymphoma (Frank et al., 1986; Goitsuka et al., 1988; Tompkins et al., 1989b).

The bone marrow in lymphoid malignancies of cats may be moderately to massively infiltrated by neoplastic lymphoid cells (Plates XIX-4 and XIX-5). Nor-

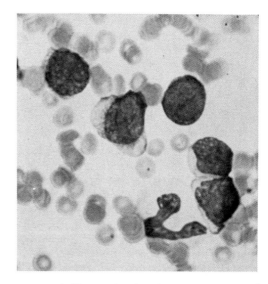

Fig. 20–2. Lymphoblasts and prolymphocytes in the bone marrow of a cat with lymphoma (× 2700). (From Jain, N.C.: Schalm's Veterinary Hematology. 4th Ed. Philadelphia, Lea & Febiger, 1986, p. 850.)

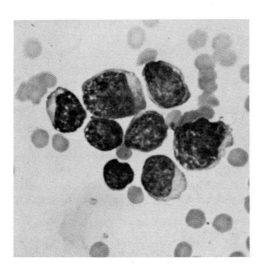

Fig. 20–3. Lymphocytes varying from normal to prolymphocytes in the bone marrow of a cat with lymphoma (×2700). (From Jain, N.C.: Schalm's Veterinary Hematology. 4th Ed. Philadelphia, Lea & Febiger, 1986, p. 851.)

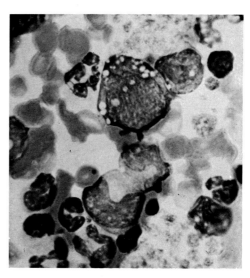

Fig. 20–5. Vacuolated reticulum cell in the bone marrow of a cat with reticulum cell sarcoma (×2700). (From Jain, N.C.: Schalm's Veterinary Hematology. 4th Ed. Philadelphia, Lea & Febiger, 1986, p. 851.)

mal feline marrow may reveal 5 to 15% small mature lymphocytes. Neoplastic infiltration of lymphoid cells is characterized by cells of varying size and maturity, ranging from mature lymphocytes to lymphoblasts (Figs. 20–2 and 20–3). Erythropoiesis is depressed and granulopoiesis is sometimes abnormal; both are common manifestations of FeLV infection rather than an effect of lymphoid infiltration. Abnormal granulopoiesis is usually characterized by the presence of giant and bizarre granulocytic cells, primarily of the neutrophil series. Cells typical of histiocytic lymphoma are also found in the bone marrow of affected cats (Fig. 20–5).

The diagnosis of lymphoid neoplasia in the cat commonly requires a combination of blood studies, bone marrow aspiration, cytologic examination of

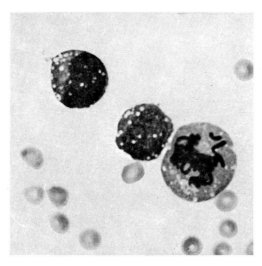

Fig. 20–4. Reticulum cells in pleural effusion in reticulum cell sarcoma of a cat (×2700). (From Jain, N.C.: Schalm's Veterinary Hematology. 4th Ed. Philadelphia, Lea & Febiger, 1986, p. 851.)

pleural effusions, and lymph node aspirates or impression smears of biopsy specimens. Only in a few instances can the blood examination by itself confirm the diagnosis. Other occasional to more common abnormal findings in cats with lymphoma or lymphocytic leukemia include hypercalcemia, as seen in the dog and horse, chromosomal abnormalities in the form of marked aneuploidies, and reduced serum complement concentration. Chromosomal abnormalities in leukemic cats included an increased number of hyperdiploid cells and the presence of double minute or morphologically abnormal chromosomes (Grindem and Buoen, 1986).

ACUTE LYMPHOBLASTIC LEUKEMIA

Cats can develop acute lymphoblastic leukemia unassociated with solid tumor masses. The incidence may vary with geographic location, but it is usually rare. Clinical signs are vague and include pallor, lethargy, weakness, anorexia, weight loss, and fever. Hepatomegaly and lymphadenopathy may be found. Hematologic findings invariably reveal anemia and leukopenia to extreme leukocytosis. The diagnosis is based on the presence of abnormal lymphocytes in the blood and/or bone marrow, and most of the lymphocytes are T cells. The bone marrow is usually hypercellular, being infiltrated with lymphoblasts or prolymphocytes. Thrombocytopenia and bleeding tendencies are infrequent, unlike the findings in human patients with acute lymphocytic leukemia (ALL). Low-dose cytosine arabinoside was used to induce a temporary remission of ALL in a cat with a persistent neutropenia due to ineffective myeloid hyperplasia (Helfand, 1987).

HODGKIN'S DISEASE

Hodgkin's disease was diagnosed in a 9-year-old female tabby cat. Splenomegaly was evident on palpation and at necropsy. The presence of numerous cells with characteristics of Reed-Sternberg cells prompted the diagnosis of Hodgkin's disease.

MULTIPLE MYELOMA

This is described in Chapter 21.

Myeloproliferative Disorders and Myelodysplastic Syndromes

A myeloproliferative disease (MPD) may involve any one or a combination of the different cell lines that are found in the bone marrow (Table 19–1). In the cat, all variants of MPD except eosinophilic leukemia are associated with FeLV infection. However, experimental inoculation of a putative *env* gene recombinant feline retrovirus (PR8) in 14 specific-pathogen free cats produced an eosinophilic leukemia in one cat and marked eosinophilic hyperplasia in another cat (Lewis et al., 1985).

Criteria for the diagnosis of an MPD in dogs and cats are based on guidelines proposed for the classification of acute myeloid leukemia (AML) in humans (Jain et al., 1991). These criteria have been described in Chapter 19 and summarized in Table 19–3 and Figure 19–2. Briefly, a diagnosis of AML is made when the bone marrow erythroid component is less 50% and more than 30% blast cells are identified as myeloblasts and monoblasts. Blast cell counts between 5 and 30% indicate a myelodysplastic syndrome (MDS), whether the erythroid component is less or more than 50%. The subclassification of AML is based on the number and types of various blast cells in bone marrow.

Myeloid leukemias involving the neutrophils, eosinophils, and basophils are the classic forms of MPD, and have been reported to occur in cats. Monocytic leukemias are rare, but myelomonocytic leukemias have been described. The proliferation of pluripotential stem cells in the bone marrow may lead to the accumulation of primitive cells that show no clear-cut differentiation toward a recognizable cell line. The term "acute undifferentiated leukemia" (AUL) is recommended to describe this form of MPD (Fig. 19–1; Table 19–3). The term "reticuloendotheliosis," which formerly described this disorder, should be discarded. Differentiation of the abnormally proliferating cells primarily into recognizable erythroid cells, without the significant participation of granulocytes, may be called erythremic myelosis, whereas an admixture of erythrocytic and granulocytic precursors suggests erythroleukemia. Both these disorders are now considered as MDSs and are, respectively, designated as MDS-Er and M6 or M6-Er under the proposed system (see Fig. 19–2 and Table 19–3). Previously, a broad diagnosis of MPD in cats implied the presence of erythremic myelosis, erythroleukemia, or reticuloendotheliosis.

Significant findings in the blood, bone marrow, and visceral organs of some of these forms of MPD in the cat are presented in Table 20–2. Additional cytologic abnormalities that may be found in some cats with MPD include phagocytosis of nucleated and mature erythrocytes by macrophages within the bone marrow, lupus erythematosus (LE) cells, agglutination of polychromatic erythrocytes and metarubricytes (Plate XXII-6), iron particles within the cytoplasm of some megaloblastic rubricytes (Plate XV-5) and macrocytic erythrocytes, reduced erythrocyte survival and total erythrocyte volume, and increased plasma volume.

Megakaryocytic leukemia is rare in cats. It is characterized by a marked increase in circulating thrombocytes, with many giant and bizarre forms, and a severe, nonregenerative anemia. Hepatosplenomegaly may be present. Megakaryocytes of abnormal morphology are present in the bone marrow, liver, and spleen, and may be FOCMA-positive. A role for megakaryocytes in the development of myelofibrosis through the production of platelet-derived growth factor has been proposed. Myelofibrosis was detected in 61% of cats with MDS and AML combined, but an association with marrow megakaryocyte count or other potential causal factors was not found (Blue, 1988). Treatment with cytosine arabinoside (100 mg/m^2, qid, for 6 days) produced a complete remission for 100 days in a case of acute megakaryocytic leukemia in a cat (Hamilton et al., 1991).

Myelofibrosis (Plate XXIII-6) may develop in some cats with MPD as a terminal event while the bizarre proliferation of hematopoietic cells continues within the vascular spaces of the liver (Plate XXIII-5), spleen, and lymph nodes (extramedullary hematopoiesis). Icterus becomes part of the syndrome when a massive accumulation of hematopoietic cells within the liver sinusoids (Fig. 20–6; Plate XXIII-5) leads to atrophy of the hepatic parenchyma. Icterus may also occur partly as a result of hemolytic anemia from marked erythrophagocytosis within the spleen and lymph nodes (Plate XVI-6).

ACUTE UNDIFFERENTIATED LEUKEMIA

As mentioned above, this disease was initially described as reticuloendotheliosis and has also been considered as acute erythremic myelosis. The designation AUL is given to this form of MPD because the predominant neoplastic cells in this disease cannot be definitively identified by methods currently available.

Typical cells have a reddish-purple nucleus and blue cytoplasm and vary somewhat in size (Plates XV-1 and XV-2). The nucleus occupies most of the cell and assumes an eccentric position. The nucleus may contain one or more nucleoli (Plate XV-1), but nucleoli are usually absent. The chromatin pattern, cytoplasmic color, and ultrastructure of some of these cells give the impression that they are closely related to erythroid precursor cells (Fig. 20–7). The cytoplasm of some cells contains a few to many reddish azurophilic granules (Plate XV-2), which is suggestive of myeloid differentiation to the promyelocyte stage (Fig. 20–8), but these granules are peroxidase-negative. Thus, some features of both erythroid and granulocytic differentiation appear among the primitive cells. In some instances, particularly in the blood, the cells may

Table 20-2. Significant Findings in the Blood, Bone Marrow, and Visceral Organs in Myeloproliferative Disorders of the Cat

Cat No.	Sex	Age	Cytologic Classification	PCV (%)	MCV (fl)	Icterus Index Units	Reticulocytes	Nucleated RBC/μl	WBC/μl	Left Shift to Include	Unclassified and Blast Cells (%)	Visceral Involvement*	
1	XM	6 yr	Undifferentiated MPD	13	63.4	2	Rare	148	14,800	Bands	34.0	LN LV SP BM	+ + + + + + + + + +
2	F	3 yr	Undifferentiated MPD	7	43.5	30	Rare	1,460	13,900	Bands	15.5	LN LV SP BM†	+ + + + + +
3	M	7 yr	Erythremic myelosis	8	50.0	2	None	16,530	11,400	Progranulocytes	10.0	LN LV SP BM†	+ + + + + + + + + +
4	M	2 yr	Erythremic myelosis	14	73.6	75	Moderate	435,000	45,100	Myelocytes	Few	LN LV SP BM†	+ + + + + + + + + +,LE
5	XF	5 yr	Erythroleukemia	12	88.9	2	Rare	110,000	48,300	Myeloblasts	Rare	LN LV SP BM†	− + − + +,F,LE
6	XM	Mature	Erythroleukemia	12	61.5	2	Moderate	26	3,500	Myelocytes	4.0	LN LV SP BM†	+ + + + + + + + + +
7	F	3 yr	Myelomonocytic Leukemia	23	57.5	2	—	None	213,000	Blasts	1.0	LN LV SP BM	− + + + + +
8	F	7 mo	Myelogenous Leukemia	22	44.0	2	None	None	4,000	Myelocytes	None	LN LV SP BM	+ + + + + +

* −, Not involved; +, slight; + +, moderate; + + +, marked enlargement or infiltration; F, myelofibrosis; LE, lupus erythematosus cells seen; LN, lymph node; LV, liver; SP, spleen; BM, bone marrow.

† C-type virus demonstrated in bone marrow cells.

‡ C-type virus in megakaryocytes.

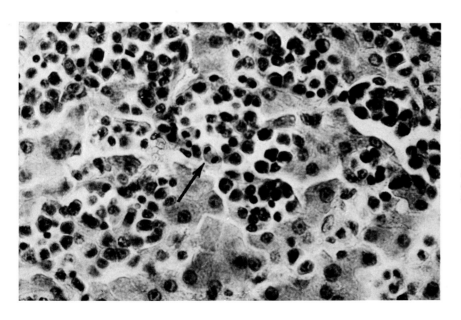

Fig. 20–6. Liver section from a cat with acute undifferentiated myeloproliferative disorder (acute undifferentiated leukemia, AUL). The liver sinusoids are packed with primitive cells. The arrow points to a cell in mitosis (H & E stain; ×400). (From Jain, N.C.: Schalm's Veterinary Hematology. 4th Ed. Philadelphia, Lea & Febiger, 1986, p. 854.)

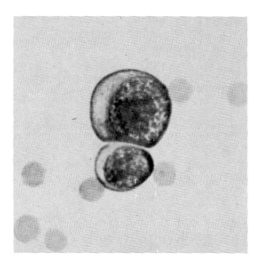

Fig. 20–7. Primitive cells in the blood of a cat with acute undifferentiated myeloproliferative disorder. The nuclear chromatin pattern is suggestive of erythroid precursor cells (×3200). (From Jain, N.C.: Schalm's Veterinary Hematology. 4th Ed. Philadelphia, Lea & Febiger, 1986, p. 856.

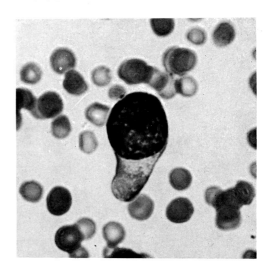

Fig. 20–9. Primitive cell with cytoplasmic pseudopod in the bone marrow of a cat with erythroleukemia (×2300). (From Jain, N.C.: Schalm's Veterinary Hematology. 4th Ed. Philadelphia, Lea & Febiger, 1986, p. 856.)

have a lighter cytoplasm, similar to that of the lymphocyte, but the nucleus retains a perfectly round shape and is eccentrically placed, so that generally more cytoplasm is evident than in the lymphocyte. Thus, the cell lineage of neoplastic cells found in AUL is difficult to ascertain by morphologic means and routine cytochemical stains are of no avail.

In the bone marrow, a monotonous pattern of round, deep blue cells is found, with an almost complete absence of recognizable maturation forms (Plate XXII-2). Some cells have a broad, pseudopod-like cytoplasmic projection (Fig. 20–9). The cytoplasmic projection may contain azurophilic granules (Plate XV-3) or vacuoles and may pinch off, forming anuclear cytoplasmic structures of varying sizes. Such cytoplasmic fragments may also be found in the blood. When

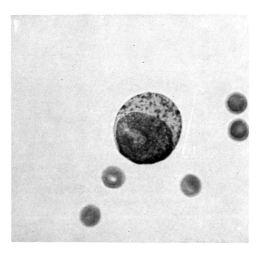

Fig. 20–8. Blast cell with large azurophilic granules in the blood of a cat with acute undifferentiated myeloproliferative disorder (×2000). (From Jain, N.C.: Schalm's Veterinary Hematology. 4th Ed. Philadelphia, Lea & Febiger, 1986, p. 856.)

the pinched-off portion contains azurophilic granules, it may resemble an enormous platelet, whereas an agranular, deep blue mass may be confused with a giant polychromatic erythrocyte. A reduction in granulopoiesis, vacuolation of granulocytic cells, and an occasional giant metamyelocyte may also be present.

Care must be taken to distinguish the bone marrow cytology of this form of MPD from that of deficiencies of vitamin B$_{12}$ and folic acid. Although deficiencies of these vitamins have not been confirmed in cats, bone marrow cytology in an occasional cat has presented megaloblastic features of erythroid cells typical of humans with these vitamin deficiencies. In such cases, erythroid cells show a maturation arrest at the prorubricyte and basophilic rubricyte stages, leading to an accumulation of deep blue erythroid cells in the marrow (compare Plates XXII-1 and XXII-2). The occurrence of large metamyelocytes in the bone marrow is also to be anticipated in these vitamin deficiencies.

ERYTHREMIC MYELOSIS

Erythremic myelosis (MDS-Er) may be suspected when, in the presence of a severe anemia, the peripheral blood morphology is characterized by marked anisocytosis without an accompanying polychromasia (Plate XXII-3). An occasional nucleated erythrocyte may exhibit asynchrony of maturation between the cytoplasm and nucleus. In other patients, the blood may be characterized by a profusion of relatively normal-appearing nucleated erythrocytes in all stages of development unaccompanied by polychromatic erythrocytes (Cat 3, Table 20–2). A cat with erythroleukemia may present a similar picture (Cat 5, Table 20–2). These nucleated red cells may be derived partly from the sites of extramedullary hematopoiesis, such as the sinusoids of the liver and spleen (Plate XXIII-5).

The examination of stained bone marrow films is essential to confirm the diagnosis. The bone marrow is generally characterized by a profusion of erythroid cells in all stages of maturation. The erythroid component is greater than 50%, myeloblasts are rare, and the total blast cell count including rubriblasts is less than 30% of all nucleated cells (Fig. 19–2). Most rubricytes may appear morphologically normal (Plate XXII-4) or megaloblastic (Plate XV-4) because of the asynchronous development of the cytoplasm and nucleus. Rarely, multiple nuclei (polyploidy) may be present in a large polychromatic cell (Plate XXIII-1). More commonly, metarubricytes with double nuclei are encountered (Plate XXII-6). When the erythropoietic activity is excessive, granulopoiesis is depressed and vacuolation of the granulocytic precursor cells may be seen. Erythrophagocytosis by abnormally proliferating erythroid cells may be seen on occasion (Plate XXIII-2).

ERYTHROLEUKEMIA

A clear separation between erythremic myelosis and erythroleukemia was not formerly made. In fact, the distinction was mostly arbitrary and was based on the finding of myeloblasts admixed with abnormal nucleated erythrocytes in the blood and/or bone marrow (Fig. 20–10). Current diagnostic recommendations are presented in Chapter 19 and outlined in Figure 19–2. Briefly, the erythroid component in bone marrow is characteristically greater than 50%. Classic erythroleukemia (M6) is considered when the blast cells (myeloblast and monoblast combined) are less than 30% of all nucleated cells but more than 30% of nonerythroid cells. Erythroleukemia with erythroid predominance (M6-Er) is considered when the blast cell count inclusive of rubriblasts is more than 30%.

Dameshek (1969) stressed the existence of three successive stages of MPD, initially involving the eryth-rocytic cell series and later the granulocytic precursor cells: (1) a period of erythremic myelosis characterized by a striking red cell hyperplasia of the bone marrow; (2) a stage of mixed erythroid and myeloid proliferation (erythroleukemia); and (3) the eventual termination of some cases in myeloblastic leukemia. In some cases, a preleukemic erythroid disorder preceded the development of an acute myelomonocytic leukemia.

Such a progression of MPD from erythremic myelosis and erythroleukemia has been observed in cats. We have observed a cat (Cat 6, Table 20–2; Table 20–3) that seemed to be in the stage of progression from erythroleukemia to acute myelogenous leukemia. In this case, two bone marrow samples taken 10 days apart presented distinctly different cytologic patterns. In the first sample, the principal cellular abnormality was referable to the erythrocytic maturation series. Rubriblasts with a single, large nucleolus (Figs. 20–11, 20–12) and megaloblastic rubricytes with normal or abnormal hemoglobinization were a prominent feature (Plate XXIII-3). Granulocytic series cells had vacuolated cytoplasm and some cells were large, with bizarre nuclei. The myeloid:erythroid (M:E) ratio was 1.26:1.0. The M:E ratio in bone marrow sampled 10 days later had increased to 14.5:1.0. This reflected the change to a predominance of atypical granulocytic precursor cells with only an occasional megaloblastic rubricyte (Plate XXIII-4). Haemobartonella felis and Toxoplasma gondii were seen (Plates XIV-8 and XIV-9). These parasites were not found in the first bone marrow sample. It was conjectured that the cat was a carrier of both parasites and that, because of its debilitated condition and FeLV-mediated immunosuppression, the parasites were beginning to multiply. Undifferentiated cells of the granulocytic series were found in the bone marrow, spleen, liver, and lymph

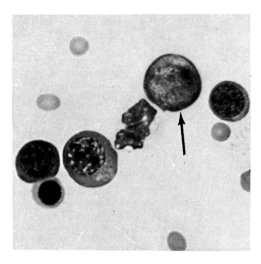

Fig. 20–10. Blood of a cat with erythroleukemia. A myeloblast *(arrow)* is shown, together with four nucleated erythrocytes in various stages of maturation (× 2700). (From Jain, N.C.: Schalm's Veterinary Hematology. 4th Ed. Philadelphia, Lea & Febiger, 1986, p. 857.)

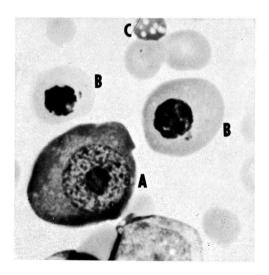

Fig. 20–11. Megaloblastoid rubriblast (A) and normochromic megaloblastoid rubricytes (B) in the bone marrow of a cat with erythremic myelosis or erythroleukemia. A vacuolated cytoplasmic fragment (C) is also shown (from Cat 6, Table 20–2; × 3600). (From Jain, N.C.: Schalm's Veterinary Hematology. 4th Ed. Philadelphia, Lea & Febiger, 1986, p. 859.)

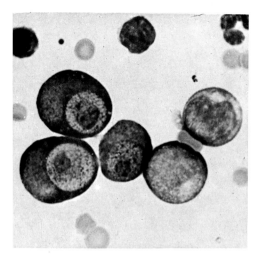

Fig. 20–12.   Bone marrow from a cat with erythroleukemia. Three abnormal rubricytes and two myelocytes are seen. The rubricytes are deficient in nuclear chromatin, and each nucleus presents a large nucleolus (from Cat 6, Table 20–2; ×2700). (From Jain, N.C.: Schalm's Veterinary Hematology. 4th Ed. Philadelphia, Lea & Febiger, 1986, p. 859.)

nodes on histopathologic examination. C-type virus particles were found budding from the plasma membrane of immature mononuclear cells examined by electron microscopy (Fig. 20–1).

MYELOGENOUS (GRANULOCYTIC) LEUKEMIA

Myelogenous or granulocytic leukemia refers to the neoplastic proliferation of myeloid cells, primarily of the neutrophilic series. The term excludes neoplasms of eosinophils and basophils, because they are singularly referred to as eosinophilic and basophilic leukemias. The blood in a typical myelogenous leukemia is characterized by a leukocytosis with a disorderly left shift up to myelocytes through myeloblasts. The WBC count in cats with myelogenous leukemia may be in the leukemic to leukopenic range (Table 20–2), with counts as high as 389,000/μl.

Clinical signs of myelogenous leukemia in cats include chronic wasting, anorexia, depression, vomiting, fever, watery and bloody diarrhea, and dehydration. Hematologic findings include reduced, normal, or elevated WBC counts, with a moderate to marked left shift to myeloblasts (Plate XXIV-1), and a moderate to marked nonregenerative anemia. Diagnosis may present a problem in the cat that has a normal WBC count or leukopenia with a left shift, including at times

Table 20-3.   Four Hemograms of a Cat with Bone Marrow Cytology Suggestive of a Progression of Erythroleukemia to Acute Myelogenous Leukemia between December 3 and December 13

Parameter	Nov. 27	Dec. 3	Dec. 12	Dec. 13
RBC ($\times 10^6$/μl)	1.95	1.89	1.30	1.25
PCV (%)	12.0	14.0	10.0	11.0
Hemoglobin (g/dl)	3.8	4.6	3.0	3.0
MCV (fl)	61.5	74.1	76.9	88.0
MCHC (%)	31.7	32.1	33.3	27.3
Icterus index (units)	2	2	—	10
Plasma proteins (g/dl)	7.6	6.9	—	6.9
Fibrinogen (g/dl)	0.20	0.20	—	0.20
Reticulocytes	Moderate	Moderate	—	Few
Polychromasia	Moderate	Moderate	Rare	Rare
Anisocytosis	Moderate	Moderate	Slight	Slight
Nucleated RBC/100 WBC	26	29	5	1
WBC/μl (corrected)	3,500	8,000	12,900	12,000
Myelocytes	175 (5.0%)	0	0	0
Metamyelocytes	35 (1.0%)	0	0	420 (3.5%)
Band neutrophils	70 (2.0%)	0	580 (4.5%)	1,920 (16.0%)
Neutrophil (mature)	2,415 (69.0%)	6,320 (79.0%)	9,739 (75.5%)	5,340 (44.5%)
Lymphocytes	420 (12.0%)	1,040 (13.0%)	516 (4.0%)	720 (6.0%)
Monocytes	245 (7.0%)	640 (8.0%)	2,064 (16.0%)	3,360 (28.0%)
Eosinophils	0	0	0	0
Basophils	0	0	0	0
Unclassified cells	140 (4.0%)	0	0	240
Parasites	—	—	Few Haemobartonella felis	Few Haemobartonella felis; rare; Toxoplasma gondii
Myeloid:erythroid ratio		1.26:1		14.5:1
Bone marrow cytology		Predominately megaloblastic erythroid cells Few myeloid precursors		Many myeloid precursors Rare megaloblastic erythroid cells

Modified from Herz, A., Theilen, G. H., Schalm, O. W., et al.: Demonstration of C-type virus particles, Toxoplasma gondii and Haemobartonella felis, in a cat with a myelo-proliferative disorder. Cal. Vet., 23:18, 1969.

myelocytes, progranulocytes, and occasionally myeloblasts (Cat 9, Table 20–2). Examination of the bone marrow aspirate is essential in such cases to make the diagnosis. The bone marrow usually reveals a predominance of myeloblasts or promyelocytes to myelocytes (Plates XXIV-2, XXIV-3, and XXIV-4). The granulocytic cells may appear abnormally large, with a bizarre nuclear pattern. Most cells are positive for cytochemical markers of myeloid cells (e.g., peroxidase). The erythrocytic maturation series may be complete, but markedly reduced. An occasional megaloblastic rubricyte may be found (Plate XXIII-4).

Necropsy findings include foci of neoplastic cells in the liver, spleen, kidneys, lymph nodes, and other body tissues or organs. Extramedullary hematopoiesis may occur at these tissues. The degree of infiltration by neoplastic myeloid cells may vary among cats with myelogenous leukemia.

The problem of diagnosing myelogenous leukemia in the cat is complicated by the fact that leukopenia with a left shift to progranulocytes and/or myeloblasts occurs frequently in association with toxemic diseases in this species. The bone marrow may be hypercellular, with many immature granulocytes having bizarre nuclei (Plates XV-8 and XV-9). This situation is transient in cats with toxemic diseases, however, and repeat bone marrow examinations about 1 or 2 weeks apart may facilitate the diagnosis. As mentioned earlier, when the bone marrow is hypercellular with myeloid cells and the blast cell count is more than 30% of all nucleated cells, AML is diagnosed, and MDS is considered with a blast cell count between 5 and 30%. Chronic myelogenous leukemia must be distinguished from MDS.

MONOCYTIC AND MYELOMONOCYTIC LEUKEMIA

A leukemic process characterized by the neoplastic proliferation of monocytes is known as monocytic leukemia, and that involving both granulocytic and monocytic cells is classified as myelomonocytic leukemia. The monoblast is derived from a stem cell (CFU-GM) in common with the myeloblast, so acute neoplastic proliferation of the monocyte is classified as an AML, but CMoL in humans is considered a MPD. Both types of leukemia have been described in cats. Many of these cats are FeLV-positive, and the clinical findings are generally nonspecific. The history reveals anorexia, depression, vomiting, and lethargy lasting days to weeks. Physical findings include fever, pale mucous membranes, mild dehydration, diarrhea, emaciation, bilateral ocular and nasal discharges, dyspnea or hyperpnea, enlarged submandibular and axillary lymph nodes, splenomegaly, and mitral valve murmur.

Hematologic findings generally consist of mild to severe anemia, with macrocytic or normochromic red cell morphology, thrombocytopenia with abnormal platelet morphology, moderate to marked leukocytosis with a left shift to promyelocytes and myeloblasts, and monocytosis with many immature cells. Immature monocytic cells, monoblasts and promonocytes, pre-

dominate in cats with AMoL. Immature monocytic cells in the blood and bone marrow contain nuclei with reticular chromatin, an irregular or clefted outline, and nuclear membrane foldings. Monocytosis is marked. Some cats may have neutrophils with a basophilic cytoplasm and Döhle bodies. Macropolycytes (giant hypersegmented neutrophils) are found on rare occasions.

The bone marrow is usually hypercellular because of increased myelopoiesis and monocytopoiesis. Erythropoiesis is diminished and the M:E ratio is increased significantly. Morphologic abnormalities in myeloid, erythroid, and megakaryocytic cells in an occasional cat indicate dyshematopoiesis or myelodysplastic changes (Raskin and Krehbiel, 1985). Erythrophagocytosis by monocytes and neutrophils in the blood and bone marrow are seen on rare occasions.

Prominent necropsy findings include splenomegaly, hepatomegaly, and lymphadenopathy. Histopathologic examination reveals diffuse infiltration with leukemic blast cells of many organs, including the lymph nodes, liver, spleen, and bone marrow. In addition, extensive perivascular hemorrhagic infarcts in the brain and hemorrhagic foci in the lungs, urinary bladder, and gastrointestinal tract are seen in a few cases.

EOSINOPHILIC LEUKEMIA

This form of granulocytic leukemia is rare in the cat, and reported cases have been in FeLV-negative cats. Cats with eosinophilic leukemia may present with a nonspecific history of anorexia, depression, vomiting, diarrhea, and weight loss.

A case of eosinophilic leukemia in a 2-year-old castrated male Maltese cat was encountered at the Veterinary Medical Teaching Hospital, University of California, Davis (VMTH-UCD). Its hemograms were characterized by neutrophilia, lymphocytosis, monocytosis, and eosinophilia, with the latter cells comprising 80 to 85% of the WBC count (range, 50,000–244,000/μl of blood). Mature eosinophils predominated in the blood and bone marrow. A few metamyelocytes were constantly seen in blood and eosinophilic bands ranged from 14 to 20%. The marrow was hypercellular, with 82% of cells in the eosinophilic series. Some eosinophilic myelocytes were considerably larger than normal and retained a deep blue cytoplasm (Plate XXIV-5). The M:E ratio was 23.8:1. Platelet counts were low on admission and again near termination, but increased to normal levels during therapy. Therapy with prednisolone and cyclophosphamide was ineffective.

An necropsy, the liver, spleen, and all visceral lymph nodes of the thoracic and peritoneal cavities were markedly enlarged. The liver had a reticulated pattern, and the spleen was dark red and of a meaty consistency. Impression smears of the lymph nodes, liver, spleen, and bone marrow revealed many eosinophils and granulocytic precursor cells, including progranulocytes and myelocytes. No evidence of virus was found in specimens of the liver, spleen, lymph nodes, and bone marrow examined by electron microscopy.

BASOPHILIC AND MAST CELL LEUKEMIAS

Basophilic and mast cell leukemias are rare in animals. A possible instance of atypical basophilic subleukemic leukemia was encountered in a 4-year-old spayed cat. The WBC count was 15,000/μl, with all stages of granulocytes from myeloblasts to mature neutrophils in the blood. Many primitive cells (44%) presented varying numbers of large, purple, cytoplasmic granules, somewhat similar to the granules of the immature basophil leukocyte of the cat. Attempts to obtain bone marrow samples were unsuccessful because of an existing myelofibrosis.

The mast cell is a tissue cell that normally lies outside the vascular system. Typically, it has a round nucleus and large, deep purple granules. Because of similarities in the staining properties of granules in the basophils, as encountered in most species other than the cat, a mast cell leukemia has at times been erroneously called basophilic leukemia. Cat mast cells have deep purple granules, whereas mature basophils are devoid of such granules and immature basophils usually contain a mixture of deep purple and grayish granules (Plates VII-6 and XII-4). Therefore, mast cell leukemia is readily distinguished from basophilic leukemia in cats. Mastocytosis associated with splenomegaly and mast cell leukemia have been described.

The most common gross lesion in mast cell leukemia is a marked splenomegaly. Ulceration of the stomach and duodenum may occur, sometimes leading to perforation and peritonitis, because of the high level of histamine in mast cells. A modest leukocytosis (25,000 to 30,000/μl) is characterized by the conspicuous presence of mast cells in the blood (Fig. 20–13), bone marrow, spleen, and liver, and with small foci of mast cells in other organs and tissues. Anemia and leuko-

penia may sometimes be seen. Erythrophagocytosis by mast cells has been observed in a few cases of mast cell leukemia. Erythrophagocytosis by primitive malignant cells in the bone marrow, but rarely in the blood, has been observed in MPD in the cat, and by well-differentiated histiocytes in the bone marrow and other organs in histiocytic medullary reticulosis (malignant histiocytosis) in the dog.

MEGAKARYOCYTIC LEUKEMIA

Megakaryocytic leukemia has been described in a few cats. The disease was characterized by severe nonregenerative anemia and marked thrombocytosis, with many giant and bizarre platelets. Hepatomegaly and splenomegaly were present in some cases. Excessive numbers of megakaryocytes of abnormal morphology were present in the bone marrow, liver, and spleen, and were FOCMA-positive in one case.

MYELODYSPLASTIC SYNDROME OR PRELEUKEMIA

Myelodysplastic syndrome (MDS), preleukemia, and "smoldering" leukemia are terms used to describe a group of hypoproliferative hematologic abnormalities that precede the development of an overt leukemia, usually AML. Prominent hematologic findings in MDS are anemia, neutropenia, and thrombocytopenia, occurring singly or in various combinations. Morphologic abnormalities are usually seen in one or more of the hematopoietic cell lines in the blood and bone marrow. An excess of leukemic blast cells in blood and bone marrow is not seen initially, and that the condition was preleukemic can be determined only in retrospect, when the hematologic picture has progressed to that of an acute leukemia. The disease progresses slowly, over a period of several months to years, before terminating in an overt leukemia. The diagnostic criteria for MDS in humans have been described by the FAB group. Similar criteria for subclassifying MDS in dogs and cats remain to be established, although a diagnosis of MDS in these species is suggested when the blast cell count in bone marrow is from 5 to 30% and dysplastic changes are present in developing hematopoietic cells (see Chap. 19). A progression to AML is considered when the blast cell count exceeds 30%.

Myelodysplastic syndrome has been observed in cats with FeLV-associated hematopoietic disturbances (Table 20–4; Blue, 1988; Blue et al., 1988). Initially, the blood picture is dominated by cytopenias with leukopenia, anemia, and thrombocytopenia in different combinations. Abnormal platelet morphology is a common finding. The anemia is usually nonregenerative, with normocytic-normochromic or macrocytic-normochromic red cell morphology. The leukopenia is the result of neutropenia and lymphopenia. No or rare blast cells are found in the blood, sometimes in association with nucleated erythrocytes (leukoerythroblastic reaction). The bone marrow often reveals a predominance of myeloid cells. The cell population consists of poorly differentiated cells, with some maturation toward myeloblasts and promyelocytes, with

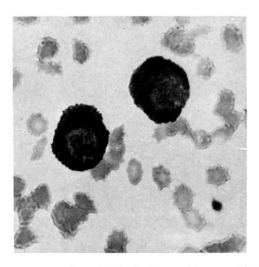

Fig. 20–13. Mast cells in the blood of a cat with mast cell leukemia (×2700). (From Jain, N.C.: Schalm's Veterinary Hematology. 4th Ed. Philadelphia, Lea & Febiger, 1986, p. 865.)

Table 20-4. Hematologic Findings in Three Cats With Myelodysplastic Syndrome

Parameter	Cat 1 Day 0	Cat 1 Day 103	Cat 2 Day 0	Cat 2 Day 347	Cat 3 Day 0	Cat 3 Day 159
RBC ($\times 10^6/\mu l$)	1.99	2.59	5.19	1.68	7.36	4.26
Hemoglobin (g/dl)	3.7	5.4	8.7	3.1	10.2	6.7
PCV (%)	11	15	27	10	30	17
MCV (fl)	55.2	57.9	52.0	59.5	40.7	39.9
MCHC (%)	33.6	36.0	32.2	31.0	34.0	39.4
MCH (pg)	18.5	20.8	16.7	18.4	13.8	15.7
Plasma protein (g/dl)	8.0	8.0	7.5	7.8	7.0	6.1
Plasma fibrinogen (g/dl)	0.1	<0.1	0.4	0.2	<0.1	0.1
Reticulocytes (%)	Rare	0	0	Few	0	Rare
Nucleated RBC (/100 WBC)	0	0	0	3	7	2
WBC*	1,900	178,400	3,400	2,700†	3,400†	40,700†
Blast cells	0	0	0	52% (1,404)	Rare	72% (29,304)
Progranulocytes	0	0	0	6% (162)	Rare	13% (5,291)
Myelocytes	0	0	0	4% (108)	Rare	6% (2,442)
Metamyelocytes	0	0	0	2% (54)	1% (34)	2% (814)
Neutrophils						
Segmented	52% (988)	1% (1,784)	34% (1,156)	0	39% (1,326)	2% (814)
Nonsegmented	2% (38)	0	0	1% (27)	1% (34)	1% (407)
Lymphocytes	42% (798)	4% (7,136)	49% (1,666)	35% (945)	48% (1,632)	4% (1,628)
Monocytes	2% (38)	0	17% (578)	0	3% (102)	0
Eosinophils	2% (38)	0	0	0	8% (272)	0
Basophils	0	0	0	0	0	0
Unclassified cells	0	95% (169,480)	0	0	0	0
Thrombocytes	Present	139,000	172,000	18,000	408,000	236,000
Platelet morphology	Pleomorphic; some very large	—	Occasional; very large	Occasional; very large	Pleomorphic; many large	Many large

From Madewell, B. R., Jain, N. C., Weller, R. E. et al.: Hematologic abnormalities preceding myeloid leukemia in three cats. Vet. Pathol., 16:510, 1979.

* Absolute values are expressed as cells/μl of blood and listed in parenthesis.

† Leukocyte counts corrected for nucleated red blood cells. Final diagnosis: Cat 1, AMMoL; Cat 2, AML-M1; Cat 3, AML-M2.

or without some monocytic differentiation. The disease progresses slowly over a few months to a year before terminating in AMMoL or AML, recognized by the predominance of blast cells in the bone marrow and as blast crisis in the blood. Cytochemical staining of blood and bone marrow smears reveals distinct populations of cells with granulocytic markers (peroxidase and alkaline phosphatase), alone or in combination with monocytic markers (α-naphthyl acetate esterase and α-naphthyl butyrate esterase).

CANINE LEUKEMIAS

Lymphoma is the most common form of lymphoproliferative neoplasia in the dog. It may occur with or without a leukemic phase. Primary lymphocytic leukemia is less common and various forms of myeloid leukemias have been described.

Lymphoproliferative Disorders

The annual incidence of lymphoma in the dog has been estimated at 24/100,000, and constitutes about 5 to 7% of all canine tumors. Lymphoma occurs pri-

marily in dogs 5 year of age and over, with no sex predilection. Breeds at relatively high risk include the boxer and Scottish terrier, whereas those at low risk include the dachshund. The cause of canine lymphoma is under investigation. Canine leukemia virus has not been demonstrated unequivocally to be a cause, although virus particles with retrovirus properties and reverse transcriptase activity have been found in the lymphoid cells of dogs with lymphoma and lymphocytic leukemia.

CLINICAL FINDINGS

The most characteristic feature of canine lymphoma is a bilateral painless swelling of the superficial nodes. Although a low-grade fever may be seen, the disease is more commonly afebrile. Edema of the face, throat, or limbs may be present in late stages of the disease. Based on clinical manifestations, canine lymphomas are grouped mainly into multicentric and alimentary types. Less common types include the cutaneous, mediastinal (thymic), and miscellaneous forms. In addition, ALL and chronic lymphocytic leukemia (CLL) may be encountered without solid tumor masses, although a slight hepatosplenomegaly may be present. A definitive diagnosis of lymphoma in the dog requires finding neoplastic cells in blood, bone marrow, and cytologic aspirates or in biopsy specimens of the lymph nodes or other tissues.

Multicentric lymphoma is the most common form. It is characterized by bilateral lymphadenopathy of most superficial nodes, hepatosplenomegaly, and involvement of almost any other tissue or organ. It may develop in stages, somewhat as follows: (1) initial lymphadenopathy in an active and relatively normal dog; (2) beginning of weight loss and mild alimentary disturbances; and (3) sudden change characterized by anorexia, listlessness, emaciation, dehydration, and death. About 75% of dogs with this form of lymphoma show abnormal thoracic radiographs and almost 50% show abnormal abdominal radiographs. Most multicentric lymphomas in the dog are of the B-cell type.

The alimentary form rarely involves the superficial lymph nodes or spleen, but the gut and mesenteric lymph nodes are regularly involved. It is characterized by a progressive wasting, diarrhea, and a palpable mass in the midabdomen.

HEMATOLOGIC AND OTHER LABORATORY FINDINGS

Hematologic data on 72 dogs with lymphoma revealed a mild to modest anemia (PCV, 24 to 26%) in approximately 40%. The anemia is often normocytic-normochromic and is generally considered an anemia of chronic disease. Other types of anemias may be found, however, including blood loss, immune-mediated, microangiopathic, diserythropoietic, and nonregenerative anemias from therapy-induced marrow hypoplasia. A moderate to marked nonregenerative anemia may develop when the bone marrow is heavily infiltrated with neoplastic lymphocytes. Hypoproteinemia (4.5 to 6.5 g/dl) relative to the age of the dog may be seen in approximately 40% of cases. Hepatosplenomegaly and generalized lymphadenopathy could result in the decreased synthesis of plasma proteins, thus causing hypoproteinemia (Table 20–5).

Elevated mean serum IgM levels have been reported in some cases.

The total and differential leukocyte counts vary in dogs with lymphoma. The mean WBC counts among 72 dogs with lymphoma were in the high normal range (15,500 to 16,500/μl), with a slight left shift and a modest monocytosis. The mean lymphocyte values fell within the normal range. Only about 21% of the dogs exhibited a lymphocytosis and 25% revealed frank lymphopenia. A frank leukemia was seen in 10% or less of the dogs. About 64% had a few to many lymphoblasts, prolymphocytes, or immature lymphocytes in the blood (Fig. 20–14; Plate XIX-1). Thus, *a blood examination is generally not diagnostic for canine lymphoma*, although lymphocyte morphology is more helpful than the lymphocyte count. Neoplastic lymphocytes may appear irregularly in small numbers in the blood, but animals in advanced stages of lymphoma often show neoplastic lymphocytes in the blood and bone marrow. Some degree of thrombocytopenia (21,000 to 135,000/μl), unassociated with bleeding problems, was seen in 53% of the dogs. Large granular lymphoma, with characteristic lymphocyte morphologic features of blood lymphocytes, has been reported in the dog (Wellman et al., 1989).

Lymph node impression smears and aspirates are generally more reliable than blood as a means of diagnosis (Plate XIX-2). A bone marrow aspirate may be of diagnostic help in some cases, and a bone marrow core biopsy can considerably improve the chances of diagnosis (Madewell, 1986; Raskin and Krehbiel, 1989). Aspirated bone marrow may also be helpful, although the bone marrow is not regularly invaded in canine lymphoma. Cytologic specimens from other organs or tissues may also be of diagnostic value because of the presence of excessive lymphoblasts or abnormal lymphocytes. Hypercalcemia is frequently observed in dogs with lymphoma, with a somewhat higher frequency in Saint Bernards and in males than in females (about 3:2). The hypercalcemia is attributed

Table 20–5. Representative Hemograms in Canine Lymphoma*

Case No.	Breed	Sex	Age (yr)	PCV (%)	ESR†	Plasma Proteins (g/dl) Total	Fibrinogen	WBC/μl	Differential Leukocyte Count (Absolute Numbers/μl) Band	Segmenters	Lymphocytes‡	Monocytes	Eosinophils	Basophils	Unclassified	Degenerated
1	Cocker Spaniel	M	6	32 (S)	13+	6.3	0.3 (H)	24,000	960	10,440	9,840++	1,080	240	0	0	1,440
2	Bulldog	F	5	46 (S)	2–	8.5	0.3	12,500	63	7,563	3,437+	1,125	250	63	0	0
3	Doberman	M	6	36 (S)	13+	5.6	0.0 (H)	15,400	0	3,619	11,550++	154	77	0	0	0
4	Collie	F	2	32	35+	9.6	0.3	8,500	510	6,035	255	510	0	0	935§	255
5	Border collie	M	9	38 (S)	14+	6.9	0.2	22,300	0	14,272	5,575++	2,119	335	0	0	0
6	Hound	M	7	33 (S)	16+	6.5	0.2 (H)	11,000	55	7,425	1,980	990	495	55	0	0
7	Vizsla	M	8	39 (S)	—	5.7	0.35 (H)	17,800	0	12,913	3,827+	979	623	0	0	178
8	Chihuahua	M	7	33	—	6.6	0.3	12,300	61	7,381	2,783+	1,149	726	0	0	0
9	Cocker	F	9	26	14+	7.0	0.3	22,700	341	15,095	5,561+	1,703	0	0	0	0
10	German shepherd	F	10	40	9+	7.0	—	16,600	0	11,703	2,324	1,411	1,079	83	0	0
11	Boxer	M	7	44 (S)	4–	7.3	0.1	3,900	0	2,535	897+	195	156	117	0	0

* All dogs exhibited lymph node enlargement, in most cases generalized. Hepatomegaly is indicated by (H) following fibrinogen value; splenomegaly is indicated by (S) following PCV value.
† Corrected erythrocyte sedimentation rate at 1 hour.
‡ +, Occasional immature lymphocyte; ++, moderate number of immature lymphocytes.
§ Large, dark neoplastic cells.

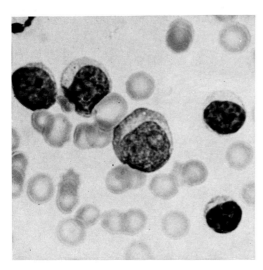

Fig. 20–14. Blood of a dog with lymphoma with a total leukocyte count of 200,000/µl with 84% lymphocytes. The two smallest cells are normal lymphocytes, the center cell is a lymphoblast with a single large nucleolus, and the two medium-sized cells are prolymphocytes (×2700). (From Jain, N.C.: Schalm's Veterinary Hematology. 4th Ed. Philadelphia, Lea & Febiger, 1986, p. 873.)

to bone-resorbing factors (e.g., osteoclast activating factor) released from tumor cells. Chromosomal abnormalities and an immune deficiency involving T cells have been described in rare cases.

HISTOPATHOLOGIC AND IMMUNOLOGIC CHARACTERIZATION

Morphologic and immunologic studies of canine lymphoma have indicated the following: (1) three distinct groups of histologic cell types are evident—lymphocytic, poorly differentiated, "histiocytic," and lymphocytic, well differentiated; (2) cells from histiocytic lymphoma are lymphocytes rather than histiocytes or macrophages; and (3) most lymphomas have a multicentric distribution and are of the B-cell type. Histologic classification of lymphoma, according to the Rappaport system, revealed nodular lymphoma in 9.7% and diffuse lymphoma in 90.3% of cases, but was of little prognostic significance (Weller et al., 1980). Immunophenotyping of canine lymphoma and leukemia using monoclonal antibodies to cell surface antigen is becoming available (Applebaum et al., 1984). It should be pursued extensively to obtain an accurate diagnosis of leukemia, provide an insight of pathophysiology of the leukemic process, and aid therapeutic management of the disease.

ACUTE AND CHRONIC LYMPHOCYTIC LEUKEMIAS

ALL and CLL have been recognized as distinct entities in the dog. CLL is a disease of middle-aged to older dogs (mean age, 9.4 years), whereas ALL is seen in relatively young dogs (mean age, 6.2 years). Both diseases are more common in females than in males, with a ratio of 3:2 for ALL and 2:1 for CLL. German shepherd dogs comprised 27% of the ALL cases reported in one study (Matus et al., 1983). The clinical course in CLL is more protracted and the physical signs are less pronounced in CLL and lymphoma than in ALL. The prognosis is more favorable for dogs with CLL than for dogs with ALL.

Acute lymphocytic leukemia is a rapidly progressive disease of sudden onset. It is characterized by high numbers of lymphoblasts in the blood and bone marrow, usually unassociated with solid tumor masses. The primary complaints include lethargy, anorexia, vomiting, and diarrhea of a few weeks' duration. Clinical signs include those of anemia, splenomegaly, and hepatomegaly. The blood shows a nonregenerative normocytic-normochromic anemia and thrombocytopenia. The bone marrow shows myelosuppression with diminished erythropoiesis and megakaryocytopoiesis. Central nervous system involvement and monoclonal gammopathy, along with hyperviscosity syndrome, may be evident in some cases.

Chronic lymphocytic leukemia is a disease with a long course that manifests over a period of several months or years. It is characterized by excessive numbers of well-differentiated mature lymphocytes in the blood and bone marrow. Clinical and other laboratory findings include lethargy, partial anorexia, nonresponsive anemia, ascites, azotemia, and proteinuria. Peripheral lymphadenopathy may be absent or mild to moderate, but the internal lymph nodes may be slightly to moderately enlarged and hepatosplenomegaly may be present. Bone marrow is usually infiltrated with small mature lymphocytes and shows mild to moderate erythroid and granulocytic hypoplasia and normal to low numbers of megakaryocytes.

Chronic lymphocytic leukemia is a disease of B lymphocytes. The serum concentrations of IgG and IgA may be increased, but hypogammaglobulinemia may occur in a few cases. Bence Jones proteinuria and hyperviscosity syndrome, associated with a monoclonal increase in IgA or IgM, may sometimes be seen (Leifer and Matus, 1986). The pathologic findings of CLL are generally similar to those of lymphoma. Chemotherapy in 17 dogs with CLL for 30 or more days resulted in survival times of 30 to 1,000 days (Leifer and Matus, 1986).

Hematologic data on seven dogs with lymphocytic leukemia, having WBC counts in excess of 100,000/µl and 85 to 97.5% lymphoid cells, are presented in Table 20–6. These dogs represented approximately 3% of all the dogs presenting with leukemias at the VMTH-UCD over a period of several years. The two dogs having no enlargement of the peripheral lymph nodes are of interest in that their diagnosis depended entirely on blood studies.

MULTIPLE MYELOMA

This is described in Chapter 21.

Table 20-6. Hemogram in Acute and Chronic Lymphocytic Leukemia in the Dog

Breed	Age (yr)	Sex	Lymphadenopathy and Organ Involvement	PCV (%)	Plasma Proteins (g/dl)	WBC/μl	Meta.	Band	Seg.	Blast	Pro	Mature	Monocytes	Eosinophils	Basophils	Degenerated
							Neutrophils			Lymphocytes						
Doberman	3	M	All nodes, splenomegaly, kidneys, and bone marrow	21	—	575,000	0	0	2.0	0	2.0	95.0	1.0	0	0	0
Boxer	8	M	No external node involved; spleen, bone marrow, and few internal nodes	24	—	580,000	0	0	0.2	0.6	6.8	89.6	0.2	0	0	2.6
Cairn terrier	10	M	Generalized with splenomegaly	23	—	120,000	0	0	12.0	+†	85.0	0	3.0	0	0	0
Boxer	6	M	Several peripheral nodes*	16	4.9	335,800	0	0.5	2.0	+†	97.5	0	0	0	0	0
Sealyham terrier	3	M	Generalized with bone marrow invasion	31	5.2	246,000	0	0	8.0	0	+†	88.5	3.0	0.5	0	0
Collie	¾	M	No peripheral node enlargement	42	7.9	131,000	0	0	4.5	0	94.5‡	0	0	0	0	1.0
Boxer	13	M	Generalized, with hepatopathy and splenomegaly	28	—	216,000	0	0.5	0	0.05	1.5	82.0 (atypical)	0	0	0	7.0

Differential Leukocyte Count (%) header spans the Neutrophils, Lymphocytes, Monocytes, Eosinophils, Basophils and Degenerated columns.

* Necropsy not authorized.
† Seen on scanning only.
‡ All cells large, atypical, in clusters.

BURKITT'S LYMPHOMA

Burkitt's lymphoma was initially considered to be a specific lymphoid tumor of children in Africa. It is a nonleukemic lymphoid tumor involving the visceral organs and bone marrow, particularly of the jaw. A characteristic feature is the scattering of phagocytic histiocytes among densely packed neoplastic lymphocytes, a pattern termed the "starry sky" effect. The lymphoid cells involved have invariably been B lymphocytes. A herpes-like virus, the Epstein-Barr virus, has been isolated from the cells of many patients with Burkitt's lymphoma and is generally regarded as the causative agent. Although starry sky pattern has been found in canine lymphomas, a true Burkitt's lymphoma has not been described.

HODGKIN'S DISEASE

Hodgkin's disease in humans is a lymphoid neoplasm recognized by its characteristic histology. The tumor in the lymph nodes begins with lymphocytic hyperplasia, followed by a gradual loss of normal architecture with replacement of the lymphocytes as the disease progresses. Binuclear or multinuclear giant cells, called Reed-Sternberg cells, are pathognomic and essential for diagnosis. In addition, the lymph node histology consists of a mixed infiltrate of lymphocytes, histiocytes, eosinophils, plasma cells, and neutrophils. Typical Hodgkin's disease has not been found in animals, although several cases of possible Hodgkin's disease in the dog have been reported.

Myeloproliferative Disorders and Myelodisplastic Syndromes

Acute and chronic myelogenous leukemias have been described in the dog (Grindem et al., 1985; Jain, 1986; Jain et al., 1991). Six dogs with histologically verified myelogenous leukemia are presented in Table 20–7. Myelogenous leukemia is more common in young dogs and lymphoma is more common in older dogs. See Chapter 19 for a general approach to the diagnosis of AML in dogs. For additional comments, see above, Feline Leukemias: MPD and MDS.

CLINICAL SIGNS

Progressive weakness and weight loss over a period of several months are common. In addition, anorexia, vomiting, polydipsia, polyuria, diarrhea, and anemia are present in various combinations. The physical examination generally reveals a slight to moderate lymphadenopathy of the peripheral nodes, splenomegaly, and sometimes hepatomegaly. Unique and misleading clinical signs may develop as a result of the neoplastic cell invasion of various tissues and organs. For example, paralysis of the lower jaw may occur because of tumorous involvement of the fifth, seventh, and ninth cranial nerve sheaths. A greenish coloration of the tumor tissue, referred to as chloroma or chloroleukemia, is encountered rarely (Table 20–7). The greenish pigmentation is ascribed to the myeloperoxidase present in the neutrophil granules. Leukostasis is a potential cause of death in leukemic dogs with

Table 20-7. Hematologic and Other Data From Dogs With Myeloid Leukemia

Breed, Sex and Age	Clinical History and Clinical Signs	PCV (%)	WBC/µl	Differential Neutrophil Count (%)						Necropsy Findings and Other Comments
				Blast	Pro.	Myelo.	Meta.	Band	Segs.	
Walker hound, male, 16 mo	Progressive weakness and depression last few months; temp. normal	7.0	37,300–132,000	6.0	1.5	0.5	4.5	4.0	73.5	Hypersegmented mature neutrophils, platelets low; spleen, liver, kidneys, and nodes enlarged
German shepherd, XF, 17 mo (Plate XXV–3)	Left eye corneal opacity, prescapular node enlarged, temp. 104° F (40° C)	26.0	86,000–127,000	25.5	0.0	0.0	0.5	6.5	8.0	In blood, 57.0% large vacuolated monocytes; bone marrow, many bizarre cell forms; gross involvement of heart, spleen, liver, and kidneys
German shepherd, XF, 2½ yr	Depression and anemia at 6 mo of age; last mo, anorexia, weakness, emaciation; temp. 103–105° F (39.4–40.6° C)	9.0	116,000	3.3	2.4	2.4	1.0	0.7	64.5	In blood, 19.7% lymphocytes and 22.6% monocytes; M:E ratio 36:1.0; spleen 30 × 13 cm, wt. 400 g, slight swelling of lymph nodes (Plate XV–4).
German shorthair pointer, XF, 5 yr	Gradual weight loss and anorexia for 1 week; temp. 102° F (39° C); hepatosplenomegaly	26.0	10,800	0.0	0.0	0.0	3.0	7.0	70.5	Liver 2½ times and spleen 3–4 times normal size, massively infiltrated by blasts to mature neutrophils; M:E ratio 2.4:1.0
Irish setter, female, 7 yr (Plate XXV–2)	Less active for 1 year; extreme weight loss last 3 mo	26.0	29,900	3.0	3.0	55.0	3.0	5.0	20.0	Platelets 107,000/µl; spleen enlarged; kidneys two times normal size, mottled red; liver mottled; greenish cast to both liver and bone marrow; * slight swelling of lymph nodes
Doberman pinscher, male, 4 yr (est.) (Fig. 20–15)	Sudden onset of conjunctivitis, vomiting, and depression; jaw paralysis 1 week later	16.0	124,000	1.0	1.5	7.5	20.0	15.0	49.0	Gross neoplastic involvement of all major organs, including trigeminal and vagus nerves; greenish cast to neoplastic tissue*

* Greenish color is said to be caused by the presence of myeloperoxidase; the condition is referred to as chloroma.

exceedingly high leukocyte counts (Hamlin and Duncan, 1990).

MYELOGENOUS LEUKEMIA

A truly leukemic blood is a common finding in the dog with myelogenous leukemia. At some phase of the disease, however, the blood may not be diagnostic for leukemia (Table 20–7), but examination of the bone marrow may reveal disorderly, left-shifted myeloid cells with an excess of myeoblasts, promyelocytes, and neutrophilic myelocytes. The diagnosis of AML or CML is based on the number and types of myeloid cells found in blood and/or bone marrow as described in Chapter 19.

The typical blood picture of myelogenous leukemia is a neutrophilia with a left shift to myeloblasts (Plate XXV-1). The neutrophils exhibit considerable variation in shape and size (Fig. 20–15) and, in some instances, hypersegmentation of the mature neutrophils is a prominent feature. Neoplastic neutrophils are susceptible to rapidly occurring degenerative changes with aging of the withdrawn blood sample. These changes consist of vacuolation of the cytoplasm and possible shrinkage of the cell. Such cells are difficult to differentiate from monocytes.

Two cell lines of neutrophilic granulocytes may be found in the blood and bone marrow, as suggested by the occurrence of neutrophils of normal morphology and by the somewhat larger basophilic cells with bizarre nuclear patterns, and at different stages of maturation (Fig. 20–16). If the neoplastic cells are too primitive or bizarre (Plates XXV-2 and XXV-3) to be classified unequivocally as granulocytes, their granulocytic origin

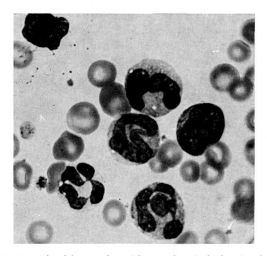

Fig. 20–15. Blood from a dog with granulocytic leukemia. The neutrophils vary in size and shape of the nucleus. Some cells have monocytoid characteristics (× 2700). (From Jain, N.C.: Schalm's Veterinary Hematology. 4th Ed. Philadelphia, Lea & Febiger, 1986, p. 878.)

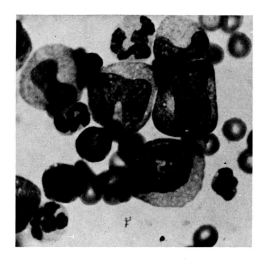

Fig. 20–16. Bone marrow from a dog with granulocytic leukemia, suggesting the existence of two separate cell lines, normal and neoplastic (× 2700). (From Jain, N.C.: Schalm's Veterinary Hematology. 4th Ed. Philadelphia, Lea & Febiger, 1986, p. 879.)

can be verified by the application of cytochemical stains (Grindem et al., 1986; Jain, 1986). Granulocytes from the progranulocytic stage onward demonstrate a profusion of peroxidase-positive granules scattered over the nucleus and cytoplasm. A peroxidase-positive reaction may also be seen in neoplastic myeloblasts because of asynchrony in their nuclear and cytoplasmic maturation. Cells of lymphocytic origin do not have peroxidase-positive granules and monocytes present only a few such granules. Rarely, neoplastic cells in the blood and bone marrow do not resemble granulocytes (Plate XXV-5) and are peroxidase-negative. A positive reaction for alkaline phosphatase (Plate XXV-6) is viewed as evidence that the cells are leukemic granulocytes.

The massive displacement of the bone marrow by neoplastic granulocytes (Plate XXV-3) leads to a marked reduction in erythropoiesis, so anemia is a common feature of myelogenous leukemia. In some instances, the anemia is so severe that the hematocrit is lower than 10% (Table 20–7). Similarly, megakaryocytopoiesis may be depressed, resulting in thrombocytopenia. Extramedullary hematopoiesis in the liver, spleen, and lymph nodes is a common finding, but it is inadequate to correct the developing anemia. Aspirates from enlarged lymph nodes may reveal large numbers of neutrophilic granulocytes in various stages of maturation. Functional studies of the peripheral blood granulocytes from a dog with chronic myelogenous leukemia revealed three neutrophil and neutrophil precursor populations of different densities compared to a single population in a control dog. Morphologic observation showed that cell density increased with cell maturity. Leukemic granulocytes also varied markedly in cytochemical composition. Their phagocytic activity, superoxide production, and release of granular enzymes (lysozyme and elastase) on activation were greatly increased (Thomsen et al., 1991).

MONOCYTIC AND MYELOMONOCYTIC LEUKEMIAS

Monocytic and myelomonocytic leukemias also occur in the dog, particularly young animals. They may occur spontaneously or can be radiation-induced. The diagnosis of acute monocytic leukemia (M5) is considered when increased numbers of mature and immature monocytes are found in the blood and bone marrow unassociated with inflammatory or other conditions known to induce monocytosis. The diagnosis of acute myelomonocytic leukemia (M4) is made when the bone marrow abounds with a mixture of myeloblasts and monoblasts and similar cells are found in the blood (Plates XXVI-1 to XXVI-4). When accurate identification of the cell type is difficult in Romanowsky-stained blood and bone marrow films, cytochemical staining for neutrophilic and monocytic markers may be helpful to establish the lineage of cellular differentiation (Plates XXVI-5 and XXVI-6).

A diagnosis of M5 in the dog should be considered when bone marrow blast cells constitute 30% of all nucleated cells, monoblasts and promonocytes comprise more than 30% of nonerythroid cells, and the granulocytic component is less than 20% (Jain et al., 1991). A diagnosis of M4 is made when myeloblasts and monoblasts together constitute more than 30% of all nucleated cells in the bone marrow, and differentiated granulocytes and monocytes each comprise more than 20% of all nucleated cells. Generally, neutrophilic differentiation exceeds monocytic differentiation in such cases (see Chap. 19 for additional criteria for distinguishing M5a and M5b).

MEGAKARYOCYTIC LEUKEMIA

Megakaryocytic leukemia is an extremely rare form of AML (Bolon et al., 1989; Cain et al., 1986). Diagnostic findings in the blood include the presence of unidentifiable blast cells or micromegakaryocytes, or cytomorphologic features suggestive of AML. The bone marrow is characterized by numerous megakaryocytes and their precursors. The primary defect seems to be an aberrant differentiation of the pluripotential stem cell, leading to the formation of bizarre and dysfunctional megakaryocytic cells. Megakaryocytic cells may also be found in other tissues such as the lymph nodes, spleen, liver, lungs, and kidneys. Cytochemical staining reveals megakaryocytic cells to be positive for acetylcholine esterase (a characteristic finding), the PAS reaction, and α-naphthyl acetate esterase (diffuse reaction).

MYELODYSPLASTIC SYNDROME

Erythremic myelosis and erythroleukemia are extremely rare in the dog as compared to the incidence in the cat. A case of erythroblastic leukemia (erythremic myelosis) in an 8-year-old male dachshund was characterized by severe refractory anemia, nucleated erythrocytes without reticulocytosis in blood, extensive proliferation of erythroid cells in the bone marrow with maturation arrest and marked splenomegaly with atrophy of follicles and diffuse infiltration by immature erythroid cells and megakaryocytes. The WBC counts varied between 5,000 and 15,250/μl, the PCV ranged from 6 to 12%, and the platelet counts varied from 126,000 to 270,000/μl. Myelofibrosis in association with erythremic myelosis was seen in another case.

A case of erythroleukemia in a 6-year-old boxer revealed a WBC count of 19,917/μl, an RBC count of 2.71 million/μl, and a platelet count of 2,000/μl. The blood was characterized by many abnormal mature and immature nucleated erythrocytes and by a left shift to promyelocytes.

Two cases of MDS in dogs were characterized by pancytopenia, bone marrow hypercellularity, and myelodysplasia (Weiss et al., 1985). Dyserythropoiesis was indicated by the presence of binuclear erythroid cells, nuclear fragmentation, and megaloblastosis. Giant metamyelocytes and band neutrophils characterized dysmyelopoiesis; small megakaryocytes with or without fragmented nuclei suggested dysmegakaryocytopoiesis.

RADIATION-INDUCED HEMATOPOIETIC NEOPLASMS

Acute erythremic myelosis was observed in a female beagle that had received a total dose of 300 R of whole body x-irradiation and died 5 years later at the age of 5 years and 8 months. Nucleated erythrocytes up to rubriblasts were seen in blood taken at necropsy. Necropsy findings included splenomegaly and multiple metastatic foci of neoplastic erythroid cells in the liver, lymph nodes, and lungs and the presence of large numbers of neoplastic erythroid cells within the blood vessels of all other major organs. A unique histologic finding in the bone marrow was the presence of multinucleated giant cells in which each nucleus was surrounded by distinct cytoplasm, giving the appearance of a cluster or colony of cells.

In a group of 24 beagles exposed to ^{60}Co–γ-irradiation (5 R/22-hour day) for the duration of life, beginning from about 13 months of age, 11 cases of MPD occurred. Of the 11 dogs, 5 showed erythroleukemia characterized by marked myeloid and erythroid hyperplasia of the bone marrow, with maturation arrest of the erythroid elements. The terminal blood picture was that of marked anemia and thrombocytopenia, with circulating erythroid precursors and abnormal red cell morphology. Hepatosplenomegaly was seen in 4 of 5 cases, although extensive leukemic infiltration was seen in all cases.

The development of a granulocytic MPD in beagles exposed to ^{90}Sr from midgestation to 1.5 years of age has been observed. A dose-related increase in incidence was noted. The most acute cases had characteristics of AML, whereas the more chronic disorders resembled myelofibrosis with myeloid metaplasia. The acute form had a clinical course of less than 100 days and was characterized by massive granulocytic proliferation in bone marrow and spleen and extensive infiltration in the liver, lymph nodes, and lungs. The blood was not leukemic, but anemia was in evidence. The more chronic disorder lasted between 240 and 624 days in 5 beagles. Clinicopathologic findings included a slight elevation in the WBC count with a left shift, anemia with prominent anisocytosis and poikilocytosis, terminal thrombocytopenia, hyperplastic bone marrow with little or no shift toward immature granulocytes, and a mild myeloid metaplasia in the spleen and elsewhere.

Micromegakaryocytes and megakaryocytes were found in blood as a preleukemic phase to myelogenous leukemia in 3 dogs exposed to continuous whole body ^{60}Co–γ-irradiation. A case of acute megakaryoblastic leukemia was seen in a young dog exposed continuously to whole body ^{60}Co-γ-radiation.

Malignant Histiocytosis

Malignant histiocytosis or histiocytic medullary reticulosis is an acute highly malignant disorder of histiocytes and their precursors. It occurs rarely in dogs, but an apparent familial predisposition has been observed in the Bernese Mountain breed involving predominantly aging male dogs. Major clinical findings include lethargy, anorexia, weight loss, and respiratory and neurologic abnormalities. Lymphadenopathy and a nonregenerative or regenerative anemia are common, but thrombocytopenia and leukopenia are rare. The lungs appear to be the chief site of pathologic involvement. Histologic examination of the lungs, spleen, bone marrow, liver, and lymph nodes reveals atypical neoplastic mononuclear or multinuclear histiocytes, some with phagocytosed tumor cells, leukocytes, and erythrocytes. Such malignant histiocytic cells can be found also in bone marrow aspirates (Plates XIII-10 through 12) and provide a diagnosis. The diagnosis in doubtful cases can be confirmed by electron microscopic examination of tissues and immunohistochemical identification of histiocytic markers on tumor cells (Rosin et al., 1986; Wellman et al., 1985).

Basophilic and Mast Cell Leukemias

Basophilic leukemia is rare compared to mast cell leukemia (Jain, 1986). Mast cells are normally found in the tissues and must be distinguished from basophils when found in the blood. They differ from basophils (Plate VII-5) in that the mast cell nucleus is round and often covered by densely stained, purplish granules that also fill the cytoplasm (Plate XII-4). In some instances of mastocytoma, the neoplastic mast cells may appear in the blood in large numbers, giving rise to a mast cell leukemia (Fig. 20–17). In such cases, the liver, spleen, and bone marrow are infiltrated with mast cells. Mast cell tumors are of common occurrence in dogs, but an accompanying mast cell leukemia is

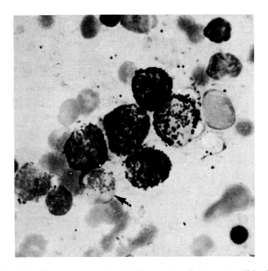

Fig. 20–17. Bone marrow invaded by mast cells in mast cell leukemia and neoplasia in a dog. The arrow points to an eosinophil (×2700). (From Jain, N.C.: Schalm's Veterinary Hematology. 4th Ed. Philadelphia, Lea & Febiger, 1986, p. 882.)

rarely seen. Mast cell leukemia with systemic masto-cytosis is more common in cats than in dogs.

Basophilic leukemia was diagnosed in an 11-year-old bitch based on the presence in the peripheral blood and bone marrow of cells with segmented nuclei and many metachromatic cytoplasmic granules (Mahaffey et al., 1987). The cells were negative for peroxidase and naphthol AS-D chloroacetate esterase activities. On electron microscopy, the cytoplasmic granules appeared to be finely granular (typical of basophils) and lacked membranous coils (found in mast cells) or crystalline lattice structures (characteristic of eosino-phils).

BOVINE LEUKEMIAS

The leukemias in cattle primarily evolve from the neoplastic proliferation of lymphocytes. A C-type on-cornavirus, designated bovine leukemia virus (BLV), is universally accepted as causing an abnormal prolif-eration of lymphocytes. This leads to a benign persis-tent lymphocytosis (PL) or a malignant tumor-forming disease referred to as enzootic bovine leukosis, or the adult form of lymphoma in cattle. BLV infection also decreases milk production, fertility, and survival. It also causes lymphoma or chronic lymphocytic leukemia in the sheep and goat (Burny et al., 1988; Djilali and Parodi, 1989). A subunit recombinant vaccine, vaccinia virus expressing gp51 and gp30 antigens of BLV, has been developed and may provide a protective immu-nity against BLV infection in cattle and sheep (Porte-telle et al., 1990, 1991).

Bovine Leukemia Virus

BLV is an exogenous B-lymphocytotropic retrovirus. It shows some nuclear sequence homology with human T lymphocytotropic viruses (HTLV-I and HTLV-II), and cross-reactive antibodies to BLV and HTLV can be found in sera of infected cattle and humans (Ma-ruyama et al., 1989). The BLV apparently infects only lymphocytes, but is not demonstrable by direct exam-ination of uncultured lymphocytes or neoplastic tissue. The virus or viral antigen, however, can be demon-strated in short term cultures of peripheral blood lymphocytes from infected cattle. BLV can infect lym-phocytes of various species in vitro, but in vivo infec-tivity or oncogenicity is relatively limited. Sheep, goats, pigs, rhesus monkeys, chimpanzees, rabbits, capybaras, and water buffaloes can be infected with BLV (Burny et al., 1988). The inoculation of virus-containing cul-tured lymphocytes into calves and sheep has produced PL, lymphocytic leukemia, or lymphoma in some an-imals. In both PL and lymphoma, the abnormally proliferating cells were glucocorticoid-sensitive B lym-phocytes.

Conflicting observations have been reported regard-ing the changes in numbers of lymphocyte subpopu-lations in BLV infected cows. In BLV-infected cows with PL, both B and T lymphocytes were found to be increased (Williams et al., 1988a), B cells were in-creased and T cells were decreased (Fossum et al., 1988; Gatei et al, 1989), or B cells were increased without significant changes in T cell numbers (Taylor et al., 1992). In BLV-infected nonlymphocytotic cows, T cells were increased without changes in B cell numbers (Williams et al., 1988a) or both B cells and T helper cells were decreased (Taylor et al., 1992). BLV-provirus has been detected in T cells (Williams et al., 1988b), including both T helper and T cytotoxic/suppressor subpopulations (Stott et al., 1991). The virus also persists in cells of the monocyte/macrophage lineage (Heeney et al., 1992).

BLV is highly prevalent in cattle with PL and lymphoma. Genetic constitution plays an important role in the development of PL and lymphoma. Al-though PL usually precedes by several years the de-velopment of lymphoma in two-thirds of cases, most cattle with PL never develop lymphoma. PL can be distinguished from transient lymphocytosis of other causes by demonstrating an increase (for at least 3 months) in the absolute number of lymphocytes more than 3 SDs above the mean normal number for the breed and age of the animal.

Natural injection by BLV can be demonstrated di-rectly in cultured lymphocytes or indirectly by serologic techniques, including immunodiffusion, immunoflu-orescence, regular and blocking ELISA, radioimmu-noassay, and DNA probe technology. Serologic tests are generally used to detect herd infections. The agar gel immunodiffusion (AGID) test using BLV glyco-protein gp51 is specific, sensitive, and simple for herd surveys and is commercially available. It is the refer-ence test for detection of antibodies against BLV.

A positive serologic test in the adult animal generally indicates BLV infection, but false-negative and false-positive results may be obtained. The results of various serologic tests and direct viral demonstration proce-dures may not correlate completely because of varia-tions in sensitivity and limitations of the techniques (Gaudi et al., 1990; Have and Hoff-Jorgensen, 1991; Hoff-Jorgensen, 1989; Platzer et al., 1990). Mono-clonal antibodies to BLV proteins (p24 and gp51) have been used to increase the sensitivity and specificity of ELISA. In one study (Molloy et al., 1990), the sensi-tivity and specificity of a p24-ELISA for detecting BLV infection compared to the gp51 AGID, were 98.1 and 96.7%, respectively. Antibodies to BLV antigens (gp51 and p24) can be detected in milk by an indirect ELISA (de Boer, et al., 1989; Florent et al., 1988). BLV proviral DNA in lymphocytotic cattle and tumor DNA from cattle at all stages of infection can be detected using the polymerase chain reaction (Naif et al., 1990). The sensitivity of this assay can be increased by hy-bridization with a BLV gene probe (Brandon et al., 1991) or by analyzing specific DNA and RNA se-quences of BLV (Naif et al., 1992; Sherman et al., 1992).

The incidence of BLV infection is low (2 to 16%) among dairy cattle in leukemia-free herds, is high (24 to 42%) in herds with a history of lymphoma, and lowest (1.2 to 2.6%) in beef herds. Infection with BLV does not mean that the animal develops PL or lymphoma. Although BLV infection is widespread, particularly in multiple-case lymphoma herds, the occurrence of tumor development or leukemia is relatively rare. Most BLV-infected cattle remain asymptomatic and economically productive. Thus, the detection of BLV infection does not constitute a diagnosis of lymphoma. The latter is demonstrated by blood, bone marrow, and other cytologic examinations.

Vertical (prenatal or congenital) and horizontal (postnatal or between animals) transmission of BLV can occur. Venereal transmission through leukocyte-free, BLV-infected semen used for artificial insemination does not occur. The risk of infection for non-pregnant cows appears to be about 3 times that for pregnant cows (Lassauzet et al., 1991b). Transfer of BLV by embryo transfer either does not occur or is rare (DiGiacomo et al., 1990). Calves may become infected by ingesting colostrum or milk from BLV-infected cows. The chances of in utero or periparturient infection are greater in calves born of cows with a blood lymphocyte count of >12,000/µl or with lymphoma (Lassauzet et al., 1991a). However, calfhood infection can be reduced by about 45% through the feeding of colostrum-containing BLV antibodies, and a further reduction in infection may be possible by feeding milk substitutes from noninfected cows (Lassauzet et al., 1989) and careful management practices to limit the mechanical transmission of infection (Thurmond, 1991).

Close physical contact between infected animals and susceptible cattle appears to be the single most important prerequisite for the transmission of BLV infection. Infection through contact exposure increases progressively with advancing age and with an increase in cattle density, as in the winter months. Infection through bloodsucking insects, such as horseflies (tabanids), is possible (Foil et al., 1989). Mechanical transmission during surgical procedures such as dehorning and castrations can also occur. Routine rectal palpation may transmit infection in susceptible cattle (Hopkins et al., 1988). Administration of as little as 1 µl of BLV-infected whole blood in Holstein calves by IM, IV,

subcutaneous, or intradermal routs has been found to transmit BLV (Evermann et al., 1986).

Lymphoproliferative Disorders

Lymphoma affects cattle of all breeds and ages, but is more common in dairy cattle and after 5 years of age. The disease has also been observed occasionally in stillborn fetuses in the eighth month of gestation, in newborns, and in growing calves. Two main forms of lymphoma have been recognized. Enzootic bovine leukosis (EBL) is the most prevalent form. It is often referred to as the adult form of lymphoma and manifests as multiple incidences in a herd. The sporadic form is rare, occurs randomly, and is comprised of three clinicopathologic forms designated calf, adolescent thymic, and cutaneous lymphomas. The adult form of lymphoma or EBL is caused by BLV, whereas all the sporadic forms are unassociated with BLV infection.

ADULT FORM OF LYMPHOMA

The adult form of lymphoma is seen in cattle 2 to 18 years of age, but almost invariably in cattle over 3 years of age and most frequently in those between 5 and 8 years of age. Most cases are encountered in herds having more than one occurrence of clinical lymphoma; such herds are called multiple-incidence herds.

Bovine lymphoma is characteristically an afebrile disease, although fever may occur. The disease is characterized by widespread lymphadenopathy with frequent involvement of the heart, abomasum, and intestine. The bone marrow, thymus, and liver are less frequently involved. Because of the marked involvement of various tissues and organs, the clinical signs may vary. Bilateral enlargement of the superficial nodes may be the first detectable abnormality, although sometimes only a single external node is involved, and in other cases no enlargement of the external lymph nodes occurs. Rectal palpation of the pelvic and abdominal organs may reveal extensive neoplastic masses. Chronic indigestion, cardiac abnormalities, and partial or complete paralysis may occur

Table 20-8. Normal Lymphocyte Counts ($\times 10^3$/µl of blood) by Age for Holstein-Frisian Cattle from California.

Age	No. of Samples	Mean ($\overline{X}$)	Standard Deviation (SD)	Coefficient Variation	95% Limits ($\overline{X} + 1.96$ SD)	99.74% Limits ($\overline{X} + 3.00$ SD)
0–6 mo	146	5.15	1.32	25.6	2.56–7.74	1.19–9.11
6–12 mo	98	6.41	1.55	24.1	3.37–9.45	1.76–11.06
1–2 yr	49	5.99	1.69	28.2	2.68–9.30	0.92–11.06
2–3 yr	64	4.29	1.16	27.0	2.01–6.57	0.81–7.77
3–4 yr	162	4.01	0.99	24.7	2.07–5.95	1.04–6.98
4–5 yr	176	3.42	1.04	30.4	1.39–5.45	0.30–6.54
Over 5 yr	488	3.08	0.96	31.2	1.19–4.97	0.20–5.96

From Theilen, G. H., Dungworth, D. L., Lengyel, J., et al.: Bovine lymphosarcoma in California. I. Epizootiologic and hematologic aspects. Health Lab. Sci., 1:96, 1964.

because of neoplastic lymphoid cell infiltration of the abomasum, myocardium, and nerves of the spinal cord, respectively. The course of the illness may vary, from a few weeks to several months. The terminal tumor phase may appear suddenly, with rapid wasting and sudden death. Cardiac failure is a major cause of death.

Specific tumor-associated antigens (TAA) appear on the surface of lymphocytes of cattle infected with EBL (Aida et al., 1987; Kitamura et al., 1990). These antigens have been detected using complement-dependent antibody cytotoxicity, indirect immunofluorescence, and ELISA tests. Various TAA antigens have been grouped as common TAA, partially common TAA, and individually distinct TAA based on the reactivity of monoclonal antibodies with tumor cells from cattle with EBL. Monoclonal antibodies to TAA also react with lymphocytes from healthy BLV-infected cows and from cows with PL. It has been suggested that monoclonal antibodies to common TAA may be used not only to detect TAA, but also to diagnose EBL and to screen BLV-infected cattle that may develop lymphoma (Aida et al., 1987).

SPORADIC FORMS OF LYMPHOMA

The calf form is seen in calves between 1 and 6 months of age. It is characterized by generalized lymphadenopathy with gross changes in the bone marrow, liver, and spleen as common additional features. Lymphocytic leukemia is often present.

The adolescent thymic form is observed in cattle 6 to 30 months of age. It is encountered more often in beef than in dairy cattle. Dyspnea and bloating are common clinical signs. The main pathologic changes are a massive infiltration of the thymus and frequent involvement of the bone marrow. The regional lymph nodes are also affected, but generalized lymphadenopathy is uncommon.

The cutaneous form is rare and occurs in cattle 1 to 3 years of age. It is characterized by a nodular leukemic infiltration of the dermis. Metastases to lymph nodes and other organs occur in latter stages.

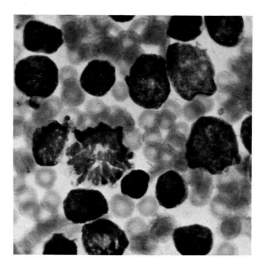

Fig. 20–18. Blood in lymphocytic leukemia in a cow with a total leukocyte count of 880,000/μl. Note the mitotic figure and marked variation in the size of lymphocytes (×2700). (From Jain, N.C.: Schalm's Veterinary Hematology. 4th Ed. Philadelphia, Lea & Febiger, 1986, p. 390.)

HEMATOLOGIC AND OTHER LABORATORY FINDINGS

The use of total and differential leukocyte counts to help diagnose bovine lymphoma requires a knowledge of the normal changes in circulating lymphocyte numbers with advancing age (Table 20-8). As already stated, infection by BLV does not mean that PL or lymphoma is present or will develop later. Similarly, the presence of PL does not mean that lymphoma will develop. Therefore, various lymphocytic parameters developed for the detection of PL now seem to be of limited value as indicators of BLV infection or lymphoma. However, the percentage of B cells was better than the absolute lymphocyte count in the peripheral blood for detection of a subclinical progression of BLV infection in individual cows (Lewin et al., 1988). The B cell percentage did not change with age.

The diagnosis of PL should be based on repeated

Table 20-9. Hemograms in Ten Cases of Bovine Lymphoma

| | | | | | \multicolumn{8}{c}{*Differential Leukocyte Count (%)*} |
Case No.	Age	Sex	PCV (%)	WBC/μl	Band	Neut.	Pro-lymph.	Lymph.	Mono.	Eos.	Bas.	D.C.*
53L40	5 wk	F	12	2,050	18.0	2.0	28.0	50.0	2.0	0	0	0
57L1672	8 mo	F	34.5	8,400	0	15.0	0	80.0	4.0	1.0	0	0
56L15	2½ yr	M	42	5,250	0	21.5	0	59.5	5.5	13.0	0.5	0
56L937	3 yr	F	28.5	6,800	0	47.5	0	33.0	14.0	5.5	0	0
961A	4 yr	F	28	175,000	0	6.0	83.0	6.0	0	0	0	5.0
53L114	5 yr	F	28	12,450	0	72.0	0	15.0	11.0	1.0	0	1.0
57L1400	Mature	F	34	20,700	0	51.5	0	42.0	6.5	0	0	0
RJO-68	Mature	F	34	19,100	0.5	3.0	16.0	79.5	0	1.0	0	0
RJO-329	Mature	F	35	145,000	0	2.0	57.0	39.0	0	0	0	2.0
UCV-65	Mature	F	25.5	198,750	0	14.0	2.5	38.5	45.0	0	0	0

* D.C. = degenerated cells

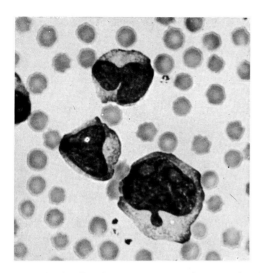

Fig. 20–19. Blood in lymphoma from a cow showing a lymphoblast and atypical lymphocytes (Reider forms) (×2700). (From Jain, N.C.: Schalm's Veterinary Hematology. 4th Ed. Philadelphia, Lea & Febiger, 1986, p. 890.)

demonstrations of a significant lymphocytosis for several weeks, mainly caused by lymphocytes of normal morphology, occurring in a clinically normal animal. Lymphoma is generally a tumor-forming disease and is not regularly associated with lymphocytosis or the occurrence of abnormal (neoplastic) lymphocytes in the blood (Figs. 20–18 and 20–19). In suspected cases, such abnormal lymphocytes should be carefully sought, because they are diagnostic. A mild to moderate leukocytosis with absolute lymphocytosis may be seen in approximately 55% of cases of lymphoma, whereas a normal hemogram is present in 10 to 30% of cases and leukemia is encountered in only 5 to 10% of cases. Lymphoblasts, lymphoid cells with multiple, asymmetrically lobed nuclei (Reider forms), and mitotic figures are frequently observed in blood during the leukemic phase. A few abnormal lymphocytes may sometimes be found in normal cattle and animals with PL. Selected hemograms illustrating variations in blood cytology in bovine lymphoma are presented in Table 20–9.

Anemia may develop when the tumor phase is protracted or when blood loss results because of an ulcerated gastrointestinal tract. Several factors tend to rule against the development of severe anemia in cattle with lymphoma: (1) the often rapid development of the terminal tumor phase; (2) the long life span (160 days) of the bovine erythrocyte; and (3) the rarity of bone marrow involvement in the adult form of lymphoma.

Some other pathologic findings may occur. The most conspicuous chromosomal abnormality in cattle with the adult form of lymphoma is hyperploidy, and BLV-seropositive cattle with PL show aneuploidy with chromosomal aberrations (Castro et al., 1988). Leukemic cattle are immunosuppressed in that they usually exhibit an absence or reduced levels of IgM, an impaired primary immune response, and defects of the cellular immune system. For example, most sera from leukemic cattle inhibit phagocytic activity of neutrophils, growth of interleukin-2-dependent bovine T cells, and mitogen-induced blastogenesis of normal bovine lymphocytes (Takamatsu et al., 1988). The antibody titer against BLV in these sera correlated with the percent inhibition of lymphocyte blastogenesis.

Leukocyte cytoplasmic fragmentation associated with lymphoid leukemia in cattle and sheep can interfere with accurate determination of platelet counts by electronic and hemocytometer methods (Weiser et al., 1989).

EQUINE LEUKEMIAS

Lymphoma is the predominant hematopoietic neoplasia in the horse, lymphocytic leukemia is infrequent, and myelogenous leukemia is extremely rare. The cause is unknown, although virus-like particles have been observed in lymphoid cells in a newborn foal with acute lymphoblastic lymphoma (Tomlinson et al., 1979).

Lymphoproliferative Disorders

Lymphoma is not as frequent in the horse as in the dog, cat, and cow. Various anatomic forms of lymphoma recognized in the horse include the multicentric (most common), alimentary, mediastinal, cutaneous, and miscellaneous types. The clinical picture of equine lymphoma is varied and the differential diagnosis may be difficult. Most cases of lymphoma in the horse could probably be diagnosed antemortem through a combination of cytologic examinations of the blood, bone marrow, and aspirated fluid from an enlarged lymph node, or an effusion fluid. Large granular lymphoma was diagnosed in a horse (Grindem et al., 1989).

Lymphoma usually occurs in horses 5 years of age and older, although the disease can occur in foals. In rare instances, lymphoma has developed in fetal life and has been diagnosed at birth. Among 39 horses diagnosed as having lymphoma at the VMTH-UCD, the mean age was 9.3 years (range, 1 to 21 years), and the various breeds affected were as follows: 14 quarter horses, 6 thoroughbreds, 3 Arabians, 1 standardbred, 1 appaloosa, and 15 crossbreeds. Although a higher incidence of lymphoma in females has been reported in some studies, no sex predilection is demonstrated when the data from various literature reports on equine lymphoma are combined.

CLINICAL SIGNS

Clinical signs may vary with the type of lymphoma. These include peripheral lymphadenopathy (generalized or limited to one or two nodes), weight loss (rapid or more protracted), ventral edema, pleural effusion, respiratory distress (ranging from coughing to frank dyspnea), fever (103 to 107° F; 39.4 to 41.7° C), pale mucous membranes in association with advanced anemia, and pelvic and abdominal masses on rectal palpation.

HEMATOLOGIC FINDINGS

Common hemogram abnormalities include modest to severe anemia, hyperproteinemia, and hyperfibrinogenemia. Immature lymphocytes indicative of ALL are present in the blood of a small number of lymphomatous horses. A leukemic WBC count is infrequent and ALL without discrete tumorous masses is rare. A moderate leukocytosis is seen in some horses and neutrophilia is a common nonspecific finding. Neutropenia and thrombocytopenia may occur from marrow displacement by neoplastic lymphocytes. The bone marrow is not regularly infiltrated by neoplastic cells in equine lymphoma. The massive displacement of normal marrow cytology by neoplastic lymphocytes may be seen in about 50% of lymphoma cases. Rare abnormalities include a monoclonal gammopathy, with β-globulin–secreting neoplastic lymphoid cells and hypercalcemia.

CYTOLOGIC AND NECROPSY FINDINGS

The lymph node cytology is usually diagnostic of lymphoma, particularly when peripheral lymphadenopathy is evident. The usual picture is of an admixture of mostly lymphoblasts and prolymphocytes, some plasma cells, and a few normal, mature lymphocytes. Mitotic figures are usually present in small numbers.

Pleural effusion, when present, may have elevated nucleated cell counts (5,700 to 103,600/µl), with 53 to 93% lymphoid cells. The lymphoid cells may vary from normal lymphocytes to large pleomorphic cells, with an occasional bizarre giant form. A small number of mitotic figures is usually present.

Prominent necropsy findings include tumor masses in the anterior mediastinal and abdominal cavities and an enlarged and/or nodular spleen. The liver and lungs are sometimes involved, with metastatic tumor foci.

MULTIPLE MYELOMA

Multiple myeloma is rare in the horse; only three cases have been described. Prominent findings in a 16-year-old thoroughbred gelding and a 22-year-old Arabian mare seen at the VMTH-UCD were hyperproteinemia, increased plasma cells in the bone marrow (Fig. 20–20), a monoclonal gammopathy involving β-globulin or IgG(T), and plasmocytic infiltration of the lymph nodes and other organs and tissues. Bence Jones protein was not detected in the urine and osteolytic lesions were not seen in the bones examined. Clinical findings were nonspecific. Other hematologic findings included a mild to severe anemia, leukopenia to leukocytosis, and slight neutrophilia. The bone marrow revealed normal to suppressed erythropoiesis, normal to decreased granulopoiesis, and adequate numbers of megakaryocytes.

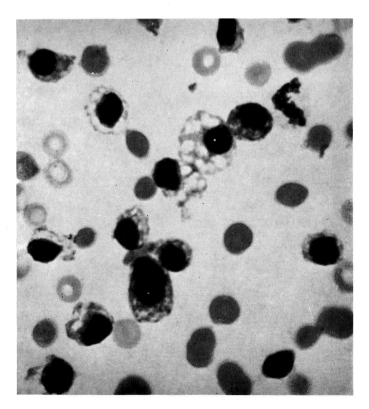

Fig. 20–20. Myelomatous plasma cells with characteristic foamy cytoplasm in bone marrow aspirated from the tuber coxae of a horse with myelomatosis (×2700). (From Cornelius, C.E., et al.: Plasma cell myelomatosis in a horse. Cornell Vet., 40:478, 1959.)

Myeloproliferative Disorders

Various types of myeloid leukemias—myelogenous, eosinophilic, monocytic, and myelomonocytic—have been reported in the horse (Blue et al., 1987; Mori et al., 1991; Spier et al., 1986).

Myelomonocytic leukemia was diagnosed in a 5-year-old quarter horse stallion at the VMTH-UCD with a history of depression and weight loss of at least 3 weeks' duration. Clinical and laboratory findings included splenomegaly, lymphadenopathy, coagulopathy, and bacteremia. Hematologic findings included a severe normocytic-normochromic anemia, thrombocytopenia, monocytosis, and a left shift, occasionally up to the promyelocyte stage. The serum lysozyme concentration was increased, suggesting an increased turnover of myelomonocytic cells. The bone marrow contained many immature cells of the myeloid series, with a myeloid:erythroid ratio of 30.5:1. Necropsy findings included generalized lymphadenopathy and hemorrhages throughout the body. Histopathologic examination revealed primitive and myeloblastic cells in several tissues, including the lymph nodes, spleen, liver, kidneys, lungs, and myocardium.

Laboratory findings in a case of monocytic leukemia in a 6-year-old Hassian gray gelding included marked normocytic-normochromic anemia, leukocytosis with marked monocytosis, latex particle phagocytosis by leukemic leukocytes, and positive staining of leukemic cells for α-naphthyl acetate esterase (a monocyte marker) and weak staining for chloroacetate esterase (a neutrophil as well as monocyte marker in the horse). Leukemic cells showed prominent ruffles and ridge-like profiles characteristic of monocytoid cells. Prominent necropsy findings were lymphadenopathy, splenomegaly, and massive infiltration with monocytoid cells of various parenchymatous organs and bone marrow.

Eosinophilic leukemia was diagnosed in a 4-year-old thoroughbred filly and a 10-month-old standardbred colt based on blood and bone marrow findings of a slight to marked eosinophilia with immature and atypical cells, and excluding possible causes of reactive eosinophilia. Additional findings were marked anemia and thrombocytopenia. The bone marrow was markedly hyperplastic, with highly aberrant eosinophils, and showed secondary myelophthisis.

LEUKEMIAS IN OTHER SPECIES

Leukemia is rare in other animal species. Sporadic cases have been reported in sheep, pigs, water buffaloes, and goats. Multiple incidences of lymphoma (enzootic leukemia) have been described in sheep. Two cases of myeloma were seen among 1.1 million sheep slaughtered. An unusual occurrence of a hereditary form of lymphoma has been reported in the pig. Lymphocytic leukemia developed in 1 of 56 pigs exposed to ^{60}Co–γ-radiation. Exposure of 665 swine to ^{90}Sr–γ-irradiation resulted in the development of lymphoproliferative disorders in 18 animals and MPD in 12 animals.

Goat

The primary clinicopathologic findings of a case of lymphoma observed in a 3-year-old female Saanen-Nubian crossbred goat at the VMTH-UCD were a moderate anemia (hemoglobin, 6.8 g/dl), a high-normal WBC count (15,100/μl) accompanied by 61% lymphocytes, with some large, atypical, and binucleate forms, and lymphadenopathy at necropsy. A Nubian goat with lymphoma had a normal WBC count and no atypical lymphocytes in blood. Myelofibrosis associated with pancytopenia has been observed in some newborn pygmy goats. Although a genetic association seems possible, its cause and myeloproliferative nature remain to be established.

Sheep

Lymphoma in sheep occurs most commonly in adult animals without sex and breed predilection. Sporadic forms and multiple-incidence herds have been described. Horizontal transmission was suspected to have occurred in a multiple-incidence herd. A pathologic study of 40 cases of ovine lymphoma revealed several anatomic forms, primarily the multicentric type, followed by the alimentary (mesenteric) form and, rarely, by thymic and skin forms (Johnstone and Manktelow, 1978). The tissues most commonly involved (in order of decreasing frequency) were the lymph nodes, spleen, liver, kidney, small intestines, and heart. Ovine lymphoma is caused by a C-type oncornavirus, and the BLV is oncogenic for sheep. Antibodies to BLV can be detected in sera of BLV-infected sheep using a bovine leukemia glycoprotein immunodiffusion kit (Green et al., 1988). T lymphocyte numbers in the peripheral blood of BLV-infected, clinically healthy and leukemic sheep were within the normal range, but B lymphocytes were increased in several cases. In addition, BLV antigen was expressed on B-lymphocytes, but not on T lymphocytes, in blood and lymph nodes of the leukemic sheep studied (Aida et al., 1989).

Pig

Lymphoma occurs mainly as a sporadic disease in young animals (less than 6 months of age) before maturity, without sex or breed predilection. Clinical signs include ataxia or paralysis, enlarged superficial lymph nodes, particularly the submandibular or prescapular lymph nodes, anorexia, loss of body weight, dyspnea, tachycardia, and sudden death. The diagnosis of lymphoma is difficult to establish from the blood examination because the WBC count is often normal and abnormal lymphocytes may not be present.

A leukemic phase may occur terminally. Among the various anatomic forms of lymphoma, the multicentric form is the most common, followed by the thymic form. The liver, spleen, and kidneys are most often infiltrated when the disease is widespread. Histologic characterization of cell types in 200 cases of porcine lymphomas revealed 42% to be lymphocytic, 34% lymphoblastic, 15% histiocytic, and 9% mixed types (Migaki, 1969).

A hereditary form of lymphoma has been described in a breeding stock of Large White pigs in great Britain (Head et al., 1974). The inheritance was autosomal recessive and all cases involved pigs under 6 months of age. The affected animals showed stunted growth, a pot belly, and some enlargement of the superficial lymph nodes. WBC counts were moderately elevated, but lymphocytes constituted up to 80% of the leukocytes, along with a variable proportion of lymphoblasts and large undifferentiated cells. Multicentric lymphoid tumors were found in the lymph nodes, particularly those draining the gut and lungs. The disease was detected as early as 6 to 12 weeks of age by the presence of abnormal cells in the blood. Thrombocytopenia and anemia developed in the terminal stages. The bone marrow was almost replaced by tumor cells and the spread of tumor cells to other organs was detected by histologic examination. The thymus was always involuted. Most of the affected animals died by 120 days, but some survived for 4 to 6 months. They rarely lived beyond 15 months of age and never attained sexual maturity. The affected animals at 10 to 24 weeks of age had increased serum γ-globulin levels and IgG heavy chain and light chain components in the serum and urine, suggestive of the B-cell lymphoma.

Single cases of myelogenous leukemia with splenomegaly, poorly differentiated myeloid leukemia, eosinophilic leukemia, and granulocytic sarcoma have been reported in pigs. A C-type virus has been found in tissues or cell lines from swine with MPD. Mast cell leukemia has been described in swine (Bean-Knudsen et al., 1989).

REFERENCES

Aida, Y., Miyasaka, M., Okada, K., et al.: Further phenotypic characterization of target cells for bovine leukemia virus experimental infection in sheep. Am. J. Vet. Res., 50:1946, 1989.

Aida, Y., Onuma, M., Kasai, N., et al.: Use of viable-cell ELISA for detection of monoclonal antibodies recognizing tumor-associated antigens on bovine lymphosarcoma cells. Am. J. Vet. Res., 48:1319, 1987.

Applebaum, F.R., Sale, G.E., Storb, R., et al.: Phenotyping of canine lymphoma with monoclonal antibodies directed at cell surface antigens: classification, morphology, clinical presentation and response to chemotherapy. Hematol. Oncol., 2:151, 1984.

Barlough, J.E., Ackley, C.D., George, J.W., et al.: Acquired immune dysfunction in cats with experimentally induced feline immunodeficiency virus infection: comparison of short-term and long-term infections. J. Acquir. Immune Defic. Syndr., 4:219, 1991.

Bean-Knudsen, D.E., Caldwell, C.W., Wagner, J.E., et al.: Porcine mast cell leukemia with systemic mastocytosis. Vet. Pathol., 26:90, 1989.

Bishop, S.A., Williams, N.A., Gruffydd-Jones, T.J., et al.: Impaired T-cell priming and proliferation in cats infected with feline immunodeficiency virus. AIDS, 6:287, 1992.

Blue, J., Perdrizet, J. and Brown, E.: Pulmonary aspergillosis in a horse with myelomonocytic leukemia. J. Am. Vet. Med. Assoc., 190:1562, 1987.

Blue, J.T.: Myelofibrosis in cats with myelodysplastic syndrome and acute myelogenous leukemia. Vet. Pathol., 25:154, 1988.

Blue, J.T., French, T.W. and Krantz, J.S.: Non-lymphoid hematopoietic neoplasia in cats: a retrospecitve study of 60 cases. Cornell Vet., 78:21, 1988.

Bolon, B., Buergelt, C.D., Harvey, J.W., et al.: Megakaryoblastic leukemia in a dog. Vet. Clin. Pathol., 18:69, 1989.

Boyce, J.T. Kociba, G.J., Jacobs, R.M., et al.: Feline leukemia virus-induced thrombocytopenia and macrothrombocytosis in cats. Vet. Pathol., 23:16, 1986.

Brandon, R.B., Naif, H., Daniel, R.C., et al.: Early detection of bovine leukosis virus DNA in infected sheep using the polymerase chain reaction. Res. Vet. Sci., 50:89, 1991.

Burny, A., Cleuter, Y., Kettmann, R., et al.: Bovine leukemia: facts and hypotheses derived from the study of an infectious cancer. Adv. Vet. Sci. Comp. Med., 32:149, 1988.

Cain, G.R., Feldman, B.F., Kawakami, T.G., et al.: Platelet dysplasia associated with megakaryoblastic leukemia in a dog. J. Am. Vet. Med. Assoc., 188:529, 1986.

Castro, N.H., Walter, J., dos Santos, R., et al.: Cytogenetic study of cattle affected by persistent lymphocytosis. Zentralbl. Veterinarmed. [A]., 35:380, 1988.

Cohen, N.D., Carter, C.N., Thomas, M.A., et al.: Epizootiologic association between feline immunodeficiency virus infection and feline leukemia virus seropositivity. J. Am. Vet. Med. Assoc., 197:220, 1990.

Cotter, S.M.: Feline leukemia virus: pathophysiology, prevention, and treatment. Cancer Invest., 10:173, 1992.

Dameshek, W.: The Di Guglielmo syndrome revisited. Blood, 34:567, 1969.

de Boer, G.F., Boerrigter, H.M., Akkermans, J.P., et al.: Use of milk samples and monoclonal antibodies directed against BLV-p24 to identify cattle infected with bovine leukemia virus (BLV). Vet. Immunol. Immunopathol., 22:283, 1989.

DiGiacomo, R.F., McGinnis, L.K., Studer, E., et al.: Failure of embryo transfer to transmit BLV in a dairy herd. Vet. Rec., 127:456, 1990.

Djilali, S. and Parodi, A.L.: The BLV-induced leukemia—lymphosarcoma complex in sheep. Vet. Immunol. Immunopathol., 22:233, 1989.

Evermann, J.F., DiGiacomo, R.F., Ferrer, J.F., et al.: Transmission of bovine leukosis virus by blood inoculation. Am. J. Vet. Res., 47:1885, 1986.

Florent, G., Delgoffe, J.C. and Zygraich, N.: Detection of antibodies to bovine leukemia virus in bovine milk samples with an ELISA involving two monoclonal antibodies. Vet. Microbiol., 18:89, 1988.

Foil, L.D., French, D.D., Hoyt, P.G., et al.: Transmission of bovine leukemia virus by Tabanus fuscicostatus. Am. J. Vet. Res., 50:1771, 1989.

Fossum, C., Burny, A., Portetelle, D., et al.: Detection of B and T cells, with lectins or antibodies, in healthy and bovine leukemia virus-infected cattle. Vet. Immunol. Immunopathol., 18:269, 1988.

Franks, P.T., Harvey, J.W., Mays, M.C., et al.: Feline large granular lymphoma. Vet. Pathol., 23:200, 1986.

Gatei, M.H., Brandon, R.B., Naif, H.M., et al.: Changes in B cell and T cell subsets in bovine leukaemia virus-infected cattle. Vet. Immunol. Immunopathol., 23:139, 1989.

Gaudi, S., Ponti, W., Agresti, A., et al.: Detection of bovine leukaemia virus (BLV) infection by DNA probe technology. Mol. Cell Probes., 4:163, 1990.

Goitsuka, R., Tsuji, M., Matsumoto, Y., et al.: A case of feline large granular lymphoma. Nippon Juigaku. Zasshi., 50:593, 1988.

Green, J.R., Herbst, I.A. and Schneider, D.J.: An outbreak of lymphosarcoma in merino sheep in the South Western Cape. J. S. Afr. Vet. Assoc., 59:27, 1988.

Grindem, C.B. and Buoen, L.C.: Cytogenetic analysis in nine leukaemic cats. J. Comp. Pathol., 101:21, 1989.

Grindem, C.B., Roberts, M.C., McEntee, M.F., et al.: Large granular lymphocyte tumor in a horse. Vet. Pathol., 26:86, 1989.

Grindem, C.B., Stevens, J.B. and Perman, V.: Morphologic classification and clinical and pathologic characteristics of spontaneous leukemia in 17 dogs. J. Am. Anim. Hosp. Assoc., 21:219, 1985.

Grindem, C.B., Stevens, J.B. and Perman, V.: Cytochemical reactions in cells from leukemic dogs. Vet. Pathol., 23:103, 1986.

Hamilton, T.A., Morrison, W.B. and DeNicola, D.B.: Cytosine arabinoside chemotherapy for acute megakaryocytic leukemia in a cat. J. Am. Vet. Med. Assoc., 199:359, 1991.

Hamlin, R.H. and Duncan, R.C.: Acute nonlymphocytic leukemia in a dog. J. Am. Vet. Med. Assoc., 196:110, 1990.

Hardy, W.D.: General principles of retrovirus immunodetection tests. J. Am. Vet. Med. Assoc., 199:1282, 1991.

Hardy, W.D. and Zuckerman, E.E.: Development of the immunofluorescent antibody test for detection of feline leukemia virus infection in cats. J. Am. Vet. Med. Assoc., 199:1327, 1991.

Have, P. and Hoff-Jorgensen, R.: Demonstration of antibodies against bovine leukemia virus (BLV) by blocking ELISA using bovine polyclonal anti-BLV immunoglobulin. Vet. Microbiol., 27:221, 1991.

Hawkins, E.C.: Saliva and tear tests for feline leukemia virus. J. Am. Vet. Med. Assoc., 199:1382, 1991.

Hawks, D.M., Legendre, A.M. and Rohrbach, B.W.: Comparison of four test kits for feline leukemia virus antigen. J. Am. Vet. Med. Assoc., 199:1373, 1991.

Hayes, K.A., Rojko, J.L. and Mathes, L.E.: Incidence of localized feline leukemia virus infection in cats. Am. J. Vet. Res., 53:604, 1992.

Head, K.W., Campbell, J.G., Imlah, P., et al.: Hereditary lymphosarcoma in a herd of pigs. Vet. Rec., 95:523, 1974.

Heeney, J.L., Valli, P.J., Jacobs, R.M., et al.: Evidence for bovine leukemia virus infection of peripheral blood monocytes and limited antigen expression in bovine lymphoid tissue. Lab. Invest., 66:608, 1992.

Helfand, S.C.: Low-dose cytosine arabinoside-induced remission of lymphoblastic leukemia in a cat. J. Am. Vet. Med. Assoc., 191:707, 1987.

Hoff-Jorgensen, R.: An international comparison of different laboratory tests for the diagnosis of bovine leukosis: suggestions for international standardization. Vet. Immunol. Immunopathol., 22:293, 1989.

Hoover, E.A. and Mullins, J.I.: Feline leukemia virus infection and diseases. J. Am. Vet. Med. Assoc., 199:1287, 1991.

Hoover, E.A., Perigo, N.A., Quackenbush, S.L., et al.: Protection against feline leukemia virus infection by use of an inactivated virus vaccine. J. Am. Vet. Med. Assoc., 199:1392, 1991.

Hopkins, S.G., Evermann, J.F., DiGiacomo, R.F., et al.: Experimental transmission of bovine leukosis virus by simulated rectal palpation. Vet. Rec., 122:389, 1988.

Jacobson, R.H.: How well do serodiagnostic tests predict the infection or disease status of cats? J. Am. Vet. Med. Assoc., 199:1343, 1991.

Jain, N.C.: Schalm's Veterinary Hematology. 4th ed. Philadelphia, Lea & Febiger, 1986, pp. 838–908.

Jain, N.C., Blue, J.T., Grindem, C.B., et al.: A report of the animal leukemia study group: Proposed criteria for classification of acute myeloid leukemia in dogs and cats. Vet. Clin. Pathol., 20:63, 1991.

Jarrett, O.: Overview of feline leukemia virus research. J. Am. Vet. Med. Assoc., 199:1279, 1991.

Johnstone, A.C. and Manktelow, B.W.: The pathology of spontaneously occurring malignant lymphoma in sheep. Vet. Pathol., 15:301, 1978.

Kensil, C.R., Barrett, C., Kushner, N., et al.: Development of a genetically engineered vaccine against feline leukemia virus infection. J. Am. Vet. Med. Assoc., 199:1423, 1991.

Kiehl, A.R., Fettman, M.J., Quackenbush, S.L., et al.: Effects of feline leukemia virus infection on neutrophil chemotaxis in vitro. Am. J. Vet. Res., 48:76, 1987.

Kitamura, R., Onuma, M., Kawakami, K., et al.: Isolation of tumor-associated antigen from sera of bovine leukemia virus-infected cattle. Microbiol. Immunol., 34:163, 1990.

Kitchen, L.W., Mather, F.J. and Cotter, S.M.: Effect of continuous oral diethylcarbamazine treatment on lymphocyte counts of feline leukemia virus-infected cats. J. Clin. Lab. Immunol., 27:179, 1988.

Lassauzet, M.L., Johnson, W.O., Thurmond, M.C., et al.: Protection of colostral antibodies against bovine leukemia virus infection in calves on a California dairy. Can. J. Vet. Res., 53:424, 1989.

Lassauzet, M.L., Thurmond, M.C., Johnson, W.O., et al.: Factors associated with in utero or periparturient transmission of bovine leukemia virus in calves on a California dairy. Can. J. Vet. Res., 55:264, 1991a.

Lassauzet, M.L., Thurmond, M.C., Johnson, W.O., et al.: Factors associated with transmission of bovine leukemia virus by contact in cows on a California dairy [published erratum appears in Am J Epidemiol 1991 May 1;133(9):965]. Am. J. Epidemiol., 133:164, 1991b.

Leifer, C.E. and Matus, R.E.: Chronic lymphocytic leukemia in the dog: 22 cases (1974–1984). J. Am. Vet. Med. Assoc., 189:214, 1986.

Lewin, H.A., Wu, M.C., Nolan, T.J., et al.: Peripheral B lymphocyte percentage as an indicator of subclinical progression of bovine leukemia virus infection. J. Dairy. Sci, 71:2526, 1988.

Lewis, M.G., Kociba, G.J., Rojko, J.L., et al.: Retroviral-associated eosinophilic leukemia in the cat. Am. J. Vet. Res., 46:1066, 1985.

Lopez, N.A. and Jacobson, R.H.: False-positive reactions associated with anti-mouse activity in serotests for feline leukemia virus antigen. J. Am. Vet. Med. Assoc., 195:741, 1989.

Lopez, N.A., Jacobson, R.H., Scarlett, J.M., et al.: Sensitivity and specificity of blood test kits for feline leukemia virus antigen. J. Am. Vet. Med Assoc., 195:747, 1989.

Lopez, N.A., Scarlett, J.M., Pollock, R.V., et al.: Sensitivity, specificity, and predictive values of ClinEase-Virastat saliva test for feline leukemia virus infection. Cornell Vet., 80:75, 1990.

Lutz, H.: Feline retroviruses: A brief review. Vet. Microbiol., 23:131, 1990.

Madewell, B.R.: Hematological and bone marrow cytoloic abnormalities in 75 dogs with malignant lymphoma. J. Am. Anim. Hosp. Assoc., 22:235, 1986.

Mahaffey, E.A., Brown, T.P., Duncan, J.R., et al.: Basophilic leukaemia in a dog. J. Comp. Pathol., 97:393, 1987.

Marciani, D.J., Kensil, C.R., Beltz, G.A., et al.: Genetically engineered subunit vaccine against feline leukemia virus: Protective immune response in cats. Vaccine, 9:89, 1991.

Maruyama, K., Fukushima, T. and Mochizuki, S.: Cross-reactive antibodies to BLV and HTLV in bovine and human hosts with retrovirus infection. Vet. Immunol. Immunopathol., 22:265, 1989.

Matus, R.E., Leifer, C.E. and MacEwen, E.G.: Acute lymphoblastic leukemia in the dog: A review of 30 cases. J. Am. Vet. Med. Assoc., 183:859, 1983.

Migaki, G.: Hematopoietic neoplasms of slaughter animals. Comparative Morphology of Hematopoietic Neoplasms: Natl. Cancer Inst. Monograph, 32:121, 1969.

Molloy, J.B., Walker, P.J., Baldock, F.C., et al.: An enzyme-linked immunosorbent assay for detection of bovine leukaemia virus p24 antibody in cattle. J. Virol. Methods, 28:47, 1990.

Mooney, S.C., Hayes, A.A., MacEwen, G., et al.: Treatment and prognostic factors in lymphoma in cats: 103 cases (1977–1981). J. Am. Vet. Med. Assoc., 194:696, 1989.

Mori, T., Ishida, T., Washizu, T., et al.: Acute myelomonocytic leukemia in a horse. Vet. Pathol., 28:344, 1991.

Mullins, J.I., Hoover, E.A., Overbaugh, J., et al.: FeLV-FAIDS-induced immunodeficiency syndrome in cats. Vet. Immunol. Immunopathol., 21:25, 1989.

Naif, H.M., Brandon, R.B., Daniel, R.C., et al.: Bovine leukaemia proviral DNA detection in cattle using the polymerase chain reaction. Vet. Microbiol., 25:117, 1990.

Naif, H.M., Daniel, R.C., Cougle, W.G., et al.: Early detection of bovine leukemia virus by using an enzyme-linked assay for polymerase chain reaction-amplified proviral DNA in experimentally infected cattle. J. Clin. Microbiol., 30:675, 1992.

Novotney, C., English, R.V., Housman, J., et al.: Lymphocyte population changes in cats naturally infected with feline immunodeficiency virus. AIDS, 4:1213, 1990.

Overbaugh, J., Donahue, P.R., Quackenbush, S.L., et al.: Molecular cloning of a feline leukemia virus that induces fatal immuno-deficiency disease in cats. Science, 239:906, 1988.

Pardi, D., Hoover, E.A., Quackenbush, S.L., et al.: Selective impairment of humoral immunity in feline leukemia virus-induced immunodeficiency. Vet. Immunol. Immunopathol., 28:183, 1991.

Platzer, C., Siakkou, H., Kraus, G., et al.: Use of monoclonal antibody against major internal protein p24 of bovine leukemia virus in capture ELISA. Arch. Exp. Veterinarmed., 44:917, 1990.

Portetelle, D., Burny, A., Desmettre, P., et al.: Development of a specific serological test and an efficient subunit vaccine to control bovine leukemia virus infection. Dev. Biol. Stand., 72:81, 1990.

Portetelle, D., Limbach, K., Burny, A., et al.: Recombinant vaccinia virus expression of the bovine leukaemia virus envelope gene and protection of immunized sheep against infection. Vaccine, 9:194, 1991.

Quackenbush, S.L., Donahue, P.R., Dean, G.A., et al.: Lymphocyte subset alterations and viral determinants of immunodeficiency disease induction by the feline leukemia virus FeLV-FAIDS. J. Virol., 64:5465, 1990.

Raskin, R.E. and Krehbiel, J.D.: Myelodysplastic changes in a cat with myelomonocytic leukemia. J. Am. Vet. Med. Assoc., 187:171, 1985.

Raskin, R.E. and Krehbiel, J.D.: Prevalence of leukemic blood and bone marrow in dogs with multicentric lymphoma. J. Am. Vet. Med. Assoc., 194:1427, 1989.

Reinacher, M.: Diseases associated with spontaneous feline leukemia virus (FeLV) infection in cats. Vet. Immunol. Immunopathol., 21:85, 1989.

Riedel, N., Hoover, E.A., Dornsife, R.E., et al.: Pathogenic and host range determinants of the feline aplastic anemia retrovirus. Proc. Natl. Acad. Sci., 85:2758, 1988.

Rojko, J.L. and Kociba, G.J.: Pathogenesis of infection by the feline leukemia virus. J. Am. Vet. Med. Assoc., 199:1305, 1991.

Rojko, J., Essex, M. and Trainin, Z.: Feline leukemia/sarcoma viruses and immunodeficiency. Adv. Vet. Sci. Comp. Med., 32:57, 1988.

Rojko, J.L., Kociba, G.J., Abkowitz, J.L., et al.: Feline lymphomas: immunological and cytochemical characterization. Cancer Res., 49:345, 1989.

Romatowski, J.: Interpreting feline leukemia test results. J. Am. Vet. Med. Assoc., 195:928, 1989.

Rosin, A., Moore, P. and Dubielzig, R.: Malignant histiocytosis in Bernese Mountain dogs. J. Am. Vet. Med. Assoc., 188:1041, 1986.

Sherman, M.P., Ehrlich, G.D., Ferrer, J.F., et al.: Amplification and analysis of specific DNA and RNA sequences of bovine leukemia virus from infected cows by polymerase chain reaction. J. Clin. Microbiol., 30:185, 1992.

Spier, S.J., Madewell, B.R., Zinkl, J.G., et al.: Acute myelomonocytic leukemia in a horse. J. Am. Vet. Med. Assoc., 1881:861, 1986.

Stott, M.L., Thurmond, M.C., Dunn, S.J., et al.: Integrated bovine leukosis proviral DNA in T helper and T cytotoxic/suppressor lymphocytes. J. Gen. Virol., 72:307, 1991.

Swenson, C.L., Kociba, G.J., Mathes, L.E., et al.: Prevalence of disease in nonviremic cats previously exposed to feline leukemia virus. J. Am. Vet. Med. Assoc., 196:1049, 1990.

Swenson, C.I., Kociba, G.J., O'Keefe, D.A., et al.: Cyclic hematopoiesis associated with feline leukemia virus infection in two cats. J. Am. Vet. Med. Assoc., 191:93, 1987.

Takamatsu, H., Inumaru, S. and Nakajima, H.: Inhibition of in vitro immunocyte function by sera from cattle with bovine leukosis. Vet. Immunol. Immunopathol., 18:349, 1988.

Taylor, B.C., Stott, J.L., Thurmond, M.A., et al.: Alteration in lymphocyte subpopulations in bovine leukosis virus-infected cattle. Vet. Immunol. Immunopathol., 31:35, 1992.

Testa, N.G., Orions, D.E. and Lord, B.I.: A feline model for the myelodysplastic syndrome: pre-leukaemic abnormalities caused in cats by infection with a new isolate of feline leukaemia virus (FeLV), AB/GM1. Haematologica, 73:317, 1988.

Theilen, G.H. and Madewell, B.R.: Veterinary cancer medicine. 2nd ed. Philadelphia, PA, Lea & Febiger, 1987, Chaps. 12 and 16.

Thomsen, M.K., Jensen, A.L., Skak-Nielsen, T., et al.: Enhanced granulocyte function in a case of chronic granulocytic leukemia in a dog. Vet. Immunol. Immunopathol., 28:143, 1991.

Thurmond, M.C.: Calf management to control bovine leukemia virus infection [editorial]. Cornell Vet., 81:227, 1991.

Tizard, I.: Use of immunomodulators as an aid to clinical management of feline leukemia virus-infected cats. J. Am. Vet. Med. Assoc., 199:1482, 1991.

Tomlinson, M.J., Doster, A.R. and Wright, E.R.: Lymphosarcoma with virus-like particles in a neonatal foal. Vet. Pathol., 16:629, 1979.

Tompkins, M.B., Nelson, P.D., English, R.V., et al.: Early events in the immunopathogenesis of feline retrovirus infections. J. Am. Vet. Med. Assoc., 199:1311, 1991.

Tompkins, M.B., Ogilvie, G.K., Gast, A.M., et al.: Interleukin-2 suppression in cats naturally infected with feline leukemia virus. J. Biol. Response Mod., 8:86, 1989a.

Tompkins, M.B., Pang, V.F., Michaely, P.A., et al.: Feline cytotoxic large granular lymphocytes induced by recombinant human IL-2. J. Immunol., 143:749, 1989b.

Tonelli, Q.J.: Enzyme-linked immunosorbent assay methods for detection of feline leukemia virus and feline immunodeficiency virus. J. Am. Vet. Med. Assoc., 199:1336, 1991.

Toth, S.R., Onions, D.E. and Jarrett, O.: Histopathological and hematological findings in myeloid leukemia induced by a new feline leukemia virus isolate. Vet. Pathol., 23:462, 1986.

Wardrop, K.J., Kramer, J.W., Abkowitz, J.L., et al.: Quantitative studies of erythropoiesis in the clinically normal, phlebotomized, and feline leukemia virus-infected cat. Am. J. Vet. Res., 47:2274, 1986.

Weijer, K., Uytdehaag, F.G. and Osterhaus, A.D.: Control of feline leukaemia virus. Vet. Immunol. Immunopathol., 21:69, 1989.

Weiser, M.G., Cockerell, G.L., Smith, J.A., et al.: Cytoplasmic fragmentation associated with lymphoid leukemia in ruminants: Interference with electronic determination of platelet concentration. Vet. Pathol., 26:177, 1989.

Weiss, D.J., Raskin, R. and Zerbe, C.: Myelodysplastic syndrome in two dogs. J. Am. Vet. Med. Assoc., 187:1038, 1985.

Weller, R.E., Holmberg, C.A., Theilen, G.H., et al.: Histologic classification as a prognostic criterion for canine lymphosarcoma. Am. J. Vet. Res., 41:1310, 1980.

Wellman, M.L., Couto, C.G., Starkey, R.J., et al.: Lymphocytosis of large granular lymphocytes in three dogs. Vet. Pathol., 26:158, 1989.

Wellman, M.L., Davenport, D.J., Morton, D., et al.: Malignant histiocytosis in four dogs. J. Am. Vet. Med. Assoc., 187:919, 1985.

Williams, D.L., Amborski, G.F. and Davis, W.C.: Enumeration of T and B lymphocytes in bovine leukemia virus-infected cattle, using monoclonal antibodies. Am. J. Vet. Res., 49:1098, 1988a.

Williams, D.L., Barta, O. and Amborski, G.F.: Molecular studies of T-lymphocytes from cattle infected with bovine leukemia virus. Vet. Immunol. Immunopathol., 19:307, 1988b.

Chapter 21

The Plasma Proteins, Dysproteinemias, and Immune Deficiency Disorders

PLASMA PROTEINS

The plasma proteins are a group of heterogeneous molecules with various characteristics and functions (Tables 21–1, 21–2, and 21–3). The total protein in the body represents a balance between anabolism and catabolism. Plasma protein concentrations reflect a balance between filtration into tissues through the capillaries and return from the tissues through the lymph. This balance depends on the colloidal osmotic pressure and circulation dynamics—the tendency for blood to attract fluids from the tissues because of colloidal osmotic pressure and the opposing hydrostatic pressure of blood, which tends to force fluids into the tissue spaces.

In disease, other signs generally become evident before changes in plasma protein concentration occur. Alterations in plasma protein levels must be examined in light of the entire complex of clinical and laboratory findings before any diagnostic or prognostic predictions can be made.

Factors Governing Concentration

The concentration of protein in the plasma is a function of the hormonal balance, nutritional status, water balance, and other factors affecting the state of health. The rate of turnover of the various proteins varies among species (Table 21–2). The half-life of a protein correlates directly with body size, with the turnover being much faster in smaller animals. The extravascular concentrations of protein are much greater than the intravascular concentrations. For example, the extravascular:intravascular ratio for albumin is 2.90 in horses, 2.58 in cattle, and 1.71 in young pigs. In addition to normal catabolism by the liver, kidney, and other tissues, plasma proteins are constantly being lost into the gut.

Table 21–1. Major Plasma Proteins and Their Functions

Plasma Protein	Function(s)
Albumin	Osmosis; amino acid pool; transporter of other anions and cations; most abundant protein in plasma
In α-globulin zone	
α1-Lipoprotein	Transports fats, lipids, fat-soluble vitamins, and hormones
α1-Acid glycoprotein	Unknown; increased in inflammatory, degenerative, and neoplastic disease
α1-Glycoprotein	Unknown
Transcortin	Binds and transports cotisol
Thyroxine-binding globulin	Binds thyroxine
Gc-globulins	Group-specific, genetically determined proteins; function unknown
Haptoglobin	Binds free hemoglobin
Ceruloplasmin	Glycoprotein that binds copper
Cholinesterase	Enzyme that degrades acetylcholine
α2-Macroglobulin	Binds insulin
α2-Lipoprotein	Transport lipids
Erythropoietin	Erythropoiesis
In β-globulin zone	
β-Lipoprotein	Transport glycerides and other lipids
Transferrin	Binds iron
Hemopexin	Binds heme
Fibrinogen	Essential to blood clotting
Plasminogen	Proenzyme form of plasmin
Partly in β-globulin zone, mostly in γ-globulin zone	Antibody activity
IgG, IgA, IgM, IgD, IgE	

Table 21–2. Half-Life of Serum Proteins of Various Animals

Species	Protein	Half-Life (days)
Sheep	Albumin	14–28
Young swine	Albumin	8.2
Cattle	Albumin	16.5
	γ-Globulin	21.2
Human	Albumin	15.0
	γ-Globulin	20.0
Dog	Albumin	8.2
	γ-Globulin	8.0
Rabbit	Albumin	5.7
	γ-Globulin	5.7
Guinea pig	Albumin	2.8
	γ-Globulin	5.4
Rat	Albumin	2.5
	γ-Globulin	5.5
Mouse	Albumin	1.9
	γ-Globulin	1.9
Baboon	Albumin	16
	γ-Globulin	12
Horse		
Normal	Albumin	19.4
Splenectomized	Albumin	17.3
Hypoalbuminemic	Albumin	14.5

The dietary protein requirements for animals vary with species, age, and physiologic status. For example, ruminants can be maintained on protein-free rations. The young need additional dietary protein for growth and additional demands are imposed during pregnancy and lactation. Dietary restrictions of protein in some animals (e.g., the dog) generally lead to hypoalbuminemia, but the globulins are not significantly affected. The absorption and utilization of dietary protein may be reduced in certain diseases, particularly those involving the gastrointestinal tract or pancreas.

A significant external hemorrhage leads to protein loss and reduced blood volume. Restoration of the plasma volume is accomplished by rapid movement of extravascular fluid into the vascular system. This intravascular movement of fluid, within a few hours of blood loss, leads to a temporary reduction in the plasma protein concentration. Thus, the hallmark of acute blood loss is a hypoproteinemia accompanying a normocytic-normochromic anemia. The existence of anemia and normal or elevated total plasma protein levels indicate that the anemia is probably not the result of external hemorrhage. In dogs, it has been shown that at least 50% of the albumin replaced within 24 hours after acute external hemorrhage appears to be from extravascular sources, principally the lymph. In addition, liver anabolism of albumin is increased and catabolism is decreased.

In contrast, a loss of body water because of dehydration leads to an elevation of total plasma protein level because of concentration in a reduced blood volume. In this instance, both albumin and globulin concentrations are elevated and, therefore, the albumin:globulin (A:G) ratio remains normal. Thus, dehydration may mask an absolute hypoproteinemia by elevating the plasma protein concentration into the normal range as a result of lowered plasma volume. Interestingly, feeding a single large meal to ponies can initiate an abrupt plasma volume loss (9 to 24%, mean 15%) with a concurrent increase (12%) in plasma protein concentration (Clarke et al., 1990). The transient change in plasma volume is attributed to copious upper alimentary secretions.

Pregnancy, parturition, and lactation can influence plasma protein concentrations, as found through studies on cows, sheep, and goats. During the latter stage of pregnancy, plasma protein concentrations decrease with the movement of blood proteins (albumin and IgG1) into the udder, particularly during colostrum formation. IgG1 is selectively transported into the mammary gland of ruminants. Serum IgA and IgM concentrations may also decrease to some extent, particularly during the first few weeks postpartum.

Plasma protein concentration increases with age in most species. It is lowest during fetal life and remarkably low at birth. An increase is apparent soon after colostrum consumption and it subsequently rises as the newborn begins to synthesize immunoglobulins (Igs). Adult concentrations are reached by about 6 months to 1 year of age, depending on the species.

Table 21–3. Characteristics of Acute Phase Proteins

Protein	Electrophoretic Mobility	Molecular Weight	Normal Serum Content* (mg/dl)	Half-Life (days)	Biologic Function
C-reactive protein	α_1-Globulin	110,000	<0.8	<1.0	Regulation of inflammatory process and microbial defense
α_1-Acid glycoprotein (orosomucoid)	α_1-Globulin	39,500	55–140	5.2	Modulation of hemostasis, binds drugs
α_1-Antitrypsin	α_1-Globulin	54,000	180–260	3.9	Protease inhibition
α_1-Antichymotrypsin	α_1-globulin	68,000	30–60	—	Protease inhibition
Serum amyloid A	α_1-Globulin	11,000	<2.0	—	Amyloid precursor
Cerulosplasmin	α_2-Globulin	151,000	15–60	4.25	Copper carrier, oxidase activity
Haptoglobin	α_2-Globulin	80,000–160,000	83–267	3.5	Binds free hemoglobin
α_2-Macroglobulin	α_2-Globulin	820,000	150–350	—	Protease inhibition, macroglobulin transport of hormones
Fibrinogen	β-Globulin	341,000	200–450	3.2	Coagulation
Transferrin	β-Globulin	76,000	200–400	8.7	Transport of iron
Hemopexin	β-Globulin	57,000	50–115	7.0	Binds oxidized heme

From Jain, N.C.: Acute phase proteins. *In* Current Veterinary Therapy 10: Small Animal Practice. Edited by R.W. Kirk. Philadelphia, W.B. Saunders, 1989, pp. 468–471.

* In humans.

Total plasma protein concentrations are comparatively high in older animals.

Colostrum ingestion and absorption by the neonate lead to increased concentrations of γ-globulins and temporary proteinuria. Electrophoresis of neonatal serum can effectively demonstrate whether the animal has absorbed colostrum, because elevations in γ-globulin levels are markedly evident in various species when colostral Igs have been absorbed (Figs. 21–1 and 21–2). Immunoglobulin concentrations in precolostral and postcolostral calf serums have been measured. The three major Igs—IgM, IgG1, and IgG2—may be detected in precolostral calf serum. Serum Ig levels peak in colostrum-fed calves at 18 to 30 hours after birth, with IgM and IgA peaking earlier than IgG1 and IgG2. A gradual decrease occurs at 1 to 5 weeks, depending on the Ig half-life, and this is followed by a gradual increase from synthesis by the young. Calves vary widely in their concentration of serum Igs. This may be related to various factors, including the amount of colostrum ingested per unit body weight, the Ig concentrations in the colostrum fed, how soon suckling commenced after birth, environmental temperature, and dietary factors.

Various Plasma Proteins

PREALBUMIN

Prealbumin (MW, 50,000 to 60,000) is found in the plasma of humans and some animals. It is synthesized

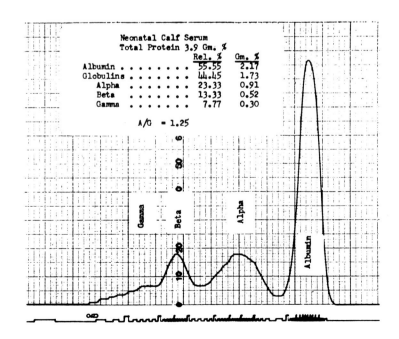

Fig. 21–1. Electrophoretic pattern of neonatal calf serum before colostrum ingestion. Note the virtual absence of γ-globulin. The calf was bled 5 minutes after parturition. (From Jain, N.C.: Schalm's Veterinary Hematology. 4th Ed. Philadelphia, Lea & Febiger, 1986, p. 946.)

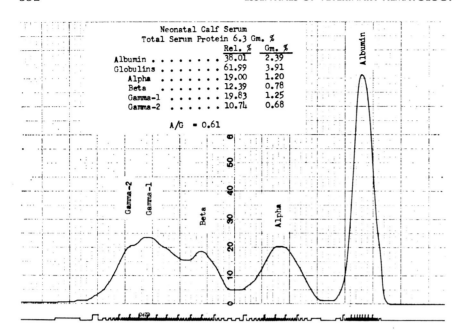

Fig. 21–2. Electrophoretic pattern of serum from the same calf shown in Figure 21–1 after colostrum ingestion and absorption. The calf was 24 hours old at the time of bleeding. (From Jain, N.C.: Schalm's Veterinary Hematology. 4th Ed. Philadelphia, Lea & Febiger, 1986, p. 946.)

by the liver and serves as a transport protein for thyroxine (both T4 and T3), therefore also called transthyretin, and retinol-binding protein involved in the transport of vitamin A. A decrease in the prealbumin concentration may suggest decreased synthesis from impaired liver function and increased loss through the kidneys, as in nephrotic syndrome. Prealbumin is found in significantly higher concentrations in healthy foals than in mares. Its concentration is elevated in horses with acute infections, laminitis, and malignant tumors.

Serum prealbumin concentration is considered an accurate indicator of nutritional status in humans; malnourished persons have reduced levels, and normal or above normal levels are attained on nutritional repletion and general improvement in health (Pleban, 1989). Prealbumin levels in humans are rapidly reduced following surgery, trauma, and infections because its half-life is short (24 hours) and because the total body pool is small. Its levels rise rapidly with clinical improvement, compared to those of albumin and transferrin concentrations, which take several days to reflect an improvement in health.

ALBUMIN

Albumin (MW, 66,300) is the most abundant of the plasma proteins. Because it is a larger molecule, it is normally retained by the capillaries, but it is the first protein to be lost from the blood during tissue injury. Albumin is important in the regulation and maintenance of the colloidal osmotic pressure of the blood. Albumin has an important transport function—it transports free fatty acids, the bile acids, bilirubin, the porphyrins, ketosteroids, many drugs, such as penicillin, aspirin, and the barbiturates, histamine, and cations and trace elements, such as calcium, copper, and zinc.

Albumin is synthesized by the liver and catabolized by various tissues. Albumin synthesis is influenced by the state of nutrition, hormonal balance, general condition of the liver, stress, and extravascular concentration of albumin. For example, its synthesis diminishes during fasting or malnutrition, hypothyroidism, and cirrhosis. The half-life of albumin varies with the species: 1.9 days for the mouse, 8.2 days for the dog, 15 days for humans, 19.4 days for the horse, and 15–21 days for the cow. Albumin synthesis appears to be inversely related to the synthesis of acute phase proteins and is regulated by interleukin-1 (IL-1) and other cytokines (Rothschild et al., 1988).

GLYCOPROTEINS AND ACUTE PHASE PROTEINS

Glycoproteins are proteins conjugated with carbohydrate, including γ-globulins, fibrinogen, ceruloplasmin, haptoglobin, α_2-macroglobulin, and α_1-acid glycoprotein or seromucoid. The functions of this heterogeneous group of proteins are not known with certainty. Marked variations in the plasma glycoprotein content may occur in both physiologic and pathologic states. Electrophoretically, glycoprotein in the α_2-globulin zone is in the highest concentration and seems to show the greatest change in the disease.

Some glycoproteins are recognized as acute phase reactants or proteins, because their plasma concentrations increase rapidly during inflammatory conditions in many species (Cooper, 1990; Eckersall and Conner, 1988; Jain, 1989; Schultz and Arnold, 1990). Table 21–3 summarizes the characteristics of some acute phase proteins and Table 21–4 lists general conditions associated with increases in such proteins.

Some components of complement, such as C3, C9, and factor B, also respond as acute phase proteins as their serum concentrations increase significantly during inflammatory responses (Adinolfi and Lehner,

Table 21–4.   Conditions Associated with Increases in Acute Phase Proteins

Acute and chronic inflammatory conditions
Bacterial infections
Endotoxemia
Surgeries
Trauma
Burns
Malignancies
Myocardial infarction
Neonatal infections
Organ transplantations
Viral infections
Certain parasitic infections
Pregnancy

From Jain, N.C.: Acute phase proteins. *In* Current Veterinary Therapy 10: Small Animal Practice. Edited by R.W. Kirk. Philadelphia, W.B. Saunders, 1989, pp. 468–471.

1988). The acute phase proteins are mainly synthesized in the liver, but some extrahepatic synthesis may occur. Synthesis of various acute phase proteins by hepatocytes (Fig. 21–5) is stimulated by endotoxin-inducible cytokines, such as IL-1, tumor necrosis factor-α and -β, and a hepatocyte stimulating factor now known to be IL-6 (di Minno and Mancini, 1992; Koj et al., 1988; Schultz and Arnold, 1990). Interferon-gamma also has a stimulatory effect. The stimulatory effect may be general or specific for certain acute phase proteins.

The acute phase proteins are nonspecific indicators of tissue damage and have a wide functional significance (Cooper, 1990; Schultz and Arnold, 1990). For example, C-reactive protein (CRP) reacts with cell surface receptors, opsonizes bacteria for efficient phagocytosis, may enhance some neutrophil functions, activates classical complement pathway, interacts with chromatin fragments in areas of tissue damage for removal by macrophages, and inhibits growth and/or metastasis of tumor cells. Serum amyloid A (SAA) acts as a precursor of amyloid A in secondary amyloidosis. The α_1-acid glycoprotein appears to be immunosuppressive and binds a number of drugs. Increased levels of acute phase proteins in cancer patients generally suggest an unfavorable prognosis (Cooper, 1988).

Surgical trauma in dogs stimulated synthesis of several acute phase proteins (Conner et al., 1988a). CRP peaked at 24 hours after surgery, while ceruloplasmin, haptoglobin, and seromucoid peaked on days 4 to 6 and α-1-antitrypsin changed insignificantly. In other studies in dogs, serum haptoglobin and ceruloplasmin concentrations correlated positively with WBC counts, segmented and band neutrophil counts, and fibrinogen concentrations (Solter et al., 1991). Both were up to 6 times more sensitive than the WBC counts and fibrinogen in detecting inflammation. Plasma concentrations of CRP and haptoglobin were increased in dogs infected with Trypanosoma brucei and CRP was useful in determining the presence of active infection and response to therapy (Ndung'u et al., 1991). Concentrations of acid soluble glycoproteins were

increased in the sera of cattle with lymphoma, glomerulonephritis associated with lymphoma, and acute mastitis, and in sera collected on the fifth day after surgery (Nagahata et al., 1989). Serum concentrations of α-1-antitrypsin, ceruloplasmin, fibrinogen, haptoglobin, and seromucoid in calves with turpentine-induced abscesses increased by 2 to 3 days, peaked by 4 to 7 days, and returned to normal levels by the seventeenth day postinoculation (Conner et al., 1988b).

Haptoglobin and α-1-glycoprotein responded as positive acute phase proteins and albumin as a negative acute phase protein (its concentration decreased) in horses with adjuvant-induced inflammatory lesions (Patterson et al., 1988). Serum concentrations of haptoglobin, orosomucoid, ceruloplasmin, and α-2-macroglobulin were increased in horses with grass sickness (Milne et al., 1991).

Plasma ceruloplasmin, plasma fibrinogen, and serum haptoglobin concentrations were measured in sheep with bronchial obstruction and pneumonia and were found to be more useful indicators of tissue injury than the numbers of circulating neutrophils (Pfeffer and Rogers, 1989).

FIBRINOGEN

Fibrinogen is a glycoprotein (MW, 341,000) primarily concerned with hemostasis; it serves as the substrate for thrombin in the formation of fibrin. The fibrinogen molecule is a dimer, with each half consisting of three polypeptide chains interconnected by disulfide bonds; its molecular formula is $(\alpha, \beta, \text{and } \gamma)_2$. The fibrinogen-fibrin transformation occurs after the removal of two acidic peptides (fibrinopeptides A and B) from the NH_2-terminal portion of the α and β chains. Fibrinogen is important in hemostasis and thrombosis primarily because of its interactions with thrombin, factor XIII, plasminogen, glycoprotein IIb/IIIa, and endothelial cells.

Fibrinogen is produced by microsomes of the hepatic parenchymal cells, where it is stored until required. Plasma fibrinogen has a much shorter half-life (2.5 to 4.5 days in the dog) than other plasma proteins and negative feedback governs its rate of formation. Studies in sheep have indicated that the half-life of fibrinogen is shorter in newborn lambs (about 2 days) compared to adults (about 5 day) (Andrew et al., 1988). Equine fibrinogen has a half-life of 4.1 to 5.2 days (Coyne et al., 1985). Normal fibrinogen concentrations in blood (g/dl) are as follows: cat, 0.05 to 0.30; dog and goat, 0.10 to 0.4; horse, sheep, and pig, 0.10 to 0.50; and cattle, 0.30 to 0.70.

TRANSFERRIN

Transferrin is the only protein in plasma that transports iron. It is a glycoprotein composed of one polypeptide chain. Species variations occur in the molecular weight (76,000 to 90,000) and in the number of iron-binding sites (one or two). Generally, each molecule of transferrin binds two Fe^{2+} through tyrosine residues. Normally, about one-third of the plasma transferrin is saturated with iron and provides about two-thirds of the iron needed for erythropoiesis. Transferrin receptors (MW, 95,000) on the cell surface bind transferrin molecules and mediate iron uptake into the cell. The plasma half-life of transferrin is 8 to 10 days. Other functions of transferrin include antiviral and antibacterial activities. It also acts as a growth factor; purified equine transferrin was found to promote the proliferation of a human monocytic leukemia cell line and two myeloid cell lines (Yoshinari et al., 1989).

Transferrin is synthesized in the liver and possibly at other sites. The total iron binding capacity is a measure of serum transferrin concentration and its level in normal animals and humans is generally 300 μg/dl. The serum transferrin concentration increases in iron deficiency states and pregnancy and decreases in diseases such as liver disease, acute and chronic infections, and leukemia. Transferrin concentrations in foals are high at birth and increase during the first 3 neonatal weeks after a transient decrease during the first 48 hours. Transferrin is selectively transported from blood to milk in lactating cows. Its concentration is highest in the first milk (1.07 mg/ml), decreases sharply during the colostral period, and then decreases slowly to stabilize (0.02 mg/ml) by the third week postpartum (Sanchez et al., 1988). A similar trend is found for lactoferrin concentration in bovine milk.

HAPTOGLOBIN AND HEMOPEXIN

Both haptoglobin and hemopexin are glycoproteins synthesized in the liver. Haptoglobin (MW, 80,000 to 160,000) consists of four polypeptide chains and has a plasma half-life of 2 to 4 days. Hemopexin (MW, 57,000) consists of one polypeptide chain and has a plasma half-life of 7 days.

Haptoglobin binds free hemoglobin released from intravascular hemolysis, as in hemolytic anemias, and the hemoglobin-haptoglobin complex is rapidly removed from the circulation by Kupffer cells (see Fig. 7–22). The half-time of hemoglobin-haptoglobin varies in different species; 10 to 30 minutes in humans (Williams et al., 1990), 1.5 hours in rats, and 4 hours in goats (Osada and Nowacki, 1989). Free hemoglobin in excess of that needed to saturate all the plasma haptoglobin is excreted by the kidneys, resulting in hemoglobinuria. Some of the excess hemoglobin breaks down in the circulation and liberates heme, which is then oxidized to hematin. This hematin binds with hemopexin and the hematin-hemopexin complex is slowly removed (half-life, 7 to 8 hours) from the plasma by the hepatocytes. Excess hematin not bound by hemopexin is bound by serum albumin, forming a complex called ferrihemalbumin (methemalbumin). This hemalbumin complex is removed from the circulation at a considerably slower rate (half-life, 22 hours) than the hematin-hemopexin complex.

Plasma haptoglobin and hemopexin concentrations are markedly reduced in hemolytic anemias and during ineffective erythropoiesis. Haptoglobin concentra-

tions in humans are age-related, being lower in the young and higher in people in their sixties (and older), and decrease during pregnancy, severe malnutrition, hyperparathyroidism, and corticosteroid therapy. Haptoglobin is an important acute phase protein, so its synthesis invariably increases during acute and chronic active inflammatory conditions. Haptoglobin migrates in the α_2-globulin region; thus, an increase of the latter in the serum electrophoretogram in many inflammatory diseases reflects changes primarily resulting from the former. It may also increase from trauma, after surgery, and because of hematopoietic malignancies.

Plasma haptoglobin concentrations are greatly elevated in infections and inflammatory conditions in horses (Kent and Goodall, 1991), cattle (Skinner et al. 1991), dogs (Solter et al., 1991), cats (Stoddart et al., 1988), and lambs (Pepin et al., 1991). For example, increases are seen in cattle with severe inflammatory diseases, such as mastitis, metritis, pyometra, traumatic reticulitis, and bacterial infection. Uncomplicated surgery in horses (castration) caused a 2- to 3-fold increase in the serum haptoglobin concentration, with levels peaking between 3 and 5 days postsurgery, whereas the concomitant presence of hematomas following surgery resulted in the disappearance of haptoglobin from the circulation (Kent and Goodall, 1991). γ-Irradiation and turpentine-induced inflammation cause increases in serum haptoglobin concentrations in sheep, goats, and cattle. Serum haptoglobin concentration is increased in cows with fatty liver, presumably because of reduced estradiol and increased glucocorticosteroid concentrations in serum (Yosino et al., 1992). In cats, recurrent intravascular hemolysis, as in autoimmune hemolytic anemia and haemobartonellosis, is associated with a transient reduction in the serum haptoglobin concentration, which becomes normal in 2 days. In comparison, an increase occurs from splenectomy, abscess formation, feline infectious peritonitis, and upper respiratory infections. A biphasic response (reduction followed by an increase) may occur with regard to haptoglobin, orosomucoid, and transferrin in cats experimentally inoculated with feline infectious peritonitis virus (Stoddart et al., 1988). In dogs, the serum haptoglobin and α_2-globulin concentrations show a positive linear correlation and increase in inflammatory conditions and after corticosteroid therapy (Harvey and West, 1987; Solter et al., 1991). Corticosteroid-induced increases in the haptoglobin level are also seen in sheep. Haptoglobin concentrations in lambs peaked by 1 to 5 days after induction of a pyogranulomatous inflammation by Corynebacterium pseudotuberculosis. Simultaneously, plasma copper levels were increased and zinc levels were decreased (Pepin et al., 1991).

CERULOPLASMIN

Ceruloplasmin (MW, 151,000) is a blue glycoprotein synthesized by the liver, with a plasma half-life of about 4 days. It transports over 90% of plasma copper and donates it to the liver and other tissues; each molecule binds six to eight atoms of copper (Cu^{3+}). The copper content of equine ceruloplasmin is estimated to be 0.31% (Medda et al., 1987). Ceruloplasmin is important in copper homeostasis and in the mobilization of iron. Ceruloplasmin has been found to prevent copper-induced lysis of erythrocytes by binding to receptors on their surface (Saenko et al., 1990). Ceruloplasmin inhibits inactivation of coagulation factors VIII and Va by activated protein C. This is because ceruloplasmin contains a decapeptide sequence that shares 60% and 40% sequence identity with the activated protein C binding sequence in factors VIII and V, respectively (Walker and Fay, 1990).

Ceruloplasmin acts as an acute phase protein, hence its synthesis in humans is increased in acute inflammatory conditions and acute bacterial, viral, and parasitic infections (Smith and Cipriano, 1987). Elevated concentrations have also been found in some other conditions, including leukemia, solid tumors, and biliary cirrhosis. Decreased ceruloplasmin concentrations may be found at birth and during malnutrition, malabsorption, nephrosis, and Wilson's disease (liver disease associated with copper toxicosis).

Equine ceruloplasmin (MW, 115,000) has been purified. Its plasma concentration in mares decreases at 24 to 48 hours before and after delivery, and in foals, its concentration increases gradually up to 2 years of age. Elevations in ceruloplasmin concentrations in horses occur several days after induction of an inflammatory response and abnormal values persist for a few weeks (Okumura et al., 1991). Increases in ceruloplasmin concentration parallel increases in non-ceruloplasmin bound plasma copper levels in horses with localized inflammatory lesions (Auer et al., 1989).

The specificity of ceruloplasmin in detecting inflammation in dogs appears comparable to that of plasma fibrinogen concentration and blood leukocyte counts (Solter et al., 1991). Ceruloplasmin levels increased in calves after endotoxin administration, but not in calves infected with Pasteurella haemolytica, although haptoglobin, α_1-proteinase inhibitor, and seromucoid levels were increased in both groups (Conner et al., 1989). Some of the calves infected with Ostertagi ostertgi showed a variable increase in the levels of these four acute phase proteins.

C-REACTIVE PROTEIN

C-Reactive protein is an acute phase protein that increases during inflammatory conditions. The name signifies its property of nonimmunologic precipitation with the somatic C polysaccharide of pneumococci in the presence of Ca^{2+}. The C-reactive protein consists of five identical subunits held together by noncovalent bonds. Each subunit has a molecular weight of about 21,000 and consists of 187 amino acids. Because of their unique structures, the C-reactive protein and serum amyloid P, which bears a nearly 60% homology to the C-reactive protein, belong to the pentraxin or pentaxin protein family (Kolb-Bachofen, 1991a). Bovine (Morimatsu et al., 1989) and equine (Takiguchi et al., 1990) C-reactive proteins have been purified

and found to be pentamers (MW, 100,000 and 118,000, respectively). Equine C-reactive protein migrates in the region between β and γ globulins. The half-life of C-reactive protein is 6 to 8 hours.

The plasma concentration of C-reactive protein increases quickly (by 6 hours), up to several hundredfold, following tissue injury, bacterial infections, inflammatory conditions, and many other pathologic conditions (Ballou and Kushner, 1992). Thus, determination of its plasma concentrations by a sensitive nephelometric method or by a simple and fast latex-agglutination method is of diagnostic importance in all types of inflammatory conditions. Synthesis of C-reactive protein is stimulated by IL-1 and IL-6 (Ganter et al., 1989). Serial quantitative measurements of C-reactive protein can be performed to monitor disease activity, response to antibiotic therapy, and postsurgical complications (Young et al., 1991). In addition, C-reactive protein may have some functional significance in the regulation of inflammatory processes and microbial defense. C-reactive protein activates the classical complement pathway, thereby promoting bacterial opsonization and phagocytosis (Cambau, 1988). A membrane-bound form of C-reactive protein functions as the recycling galactose-specific particle receptor in rat kupffer cells and mediates endocytosis (Kolb-Bachofen, 1991b). It is speculated that C-reactive protein modifies the functions of neutrophils, macrophages, lymphocytes, and platelets and thereby regulate the inflammatory response (Gotschlich, 1989).

Serum concentrations of C-reactive protein in dogs have been measured by specific immunoassay (Caspi et al., 1987). Healthy dogs generally have less than 5 mg/L, whereas those with inflammatory and noninflammatory disorders have up to 246 mg/L. Markedly increased concentrations were found 24 hours after the injection of casein to induce acute inflammation and in dogs subjected to ovariohysterectomy or elective, nonacute, orthopedic surgery. Increased concentrations of C-reactive protein are found in horses with pneumonitis, enteritis, and arthritis, and after the intramuscular injection of turpentine (to induce inflammation) or castration (Takaguchi et al., 1990). C-reactive protein concentrations in horses vary with age and in mares during the perinatal and postnatal periods (Yamashita et al., 1991). Inflammatory stimuli in horses stimulate synthesis of C-reactive protein by 24 hours and peak values of 3 to 6 times the base values are reached by 3 to 5 days. Interestingly, C-reactive protein does not act as an acute phase protein in ruminants (Boosman et al., 1989). However, lactation might stimulate C-reactive protein synthesis; its concentrations are higher in sera from lactating cows (76.0 ± 13.6 μg/ml) than from nonlactating cows (20.6 ± 1.4 μg/ml) (Morimatsu et al., 1991).

SERUM AMYLOID A

Serum amyloid A (MW, 11,000) is an acute phase protein that migrates in the α_1-globulin region. It is one of the major acute phase proteins in humans and mice and is synthesized predominantly by the liver under the regulation of IL-1 (Rienhoff et al., 1990). Its concentration in equine serum has been measured by a sensitive electroimmunoassay (Pepys et al., 1989). Among 46 healthy adult horses, 29 had no detectable serum amyloid A and 15 had a mean value of 1.2 units/L. Among 11 healthy newborn foals, only one had detectable serum amyloid A (4.1 units/L). Surgery was associated with an acute phase response in circulating serum amyloid A, with peaks at 2 to 3 days postsurgery and a decline to normal levels by 7 to 14 days. High values were found in horses with acute bacterial infections. The serum amyloid A response of cattle is similar to that of other species; its concentration increases as soon as 5 hours after an intravenous injection of endotoxin, with maximal concentration at 17 to 20 hours (Boosman et al., 1989). The mean serum amyloid A concentration in Abyssinian cats with systemic amyloidosis was significantly higher than mean values in healthy Abyssinian cats, although the ranges overlapped in both groups (DiBartola et al., 1989). Healthy Abyssinian cats had higher values than clinically healthy non-Abyssinian cats.

α_1-ACID GLYCOPROTEIN

Purified α_1-acid glycoprotein (orosomucoid; MW, 31,000 to 42,000) has a circulating half-life of about 5 days. Its sialic acid content is the highest among various acute phase proteins. Because it is an acute phase protein, its concentration increases in human and animal sera in inflammatory and neoplastic conditions and following trauma (Routledge, 1989). Elevated values are found in cattle with traumatic pericarditis, arthritis, mastitis, pneumonia, lymphoma and leukemia, hepatitis and hepatic abscesses, "downer" cow syndrome, and mesenteric liponecrosis (Motoi et al., 1992; Tamura et al., 1989). Although the finding of an increased serum concentration of this protein provides no specific diagnosis, its value seems to correlate with the extent of the disease. The mechanism of increased synthesis of this acute phase protein is unknown, but may involve increased synthesis by hepatocytes in response to cytokines (IL-1 and tumor necrosis factors) secreted by activated macrophages (see Fig. 21-5).

Determination of serum α_1-acid glycoprotein by a radial immunodiffusion method has been used for the diagnosis of hepatic abscesses in cattle. In cattle with experimentally induced hepatic abscesses from inoculation with Fusobacterium necrophorum, α_1-acid glycoprotein concentration increased in parallel with serum sialic acid content (Motoi et al., 1992). Increased serum levels were seen by 4 to 6 days postinoculation, peak values in most cases were attained by 6 to 8 days, and greater than normal values persisted for several weeks. Similar observations were made in naturally affected cattle. Serums from both groups of cattle suppressed mitogen-induced in vitro blastogenesis of bovine lymphocytes, and the suppressive effect paralleled the serum α_1-acid glycoprotein content.

Serum α_1-acid glycoprotein concentration is increased in horses with inflammatory conditions (Taira et al., 1992). Its level in pregnant mares changes in relation to the stage of pregnancy and the concentration of progesterone in blood during pregnancy.

α-FETOPROTEIN

Human α-fetoprotein (AFT) is a single-chain glycoprotein (MW, 60,000 to 70,000). It is one of the most prominent plasma proteins found in early fetal life, reaching peak concentrations at about the middle trimester. Its concentration then declines considerably by birth, so it is present only in trace amounts during neonatal life. It is synthesized by various tissues, including the yolk sac, liver, gastrointestinal tract, and placenta. Based on its structural, immunologic, and certain functional similarities to albumin, it has been suggested that α-fetoprotein during fetal life may serve functions similar to those of serum albumin in adult life. A possible role in the regulation of immune response is also proposed (Deutsch, 1991). In adult life, its concentration increases remarkably in primary carcinoma of the liver. A slight but transient increase may also occur during metastatic malignancies of the liver and inflammatory liver and gastrointestinal diseases. AFT of fetal origin is also found in the serum of healthy pregnant women, with the highest concentration being detected during the middle trimester, and increased concentrations are found when there are abnormalities of placenta and fetal development (Thomas and Blackmore, 1990).

α-Fetoprotein is present in the fetal plasma of various animal species, including the cow, horse, sheep, and pig. Two molecular variants of AFT are found in cattle. One of these, α_1-fetoprotein (MW, 68,000), has amino acid composition similar to that of other mammalian α_1-fetoproteins, and it is related immunochemically to human α_1-fetoprotein. Equine AFT (MW, 70,000 to 75,000) migrates in the α_2 region. It cross-reacts with bovine and porcine AFT. In the sheep, cow, horse, and pig, the fetal AFT concentration is highest during early to midgestation and then declines rapidly before birth, irrespective of fetal weight or maturity. α-Fetoprotein, measured by an enzymatic procedure, was more than 250 ng/ml in the serum of dogs with cholangiocarcinoma or hepatocellular carcinoma, and, in two of three dogs with primary hepatic lymphoma, the normal range was 14 to 148 ng/ml (Lowseth et al., 1991). A yearling Arabian-type filly with a metastatic erythropoietin-secreting hepatic carcinoma developed erythrocytosis (PCV, 60 to 66%), persistent hypoglycemia with a normal serum insulin level, and α-fetoproteinemia (Roby et al., 1990).

LIPOPROTEINS

The plasma lipids include glycerides, cholesterol and its esters, and phospholipids. They are transported combined with specific proteins (apolipoproteins) as micellar or macromolecular lipoproteins (LPs). It is generally accepted that LPs are spherical particles having a membrane composed of phospholipids, free cholesterol, and protein (apolipoprotein), and a "nucleus" of triglycerides and esterified cholesterol.

Lipoproteins can be separated into several classes based on their density, which mainly results from their lipid content, or electrophoretic mobility, a function of their structural protein. Four major LP classes are recognized: high-density LP, low-density LP, very low-density LP, and chylomicra. Electrophoretically, the first three separate into α-LP, β-LP, and pre-β-LP, respectively, whereas chylomicra do not migrate and remain at the origin. The electrophoretic mobilities of α-LP, β-LP, and pre-β-LP are determined by the three predominant apoproteins, apo-A, apo-B, and apo-C, respectively. High-density LPs are composed primarily of cholesterol, low-density LPs are mainly composed of cholesterol and some triglycerides, very low-density LPs are composed mostly of triglycerides and some cholesterol, and chylomicra are composed principally of triglycerides.

Lipoproteins are synthesized in the liver and/or intestine. An association between disease states and changes in the LP profile has been found in humans and acquired and genetic LP abnormalities have been described. In normal animals (horse, sheep, pig, dog), the α-LPs are found in a higher concentration than the β-LPs. Species and individual variations in LP profiles have been observed, and changes in LP and lipid profiles have been reported for developing pigs. Lipoprotein distribution is altered in dogs, rats, and humans with obstructive jaundice and cholestasis and in horses with obstructive jaundice induced by surgical ligation (Bauer et al., 1990). Dogs with acute pancreatitis may have a turbid or lipemic plasma because of hypertriglyceridemia and hypercholesterolemia. Such plasmas contain increased concentrations of low density (β) LP and decreased concentrations of high density (α) LP (Whitney et al., 1987).

Immunoglobulins

BASIC STRUCTURE

Immunoglobulins are glycoproteins comprised of 82 to 96% protein and 4 to 18% carbohydrate. The biologic properties of Ig molecules are primarily ascribed to their polypeptide structure. An Ig molecule is basically bilaterally symmetric and appears to be Y-shaped (Fig. 21–3). It is comprised of four polypeptide chains held together by covalent and disulfide bonds. Two of the chains are long (MW of each, 50,000) and are comprised of 446 amino acid residues in an identical sequence; these are called heavy chains. In comparison, the other two chains are small (MW of each, 25,000) and have identical sequences of 214 amino acid residues; these are called light chains. The entire Ig monomer is a 7S molecule (MW, 180,000).

Based on the relative variability or heterogeneity of their amino acid sequences, each light chain has a variable region, comprised of about a half-chain length toward the amino terminal and a constant region of equal length toward the carboxyl end. Similarly, each heavy chain is comprised of one variable region and

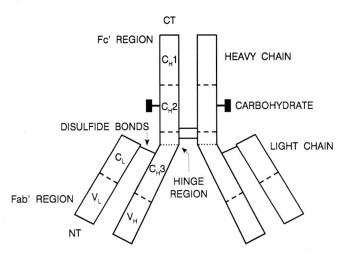

Fig. 21–3. Schematic representation of the basic structure of an IgG molecule. The molecule is composed of two heavy (H) and two light (L) chains joined by disulfide bonds. Each heavy and light chain has structurally variable (V) and constant (C) regions, or domains. Antigen-binding (Fab') sites are located in the variable regions of both the light and heavy chains toward amino terminal (NT), complement-binding (Fc') sites are located on the carboxy terminal (CT) constant regions of the heavy chains, and sites of glycosylation are located in the C$_H$2 region. The hinge region provides flexibility to the IgG molecule so it can bind to two antigens located at variable distances on the cell surface. The IgM and IgE molecules have an extra constant heavy chain domain at the CT end.

three constant regions of approximately equal lengths. Within the variable regions, certain portions have exceedingly variable amino acid sequences; these are called hypervariable regions. These various regions contribute to the structural and functional heterogeneity of Ig molecules. The hypervariable regions of the light and heavy chains, at the amino terminal ends, together carry the antigen-binding sites. Thus, the antigenic specificity of an Ig molecule is determined by innumerable amino acid sequences in the hypervariable region. Secondary functions of the Ig molecule, such as complement fixation, are the property of the terminal constant region of the heavy chains. The hinge region has a high protein content and facilitates the extension of the antigen-binding portions of the Ig molecule.

Papain, a proteolytic enzyme, splits the Ig molecule so that two Fab (antigen-binding) fragments and one Fc (crystallizable) fragment are obtained. In contrast, pepsin splits the molecule at a slightly higher location, resulting in two Fab fragments held together, the F(ab)'$_2$ fragment, and breaks down the Fc region into small peptides.

Five major classes of Igs have been identified in humans and various animal species (Tables 21–5 and 21–6). These Igs have been defined by antigenic differences in the constant region of the heavy chains. The specific heavy chains are designated as gamma (γ), mu (μ), alpha (α), delta (δ), and epsilon (ε) for the IgG, IgM, IgA, IgD, and IgE molecules, respectively. The light chains are divided into two classes, kappa (κ) and lambda (λ). An Ig molecule contains only a single type of light chain, but never both. Both types

Table 21–5.   Classes and Subclasses of Immunoglobulins in Domestic Animals and Humans

Species	IgG	IgA	IgM	IgE	IgD
Horses*	Ga, Gb, Gc, G(B), G(T)a, G(T)b	A	M	E	?
Cattle	G1, G2(G2a, G2b?), G3	A	M	E	?
Buffaloes	G1, G2, G3	A1, A2	M	?	?
Sheep	G1, G1a, G2, G3	A1, A2	M	E	?
Goats	G1, G2, G3				
Pigs†	G1, G2, G3, G4	A1, A2	M	E	D
Dogs	G1, G2a, G2b, G2c	A	M	E	?
Cats	G1, G2	A	M	E	?
Chickens	G1, (G2, G3)?	A	M	?	D
Humans	G1, G2, G3, G4	A1, A2	M	E	D

Modified from Tizard, I.: Veterinary Immunology. An Introduction. 3rd Ed. Philadelphia, W.B. Saunders, 1987, p. 44.

* A γ-10S molecule and two immunoglobulins of fast mobility have been reported.

† γ-18S molecule and a 4S "half" Ig molecule have also been reported.

are found in the same individual, but their ratio may vary among species (e.g., 2:1 in humans). Antigenic determinants (differences) of the heavy and light chains are responsible for the isotypes of Igs found in all animals of the same species. Similarly, antigenic determinants of the constant region of the polypeptide chains form the basis of the Ig allotypes found in some individuals of the same species, whereas antigenic determinants of the variable regions (antigen-combining sites) form the basis of the Ig idiotypes found in an individual animal.

CLASSES

The various classes of Igs are characterized according to their physicochemical, electrophoretic, immunochemical, and functional properties. Current and more detailed information about various Igs can be found in recent immunology texts.

IgG. IgG is the major Ig of blood in the adult of various species. It is responsible for most of the humoral immunity of the organism. The IgG is a 7S molecule (MW, 180,000), with electrophoretic mobility

in the γ region and a biologic half-life of approximately 20 days. It is found in various body fluids in minute quantities in health and in larger amounts during inflammatory conditions. It is the only Ig that can cross the placenta and is found in fetal serum in humans and certain animals (dog, cat, and rodents). It is the primary Ig in colostrum and is responsible for natural passive immunity in the neonatal calf, foal, lamb, kid, and piglet.

IgG molecules have several biologic activities, including opsonization, agglutination, precipitation, and complement fixation. They contain most of the antibacterial, antiviral, and antitoxic antibodies. Neutrophils and macrophages have receptors to bind the Fc region of the IgG molecule. Effective complement fixation requires the binding of IgG molecules to specific antigens in close proximity to form dimers, and it has become apparent that certain subclasses of IgG either do not fix complement or are less efficient in this regard. Various subclasses of IgG have been recognized on the basis of serologic and physicochemical differences in the constant region of the light chain, and they also differ in biologic activities.

IgM. IgM is a 19S molecule (MW, 900,000) with electrophoretic mobility in the β to fast γ regions, and a biologic half-life of about 5 days. It typically exists as a pentamer composed of five 7S subunits, similar to IgG. The heavy chain ends of the subunits are interconnected by disulfide bonds and a glycopeptide J chain unites two of the subunits to complete a circular structure. The J chains (MW, 15,000) are synthesized by the plasma cells. An intact IgM molecule is elaborated by the plasma cells. It is found in fetal and precolostral foal serum.

IgM is the second major Ig of serum, and remains confined primarily to the vascular system because of its molecular size. It is usually the first Ig to increase in concentration in serum during the primary immune response. It also increases during the secondary immune response, but its concentration is usually exceeded by that of the IgG synthesized during this phase of the immune response.

Various biologic activities of IgM are similar to those of IgG. As a pentamer, though, it has 10 binding sites

Table 21–6.   Serum Immunoglobulin Levels (mg/dl) in Domestic Animals and Humans*

Species	IgG	IgM	IgA	IgG(T)	IgG(B)	IgE
Horse	1000–1500	100–200	60–350	100–1500	10–1000	—
Bovine†	1700–2700	250–400	10–50	—	—	<50‡
Buffaloes	2331	253	—	—	—	—
Sheep	1700–2000	150–250	10–50	—	—	—
Pigs	1700–2900	100–500	50–500	—	—	—
Dogs	1000–2000	70–270	20–150	—	—	2.3–42
Chickens	300–700	120–250	30–60	—	—	—
Humans	800–1600	50–200	150–400	—	—	0.002–0.05

* All data, except bovine IgE, and buffalo Igs, from Tizard, I.: Veterinary Immunology. An Introduction. 3rd Ed. Philadelphia, W.B. Saunders, 1987, p. 41.

† Cattle show very significant seasonal differences in serum Ig levels.

‡ 6-months-old, parasite-free calves, <50 U/ml; adult daily cattle, <40 U/ml.

and is functionally more efficient—one molecule of IgM can fix complement. Some noncomplement-fixing IgM, however, has been found in humans under certain conditions.

IgM molecules contain "natural" antibodies for gram-negative bacteria, blood group isoantibodies, rheumatoid factors, and antinuclear and other antibodies. They are of minor importance in toxin neutralization. IgM monomers (7S) have been found on antigen-responsive B and T lymphocytes, where they are thought to regulate the immune response. Secretory IgM with bound secretory component has been found in body secretions. It may play a compensatory role in disorders associated with IgA deficiency, because increased synthesis of secretory IgM has been found in such conditions.

IgA. IgA forms a minor component of the serum, but is a major component of various external secretions (tears, saliva, and respiratory and gastrointestinal secretions) in most species. It exhibits electrophoretic mobility in the β to fast γ regions and has a biologic half-life of 6 days. The IgA monomer is a 7S molecule (MW, 160,000), but tends to polymerize to form 11S dimers, 13S trimers, and higher polymers.

The dimeric form, interconnected by a J chain, predominates in the sera of most animal species in contrast to the monomeric form, which constitutes about 90% of human serum IgA. Secretory IgA is an 11S molecule (MW, 400,000) composed of two monomers, a J chain, and a secretory component. The secretory component (MW, 70,000) is synthesized by intestinal epithelial cells near the mucous membranes and also by the hepatocytes. It enables the IgA molecules elaborated locally in the intestinal lymphoid tissue to be transported across the mucosa into the gut. It also renders the IgA molecule resistant to proteolysis by digestive enzymes. The hepatic secretory component allows the secretion of serum IgA into the bile. The secretory component is not essential for the transport of IgA into the circulation. The secretory component may be found free and also bound to IgM, but not to IgG and IgE, in body secretions.

IgA is important in local defense because it protects various body surfaces (e.g., the intestinal, respiratory, and urogenital tracts, the mammary gland, and the eye) from bacterial and viral invasion. It prevents bacterial adherence by binding to glycoproteins essential for colonization. IgA has virus neutralization and agglutinating activities, can fix complement (only by the alternate pathway), has no or limited opsonic activity, and is not bactericidal. Specific IgA antibodies present in colostrum provide passive immunity to the newborn against neonatal bacterial and viral infections.

IgD. IgD is a 7 to 8S molecule (MW, 180,000) with electrophoretic mobility in the fast γ region, and a biologic half-life of 2.8 days. It is found in trace amounts in human serum and on about 15% of B lymphocytes. It is found in chickens and pigs but has not been detected in other species. Its function is unknown, although it has been shown to have some antibody activity and is thought to be involved in the differentiation of B lymphocytes.

IgE. IgE is an 8S molecule (MW, 190,000) with electrophoretic mobility in the fast γ region, and a biologic half-life of 1 to 5 days. IgE occurs in extremely low concentration in serum, so it is difficult to detect. Its concentration in nasopharyngeal secretions, however, is higher than in the serum. Increasing amounts of IgE are produced in response to many parasitic infestations and allergens (antigens stimulating the production of IgE). Most cattle infested with gastrointestinal nematodes and cestodes have total serum IgE concentrations higher than those of normal controls. Passive transfer of maternal IgE through colostrum consumption occurs in bovine calves and may provide an early protection against parasitic infections (Thatcher and Gershwin, 1989).

IgE mediates the type I hypersensitivity reaction (allergies and anaphylaxis) and is referred to as a reagin or reaginic antibody. It is a noncomplement-fixing antibody, but its Fc region uniquely binds to mast cells and basophils (i.e., it is homocytotropic), and it triggers an immediate degranulation of these cells after combining with specific antigens. The IgE is also unique in that it is destroyed when serum is heated at 56°C for 30 minutes.

β₂-*Microglobulin.* β₂-Microglobulin is a polypeptide (MW, 118,000) found free in serum and in body fluids such as milk, colostrum, and urine. It is bound to the surface membrane of many cells in several species. Its molecular structure is related to both immune and histocompatibility antigen systems. In part, it resembles IgG. Thus, it can fix complement and bind to Fc receptors on cells of the mononuclear phagocyte system. The amount of β₂-microglobulin in body fluids is several times greater than that in normal serum, and its concentration may increase in disease.

SPECIES DIFFERENCES

All animals contain species-specific IgG, IgM, and IgA, whereas IgE has so far been identified in some species and IgD in the chicken only. Species differences (Table 21–5) have been found in the number and types of subclasses of various Igs. In general, Ig concentrations in serum (Table 21–6) and body fluids vary with the species and age. Newborn animals differ from adults in that they are hypogammaglobulinemic.

Species differences have also been noted with regard to biologic activities and body distribution of some Igs. For example, equine IgG(T) does not fix complement and is found in body secretions in high concentrations. Its half-life is about 20 days in the newborn foal, which is similar to that of IgG. Bovine IgG₁ constitutes about half of serum IgG and is the major secretory Ig in milk. It migrates faster than IgG₂ toward the anode in agar gel electrophoresis. Biologic activities of bovine IgG₁ and IgG₂ are essentially similar, but the former does not promote phagocytosis by monocytes and neutrophils and the latter does not fix complement.

Cattle have genetically high or low serum concentrations of IgG_2. Breed differences exist in Ig concentrations of newborn lambs and horses.

Because of the selective transfer of Igs from the circulation into the mammary glands, the colostrum of all the major domestic animals contains higher amounts of Igs than milk, and it is particularly rich in IgG. In comparison, milk predominantly contains IgG (specifically IgG_1) in ruminants and IgA in humans, primates, and some nonruminant domestic animals. In cats, IgG predominates in the serum, colostrum, and milk, and IgA forms a major component in other body secretions.

Laboratory Determination

Plasma or serum protein concentrations can be determined by various methods. The total plasma protein concentration in a diagnostic laboratory can be determined by the biuret, Lowery, refractometric, and other calorimetric methods. The concentrations of individual proteins can be determined by electrophoretic and immunochemical procedures. Specific techniques are also available to determine the concentrations of particular plasma or serum proteins (e.g., albumin, transferrin, ceruloplasmin, haptoglobin).

TOTAL PLASMA PROTEIN CONCENTRATION

The biuret method requires a larger volume of serum or plasma than the Lowery method, and is relatively less sensitive. The refractometric method is perhaps the most practical, because only one drop of sample is required, and a determination can be made in seconds. Although it is the least sensitive method, measuring 100 mg/dl of proteins or more, the refractometric method provides satisfactory results for routine diagnostic work.

A rough estimate of the globulin content of serum can be obtained by salt precipitation. Depending on the animal species, a certain amount of sodium, ammonium, or zinc sulfate is added to serum. This precipitates globulins, but not albumin. The amount of globulins can then be estimated calorimetrically using a suitable standard. This procedure has been refined to estimate Ig concentration in the sera of newborn calves, foals, and lambs to detect immunoglobulins. A simple glutaraldehyde coagulation test has been used as a screening test to detect hypogammaglobulinemia in foals (Clabough et al., 1989).

PROTEIN ELECTROPHORESIS

At an alkaline pH (usually 8.6), serum proteins have a net negative charge; hence, they migrate from the cathode to anode in an electric field. Because the charge density of individual proteins varies, they can be separated from each other using the technique of electrophoresis. The most common method in clinical medicine is zone electrophoresis, in which the serum is placed on a supporting medium such as cellulose acetate, agarose, starch, or polyacrylamide gel.

Cellulose acetate electrophoresis is simple, accurate, and commonly used, but agarose electrophoresis is claimed to provide better resolution and yields more fractions. After electrophoretic separation, the proteins are treated with specific stains. One can also stain selectively for glycoproteins and lipoproteins. After rinsing and destaining, the proteins appear as bands (zones) representative of albumin and the various globulins (Fig. 21–4). Except for albumin, the bands are comprised of a group of individual proteins (see Table 21–1). The proteins are quantitated by a recording and integrating spectrophotometer (Fig. 21–1).

Albumin, because it is strongly electronegative, migrates farthest toward the anode, whereas globulins, which are weakly electronegative, move in succession as α, β, and γ globulins. The value for each component is calculated as a percentage of the total. This is converted to an absolute amount after determination of the total serum protein concentration by a standard method. The mobility of the albumin and globulin fractions varies among species, particularly in zoo animals (Fig. 21–4A to D).

Immunochemical methods are highly specific and sensitive, but require monospecific reagents (antibodies) for each of the proteins to be detected for the species concerned. Immunoelectrophoresis, which is gel electrophoresis followed by immunodiffusion, is a simple procedure for demonstrating the presence of plasma proteins, particularly Igs, but it is not a quantitative procedure. The single radial immunodiffusion technique (Mancini's method) is a simple and sensitive procedure for quantitating proteins, particularly Igs, and the results are available within 24 to 72 hours. Rocket immunoelectrophoresis (electroimmunodiffusion) is another simple and rapid quantitative proce-

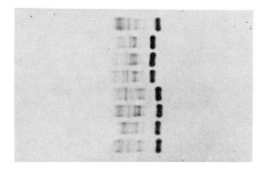

Fig. 21–4. Cellulose acetate strip on which eight serum samples have been applied, separated by electrophoresis, and stained for protein. These particular samples are from animals from the Los Angeles zoo. Migration is from left to right. (*Top to bottom*: African lion, white-handed gibbon, another white-handed gibbon, gorilla, cheetah, jaguar, leopard, and domestic cat). Note the faster migration of the albumin band (dark band on the extreme right) of the Felidae. Note also the heterogeneity with regard to the concentration and relative mobility of the various globulins. (For additional information see Carroll, E.J., Sedgwick, C.J., and Schalm, O.W.: Hematology of Zoo Animals. II. Serum Proteins. Am. J. Vet. Clin. Pathol., *1:115*, 1967.)

dure; it is as or more accurate than the radial immunodiffusion method. Radioimmunoassay and the enzyme-linked immunosorbent assay (ELISA) are sensitive tests for detecting minute quantities of various proteins.

DYSPROTEINEMIAS

The term "dysproteinemia" literally means a derangement of the protein content of the blood. It includes an abnormality of the total protein content and that of individual proteins. An appreciation of the derangement requires a determination of the total plasma or serum protein concentration, plasma fibrinogen concentration, serum protein electrophoresis, and the A:G ratio. A classification of dysproteinemias based on the A:G ratio and serum protein electrophoretic profile is given in Table 21–7 (Kaneko, 1989).

Hypoproteinemia is a reduction in the plasma protein concentration below the minimum level that is normal for the species. The converse is hyperproteinemia. The relative concentration of individual proteins may, however, change without an alteration in the total amount (normoproteinemia). A rise in globulin levels is generally accompanied by a concomitant drop in albumin concentration. The exact mechanism whereby this occurs has not been satisfactorily explained. An absolute rise in the albumin level is rarely, if ever, seen.

Before it can be determined whether a given animal is hyperproteinemic or hypoproteinemic, several factors must be considered. The age of the animal is of particular importance. The total plasma protein concentration is low in the newborn of most species, usually less than 5 g/dl. Colostrum consumption causes a temporary elevation (Figs. 21–1 and 21–2). Thereafter, the total plasma protein level increases gradually and is within the normal range of 6.0 to 8.0 g/dl by 6 months to 1 year of age in most species. The total protein level is toward the high end of normal in older animals as a result of increased Ig synthesis because of exposure to varied antigens over the years. Thus, an older animal with a total plasma protein level of approximately 6.5 g/dl or less should be classed as hypoproteinemic. In lactating cows, a concentration of 8.0 to 8.5 g/dl is not uncommon, especially in the summer.

The state of hydration of an animal is also an important consideration. It is imperative that the plasma protein concentration be considered along with the hematocrit. If a hyperproteinemia with a normal A:G ratio and a significantly elevated PCV are present, the high protein concentration is probably a consequence of dehydration. An increase in total plasma protein concentration, however, appears to be a better indicator of hydration status than an increase in PCV (Genetzky et al., 1987; Hardy and Osborne, 1979), possibly because the spleen normally sequesters a portion of the intravascular red cell mass. When the PCV is significantly elevated and the total plasma

Table 21–7. Classification of the Dysproteinemias Based on the Albumin-to-Globulin (A:G) Ratio and the Serum Protein Electrophoretic (SPE) Profile

Normal A:G—normal SPE profile
  Hyperproteinemia: dehydration
  Hypoproteinemia
    Overhydration
    Acute blood loss
    External plasma loss: extravasation from burns, abrasions, exudative lesions, exudative dermatopathies, external parasites; gastrointestinal disease, diarrhea
    Internal plasma loss: gastrointestinal disease, internal parasites
Decreased A:G—abnormal SPE profile
  Decreased albumin
    Selective loss of albumin: glomerulonephritis, nephrotic syndrome, gastrointestinal disease, internal parasites
    Decreased synthesis of albumin: chronic liver disease, malnutrition, chronic inflammatory disease
  Increased globulins
    Increased α_1-globulin
      Acute inflammatory disease: α_1-antitrypsin, α_1-acid glycoprotein (orosomucoid, seromucoid)
    Increased α_2-globulin
      Acute inflammatory disease: α_2-macroglobulin, ceruloplasmin, haptoglobin
      Severe active hepatitis: α_2-macroglobulin
      Acute nephritis: α_2-macroglobulin
      Nephrotic syndrome: α_2-macroglobulin, α_2-lipoprotein (VLDL)
    Increased β-globulin
      Acute hepatitis: transferrin, hemopexin
      Nephrotic syndrome: β_2-lipoprotein (LDL), transferrin
      Suppurative dermatopathies: IgM, C3
    β–γ Bridging
      Chronic active hepatitis: IgA, IgM
    Increased γ-globulin (broad increases)—polyclonal gammopathies: IgG, IgM, IgA
      Chronic inflammatory disease, infectious disease, collagen disease
      Chronic hepatitis
      Hepatic abscess
      Suppurative disease: feline infectious dermatitis, suppurative dermatitis, tuberculosis
      Immune-mediated disease: autoimmune hemolytic anemia, autoimmune thrombocytopenia, Aleutian disease of mink, equine infectious anemia, systemic lupus erythematosus, autoimmune polyarthritis, autoimmune glomerulonephritis, autoimmune dermatitis, allergies
      Tumors of the reticuloendothelial system (RES): lymphoma
    Increased γ-globulin (sharp increases)—monoclonal gammopathies: IgG, IgM, IgA
      Tumors of the reticuloendothelial system (RES): lymphoma
      Plasma cell dyscrasia: multiple myeloma, Aleutian disease of mink
      Macroglobulinemia
      Canine ehrlichiosis
      Benign
Increased A:G—abnormal profile
  Increased albumin: does not occur except in dehydration
  Decreased globulins
    Fetal serum
    Precolostral neonate
    Combined immunodeficiency of Arabian foals
    Aglobulinemia

From Kaneko, J.J. (ed.): Clinical Biochemistry of Domestic Animals. 4th Ed. San Diego, Academic Press, 1989, p. 158.

protein level remains within the normal range, splenic contraction is strongly indicated. In contrast, hypoproteinemia with a normal A:G ratio and a significantly diminished PCV is a consequence of either fluid therapy or acute blood loss. Hypoproteinemia from fluid loss only could have normal to elevated PCV values, depending on the degree of fluid loss.

Changes in Plasma Protein Levels

ALBUMIN

Albumin constitutes about 35 to 50% of the total serum protein in various animals, in contrast to 60 to 67% in humans and nonhuman primates. Hypoalbuminemia is more common than hyperalbuminemia. Hypoalbuminemia may be a result of decreased synthesis, increased loss (through the intestine, urine, or skin), increased catabolism, or pathologic distribution in body spaces (Table 21–7). The most common cause of hypoalbuminemia in horses include parasite infestation, chronic infection and inflammation, and neoplasia. About 50% of equine patients with hypoalbuminemia have normal plasma protein concentrations (Pearson, 1990). Similar causes may be associated with hypoalbuminemia in other species. Hyperalbuminemia is usually a result of hemoconcentration because a true elevation in the serum albumin level from increased synthesis does not occur.

A marked correlation has been found between hypoalbuminemia (<3.0 g/dl) and the incidence of morbidity and mortality in hospitalized human patients (Doweiko and Nompleggi, 1991; Pleban, 1989). This may be because of various pathophysiologic roles ascribed to albumin. Hypoalbuminemia may delay wound healing, interfere with the normal functioning of the gastrointestinal tract, and adversely affect the coagulation system.

FIBRINOGEN

Plasma fibrinogen concentrations are not appreciably affected by age, sex, exercise, repeated bleeding, or hemorrhage, but they can be altered by only moderately inflammatory states. Fibrinogen behaves as an acute phase protein in most species, including birds. Therefore, its plasma concentration usually increases in inflammatory, suppurative, traumatic, and neoplastic conditions. This is because of increased synthesis by hepatocytes, probably the result of stimulation by IL-1, IL-6, and tumor necrosis factors (Fig. 21–5). Inflammatory stimuli are believed to induce the activation of the mononuclear phagocyte system, leading to an increased elaboration of these factors. Increase in fibrinogen level in inflammatory and suppurative disease is, however, not always in direct relationship to the severity of the disease process. The fibrinogen concentration is also elevated in moderate liver damage, but severe liver damage causes a decrease in association with hypoproteinemia resulting from reduced hepatic protein synthesis. In disseminated intravascular coagulation and fibrinolysis, the fibrinogen

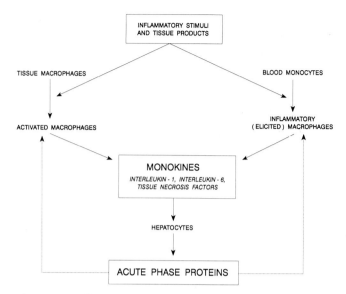

Fig. 21–5. Cellular and molecular mechanisms involved in the synthesis of acute phase proteins. Negative feedback regulation of acute phase protein synthesis is also shown (broken line).

concentration declines because of increased consumption and catabolism, respectively. This may occur whenever intravascular activation of procoagulants or a release of thromboplastin into the circulation occurs. Congenital afibrinogenemia, hypofibrinogenemia, and functionally defective fibrinogen (dysfibrinogenemia) are rare conditions in humans.

The plasma protein:fibrinogen ratio (PP:F) is useful in distinguishing hyperfibrinogenemia caused by disease from that associated with dehydration (Jain, 1986). This is because hemoconcentration produces a relative increase in all components of plasma proteins, including fibrinogen, whereas the increased synthesis of fibrinogen is usually unaccompanied by elevations in other plasma protein levels. The PP:F ratio is obtained by subtracting the fibrinogen concentration [Fib] from the total plasma protein concentration [TPP] and then dividing the remainder by the concentration of fibrinogen:

$$PP:F = \frac{[TPP] - [Fib]}{[Fib]}$$

Normal values for fibrinogen and the PP:F ratios for some species are given in Table 21–8. Generally, a PP:F ratio lower than 15:1 indicates a relative increase in the fibrinogen over the plasma protein level. A ratio below 10:1 indicates a marked increase in the fibrinogen level. The ratio rises steadily with age because of increasing concentrations of plasma proteins, whereas fibrinogen concentrations remain relatively constant. Hemoconcentration alone would not significantly alter the normal PP:F ratio.

Hyperfibrinogenemia is a better indicator of inflammatory disease in cattle than neutrophilia, because it is encountered more frequently. Similarly, a greater proportion of horses with an intra-abdominal abscess show hyperfibrinogenemia and neutrophilia than horses with intra-abdominal neoplasms (Zicker et al.,

Table 21-8. **Total Plasma Protein and Fibrinogen Concentrations in Normal Dogs, Calves, Cows, Foals, and Horses**

Animal	Number	Age	Plasma Proteins (g/dl)		Fibrinogen (g/dl)		Protein:Fibrinogen Ratio	
			Range	Mean	Range	Mean	Range	Mean
Dog	11	8 wk	5.0–6.5	5.7	0.1–0.3	0.2	19–50:1	27.5:1
	11	10–12 wk	5.5–6.5	6.2	0.2–0.4	0.23	15–31:1	29.8:1
	9	4–6 mo	6.3–7.0	6.7	0.1–0.3	0.22	20–68:1	30.5:1
	9	1–1½ yr	6.5–7.7	7.1	0.1–0.4	0.23	17–66:1	34.5:1
	9	2–3½ yr	6.9–7.8	7.5	0.1–0.3	0.2	25–74:1	36.4:1
Cattle								
Calf	16*	Newborn	4.0–5.3	4.7	0–0.4	0.19	10–52:1	19.0:1
	5	2–7 days	4.7–5.3	4.9	0.2–0.4	0.3	12–30:1	15.3:1
Cow	6†	Mature	6.8–8.0	7.3	0.2–0.6	0.4	10–37:1	18.2:1
Horse								
Thoroughbred	12	1 day	5.1–6.8	5.7	0.2–0.4	0.27	17–30:1	22.9:1
Foal	12	1 wk	5.4–6.9	6.2	0.3–0.5	0.37	12–22:1	17.5:1
	10‡	1 mo	5.5–7.0	6.9	0.3–0.5	0.43	10–20:1	13.9:1
	4‡	2 mo	6.2–6.8	6.5	0.5	0.5	11–13:1	12.1:1
Thoroughbred	7	1½–7 yr	6.8–7.8	7.2	0.2–0.4	0.27	18–34:1	26.7:1
Quarter horse	5	2–7 yr	6.6–7.1	6.8	0.2–0.3	0.22	21–34:1	31.8:1
Appaloosa	1	3 yr	7.2	—	0.2	—	35:1	—

Modified from Schalm, O.W., Smith, R., Kaneko, J.J., et al.: Plasma protein:Fibrinogen ratios in dogs, cattle, and horse. Part I. Influence of age on normal values and explanation of use in disease. Cal. Vet., 24:9, Feb., 1970.
* Newborn calves were colostrum-deprived and mostly taken by cesarean section at term.
† 37 separate determinations on the six cows.
‡ A number of the original 12 foals developed a mild respiratory disease with increases of fibrinogen to between 0.60 and 0.8 g/dl.

1990). Lymphopenia and normocytic normochromic anemia are more common in horses with neoplasms than in horses with abscesses.

Studies of the plasma fibrinogen concentration and neutrophil counts in blood from many nondomestic mammals have indicated that the fibrinogen level is more often abnormal than the neutrophil count in Perissodactyla, Artiodactyla, and Proboscidea. The two tests provided positive confirmation of infection in a greater percentage of samples than did the results of either test alone (Hawkey and Hart, 1987). Thus, fibrinogen estimation is also a valuable hematologic screening procedure in nondomestic mammals.

α- AND β-GLOBULINS

A decrease in albumin and an increase in α-globulin are often noted. Because it is an acute phase protein, α-globulin is increased in acute inflammatory conditions, nephrotic syndrome, fractures, infections, and certain tumors (Jain, 1986). A selective, 2-fold increase in α_2-globulin was observed in dogs given cortisone or cortisone and cholesterol, and the increase was attributed to the lipoprotein component.

Increases in serum α_2 and β-globulins have been reported in dogs with various neoplasms (Jain, 1986). Elevated concentrations of α_2-globulins with normoproteinemia have been reported in dogs with mastocytoma. The increased protein was a glycoprotein, and a direct correlation between the concentration of the glycoprotein and the extent of tumor development was found. Dogs with lymphoma may have increased concentrations of IgM. A moderate increase in the α_2-globulin level may occur in leukemic cattle, and IgM production is often significantly impaired, although an increase may sometimes be seen, particularly in

animals with a high number of lymphocytes. Cows with lymphoma may have lower serum albumin and variable globulin concentrations.

Increases in β-globulins have been observed in active liver disease, suppurative dermatologic conditions, and occasionally in nephrotic syndrome. Polyclonal gammopathy may involve increases of IgM.

An increase in both γ- and β_2-globulins, leading to what has been termed "β-γ bridging," is considered almost pathognomic for chronic active hepatitis and is occasionally seen in lymphoma (Kaneko, 1989). It results from an increase in the level of IgA, IgM, or both.

γ-GLOBULINS

Hypogammaglobulinemia is natural during fetal life and in the newborn. Low Ig concentrations are found in postcolostral serum and during the first few months of life. Animals with immune deficiency disorders are particularly hypogammaglobulinemic. Calves with a total plasma protein concentration of less than 6.0 g/dl before weaning have a higher frequency of disease. Also, calves with a low serum IgG level (1267 mg/dl) have higher morbidity, requiring early and frequent treatments, when compared to calves with a high IgG concentration (2698 mg/dl). Decreased γ-globulin concentrations in the adult animal may be physiologic (as before parturition in the cow) or pathologic (as in immunodeficiencies of various types).

Hypergammaglobulinemia is discussed below (gammopathies). A simple test for hypergammaglobulinemia in cattle is as follows:

1. Mix 2.5 ml of a 1.2% glutaraldehyde solution with 1 mg/ml of Na_2EDTA and an equal quantity of fresh blood, directly from the vein.

Table 21–9. Plasma Cell Dyscrasias

Primary monoclonal gammopathies
  Myeloma
  Waldenström's macroglobulinemia
  Solitary plasma cell tumor or plasmacytoma
  Heavy chain disease
  Light chain disease
  Lymphoma
  Chronic lymphocytic leukemia
Secondary monoclonal gammopathies
  Nonlymphoid malignancies
  Monocytic leukemias
  Hepatobiliary diseases
  Rheumatoid diseases
  Chronic inflammation
Benign monoclonal gammopathy
  Transient
  Persistent

Modifed from Stites, D.P., Stobo, J.D., Fudenberg, H.H., et al.: Basic and Clinical Immunology. 5th Ed. Los Altos, Cal., Lang Medical Publications, 1984, p. 454.

2. After 15 minutes at room temperature, the blood with hypergammaglobulinemia coagulates, whereas normal blood flows on tilting the tube.

One serious disadvantage of the test is that gelling times of blood can vary with the glutaraldehyde solution used (Mahin et al., 1985).

Gammopathies

Gammopathies are a heterogeneous group of diseases characterized by the presence of highly elevated concentrations of Igs in the blood. The gammopathies are classified as monoclonal or polyclonal on the basis of the relative spreading of the γ-globulin zone on electrophoresis. An abnormally elevated, heterogeneous, broad-based sawtooth pattern indicates a polyclonal gammopathy, whereas a sharp, narrow-based, church spire pattern indicates a monoclonal gammopathy. Polyclonal gammopathies are generally characteristic of benign plasma cell proliferation in response to a persistent antigenic stimulation. Polyclonal gammopathies are seen in chronic infections, chronic inflammatory diseases, immune-mediated diseases, and occasionally in lymphoma. In contrast, monoclonal gammopathies are usually found in association with various plasma cell and lymphocytic neoplasms, and sometimes in other plasma cell dyscrasias (Table 21–9). Monoclonal gammopathies are seen in about 5% of dogs with lymphoproliferative disorders. Clinicopathologic manifestations of monoclonal gammopathy vary with the degree of plasma cell proliferation, tissue infiltration, and paraproteinemia.

A monoclonal gammopathy results from a malignant or "benign" proliferation of a single clone of lymphoid cells that characteristically secrete massive amounts of a single protein. Gammopathies involving the malignant proliferation of more than one clone of cells have been reported in humans, but are extremely rare.

The terms "paraprotein" and "paraproteinemia" were coined to indicate the presence of foreign proteins in patients with various plasma cell dyscrasias. The protein has also been called myeloma protein, M protein, or M component. Chemical analysis of the abnormally increased protein has revealed that the molecules are structurally homogeneous and similar to normal γ-globulin. Although the conditions are called gammopathies, it must be emphasized that the increased globulin may migrate in the β zone or even in the slow α zone on electrophoresis (Figs. 21–6, 21–7 and 21–8). Electrophoretically, IgG migrates in the

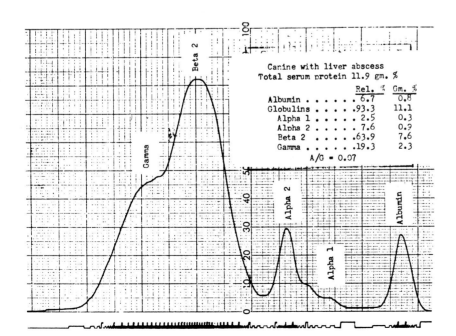

Canine with liver abscess
Total serum protein 11.9 gm. %

	Rel. %	Gm. %
Albumin	6.7	0.8
Globulins	93.3	11.1
Alpha 1	2.5	0.3
Alpha 2	7.6	0.9
Beta 2	63.9	7.6
Gamma	19.3	2.3

A/G = 0.07

Fig. 21–6. Electrophoretic tracing of serum of a dog with a liver abscess showing a polyclonal gammopathy. (From Jain, N.C.: Schalm's Veterinary Hematology. 4th Ed. Philadelphia, Lea & Febiger, 1986, p. 965.)

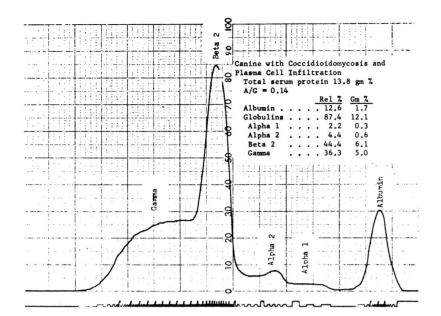

Canine with Coccidioidomycosis and
Plasma Cell Infiltration
Total serum protein 13.8 gm %
A/G = 0.14

	Rel %	Gm %
Albumin	12.6	1.7
Globulins	87.4	12.1
Alpha 1	2.2	0.3
Alpha 2	4.4	0.6
Beta 2	44.4	6.1
Gamma	36.3	5.0

Fig. 21–7. Electrophoretic tracing of serum of a dog with coccidioidomycosis and plasma cell infiltration of internal organs, leading to a diagnosis of myelomatosis. (From Jain, N.C.: Schalm's Veterinary Hematology. 4th Ed. Philadelphia, Lea & Febiger, 1986, p. 966.)

γ region, IgA in the β region, IgM in the β to fast γ regions, and IgD and IgE in the fast γ region. Serum protein abnormalities in gammopathies may also include excessive amounts of free κ or λ chains or fragments of heavy chains that may not be recognized on electrophoresis. Paraproteinemias have been described in the dog, cat, and horse.

The laboratory investigation of a patient suspected to have a monoclonal gammopathy should include hematologic examination of blood and bone marrow aspirates, bone marrow biopsy, serum chemistries, hemostatic profile, serum viscosity measurement, radiographic examination, urinalysis, and immunologic tests. Serum protein electrophoresis should be fol-

lowed by immunoelectrophoresis to identify the abnormal Ig and then by single radial immunodiffusion to quantitate various Igs. Serum should be separated at 37°C to avoid the cryoprecipitation of certain Igs. In rare cases of nonsecretory myeloma, serum protein analyses may be nondiagnostic. In such cases, bone marrow smears should be examined by immunofluorescence to define the intracellular location of the monoclonal Ig. Plasma cell infiltration of the bone marrow is focal in various plasma cell dyscrasias, so a random marrow aspirate may appear nondiagnostic.

Bence Jones proteins may be found in the urine in plasma cell myeloma, but not in Waldenström's macroglobulinemia. Bence Jones proteins consist of mon-

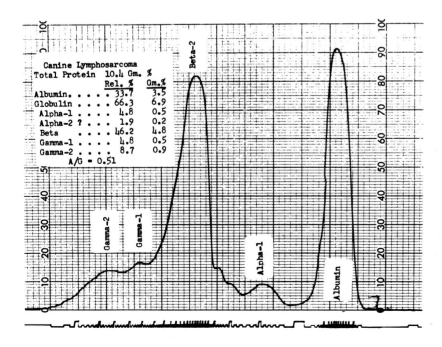

Canine Lymphosarcoma
Total Protein 10.4 Gm. %

	Rel. %	Gm.%
Albumin	33.7	3.5
Globulin	66.3	6.9
Alpha-1	4.8	0.5
Alpha-2 ?	1.9	0.2
Beta	46.2	4.8
Gamma-1	4.8	0.5
Gamma-2	8.7	0.9
A/G = 0.51		

Fig. 21–8. Electrophoretic tracing of serum from a dog with lymphoma. (From Jain, N.C.: Schalm's Veterinary Hematology. 4th Ed. Philadelphia, Lea & Febiger, 1986, p. 966.)

oclonal κ or λ light chains. Although Bence Jones proteins in urine can be demonstrated by heat precipitation (precipitating when heated to 50 to 60°C at pH 4.5 to 5.0, and redissolving at 90 to 100°C), they are best demonstrated by electrophoretic techniques. The urine sample often needs to be concentrated before analysis. Bence Jones proteins are present in the urine of 55 to 80% of human patients, in less than 10% of canine patients, and in some cats with myeloma.

MULTIPLE MYELOMA

In humans, multiple myeloma is characterized by increased concentrations of a monoclonal protein in the serum (or urine) associated with increased numbers (15 to 20% or more) of plasma cells in the bone marrow and typical lytic bone lesions. The paraprotein is usually IgG, and in some cases IgA or only light chains, and rarely IgD.

Multiple myelomas involving IgG or IgA have been described in the dog, cat, and horse (Geisel et al., 1990; Hawkins et al., 1986; Jain, 1986; Kirschner et al., 1988; MacAllister et al., 1987; Matus et al., 1986). Multiple myeloma in 60 dogs was confirmed by detecting a monoclonal gammopathy of IgG or IgA and finding greater than 5% plasma cells in bone marrow aspirates from each case (Matus et al., 1986). Multiple myeloma was detected as early as 3 months of age in a foal (Henry et al., 1989) and an α chain (IgA) myeloma that responded to prednisolone therapy was described is a dog (Hoenig, 1987). Although marked increases in monoclonal γ-globulin concentrations and plasma cells in bone marrow were apparent in these cases, Bence Jones proteinuria was found only in some animals. Extramedullary plasmocytomas are rare in animals. Extramedullary plasmocytoma in a cat was associated with a monoclonal gammopathy in the gamma region and a systemic AL (amyloid light chain) amyloidosis (Carothers et al., 1989). Multiple myeloma usually develops from the neoplastic clonal proliferation of plasma cells in the bone marrow. In rare instances, the tumor may arise at extramedullary sites as solitary plasmocytoma and may later metastasize.

Many other laboratory and clinical abnormalities may be found in multiple myeloma. The concentration of Igs other than paraprotein generally decreases because of a diminished immune response. Anemia (nonresponsive), azotemia, and hypercalcemia are common. Thrombocytopenia and hemostatic defects may be found. Leukopenia caused by neutropenia may be encountered. The erythrocyte sedimentation rate is generally elevated. Splenomegaly and hepatomegaly may be present. Abnormalities of plasma cell morphology may be evident in the bone marrow. Plasma cells with distinct nucleoli, excessive cytoplasm, or multiple nuclei may be evident in clusters or singly. Flame cells—plasma cells with reddish cytoplasmic staining at the periphery (Plates XIII–7, XIII–8, and XIII–9)—and "thesaurocytes" (storage cells) may occur in IgA myeloma. Plasma cell leukemia in multiple myeloma is extremely rare and probably indicates a terminal event.

Various pathologic changes occur in patients with multiple myeloma. Frequent complications include recurrent infections from a diminished immune response and impaired phagocytic activity. Acute or chronic renal failure occurs primarily from the excretion of myeloma proteins. Lameness, bone pain, and pathologic fractures from bone marrow infiltration by malignant plasma cells and osteolysis can occur. Hypercalcemia results from the release of an osteoblast-activating factor secreted by tumor cells. Spinal cord compression and peripheral neuropathy may develop as a result of plasma cell infiltration. Hyperviscosity syndrome may be seen if excessive paraproteins in the blood are present. Blindness developed in a dog with IgA myeloma because of bilateral detachment of retina. A bleeding tendency develops as a result of thrombocytopenia and hemostatic defects. The disease may progress to a myelogenous or myelomonocytic leukemia in some cases. Renal insufficiency and neurologic manifestations are more common in humans than in dogs.

Although plasma cell myeloma cannot be cured, about 70% of human patients respond to irradiation and chemotherapy with melphalan, cyclophosphamide, and prednisone, and have a mean life span of 30 months (Williams et al., 1990). Supportive treatment is crucial for patient survival. Allogeneic and autologous bone marrow transplantations have been performed to avoid irreversible hematopoietic stem cell damage resulting from intensive chemotherapy and radiation (Barlogie and Gahrton, 1991). Interferon therapy has been found to prolong duration of chemotherapy-induced remissions and alter the course of disease (Bergsagel, 1991). Clodronate, a potent inhibitor of osteoclast activity, may inhibit the progression of osteolytic lesions in multiple myeloma. In one study it was found to normalize the serum calcium level and decrease the incidence of pathologic fractures (Delmas, 1991).

Multiple myeloma dogs treated with melphalan, cyclophosphamide, and prednisone had a long term median survival of 540 days (Matus et al., 1986). A similar treatment with cytotoxic drugs combined with plasmapheresis was instituted for monoclonal gammopathy associated with canine ehrlichiosis (Matus et al., 1987).

WALDENSTRÖM'S MACROGLOBULINEMIA

A monoclonal increase in IgM is referred to as macroglobulinemia. Waldenström's macroglobulinemia is a primary disorder of this nature. It may also occur secondary to lymphoma, infections, and inflammation, and sometimes as a benign monoclonal gammopathy.

Waldenström's macroglobulinemia has been described in the dog. The disease is characterized by lassitude, bleeding, distention of the retinal veins, retinal hemorrhage, and enlarged lymph nodes and spleen. The bleeding tendency is thought to be the result of the effects of anoxia, clotting abnormalities, and thrombocytopenia. Laboratory findings include a marked hyperproteinemia with a sharply defined β or γ peak on electrophoresis and plasmacytic or lymphocytic infiltration of bone marrow and other tissues. The plasma is viscous, which contributes to the eye problem. Macroglobulinemia secondary to extensive suppurative inflammation, Coccidioides immitis infection, and lymphoma have been observed in dogs (Figs. 21–6, 21–7, 21–8, 21–9).

Bone marrow aspirates of human patients with this disease may yield a "dry tap" or contain lymphocytoid rather than plasmacytic cells. The disease differs from myeloma in that no bone lesions are present. Bence Jones proteinuria is less common. Patients are given frequent plasmapheresis and treated with low doses of chlorambucil. A combination chemotherapy including cyclophosphamide, melphalan, and prednisolone can be instituted in nonresponsive cases. Death is commonly caused by infection resulting from the depression of normal antibody production.

HYPERVISCOSITY SYNDROME

Hyperviscosity syndrome (HVS) has been observed in the dog and cat. In the dog, as in humans, it is primarily associated with IgM, less commonly with IgA, and rarely with IgG paraproteins. Thus, HVS is not only a manifestation of Waldenström's macroglobulinemia, but may also be seen in certain cases of multiple myeloma, particularly those having polymeric IgA, and in lymphoma and lymphocytic leukemia with macroglobulinemia (Jain, 1986). HVS associated with IgG, IgM, and IgA myelomas has been reported in cats (Forrester et al., 1992). Bence Jones proteinuria was evident in 2 cats with HVS associated with IgG myeloma. HVS may also accompany benign monoclonal gammopathy and cryoglobulinemia.

The hematocrit is the most important single factor influencing whole blood viscosity. Plasma fibrinogen and certain Igs influence plasma and, in turn, whole blood viscosity. Flow characteristics of blood are therefore affected by the red cell count and plasma viscosity. In paraproteinemia, increased plasma viscosity and aggregation of erythrocytes may significantly alter blood flow. Plasma viscosity in macroglobulinemias and myelomatosis is elevated because of extremely high concentrations of serum paraproteins and the physical properties of the Igs involved. IgM is not only a macromolecule, but also has a high intrinsic viscosity. IgA and, to some extent, IgG3 in humans tend to form high-molecular-weight complexes (polymers) and to raise the plasma viscosity at relatively lower concentrations than IgM.

Increased plasma viscosity and the aggregation of erythrocytes decrease blood flow and tissue perfusion. This is associated with a spectrum of clinical signs, including abnormalities of cardiovascular, neurologic, and renal functions and of hemostasis and immune mechanisms. For example, cardiomegaly, a distended tortuous appearance of the retinal veins, and neurologic manifestations may be present to a varying degree at admission. The paraproteins may interact with various coagulation factors and may also interfere with platelet functions, thus adding to a bleeding tendency from clotting defects and thrombocytopenia. Retinal hemorrhages and bleeding from the mucous membranes are common.

The long-term prognosis in HVS is poor, but some advances have been made in treatment. Weekly or biweekly plasmapheresis, chemotherapy, and treatment with penicillamine or other agents to reduce paraprotein aggregation are palliative measures. Frequent plasmapheresis and therapy with melphalan and cyclophosphamide induced sustained remission in three dogs with HVS associated with IgA monoclonal gammopathy (Matus et al., 1983). Clinical signs associated with HVS resolved, and normal serum protein concentrations were attained.

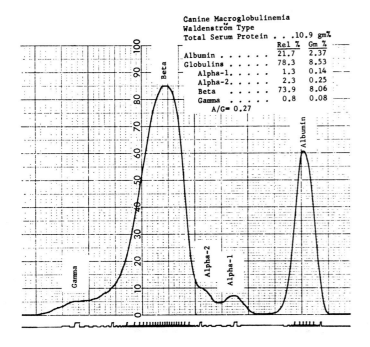

Canine Macroglobulinemia
Waldenström Type
Total Serum Protein . . . 10.9 gm%

	Rel %	Gm %
Albumin	21.7	2.37
Globulins	78.3	8.53
Alpha-1.	1.3	0.14
Alpha-2.	2.3	0.25
Beta	73.9	8.06
Gamma	0.8	0.08

A/G= 0.27

Fig. 21–9. Serum protein profile from a dog with lymphoma. (From Jain, N.C.: Schalm's Veterinary Hematology. 4th Ed. Philadelphia, Lea & Febiger, 1986, p. 970.)

ALEUTIAN DISEASE IN MINK

Aleutian disease of mink is characterized by plasma cell infiltration of the liver, kidney, and other organs, hyperproteinemia, and widespread immune-complex periarteritis and glomerulonephritis. Progression of the disease appears to be under genetic influence (Aastead and Hauch, 1988). The electrophoretic patterns in this disease are striking in that they appear as tracings of normal serum, only in reverse order; the γ-globulin concentration is similar to that of the albumin of normal serum, as found in monoclonal gammopathy. Marked hypoalbuminemia accompanies the hypergammaglobulinemia. Sera of affected minks also have autoantibodies to several tissue components such as double stranded DNA, thyroglobulin, cardiolipin, and mitochondrial antigens (Mouritsen et al., 1989). The number of CD8 + T lymphocytes approximately doubles as the disease develops, but the number of B lymphocytes does not change remarkably (Aasted, 1989). Severely affected minks also show profound blockade of the mononuclear phagocyte system (Lodmell et al., 1990). Neither Bence Jones proteinuria nor lytic bone lesions are seen. The disease is caused by a parvovirus (Aleutian disease virus, ADV) that replicates in macrophages. Although viral DNA can be demonstrated in many tissues of infected mink by in situ hybridization (Haas et al., 1988), virus-specific B lymphocytes are probably the primary targets for ADV (Aasted and Leslie, 1991). A similar disease has also been described in ferrets (Palley et al., 1992).

Neonatal infection of mink kits by a highly virulent strain of ADV causes 100% mortality from interstitial pneumonia. The severity of clinical disease and mortality is reduced by 50 to 75% when infected kits are treated with either a mink anti-ADV gamma-globulin or mouse monoclonal antibodies against ADV structural proteins (Alexandersen et al., 1989).

BENIGN MONOCLONAL GAMMOPATHY

In humans, benign monoclonal gammopathy is characterized by the presence of a monoclonal protein in the serum or urine unassociated with other manifestations of a plasma cell dyscrasia (Williams et al., 1990). The number of plasma cells in the bone marrow is normal to below 10%, and they have a typical morphology. Such patients are prone to develop multiple myeloma, which may take more than two decades, but this does not always occur. Patients with high or increasing serum paraprotein levels, low serum concentrations of normal Igs, and significant Bence Jones proteinuria are more likely candidates. In more than 95% of cases, the amount of M protein does not change significantly over the years. Most cases of benign monoclonal gammopathy are secondary to various other conditions, including chronic suppurative processes, autoimmune diseases, immunodeficiency states, hematologic malignancies, and other tumors. Some age relationship has been noted, and genetic influences may also be a factor.

Selected Conditions

Studies on different profiles of serum proteins have indicated that an acute inflammation, especially in the dog, pig, and cattle, is reflected in an increase in the α-globulin level, a subacute inflammation is seen with an increase in the α- and γ-globulin levels, and a chronic inflammation is accompanied by an increase in the γ-globulin level. A decrease in the albumin fraction was noted with a simultaneous increase in globulin levels, mainly γ-globulins. Such deviations in plasma protein concentrations may manifest as various diseases (Table 21–7). Severe thermal injury in a dog resulted initially in hypoalbuminemia from protein-losing dermatopathy and reduced synthesis by the liver, and later increases occurred in α_2-, β_2-, and γ-globulin concentrations (Kern et al., 1992).

GASTROINTESTINAL DISORDERS

Excessive loss of protein into the gut is one of the major pathophysiologic disorders in several conditions in which the gastrointestinal (GI) tract is involved. Hypoproteinemia is invariably seen in protein-losing enteropathy. Loss of plasma proteins into the GI tract may markedly increase secondary to conditions leading to obstruction of the GI lymphatics, which produces a loss of lymph into the intestinal lumen, or in disorders of the mucosal cells, such as inflammation or ulceration. Various conditions are associated with excessive protein loss into the GI tract, including ulcerative gastritis, stomach polyps or cancer, idiopathic steatorrhea or sprue, malabsorption syndrome, intestinal lymphangiectasia, enteritis, colitis, lymphoma and hemangiosarcoma involving the gut, and congestive heart failure.

Inflammation or ulceration of the GI tract could lead to impaired absorption of dietary protein and to increased protein loss because of injured mucosal cells. This mechanism may be potentiated by intestinal parasites. A preferential loss of globulins may also occur from the GI tract. For example, a diminished total serum protein concentration in diarrheic calves was associated with decreases in both β- and γ-globulins up to 2 weeks of age and with the loss of only β-globulins at 3 to 6 weeks of age.

Dilated lymphatic channels of the bowel wall are characteristically seen in intestinal lymphangiectasia. In this instance, protein, lipid, and lymphocyte-rich lymph (chyle) are lost into the intestinal tract and serous cavity because of obstruction of lymphatic ducts and retrograde distention of lacteals and subsequent leakage. Lymphocytopenia is common, probably because of both interrupted recirculation of lymphocytes into the peripheral blood and loss in chyle. Although rare in animals, such cases have been reported in dogs and cattle. Johne's disease of cattle leads to intestinal protein loss, particularly of albumin, although a fairly good plasma protein level may be maintained by a modest hypergammaglobulinemia from the immune response. Part of the protein loss in this disease has been ascribed to lymphangiectasia, because dilation and occlusion of the submucosal and subserosal lymphatics was found to occur.

Congestive heart failure and other cardiac problems lead to GI protein loss because of dilated intestinal lymphatic channels resulting from abnormal blood pressure changes. In addition, a significant concomitant alteration of liver function may occur.

PARASITISM

Parasitic infestations of ruminants have a profound effect on plasma proteins in addition to causing a blood loss or depression anemia. Apart from frank blood loss by bloodsucking parasites, such as Haemonchus and Ostertagia, parasites common to calves, lambs, and adult cattle and sheep produce nutritional hypoproteinemia caused by the animal's decreased food and water consumption. Excessive water loss in the feces reduces the amount of protein resorbed from the gut. Haemonchosis causes a mild gastritis, whereas Trichostrongylus axei larvae can cause acute catarrhal gastritis; thus, all degrees of protein loss can occur from the abomasum. Oesophagostomiasis causes loss of albumin and of α- and β-globulins into the cecum and colon. Experimental infestations with T. axei, H. placei, Oesophagostomum radiatum, and Bunostomum phlebotomum and ostertagiasis in cattle induced hypoproteinemia and hypoalbuminemia.

The total serum protein concentration increases in horses with helminthiasis, probably as a result of an increase in the β-globulin level, although the albumin concentration is decreased. IgG(T) is increased fourfold in ponies chronically infected with Strongylus vulgaris and significantly increased in horses and ponies grazing on pastures contaminated with eggs and larvae of intestinal parasites.

Broad fluctuations in serum protein concentrations were observed in leishmaniasis in dogs. The albumin concentration decreased as much as 30% of normal and the γ-globulin level increased as much as 31% of normal, with the total protein concentration remaining within normal limits. In some cases of leishmaniasis, however, a moderate to marked hyperproteinemia was a consistent feature for several months. Dogs naturally infected with Dirofilaria immitis may have significantly higher serum β-globulin levels than uninfected dogs.

Serum Ig and complement levels may also be altered during parasitism. For example, in cattle with trypanosomiasis serum concentrations of IgG and IgM may increase, whereas IgA, IgE, C1, and C3 levels may decrease.

LIVER DISEASE

Because the liver plays a central role in the anabolism and catabolism of plasma proteins, it is not unreasonable to expect the plasma protein concentration to change in liver disease. These changes, however, appear late in the disease process.

In hepatitis, cirrhosis, and carcinoma, characteristic findings include a reduction in the albumin and elevation in γ-globulin concentrations. The fall in the albumin level is caused by the failure of synthesis by the hepatic parenchyma. The remarkable regenerative power of the liver is such, though, that significantly depressed albumin synthesis is generally found only in a chronic process, such as diffuse fibrosis or chronic hepatitis. The reason for the elevated γ-globulin levels has not been determined, although an immune response might be involved. Puppies infected with canine infectious hepatitis virus may show increases in α- or in both α- and β-globulin level and a decrease in the albumin level.

KIDNEY DISEASE

The potential for the loss of protein in kidney disease is substantial. The rate of urinary protein excretion depends on the glomerular filtration rate, the permeability of the glomerular membrane, the rate of absorption through the glomerular membrane, the rate of absorption in the tubules, and the rate at which the tubules dispose of absorbed protein. The first proteins to leak through the glomerular membranes are albumin and α-globulin. The β- and γ-globulins leak through when the damage is greater.

In dogs, chronic interstitial nephritis (end-stage kidney disease) is a common finding. Significant changes in plasma protein levels are not found, however, except that an unexplained hyperfibrinogenemia is a common finding and hyperproteinemia may occur because of dehydration. Conversely, glomerulonephritis results in a significant loss of protein, particularly albumin, and hypoproteinemia is the usual finding.

Hypoproteinemia associated with proteinuria is common in the nephrotic syndrome from various causes. The electrophoretic pattern is one of marked reduction in serum albumin and elevation of α2-globulin levels. The former results from proteinuria despite the enhanced production of serum albumin, whereas the latter is caused by an increase in α-lipoprotein. An increase in the γ-globulin and β-globulin levels may also sometimes be present and may be related to increased synthesis of IgG and IgM, respectively (Kaysen and Bander, 1990). The nephrotic syndrome occurs in the dog. Hypoalbuminemia in dogs and humans with nephrotic syndrome may increase platelet aggregability and risk for thrombosis (Green et al., 1985).

EFFECT OF INFECTION ON SERUM PROTEINS

The immune response to infection may not be associated with elevations in the total plasma protein or Ig concentrations. In acute febrile infections, the principal changes are a decrease in the albumin level and, most frequently, an increase in the α-globulin level. These changes are observed after injury, surgery, or neoplastic disease and are probably related to adrenal stimulation from stress that leads to the endogenous release of corticosteroids and increased protein catabolism. In chronic infections, especially if abscess formation occurs to provide a constant and potent source of antigen, a marked rise in the γ-globulin level and hyperproteinemia can be seen. In this event, a concomitant decrease in the albumin level is invariably present. A good example is Corynebacterium pseudotuberculosis infection in horses and goats.

Generally, viral and rickettsial infections do not produce significant changes in either the relative or absolute amount of plasma proteins, even though antibody titers may be elevated. Examples include western or Venezuelan equine encephalomyelitis, Japanese B encephalitis, influenza, foot-and-mouth disease, vascular stomatitis, and Newcastle disease.

Persistent viremia in equine infectious anemia is associated with hypergammaglobulinemia caused by elevated IgG and IgG(T) levels. Early in the course of infection, increases in globulin concentration are associated with IgM, which decreases to normal levels during the infection.

In feline infectious peritonitis (FIP), total serum proteins can attain high levels (Fig. 21–10) and the peritoneal fluid may be unusually hyperproteinemic (Fig. 21–11). Hypergammaglobulinemia from increases in both the β- and γ-globulin levels is characteristic of FIP. In 35 cats with FIP, plasma protein levels averaged 8.3 ± 1.1 g/dl and ranged from 6.4 to 11.0 g/dl (Table 21–10). The fibrinogen level was elevated (400 to 700 mg/dl) in over 50% of the cats examined. Many of the infected cats developed a normocytic normochromic anemia from depressed erythropoiesis. The icterus index was elevated (10 to 50 units) in nearly 50% of the cats, and was of hepatic origin. Clotting abnormalities suggestive of DIC may occur.

Tropical canine pancytopenia, caused by Ehrlichia canis, in the terminal stages is characterized by a marked elevation in the γ-globulin concentration concomitant with a decrease in the albumin level. In experimentally infected puppies, elevated α2-glycoprotein levels were observed during the febrile stage, followed by a gradual rise in the γ-globulin level.

GERM-FREE ANIMALS

The intestinal flora contribute significantly to serum protein concentrations, as evidenced by a comparison of germ-free animals with normally raised animals. Germ-free rats and piglets have comparatively lower globulin concentrations. Exposing them to normally raised animals for 1 week caused an elevation in the α2-globulin level, followed in the second week by an increase in the β fraction. Only after more than 2 weeks did the serum γ-globulin level increase, with a concomitant decrease in the serum albumin concentration. In germ-free and normally raised ruminants (goats and sheep), no significant differences were found in albumin and α- and β-globulin concentrations, whereas a significant increase in the γ-globulin level occurred with age in normally raised animals but not in germ-free animals. Thus, the total protein concentration is lower in germ-free animals during the first few weeks of life.

IMMUNE DEFICIENCY DISORDERS

The importance of humoral and cellular defense mechanisms for the well-being of an individual has been amply demonstrated. Inadequacies of phagocytic cells, lymphocytes, and complement components are associated with increased susceptibility to infections and sometimes death. Allogeneic bone marrow transplantation and cytokine administration are newer approaches for the treatment of immune deficiency states (Lenarsky and Parkman, 1990). Immune deficiency disorders, in the broadest sense, include disorders of these cellular and humoral defense systems. A restricted consideration includes only disorders associated with the immune system—the lymphocytes and

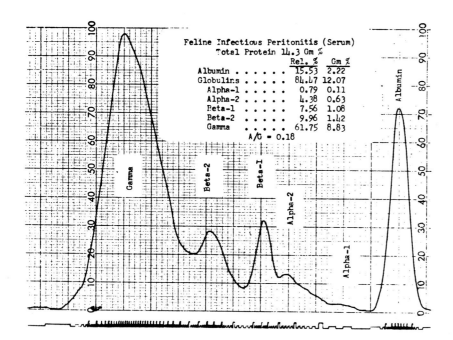

Fig. 21–10. Electrophoretic pattern of serum from a cat with feline infectious peritonitis. (From Jain, N.C.: Schalm's Veterinary Hematology. 4th Ed. Philadelphia, Lea & Febiger, 1986, p. 976.)

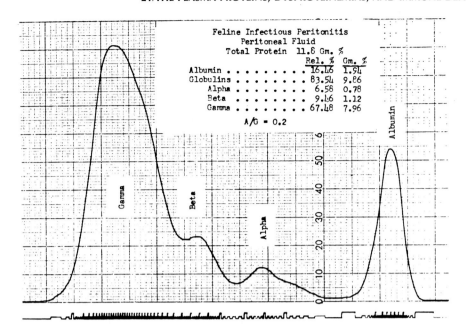

Fig. 21–11. Electrophoretic pattern of peritoneal fluid from a cat with feline infectious peritonitis (same cat as in Fig. 21–10). (From Jain, N.C.: Schalm's Veterinary Hematology. 4th Ed. Philadelphia, Lea & Febiger, 1986, p. 977.)

complement components. This more restrictive approach is used in the following discussion.

Clinical Signs and Diagnostic Approach

Primary immune deficiencies arise as a result of hereditary defects in the immune system, and immune deficiencies associated with or developing as a result of a known disease are considered secondary. The former usually manifest at birth or during early postnatal life, but the latter may occur at any age. Primary immune deficiencies have been reported in horses and cattle and secondary immune deficiencies from a number of causes, including drug therapy, are being increasingly recognized in various species.

Clinical signs most commonly associated with a disturbance of the immune system include infections during neonatal life, particularly during the first 6 to 8 weeks, recurrent infections or a poor response to

Table 21–10. Hemogram in Feline Infectious Peritonitis (35 Cats)

Parameter	Minimum	Maximum	Median	Mean	Standard Deviation	No. of Cats
Erythrocytes ($\times 10^6/\mu$l)	3.21	9.88	5.50	5.71	1.64	34
Hemoglobin (g/dl)	4.6	15.1	8.5	8.2	2.3	34
PCV (%)	12.0	50.0	26.5	26.2	7.5	35
MCV (fl)	37.3	58.5	45.6	46.2	4.4	34
MCH (pg)	11.2	17.4	14.3	14.5	1.4	34
MCHC (%)	28.3	38.3	31.0	31.4	1.9	34
Icterus index (units)	2.0	50.0	5.0	7.5	10.0	29
Plasma proteins (g/dl)	6.4	11.0	8.0	8.3	1.1	26
Fibrinogen (g/dl)	0.10	0.70	0.40	0.40	0.18	26
Leukocytes/μl	1,700	52,000	12,800	18,000	11,500	34
Band neutrophils	0	13,450	1,000	1,750	2,600	33
Mature neutrophils	1,088	40,300	11,500	15,400	9,300	33
Lymphocytes	0	3,750	450	769	770	33
Monocytes	0	1,470	250	384	382	33
Eosinophils	0	294	0	34	79	33
Basophils	0	220	0	13	42	33
Leukocytes (%)						
Band neutrophils	0	38.0	6.0	8.9	9.2	33
Mature neutrophils	50.0	96.0	82.5	83.3	11.3	33
Lymphocytes	0	20.5	3.5	4.8	4.7	33
Monocytes	0	8.0	1.5	2.5	2.3	33
Eosinophils	0	2.0	0	0.2	0.5	33
Basophils	0	0.5	0	0.06	0.16	33

From Schalm, O.W.: Feline infectious peritonitis: Vital statistics and laboratory findings. Ca. Vet., 25:6, 1971.

appropriate antibiotic therapy, increased susceptibility to minor pathogens or unusual organisms such as Pneumocystis carinii, and systemic illness following vaccination with a live virus vaccine.

Diagnostic evaluation of the suspected immune deficient patient should be directed at defining the possible cellular or humoral defect. A minimum initial laboratory evaluation should include a hematologic examination, estimation of the total serum protein concentration, and protein electrophoresis. Both B- and T-lymphocyte functions should be evaluated to determine humoral and cell-mediated defects of the lymphoid system. Whenever possible, histologic examination of the lymphoid tissues, particularly the thymus, spleen, lymph nodes, and gut-associated lymphoid tissue, should be carried out. Total hemolytic complement may be determined and single radial immunodiffusion may be performed to evaluate any deficiency of complement components. Evaluation of the phagocytic system requires the quantitation of neutrophils in the blood and bone marrow and an assessment of their functional capabilities, such as adherence, chemotaxis, phagocytosis, and bactericidal activity.

Primary Immune Deficiency Disorders

COMBINED IMMUNE DEFICIENCY IN HORSES, CATTLE, AND DOGS

Combined immune deficiency (CID) is a hereditary functional disorder of T and B lymphocytes. In pure or part Arabian foals, it is inherited as an autosomal recessive trait. The natural incidence is estimated at 2.3 to 2.7%, without any sex predilection. The newborn foal appears normal at birth and remains healthy up to 2 months of age. The foal becomes susceptible to infection as the level of circulating globulins that had been acquired through colostrum consumption diminishes. Death usually occurs within 5 months, frequently from bacterial infections, equine adenovirus, and the protozoan Pneumocystis carinii. Necropsy findings characteristically reveal a poorly developed lymphoid system. Grossly, the thymus appears poorly developed and the spleen may be normal to subnormal. Histologically, the thymus, spleen, and lymph nodes show an absence of lymphoid cells, including plasma cells. Rarely, CID may occur in other breeds of horses (e.g., Appaloosa).

The pathogenesis of CID remains to be elucidated. About 50% of the cases of autosomal recessive severe CID in humans are associated with abnormalities of purine metabolism because of an inherited deficiency of adenosine deaminase (Hirschhorn, 1990). An abnormality of purine metabolism was detected in Arabian foals with CID, but disease association was not established (Splitter et al., 1980).

CID can be diagnosed at birth by finding at least two of the following three criteria: (1) lymphopenia (less than 1000/µl); (2) the absence of circulating IgM; and (3) hypoplastic lymphoid tissues (e.g., the thymus). Hematologic examination reveals a marked lymphopenia, with counts usually less than 500/µl of blood (Table 21–11). The normal number of lymphocytes at birth to 21 days of age is much higher (4119 ± 1,649/µl). The lymphopenia is not corticosteroid-induced, because plasma corticosteroid levels are not elevated. Although the production of mature B and T lymphocytes is inhibited in foals with severe CID, formation of cytotoxic large granular lymphocytes remains unaffected (Perryman et al., 1988).

The normal equine fetus begins to synthesize IgM at 190 days of gestation so that a small amount (0.08 to 0.2 mg/ml) is present in serum at birth and slightly higher (0.1 to 0.5 mg/ml) levels are detected at 1 to 21 days of life. The absence of IgM in precolostral foal serum is diagnostic of primary immune deficiency (Table 21–11). In suckled CID foal serum, IgM and IgA concentrations decline rapidly because of a shorter half-life; hence, an absence or low levels of IgM and IgA at a later date are also diagnostic. Secretory IgA is not found in CID foals over 2 months of age.

An acquired CID was detected in a 7-year-old Appaloosa gelding (Freestone et al., 1987). The immunodeficiency was characterized by lymphopenia, low serum IgM and IgA concentrations, marginally low serum IgG concentrations, low antibody response to Rhodococcus equi infection, negligible mitogen-induced lymphocytic stimulation, and histologic evidence of depleted lymphoid tissue.

Combined immunodeficiency was detected in a 6-week-old male Angus calf (Bartram et al., 1989). The characteristic findings included a marked lymphopenia, hypoproteinemia, diminished serum IgG levels, absence of IgM and IgA in serum, lack of intestinal

Table 21–11. Hematologic Findings in a Newborn Male Arabian Foal with Combined Immunodeficiency

Parameter	Values
Erythrocytes	
RBC ($\times 10^6$/µl)	8.66
Hemoglobin (g/dl)	11.7
PCV (%)	36
MCV (fl)	41.6
MCHC (%)	32.5
MCH (pg)	13.5
Anisocytosis	Slight
Leukocytes	%
WBC/µl	12,300
Neutrophils	11,316 92
Lymphocytes	rare, seen on scanning
Monocytes	984 8
Eosinophils	0 0
Platelets/µl	Present in adequate numbers
Plasma	
Icterus index (unit)	5
Total protein (g/dl)	6.6
Fibrinogen (g/dl)	0.8
Serum IgG (mg/dl)	355
Serum IgM (mg/dl)	0

associated lymphoid tissue, and systemic fungal infection.

Basset hounds were reported to develop an X-linked CID by a recessive mode of inheritance (Felsburg et al., 1982). The primary features included lymphopenia, impaired T-cell function, reduced serum IgG and IgA concentrations, and variable serum IgM levels. Skin, ear, and oral infections were common in affected dogs and death occurred from systemic viral infections by 4 months of age. Basset hounds also show an apparent predisposition to avian tuberculosis, probably because of a similar or undefined defect of cellular immunity (Carpenter et al., 1988). IgA deficiency may diminish mucosal resistance against bacterial and viral infections. For example, IgA deficiency in a pup was believed to be a factor in the development of immunosuppression by distemper virus and secondary cryptosporidiosis (Turnwald et al., 1988).

LETHAL TRAIT A-46 IN BLACK-PIED DANISH CATTLE

A lethal primary immune deficiency of T cells has been described in black-pied Danish cattle of Frisian ancestry. It is an autosomal recessive trait. The calves are normal at birth, but develop characteristic skin lesions at 4 to 8 weeks of age and die by the age of 4 months. These skin lesions include exanthema, alopecia, and parakeratosis. The animals are highly susceptible to infection. Generalized hypoplasia of the lymphoid tissue, particularly of the T regions, is seen in the thymus, spleen, lymph nodes, and gut-associated lymphoid tissue. Cellular immunity is markedly reduced, whereas humoral immune response is undisturbed. A unique characteristic of the disorder is that affected calves recover by zinc therapy.

COMPLEMENT DEFICIENCY

A deficiency of several complement components has been detected in humans and in inbred strains of certain laboratory animals, including mice, guinea pigs, rabbits, rats, and hamsters. Complement-deficient animals are valuable for research on the pathogenesis of disease processes because complement is important in host defense. An inherited deficiency of C3 was reported in some Brittany spaniel dogs bred to develop a colony for the study of canine spinal muscular dystrophy. This deficiency was inherited as an autosomal recessive trait unrelated to the primary disease. Recurrent bacterial infections were common in these dogs, and their susceptibility to renal disease increased. Hematologic parameters were normal. Humoral immune response to both T-cell dependent and T-cell independent antigens is defective in dogs homozygous for C3 deficiency (O'Neil et al., 1988).

Secondary Immune Deficiency Disorders

Several conditions have been recognized in various species, but only a few are described here.

FAILURE OF PASSIVE TRANSFER OF MATERNAL IMMUNOGLOBULIN

Failure of passive transfer of maternal Ig is the most common form of immune deficiency in foals (Clabough et al., 1989; LeBlanc et al., 1992; Stoneham et al., 1991). It is also reported in calves, lambs, piglets, and goat kids. It may be complete or partial. It is the most common cause of neonatal infection and early death of the young in most species, particularly the horse and cattle. It has been estimated that about 3 to 24% of foals born on a given farm may be affected by failure of passive transfer (Liu et al., 1991). Affected foals may develop omphalophlebitis, septic arthritis, and respiratory infections. Neonatal septicemia and diarrhea are common in calves. Failure of passive transfer was found to be the major cause of mortality in newborn alpacas (Garmendia et al., 1987).

Some knowledge of the normal immune status of the newborn is essential for understanding problems associated with this type of immune deficiency. Maternal antibodies are acquired by the newborn foal, calf, lamb, piglet, and goat kid through the consumption of colostrum within the first 24 hours of birth. In utero transfer of maternal antibodies does not occur in these animals because of their unique placental patterns and surface receptors, and probably also for unknown reasons. Therefore, colostrum consumption and the absorption of Igs are essential for the passive transfer of maternal immunity.

The intestinal epithelium of the newborn absorbs all Igs, predominantly during the first 6 hours, and at gradually diminishing rates up to 24 to 48 hours of age. Some selectivity of absorption among individual classes of Igs has been observed in different species and discontinuance of absorption occurs at different times, depending on the Ig type. The subsequent nonabsorption of Igs is associated with the rapid replacement of intestinal epithelial cells during this period. The transfer process is mediated by membrane receptors for IgG and its Fc fragment on absorptive cells of the fetal membranes and neonatal gut.

Normally, serum Ig levels of the 24-hour-old foal are comparable to adult levels. The foal begins to synthesize its own Igs by 2 weeks of life and gradually replaces the diminishing maternal antibodies, which catabolize at varying rates. Thus, the serum Ig levels of the foal initially decline, reaching a nadir by 2 months of age and then increasing again to adult levels by 6 months. Similar observations have been reported for the calf and lamb.

Mare's colostrum is rich in IgG and IgG(T) and contains some IgM and IgA. Immunodeficient foals have low serum levels of both IgG and IgG(T). Serum levels of 400 mg/dl or higher indicate adequate absorption of colostral Igs in the foal, levels of 0 to 200 mg/dl constitute failure of transport, and values between 200 and 400 mg/dl suggest partial failure. Inadequate transfer of maternal Igs to the newborn can have various causes. The most common cause in foals is colostrum that is deficient or low in IgG (less than 1000 mg/dl), as from dripping mares. An inability to ingest sufficient colostrum within the first 24 hours or delayed ingestion is another cause. Malabsorption may also account for some failure of transfer of sufficient Igs. In one study, this was found to occur in 14% of lambs.

Farm management, premature birth, and birth after 345 days of gestation may adversely affect colostral IgG absorption in foals. Similarly, foals from mares >15 years of age and foals born in a cold, wet environment may not attain adequate serum IgG concentration (LeBlanc et al., 1992). Colostrum supplementation of foals may be required under these circumstances to prevent adverse effects of failure of passive transfer.

Prompt diagnosis and management of immune deficient animals is important to provide protection from possible infection. Immunoglobulin deficiency from passive transfer in the newborn can be detected by the quantitation of postcolostral serum Ig levels, which can be done by single radial immunodiffusion, serum electrophoresis and immunoelectrophoresis, refractometry, the zinc sulfate turbidity test, ELISA, and the latex agglutination test. Single radial immunodiffusion is the most accurate method of quantitation of serum IgG, but it is complex and time consuming. However, the glutaraldehyde coagulation test is considered a preferred screening test for detection of failure of passive transfer in equine neonates (Clabough et al., 1989).

Once a failure of Ig transfer problem has been diagnosed, forced colostrum feeding (200 to 300 ml) can be attempted or plasma or serum rich in Igs (maternal or frozen pool) can be given intravenously (20 ml/kg body weight). The intravenous administration of 10% purified IgG solution is considered a satisfactory treatment for foals with failure of passive transfer diagnosed later than 24 hours after birth (Liu et al., 1991). The colostrum and serum should be checked for antierythrocyte antibodies to avoid a fatal incompatible hemolytic transfusion reaction.

AGAMMAGLOBULINEMIA

Agammaglobulinemia was found in two male thoroughbreds and a standardbred horse. A sex-linked inheritance was suggested, because all three cases were males. B-lymphocyte deficiency was detected by extremely low or no serum Ig levels, a functional evaluation of lymphocytes, and the absence of plasma cells and germinal centers in lymphoid tissues. Normal T-lymphocyte functions were indicated by adequate responses to phytohemagglutinin and skin sensitization. Repeated infections and a poor response to therapy were common. Death occurred by 17 to 18 months of age.

SELECTIVE IMMUNOGLOBULIN DEFICIENCIES

Several cases of selective IgM deficiency have been described in Arabian and quarter horses. Low or no serum IgM was found, but levels of IgG and comple-

ment components, numbers of B and T lymphocytes, and response to phytohemagglutinin were normal. Clinical manifestations included poor growth and recurrent respiratory infections, beginning within the first month of life, with death usually at 4 to 8 months of age and occasionally by 2 years. Acquired IgM deficiency has been observed in horses with lymphoma; in some cases IgA values were low and suppressor T cell activity was increased in one case (Furr et al., 1992).

Selective IgM deficiency was found in two Doberman pinschers, but an association with clinical disease was not seen if the IgG and IgA levels were within the normal range. A deficiency of IgA has been detected in German shepherds as a breed characteristic (Whitbread et al., 1984), in many normal Chinese Shar-pei dogs (Moroff et al., 1985), and in Beagles (IgA, less than 30 mg/dl) from a large breeding colony (Glickman et al., 1988). The Beagles were found to have an immunologic defect in maturation or terminal differentiation of IgA-positive B cells into IgA-secreting plasma cells (Shofer et al., 1990). A decrease in serum IgA concentration in immunosuppressed Airedale Terrier dogs was thought to contribute to a bacterial infection leading to diskospondylitis. These dogs also had increased serum β_1-globulin levels and undefined serum factors inhibiting mitogen-induced blastogenesis of T lymphocytes (Barta et al., 1985).

A selective deficiency of IgG was described in red Danish milk cattle. The affected cattle showed increased susceptibility to gangrenous mastitis and pyogenic bacterial infections such as bronchopneumonia, peritonitis, and abomasoenteritis.

TRANSIENT HYPOGAMMAGLOBULINEMIA

A delayed onset of postnatal Ig synthesis leading to hypogammaglobulinemia has been observed in Arabian foals. Serum IgG and IgG(T) levels were low at 2 months of age and significant synthesis did not occur until 3 months of age, with a normal response being evident by 3.5 months. Systemic bacterial and adenovirus infections were common during this undefined hypogammaglobulinemic state.

Kittens receiving inadequate colostrum from their mothers are particularly susceptible to infection after 5 weeks of age because of the loss of all maternal Igs acquired by them, and an inability to synthesize their own immunoglobulins completely (Yamada et al., 1991).

SIMIAN ACQUIRED IMMUNE DEFICIENCY SYNDROME

A naturally occurring immunodeficiency syndrome having certain clinicopathologic and immunologic features in common with acquired immune deficiency syndrome (AIDS) in humans occurs in macaque and rhesus monkeys (Gardner and Luciw, 1989; King, 1986). It is known as Simian immunodeficiency syndrome (SIDS), and it is caused by a type D retrovirus termed simian immunodeficiency virus (SIV). AIDS is caused by a lentivirus, human immunodeficiency virus (HIV). Patients with this disease complex develop immunosuppression, infection with opportunistic organisms, and neurologic, pulmonary, and gastrointestinal dysfunction. Hematologic abnormalities include anemia, leukopenia from neutropenia and lymphopenia, and thrombocytopenia (Zon and Groopman, 1988). Neutropenia and anemia may be caused by decreased proliferation of specific committed hematopoietic stem cells (colony forming unit granulocyte-macrophage and burst forming unit-erythroid) in the bone marrow. Various pathologic abnormalities become more severe as the disease enters the chronic phase.

Animals naturally infected with SIV develop chronic diarrhea and wasting and exhibit hematologic abnormalities such as anemia, neutropenia and bizarre immature monocytes in peripheral blood, abnormal liver function tests, and diminished T-cell responses. Death occurs from unusual disease, neoplasia, or opportunistic infections. Experimental infection of rhesus macaques with SIV produces decreases in hemoglobin concentration, total leukocyte count, and neutrophil, lymphocyte, and platelet numbers and a transient eosinophilia, in association with bone marrow viral infection (Mandell et al., 1991). Neutropenia and thrombocytopenia observed during SIV-infection may result from defective hematopoiesis because bone marrow hematopoietic progenitor cell growth is inhibited by SIV (Watanabe et al., 1990). The mechanisms of lymphopenia and T-cell deficiency remain unknown.

FELINE IMMUNE DEFICIENCY SYNDROME

Feline AIDS is caused by the feline immunodeficiency virus (FIV), a lentivirus, first isolated in 1986 from a large, multiple-cat household in California (Pedersen et al., 1987). FIV is an RNA virus and has tropism for T-lymphocytes and macrophages from various tissues. Infection of cats with the FIV has now been found in many countries and clinical and epidemiologic findings have been described (Fleming et al., 1991; Pedersen and Barlough, 1991; Yamamoto et al, 1989). These infected cats develop antibodies to all protein components of the virus, signifying persistent viral infection, but the antibodies are nonprotective. A higher incidence of infection occurs in males, older (>6 years) cats, domestic cats compared to pure-bred cats, and in free-roaming cats compared to confined cats. In FIV-infected cats, coinfection with feline syncytium-forming virus (FeSFV) was much greater (74%) than with FeLV (16%). Clinically ill cats shed more virus in saliva than healthy carriers and biting appears to be an important natural mode of FIV transmission. Infected cats have a higher incidence of abscesses or cellulitis and neoplasia than FIV-negative cats, a finding compatible with immune suppression of FIV-infected cats. Neoplasias associated with FIV infection include myeloproliferative disorders, lymphoma, and squamous cell carcinoma (Hutson et al., 1991). Infected cats often show signs of a severe

chronic inflammatory disease, but may also exhibit no clinical signs of disease. The mean survival was 24.4 months from the time of diagnosis (Fleming et al., 1991).

The major clinical abnormalities in naturally infected cats include chronic oral cavity infections, chronic upper respiratory infections, chronic enteritis, anemia, weight loss, chronic skin disease, and chronic conjunctivitis. Other clinical findings in some affected cats may include fever of unknown origin, anorexia, lethargy, diarrhea, vomiting, neurological dysfunction, lymphoma and myeloproliferative disease. Secondary infection with opportunistic organisms such as Toxoplasma gondi may occur (Witt et al., 1989).

Common hematologic abnormalities in FIV-infected cats are a normocytic normochromic anemia and leukopenia because of neutropenia and/or lymphopenia, but thrombocytopenia is rare (Hopper et al., 1989; Shelton et al., 1990, 1991). Serum from a neutropenic cat inhibited in vitro proliferation of GM-CFU progenitors (Shelton et al., 1989). Lymphopenia in both naturally and experimentally infected cats is associated with decreases in CD4+ T lymphocytes, CD4+/CD8+ ratio, and mitogen-induced blastogenic response of T-cells. Some cats develop lymphocytosis and monocytosis and about one third of the FIV-infected clinically ill cats develop hyperproteinemia from increases in IgG concentration (Hopper et al., 1989).

Cats experimentally infected with FIV develop an acute phase of the disease characterized by fever and lymphadenopathy. This is followed by a long asymptomatic phase, which lasts from months to years, before a chronic disease develops. Hematologic changes during experimental FIV infection in cats have been studied (Fig. 21–12) (Mandell et al., 1992). A moderate to severe leukopenia, neutropenia, and eosinopenia developed during the period of acute infection between weeks 5 and 13 postinoculation (PI). Bone marrow findings during the neutropenic phase were characterized by normal myeloid activity or mild myeloid hyperplasia with a left shift to promyelocytes. Chronic infection was characterized by an intermittent neutropenia in three out of six FIV-infected cats beginning after week 50 PI and lymphopenia in two cats beginning week 66 PI. The severity of neutropenia and lymphopenia varied among cats. Anemia and thrombocytopenia did not manifest in these cats, unlike cats with natural FIV infection.

Diagnosis of FIV infection is made by detection of specific antibodies in serum by an indirect immunofluorescence assay (IFA), ELISA, radioimmunoassay, or immunoblot (western blot) (Barr et al., 1991; Egberink et al., 1991a; Pedersen and Barlough, 1991). The ELISA is more sensitive, but less specific compared to IFA and immunoblot. The virus can be cultured from bone marrow cells, blood mononuclear cells, and peritoneal macrophages. FIV proviral DNA in tissues can be detected by the polymerase chain reaction.

Treatment of clinically ill cats is generally empirical and symptomatic. Zidovudine (3′-acido-3′deoxythy-

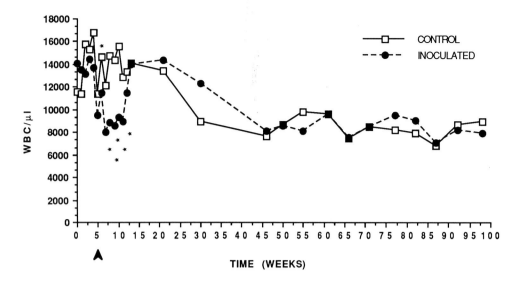

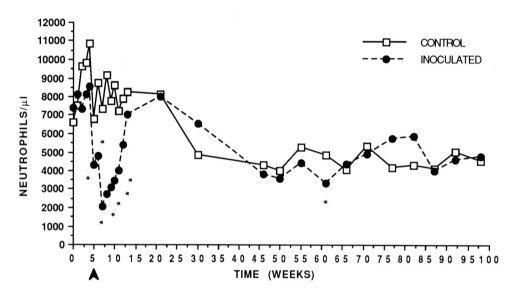

Fig. 21–12. Mean WBC (A), neu-trophil (B), and platelet (C) counts/μl of blood of 6 kittens (14.5–27 weeks old) experimen-tally infected with feline immu-nodeficiency virus (FIV). In all fig-ures, the arrow indicates the day by which all cats seroconverted for antibody to FIV. Asterisk indicates statistical significance ($p < .05$) between control and inoculated groups for the given time period. An age-related decline in WBC, neutrophil, and platelet counts is evident in both control and inoc-ulated groups during the study pe-riod. (Courtesy of Dr. Carol Man-dell; for details see Mandell et al., Comp. Haematol. Int., 2:8, 1992).

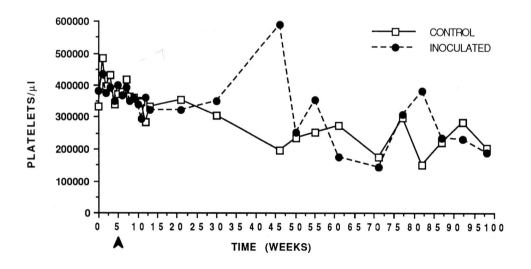

midine or AZT) and the acyclic purine nucleoside analogue 9-(2-phosphonomethoxyethyl) adenine appear to be of some clinical benefit. Although these drugs prevent replication of FIV by blocking the activity of reverse transcriptase, they do not eliminate FIV from infected cats (Egberink et al., 1991b). Efforts are being made to develop a safe and effective vaccine (Lehmann et al., 1991; Yamamoto et al., 1991).

OTHER CONDITIONS

Several infectious diseases have been found to induce secondary immune deficiencies of T- or B-cell functions, or both. For example, equine herpes virus I infection of thoroughbred foals during the later part of gestation may destroy lymphoid tissues, resulting in secondary immune deficiency at birth. Bovine viral diarrhea in calves suppresses both T- and B-cell functions, whereas cattle with Johne's disease and calves with lymphoma primarily develop reduced T-cell activity. Canine distemper is associated with suppression of both T- and B-cell functions, whereas Demodex canis inhibits T-cell function. A serum factor was found to be responsible for the development of immune deficiencies associated with Johne's disease in cattle and demodicosis in dogs. Immunosuppression has been observed in cats infected with FeLV and panleukopenia virus.

REFERENCES

Aasted, B.: Mink infected with Aleutian disease virus have an elevated level of CD8-positive T-lymphocytes. Vet. Immunol. Immunopathol., 20:375, 1989.

Aasted, B. and Hauch, H.: Studies on the progression of Aleutian disease in mink. Acta Vet. Scand., 29:315, 1988.

Aasted, B. and Leslie, R.G.: Virus-specific B-lymphocytes are probably the primary targets for Aleutian disease virus. Vet. Immunol. Immunopathol., 28:127, 1991.

Adinolfi, M. and Lehner, T.: C9 and factor B as acute phase proteins and their diagnostic and prognostic value in disease. Exp. Clin. Immunogenet., 5:123, 1988.

Alexandersen, S., Larsen, S., Cohn, A., et al.: Passive transfer of antibiral antibodies restricts replication of Aleutian mink disease parvovirus in vivo. J. Virol., 63:9, 1989.

Andrew, M., Mitchell, L., Berry, L.R., et al.: Fibrinogen has a rapid turnover in the healthy newborn lamb. Pediatr. Res., 23:249, 1988.

Auer, D.E., Ng, J.C., Thompson, H.L., et al.: Acute phase response in horses: changes in plasma cation concentrations after localised tissue injury. Vet. Rec., 124:235, 1989.

Ballou, S.P. and Kushner, I.: C-reactive protein and the acute phase response. Adv. Intern. Med., 37:313, 1992.

Barlogie, B. and Gahrton, G.: Bone marrow transplantation in multiple myeloma. Bone Marrow Transplant., 7:71, 1991.

Barr, M.C., Pough, M.B., Jacobson, R.H., et al.: Comparison and interpretation of diagnostic tests for feline immunodeficiency virus infection. J. Am. Vet. Med. Assoc., 199:1377, 1991.

Barta, O., Turnwald, G.H., Shaffer, L.M., et al.: Blastogenesis-suppressing serum factors decreased immunoglobulin A, and increased β1-globulins in Airedale Terriers with diskospondylitis. Am. J. Vet. Res., 46:1319, 1985.

Bartram, P.A., Smith, B.P., Holmberg, C., et al.: Combined immunodeficiency in a calf. Am. J. Vet. Med. Assoc., 195:347, 1989.

Bauer, J.E., Meyer, D.J., Campbell, M., et al.: Serum lipid and lipoprotein changes in ponies with experimentally induced liver disease. Am. J. Vet. Res., 51:1380, 1990.

Bergsagel, D.E.: Plasma cell myeloma: biology and treatment. Ann. Rev. Med., 42:167, 1991.

Boosman, R., Niewold, T.A., Mutsaers, C.W.A.A.M., et al.: Serum amyloid A concentrations in cows given endotoxin as an acute phase stimulant. Am. J. Vet. Res., 50:1690, 1989.

Cambau, E.: [C-reactive protein: general review and role in the study of infections]. Pathol. Biol. (Paris), 36:1232, 1988.

Carothers, M.A., Johnson, G.C., DiBartola, S.P., et al.: Extramedullary plasmacytoma and immunoglobulin-associated amyloidosis in a cat. Am. J. Vet. Med. Assoc., 195:1593, 1989.

Carpenter, J.L., Myers, A.M., Conner, M.W., et al.: Tuberculosis in five basset hounds. A. J. Vet. Med. Assoc., 192:1563, 1988.

Caspi, D., Snel, F.W.J.J., Batt, R.M., et al.: C-reactive protein in dogs. Am. J. Vet. Res., 48:919, 1987.

Clabough, D.L., Conboy, H.S. and Roberts, M.C.: Comparison of four screening techniques for the diagnosis of equine neonatal hypogammaglobulinemia. Am. J. Vet. Med. Assoc., 194:1717, 1989.

Clarke, L.L., Argenzio, R.A. and Roberts, M.C.: Effect of meal feeding on plasma volume and urinary electrolyte clearance in ponies. Am. J. Vet. Res., 51:571, 1990.

Conner, J.G., Eckersall, P.D., Ferguson, J., et al.: Acute phase response in the dog following surgical trauma. Res. Vet. Sci., 45:107, 1988a.

Conner, J.G., Eckersall, P.D., Wiseman, A., et al.: Bovine acute phase response following turpentine injection. Res. Vet. Sci., 44:82, 1988b.

Conner, J.G., Eckersall, P.D., Wiseman, A., et al.: Acute phase response in calves following infection with Pasteurella haemolytica, Ostertagia ostertagi and endotoxin administration. Res. Vet. Sci., 47:203, 1989.

Cooper, E.H.: Acute phase reactant proteins as prognostic indicators in cancer. Tokai J. Exp. Clin. Med., 13:361, 1988.

Cooper, E.H.: Acute phase reactant proteins. Immunol. Ser., 53:521, 1990.

Coyne, C.P., Hornof, W.J., Kely, A.B., et al.: Extraction, radioiodination, and in vivo catabolism of equine fibrinogen. Am. J. Vet. Res., 46:2572, 1985.

Delmas, P.D.: The use of clodronate in multiple myeloma. Bone, 12Suppl., 1:S31, 1991.

Deutsch, H.F.: Chemistry and biology of alpha-fetoprotein. Adv. Cancer Res., 56:253, 1991.

di Minno, G. and Mancini, M.: Drugs affecting plasma fibrinogen levels. Cardiovasc. Drugs Ther., 6:25, 1992.

DiBartola, S.P., Reiter, J.A., Cornacoff, J.B., et al.: Serum amyloid A protein concentration measured by radial immunodiffusion in Abyssinian and non-Abyssinian cats. Am. J. Vet. Res., 50:1414, 1989.

Doweiko, J.P. and Nompleggi, D.J.: The role of albumin in human physiology and pathophysiology, Part III: Albumin and disease states. JPEN, 15:476, 1991.

Eckersall, P.D. and Conner, J.G.: Bovine and canine acute phase proteins. Vet. Res. Commun., 12:169, 1988.

Egberink, H.F., Hartman, K. and Horzinek, M.C.: Chemotherapy of feline immunodeficiency virus infection. Am. J. Vet. Med. Assoc., 199:1485, 1991a.

Egberink, H.F., Lutz, H. and Horzinek, M.C.: Use of western blot and radioimmunoprecipitation for diagnosis of feline leukemia and feline immunodeficiency virus infections. Am. J. Vet. Med. Assoc., 199:1339, 1991b.

Felsburg, P.J., Jezyk, P.F. and Haskins, M.E.: A canine model for variable combined immunodeficiency. Clin. Res., 30:347A, 1982.

Fleming, E.J., McCaw, D.L., Smith, J.A., et al.: Clinical, hematologic, and survival data from cats infected with feline immunodeficiency virus: 42 cases (1983–1988). Am. J. Vet. Med. Assoc.,199:913, 1991.

Forrester, S.D., Greco, D.S. and Relford, R.L.: Serum hyperviscosity syndrome associated with multiple myeloma in two cats. Am. J. Vet. Med. Assoc., 200:79, 1992.

Freestone, J.E., Hietala, S., Moulton, J., et al.: Acquired immunodeficiency in a seven-year-old horse. Am. J. Vet. Med. Assoc., 190:689, 1987.

Furr, M.O., Crisman, M.V. and Robertson, J.: Immunodeficiency associated with lymphosarcoma in a horse. J. Am. Vet. Med. Assoc., 201:307, 1992.

Ganter, U., Arcone, R., Toniatti, C., et al.: Dual control of C-reactive protein gene expression by interleukin-1 and interleukin-6. EMBO J., 8:3773, 1989.

Gardner, M.B. and Luciw, P.A.: Animal models of AIDS. FASEB J, 3:2593, 1989.

Garmendia, A.E., Palmer, G.H., DeMartini, J.C., et al.: Failure of passive immunoglobulin transfer: A major determinant of mortality in newborn alpacas (Lama pacos). Am. J. Vet. Res., 48:1472, 1987.

Geisel, O., Stiglmair-Herb, M. and Linke, R.P.: Myeloma associated with immunoglobulin lambda-light chain derived amyloid in a dog. Vet. Pathol., 27:374, 1990.

Genetzky, R.M., Loparco, F.V. and Ledet, A.E.: Clinical pathologic alterations in horses during a water deprivation test. Am. J. Vet. Res., 48:1007, 1987.

Glickman, L.T., Shofer, F.S., Payton, A.J., et al.: Survey of serum IgA, IG, and IgM concentrations in a large beagle population in which IgA deficiency had been identified. Am. J. Vet. Res., 49:1240, 1988.

Gotschlich, E.C.: C-reactive protein. A historical overview. Ann. N.Y. Acad. Sci., 557:9, 1989.

Green, R.A., Russo, E.A., Greene, R.T., et al.: Hypoalbuminemia-related platelet hypersensitivity in two dogs with nephrotic syndrome. Am. J. Vet. Med. Assoc., 186:485, 1985.

Haas, L., Lochelt, M. and Kaaden, O.R.: Detection of Aleutian disease virus DNA in tissues of naturallyl infected mink. J. Gen. Virol., 69:705, 1988.

Hardy, R.M. and Osborne, C.A.: Water deprivation test in the dog: Maximal normal values. Am. J. Vet. Med. Assoc., 174:479, 1979.

Harvey, J.W. and West, C.L.: Prednisone-induced increases in serum alpha-2-globulin and haptoglobin concentrations in dogs. Vet. Pathol., 24:90, 1987.

Hawkey, C.M. and Hart, M.G.: Fibrinogen levels in mammals suffering from bacterial infections. Vet. Rec. 121:519, 1987.

Hawkins, E.C., Feldman, B.F. and Blanchard, P.C.: Immunoglobulin A myeloma in a cat with pleural effusion and serum hyperviscosity. Am. J. Vet. Med. Assoc., 188:876, 1986.

Henry, M., Prasse, K. and White, S.: Hemorrhagic diathesis caused by multiple myeloma in a three-month-old foal. Am. J. Vet. Med. Assoc., 194:392, 1989.

Hirschhorn, R.: Adenosine deaminase deficiency. Immunodefic. Rev., 2:175, 1990.

Hoenig, M.: Multiple myeloma associated with the heavy chains of immunoglobulin A in a dog. Am. J. Vet. Med. Assoc., 190:1191, 1987.

Hopper, C.D., Sparkes, A.H., Gruffydd-Jones, T.J., et al.: Clinical and laboratory findings in cats infected with feline immuno-deficiency virus. Vet. Rec., 125:341, 1989.

Hutson, C.A., Rideout, B.A. and Pedersen, N.C.: Neoplasia associated with feline immunodeficiency virus infection in cats of Southern California. Am. J. Vet. Med. Assoc., 199:1357, 1991.

Jain, N.C.: Schalm's Veterinary Hematology. 4th ed. Philadelphia, Lea & Febiger, 1986, pp. 350–387, 940–989.

Jain, N.C.: Acute phase proteins. In Current veterinary Therapy 10: Small animal practice. Edited by R.W. Kirk. Philadelphia, W.B. Saunders, 1989, pp. 468–471.

Kaneko, J.J.: Serum proteins and the dysproteinemias. In Clinical Biochemistry of Domestic Animals. Edited by J.J. Kameko. San Diego, Academic Press, 1989, pp. 142–165.

Kaysen, G.A. and al Bander, H.: Metabolism of albumin and immunoglobulins in the nephrotic syndrome. Am. J. Nephrol., 10Suppl, 1:36, 1990.

Kent, J.E. and Goodall, J.: Assessment of an immunoturbidimetric method for measuring equine serum haptoglobin concentrations. Equine Vet. J., 23:59, 1991.

Kern, M.R., Stockham, S.L. and Coates, J.R.: Analysis of serum protein concentrations after severe thermal injury in a dog. Vet. Clin. Pathol., 21:19, 1992.

King, N.W.: Simian models of acquired immunodeficiency syndrome (AIDS): A review. Vet. Pathol., 23:345, 1986.

Kirschner, S.E., Niyo, Y., Hill, B.L., et al.: Blindness in a dog with IgA-forming myeloma. Am. J. Vet. Med. Assoc., 193:349, 1988.

Koj, A., Magielska-Zero, D., Bereta, J., et al.: The cascade of inflammatory cytokines regulating synthesis of acute phase proteins. Tokai J. Exp. Clin. Med., 13:255, 1988.

Kolb-Bachofen, V.: A review on the biological properties of C-reactive protein. Immunobiology, 183:133, 1991a.

Kolb-Bachofen, V.: A membrane-bound form of the acute-phase protein C-reactive protein is the galactose-specific particle receptor on rat liver macrophages. Pathobiology, 59:272, 1991b.

LeBlanc, M.M., Tran, T., Baldwin, J.L., et al.: Factors that influence passive transfer of immunoglobulins in foals. Am. J. Vet. Med. Assoc., 200:179, 1992.

Lehmann, R., Franchini, M., Aubert, A., et al.: Vaccination of cats experimentally infected with feline immunodeficiency virus, using a recombinant feline leukemia virus vaccine. Am. J. Vet. Med. Assoc., 199:1446, 1991.

Lenarsky, C. and Parkman, R.: Bone marrow transplantation for the treatment of immune deficiency states. Bone Marrow Transplant., 6:361, 1990.

Liu, I.K.M., Brown, C., Myers, R.C., et al.: Evaluation of intravenous administration of concentrated immunoglobulin G to colostrum-deprived foals. Am. J. Vet. Res., 52:709, 1991.

Lodmell, D.L., Bergman, R.K., Bloom, M.E., et al.: Impaired phagocytosis by the mononuclear phagocytic system in sapphire mink affected with Aleutian disease. Proc. Soc. Exp. Biol. Med., 195:75, 1990.

Lowseth, L.A., Gillett, N.A., Chang, I.-Y., et al.: Detection of serum α-fetoprotein in dogs with hepatic tumors. Am. J. Vet. Med. Assoc., 199:735, 1991.

MacAllister, C., Qualls, C., Jr., Tyler, R., et al.: Multiple myeloma in a horse. Am. J. Vet. Med. Assoc., 191:337, 1987.

Mahin, L., Chadli, M., Marzou, A., et al.: Differences in coagulability of three glutaraldehyde solutions in the glutaraldehyde test on bovine whole blood. Zentralbl. Veterinarmed. [A]., 32:151, 1985.

Mandell, C.P., Jain, N.C., Lackner, A.A., et al.: Hematologic changes in rhesus macaques experimentally infected with simian immunodeficiency virus (SIV) (Abstract). Proceedings of the ninth annual symposium on nonhuman primate models for AIDS. Seattle, Washington, Nov. 6–9, 1991, p. 67.

Mandell, C.P., Sparger, E., Pedersen, N.C., et al.: Long-term haematological changes in cats experimentally infected with feline immunodeficiency virus (FIV). Comp. Haematol. Intl., 2:8, 1992.

Matus, R.E., Leifer, C.E., Gordon, B.R., et al.: Plasmapheresis and chemotherapy of hyperviscosity syndrome associated with monoclonal gammapathy in the dog. J. Am. Vet. Med. Assoc., 183:215, 1983.

Matus, R.E., Leifer, C.E. and Hurvitz, A.I.: Use of plasmapheresis and chemotherapy for treatment of monoclonal gammopathy associated with Ehrlichia canis infection in a dog. Am. J. Vet. Med. Assoc., 190:1302, 1987.

Matus, R.E., Leifer, C.E., MacEwen, G., et al.: Prognostic factors for multiple myeloma in the dog. Am. J. Vet. Med. Assoc., 188:1288, 1986.

Medda, R., Cara, N. and Floris, G.: Horse plasma ceruloplasmin molecular weight and subunit analysis. Preparative Biochemistry, 17:447, 1987.

Milne, E.M., Doxey, D.L., Kent, J.E., et al.: Acute phase proteins in grass sickness (equine dysautonomia). Res. Vet. Sci., 50:273, 1991.

Morimatsu, M., Sakai, H., Yoshimatsu, K., et al.: Isolation and characterization of C-reactive protein and serum amyloid P component from bovine serum. Nippon Juigaku Zasshi, 51:723, 1989.

Morimatsu, M., Watanabe, A., Yoshimatsu, K., et al.: Elevation of bovine serume C-reactive protein and serum amyloid P component levels by lactation. J. Dairy Res., 58:257, 1991.

Moroff, S.D., Hurvitz, A.I., Peterson, M.E., et al.: IgA deficiency in the dog. Vet. Immunol. Immunopathol., 36:1, 1985.

Motoi, Y., Itoh, H., Tamura, K., et al.: Correlation of serum concentration of α1-acid glycoprotein with lymphocyte blastogenesis and development of experimentally induced or naturally acquired hepatic abscesses in cattle. Am. J. Vet. Res., 53:574, 1992.

Mouritsen, S., Aasted, B. and Hoier-Hadsen, M.: Mink with Aleutian disease have autoantibodies to some autoantigens. Vet. Immunol. Immunopathol., 23:179, 1989.

Nagahata, H., Taguchi, K. and Noda, H.: Preliminary studies on the acid soluble glycoproteins in serum and their diagnostic value for acute inflammatory diseases in cattle. Vet. Res. Commun., 13:257, 1989.

Ndung'u, J.M., Eckersall, P.D. and Jennings, F.W.: Elevation of the concentration of acute phase proteins in dogs infected with Trypanosoma brucei. Acta Trop. (Basel), 49:77, 1991.

O'Neil, K.M., Ochs, H.D., Heller, S.R., et al.: Role of C3 in humoral immunity. Defective antibody production in C3-deficient dogs. J. Immunol., 140:1939, 1988.

Okumura, M., Fujinaga, T., Yamashita, K., et al.: Isolation, characterization, and quantitative analysis of ceruloplasmin from horses. Am. J. Vet. Res., 52:1979, 1991.

Osada, J. and Nowacki, W.: Elimination of goat haemoglobin and its complexes with goat haptoglobin from goat and rat circulation. Acta Biochim. Pol., 36:365, 1989.

Palley, L.S., Corning, B.F., Fox, J.G., et al.: Parvovirus-associated syndrome (Aleutian disease) in two ferrets. J. Am. Vet. Med. Assoc., 201:100, 1992.

Patterson, S.D., Auer, D. and Bell, K.: Acute phase response in the horse: plasma protein changes associated with adjuvant induced inflammation. Biochem. Int., 17:257, 1988.

Pearson, E.G.: Hypoalbuminemia in horses. Compend. Contin. Educ. Pract. Vet., 12:555, 1990.

Pedersen, N.C. and Barlough, J.E.: Clinical overview of feline immunodeficiency virus. Am. J. Vet. Med. Assoc., 199:1298, 1991.

Pedersen, N.C., Ho, E.W., Brown, M.L., et al.: Isolation of a T-lymphotropic virus from domestic cats with an immunodeficiency-like syndrome. Science, 235:790, 1987.

Pepin, M., Pardon, P., Lantier, F., et al.: Experimental Corynebacterium pseudotuberculosis infection in lambs: kinetics of bacterial dissemination and inflammation. Vet. Microbiol., 26:381, 1991.

Pepys, M.B., Baltz, M.L., Tennent, G.A., et al.: Serum amyloid A protein (SSA) in horses: Objective measurement of the acute phase response. Equine Vet. J., 21:106, 1989.

Perryman, L.E., Wyatt, C.R., Magnuson, N.S., et al.: T lymphocyte development and maturation in horses. Anim. Genet., 19:343, 1988.

Pfeffer, A., and Rogers, K.M.: Acute phase response of sheep: changes in the concentrations of ceruloplasmin, fibrinogen, haptoglobin and the major blood cell types associated with pulmonary damage. Res. Vet. Sci., 46:118, 1989.

Pleban, W.E.: Prealbumin: a biochemical marker of nutritional support. Conn. Med., 53:405, 1989.

Reinhoff, H.Y., Jr., Huang, J.H., Li, X.X., et al.: Molecular and cellular biology of serum amyloid A. Mol. Biol. Med., 7:287, 1990.

Roby, K.A., Beach, J., Bloom, J.C., et al.: Hepatocellular carcinoma associated with erythrocytosis and hypoglycemia in a yearling filly. Am. J. Vet. Med. Assoc., 196:465, 1990.

Rothschild, M.A., Oratz, M. and Schreiber, S.S.: Serum albumin. Hepatology, 8:385, 1988.

Routledge, P.A.: Clinical relevance of alpha 1 acid glycoprotein in health and disease. Prog. Clin. Biol. Res., 300:185, 1989.

Saenko, E.L., Skorobogat'ko, O.V. and Yaropolov, A.I.: Protective action of blood ceruloplasmin obtained from normal individuals on red blood cells compared with that from patients with Wilson's disease. Biomed. Sci., 1:453, 1990.

Sanchez, L., Aranda, P., Perez, M.D., et al.: Concentration of lactoferrin and transferrin throughout lactation in cow's colostrum and milk. Biol. Chem. Hoppe Seyler, 369:1005, 1988.

Schultz, D.R. and Arnold, P.I.: Properties of four acute phase proteins: C-reactive protein, serum amyloid A protein, alpha 1-acid glycoprotein, and fibrinogen. Semin. Arthritis Rheum., 20:129, 1990.

Shelton, G.H., Abkowitz, J.L., Linenberger, M.L., et al.: Chronic leukopenia associated with feline immunodeficiency virus infection in a cat. Am. J. Vet. Med. Assoc., 194:253, 1989.

Shelton, G.H., Linenberger, M.L., Grant, C.K., et al.: Hematologic manifestations of feline immunodeficiency virus infection. Blood, 76:1104, 1990.

Shelton, G.H., Linenberger, M.L., and Abkowitz, J.L.: Hematologic abnormalities in cats seropositive for feline immunodeficiency virus. Am. J. Vet. Med. Assoc., 199:1353, 1991.

Shofer, F.S., Glickman, L.T., Payton, A.J., et al.: Influence of parental serum immunoglobulins on morbidity and mortality of Beagles and their offspring. Am. J. Vet. Res., 51:239, 1990.

Skinner, J.G., Brown, R.A., and Roberts, L.: Bovine haptoglobin response in clinically defined field conditions. Vet. Rec., 128:147, 1991.

Smith, J.E. and Cipriano, J.E.: Inflammation-induced changes in serum iron analytes and ceruloplasmin of shetland ponies. Vet. Pathol., 24:354, 1987.

Solter, P.F., Hoffmann, W.E., Hungerford, L.L., et al.: Haptoglobin and ceruloplasmin as determinants of inflammation in dogs. Am. J. Vet. Res., 52:1738, 1991.

Splitter, G.A., Perryman, L.E., Magnuson, N.S., et al.: Combined immunodeficiency of horses: A review. Dev. Comp. Immunol., 4:21, 1980.

Stoddart, M.E., Whicher, J.T. and Harbour, D.A.: Cats inoculated with feline infectious peritonitis virus exhibit a biphasic acute phase plasma protein response. Vet. Rec., 123:622, 1988.

Stoneham, S.J., Digby, N.J. and Ricketts, S.W.: Failure of passive transfer of colostral immunity in the foal: incidence, and the effect of stud management and plasma transfusions. Vet. Rec., 128:416, 1991.

Taira, T., Fujinaga, T., Tamura, K., et al.: Isolation and characterization of α_1-acid glycoprotein from horses, and its evaluation as an acute-phase reactive protein in horses. Am. J. Vet. Res., 53:961, 1992.

Takiguchi, M., Fujinaga, T., Naiki, M., et al.: Isolation, characterization, and quantitative analysis of C-reactive protein from horses. Am. J. Vet. Res., 51:1215, 1990.

Tamura, K., Yatsu, T., Itoh, H., et al.: Isolation, characterization, and quantitative measurement of serum α_1-acid glycoprotein in cattle. Jpn. J. Vet. Sci., 51:987, 1989.

Thatcher, E.F. and Gershwin, L.J.: Colostral transfer of bovine immunoglobulin E and dynamics of serum IgE in calves. Vet. Immunol. Immunopathol., 20:325, 1989.

Thomas, R.L. and Blakemore, K.J.: Evaluation of elevations in maternal serum alpha-fetoprotein: a review. Obstet. Gynecol. Surv., 45:269, 1990.

Turnwald, G.H., Barta, O., Taylor, H.W., et al.: Cryptosporidiosis associated with immunosuppression attributable to distemper in a pup. Am. J. Vet. Med. Assoc., 192:79, 1988.

Walker, F.J. and Fay, P.J.: Characterization of an interaction between protein C and ceruloplasmin. J. Biol. Chem., 265:1834, 1990.

Watanabe, M., Ringler, D.J., Nakamura, M., et al.: Simian immunodeficiency virus inhibits bone marrow hematopoietic progenitor cell growth. J. Virol., 64:656, 1990.

Whitbread, T.J., Batt, R.M. and Garthwaite, G.: Relative deficiency of serum IgA in the German Shepherd dog: A breed abnormality. Res. Vet. Sci., 37:350, 1984.

Whitney, M.S., Boon, D., Rebar, A.H., et al.: Effect of acute pancreatitis on circulating lipids in dogs. Am. J. Vet. Res., 48:1492, 1987.

Williams, W.J., Beutler, E., Erslev, A.J., et al.: Hematology. 4th ed. New York, McGraw-Hill, 1990.

Witt, C.J., Moench, T.R., Gittelsohn, A.M., et al.: Epidemiologic observations on feline immunodeficiency virus and Toxoplasma gondii coinfection in cats in Baltimore, Md. Am. J. Vet. Med. Assoc., 194:229, 1989.

Yamada, T., Nagai, Y. and Matsuda, M.: Changes in serum immunoglobulin values in kittens after ingestion of colostrum. Am. J. Vet. Res., 52:393, 1991.

Yamamoto, J.K., Hansen, H., Ho, E.W., et al.: Epidemiologic and clinical aspects of feline immunodeficiency virus infection in cats from the continental United States and Canada and possible mode of transmission. Am. J. Vet. Med. Assoc., 194:213, 1989.

Yamamoto, J.K., Okuda, T., Ackley, C.D., et al.: Experimental vaccine protection against feline immunodeficiency virus. AIDS Res. Hum. Retroviruses, 7:911, 1991.

Yamashita, K., Fujinaga, T., Okumura, M., et al.: Serum C-reactive protein (CRP) in horses: the effect of aging, sex, delivery and inflammations on its concentration. J. Vet. Med. Sci., 53:1019, 1991.

Yoshinari, K., Yuasa, K., Iga, F., et al.: A growth-promoting factor for human myeloid leukemia cells from horse serum identified as horse serum transferrin. Biochim. Biophys. Acta, 1010:28, 1989.

Yoshino, K., Katoh, N., Takahashi, K., et al.: Purification of a protein from serum of cattle with hepatic lipidosis, and identification of the protein as haptoglobin. Am. J. Vet. Res., 53:951, 1992.

Young, B., Gleeson, M. and Cripps, A.W.: C-reactive protein: a critical review. Pathology., 23:118, 1991.

Zicker, S.C., Wilson, D. and Medearis, I.: Differentiation between intra-abdominal neoplasms and abscesses in horses, using clinical and laboratory data: 40 cases (1972–1988). Am. J. Vet. Med. Assoc., 196:1130, 1990.

Zon, L.I. and Groopman, J.E.: Hematologic manifestations of the human immune deficiency virus (HIV). Semin. Hematol., 25: 208, 1988.

Immunohematology

Immunohematology is the branch of medicine that deals with the antigenic structure of blood cells and with diseases of the blood resulting from antigen-antibody reactions. It is a distinct discipline in human medicine and is becoming important in veterinary medicine, mainly because of extensive investigations of blood group systems and transplantation antigens and recognition of the immunologic basis of disease. Originally, the field of immunohematology was primarily concerned with blood groups and related phenomena, such as blood transfusion and hemolytic disease of the newborn. It has now expanded to encompass tissue or organ transplantation and immune-mediated hematologic disorders. Blood groups and leukocyte and platelet antigens are being extensively studied as the disciplines of organ transplantation and immunogenetics continue to expand. The development of extremely sensitive serologic techniques, together with advances in understanding the role of complement and antibody in the pathogenesis of disease, have established the immunologic basis of certain hematologic disorders. Autoimmune hemolytic anemia is the classic example.

RED CELL ANTIGENS AND BLOOD GROUPS

The present knowledge of blood group antigens dates back to 1900, when Landsteiner discovered the ABO antigens in humans and Ehrlich and Morgenroth reported antigenic dissimilarities of goat red cells. Numerous red cell antigens have since been discovered in humans and animals.

The erythrocytes of common domestic animals possess several species-specific antigens belonging to many blood group systems (Table 22–1). These antigens, in different species, are arbitrarily designated by the same letters, but this does not imply that the antigens are related—for example, antigen A of the dog is not the same as the A antigen of humans. Blood group antigens characteristic of a species, however, may sometimes also be found on the red cells of another species (e.g., human blood group A- and H-antigens have been found on the red cells of pigs) (Sako et al., 1990).

Blood groups are usually inherited as simple mendelian dominant characters. All blood group genes except one are located on autosomes; the exception is the gene for a sex-linked antigen of humans (X_ga), which is located on the X chromosome. Antigens believed to be the products of allelic or closely linked genes are classified together in a blood group system. The B system of cattle, with over 1000 different alleles, is the most complex blood group system known in any species. The B system of goat, like its homologue in the sheep, is very complex (Nguyen, 1990). In the dog, it is only the A blood group which has subtypes; 4 alleles coding for 3 factors were recognized recently with the frequency of 0.224 (A^{a1}), 0.042 (A^{a2}), 0.045

Table 22–1. Blood Group Systems and Related Phenomena in Humans and Animals

Species	Blood Group Systems	Blood Group Factors	Techniques Generally Used for Blood Typing	Soluble Blood Group Factors in Body Fluids	Natural Alloantibodies in Serum	Transfer of Antibodies to the Young	Causes of Isoimmune Hemolytic Anemia
Bison	7	15+	Hemolytic	?	?	?	ND
Cats	2	2	Hemolytic Agglutination	?	Anti-A Anti-B	Colostrum	Pregnancy Experimental
Cattle	12	80+	Hemolytic	J	Anti-J	Colostrum	Vaccination
Chickens	12	30+	Agglutination	?	?	?	ND
Dogs	11	15+	Agglutination Hemolytic Antiglobulin	Tr, O	Anti-B Anti-D Anti-Tr	Colostrum	Experimental only
Goats	6	28+	Hemolytic Agglutination	?	?	?	ND
Horses	8	30+	Hemolytic Agglutination	ND*	Anti-A	Colostrum	Vaccination Pregnancy Transfusion
Humans	14	100+	Agglutination	A, B, H, Lewis	Anti-A Anti-B	In utero	Pregnancy Transfusion
Pigs	15	65+	Agglutination Hemolytic Antiglobulin	A, O	Anti-A Anti-E	Colostrum	Vaccination Bleeding Transfusion
Sheep	8	30+	Hemolytic Agglutination	R, O	Anti-R Anti-O	Colostrum	ND
Turkeys	7	12+	Agglutination	?	?	?	ND

* ND, not described.

(A^{a3}), and 0.669 (A^-) in various breeds of dogs from Australia (Symons and Bell, 1991). The existence of a new subtype A^{a3} in the canine A system has importance in blood transfusion. A_{a3} cells injected into an A negative dog can induce an immune response and hemolyze types a_1 and a_2 cells.

Antigens of all blood group systems in an individual are present on every one of its erythrocytes, with each blood group system occupying innumerable separate locations on the erythrocyte surface. Some of the erythrocyte antigens are also present on platelets, leukocytes, and other body tissues, although in weaker concentrations.

Certain blood group substances can be found in soluble form in blood plasma, saliva, milk, gastric juice, meconium, seminal fluid, and ovarian cyst fluid. Notable examples are the J antigen of cattle, the R and O antigens of sheep, the A and O antigens of pigs, the Tr and O antigens of dogs, and the Lewis antigen in humans (Table 22–1). Human blood group A and H substances have been found in the gastric mucin of pigs (Sako et al., 1990). Soluble blood group substances are produced in the tissues, secreted into the blood plasma, and then secondarily acquired by red cells in the circulation.

The isolation of blood group factors from bloody fluids in pure form has made it possible to characterize their chemical structures. The structures of A, B, H, and Lewis substances from human red cells have been determined and compared (Williams et al., 1990). The A and B antigens from red cells appear to be glycolipids, whereas those from secretions are glycoproteins. The serologic specificity in each case is determined by the carbohydrate component. Similar studies of animal blood groups have revealed the J blood group sub-

stance of bovine red cell membranes to be a glycosphingolipid with a terminal N-acetyl-D-galactosamine residue. The J substance in plasma occurs as a glycosphingolipid as well as a glycoprotein, but only the soluble lipidic J substance is secondarily acquired by the erythrocytes of cattle (Thiele, 1988). The form of neuraminic acid present on the major feline erythrocyte membrane glycolipid differs between types A and B cats, and may be responsible for the variation in reactivity of feline erythrocytes with wheat germ lectin (type B cells agglutinate, but type A do not). It may also be involved in determining the antigenic nature of the feline A and B blood types (Andrews, 1992; Butler et al., 1991).

Blood group substances vary in antigenicity. Naturally occurring antibodies (alloantibodies) to some red cell antigens can be found, although irregularly, in normal animals that lack the respective antigens. Examples are anti-J in cattle, anti-R in sheep, and anti-A in pigs (Table 22–1). These antibodies are believed to be produced from natural exposure of the animal to similar or identical antigenic determinants in nature. Seasonal variations may occur in the levels of natural alloantibodies. Specific antisera or reagents for blood typing purposes can be prepared from such natural sources, but natural antibodies in animals are found against only a few antigens and are generally present in low concentrations. Hence, most reagents for blood grouping in animals are obtained by planned alloimmunization and a few are obtained by heteroimmunization. Monospecific typing reagents are prepared by proper absorption with tissue cells or material to eliminate undesirable cross-reactive antibodies.

Regional differences may occur in the frequency of blood groups and alloantibodies against them. The

Table 22–2. Frequency of Blood Groups in Cats from Different Countries

Location	No. Sampled	Blood Type (%)*			Serum (%)**		Reference
		A	B	AB	Anti-A	Anti-B	
England	477	97.0	3.0	—	—	—	Holmes, 1950
France	350	85.0	15.0	—	66.7	27.3	Eyquem et al., 1962
Australia	1895	73.0	26.3	0.4	95.0	35.0	Auer and Bell, 1981
Japan	299	89.3	1.0	9.7	—	—	Ikemoto et al., 1981
Japan	207	90.3	9.7	—	—	—	Ejima et al., 1986
United States	485	99.6	0.4	0	100.0	30.0	Giger et al., 1989
United States	1100[a]	78.5	21.5	0	100.0	†	Giger et al., 1991
	1072[b]	99.7	0.3	0	100.0	†	

* Cats lacking blood types A and B have not been found, and A + B + cats are very rare.
** Blood group A cats contain weak isoagglutinins against type B cells (anti B), whereas blood group B contain strong anti-A.
† No or weak isoagglutinins found, but percentage data not described.
[a] Purebred cats.
[b] 964 domestic shorthair and 108 domestic longhair cats.

frequency of blood types A and B has been found to vary among cats from different countries, although type A cats predominated in each survey (Table 22–2). These studies show that anti-A alloantibodies are more frequent, act as strong agglutinins (titers, more than 1:8), and can cause serious incompatible transfusion reactions in type B cats. Anti-A isoagglutinins appear to be predominantly IgM and some IgG, whereas anti-B is comprised of low titers of the IgG and IgM types (Giger and Bucheler, 1991; Wilkerson et al., 1991). Anti-B antibodies are less frequent, usually act as weak agglutinins (titers, rarely more than 1:4), may occasionally have strong hemolytic activity, and do not cause any major clinical problems (Giger et al., 1989, 1991). No sex or breed preference was recorded for domestic shorthair cats. In a survey involving 400 purebred cats in the United States, Abyssinian, Birman, British shorthair, Devon Rex, Himalayan, Persian, and Somali cats were found to have a markedly higher proportion of type B blood than the less than 1% found in domestic shorthair cats (Giger, 1990). These observations were confirmed in a more recent similar survey involving 1100 purebred cats (Giger et al., 1991). In certain breeds as many as 50% had type B blood, but all Siamese cats had type A blood. Family studies have suggested that feline blood types A and B result from the action of two different alleles at the same gene locus, and that A is completely dominant over B. Neonatal isoerythrolysis was found in several purebred catteries with type B queens.

Techniques used for animal blood typing vary with the species (Table 22–1). Saline agglutination, a satisfactory method for typing human blood, is of limited use in animal blood typing. The hemolytic test system is the method of choice for typing cattle, sheep, and goat blood because red cells of these species are not prone to agglutinate. Fresh rabbit serum is generally used as a source of complement in the hemolytic test. Saline agglutination, however, can be used for grouping dog and pig red cells. Agglutination can be enhanced by incorporating dextran and serum albumin in the test system or by using papainized or trypsinized red cells. Hemolytic and saline agglutination tests are used simultaneously in some species, such as the horse. The antiglobulin test may also be used for blood typing in some animals, such as the pig and dog.

The importance of blood groups in genetics and breeding is well known. Monozygotic twins can be differentiated from dizygotic twins by the demonstration of blood group chimerism in the latter but not in the former. Blood groups may also serve as markers for the inheritance of certain biochemical and physiologic characteristics. For example, sheep with the gene for red cell antigen M also have the gene for high K^+ content in the erythrocyte, and stress susceptibility and hemorrhagic diathesis in pigs were associated with H blood types. The significance of human ABO antigens in transplantation has been established. The significance of blood groups in blood transfusion and in hemolytic disease of the newborn is well known, and is discussed below.

BLOOD TRANSFUSION

Transfusion therapy is basically an attempt to replace blood or its components when life is threatened without such a restoration. Although it is often a life-saving measure, it can be potentially dangerous; hence, transfusion should be instituted with extreme caution and care. An effective and safe transfusion requires accurate knowledge of the condition to be treated, determination of specific transfusion requirements, and awareness of the hazards and benefits associated with such therapy (Cotter, 1991; Giger and Bucheler, 1991; Slappendel, 1992; Stone et al., 1992). Appropriate whole blood, red cell, platelet, neutrophil, or plasma or component transfusion therapy is given when needed (Williams et al., 1990). Fluoro-carbon and hemoglobin solutions have been introduced as blood substitutes for oxygen transport, but an ideal substitute is not yet available (Vlahakes et al., 1990).

Generally, freshly collected neutrophils and platelets, fresh or stored whole blood or red cells (3 to 6 weeks at 4°C), and fresh or frozen plasma (up to 1 year at −40 to −70°C) are transfused.

Blood for transfusion may be collected in acid-citrate-dextrose (ACD) or citrate-phosphate-dextrose (CPD) solution and used fresh or stored in cold (lower than 10°C) up to 3 weeks for use as needed. Although canine-packed RBCs may be stored in citrate-phosphate-dextrose-adenine (CPDA-1) solution for 35 days, storage for longer than 20 days is not recommended based on the post-transfusion survival of transfused red cells (Price et al., 1988). CPDA-1 is composed of 1.66 g sodium citrate, 206.0 mg citric acid, 140.0 mg sodium dihydrogen phosphate, 2.0 g dextrose, and 17.3 mg adenine in water. Canine blood preserved in a special medium containing ascorbate phosphate, citric acid, sodium citrate, sodium phosphate, and dextrose and stored at 4°C can be safely used for up to 6 weeks (Smith et al., 1978). The survival and functional usefulness of erythrocytes decrease with increases in storage temperature and time because of glucose consumption and the depletion of ATP and 2,3-diphosphoglycerate. Donor animals may be maintained as a ready source of fresh blood. Donor dogs and cats should be splenectomized and blood typed to avoid incompatibility, at least of the major blood groups. They should be kept in excellent health and current on necessary vaccinations. Cats should be screened for FeLV and FIV infections. A nutritious diet and hematinics should be provided for optimum erythropoiesis. Frequent bleeding should be avoided to prevent the development of iron deficiency anemia. Dogs can tolerate repeated withdrawal of 13 to 17 ml blood/kg body weight every 3 to 4 weeks.

The transfusion of fresh, compatible whole blood or erthrocytes provides the full benefit of the therapy in that infused red cells circulate in the recipient for almost their normal life span. Conversely, incompatible erythrocytes are quickly destroyed by antibodies in the recipient at the time of transfusion or by antibodies that develop shortly thereafter. An acute hemolytic transfusion reaction or intravenous hemolysis occurs when highly incompatible red cells are infused. This process is complement-mediated and occurs within minutes of transfusion. It is recognized by the immediate appearance of mild to severe signs of anaphylactic shock, followed by hemoglobinemia and hemoglobinuria. A massive hemolysis may be accompanied by abnormal bleeding because of consumption coagulopathy. In minor incompatibilities, the erythrocytes are slowly destroyed as antibodies against them are produced by the recipient over a period of 4 to 14 days. This delayed transfusion reaction is accompanied by a progressive anemia, icterus, and a positive direct antiglobulin test. Clinical signs and laboratory findings in either event vary with the degree of incompatibility, amount of blood transfused, and animal species involved.

Excessive and rapid injection of blood or plasma can lead to circulatory overload and heart failure. The amount of blood to be transfused should be determined according to the body weight, estimated blood volume, and hematocrit of the recipient, hematocrit of the donor blood, and goal of the transfusion therapy. Blood should be warmed to body temperature prior to transfusion and should be given slowly, particularly when stored blood is used. Patients should be watched carefully for early signs of anaphylaxis, in which case the transfusion should be stopped immediately and adequate therapy instituted. In field situations involving ruminants, in the absence of crossmatching, a small amount of donor blood may be injected into the recipient. If no adverse reactions occur within 10 minutes, the rest of the blood can probably be given safely as long as circulatory overload problems are avoided (Hunt and Moore, 1990). Similarly, frozen plasma should be warmed and the appropriate amount should be administered slowly, avoiding anaphylactic reactions and cardiovascular overload.

Sensitivity to plasma proteins is generally responsible for allergic reactions seen following a transfusion. A sensitivity to leukocytes and platelets is the most common cause of fever following transfusion. The transmission of infection is a serious complication of blood transfusion. Examples include parasitic diseases, such as haemobartonellosis, toxoplasmosis, anaplasmosis, babesiasis, trypanosomiasis, theileriasis, and sarcocystosis, and viral diseases, such as infectious canine hepatitis and FeLV infection.

Blood typing and crossmatching to select a proper donor-recipient pair is a step to safeguard against a severe transfusion reaction (Jain, 1986). Blood typing may not be feasible in general veterinary practice because of a lack of suitable reagents. Crossmatching is the most practical approach. A common procedure is to perform saline agglutination, but this may be inadequate for certain species or under certain circumstances. For instance, the saline agglutination test is usually suitable for selecting donor dogs and cats, but hemolytic tests should be used for horses and cattle. It may be necessary to use direct and indirect antiglobulin tests to demonstrate the presence of nonagglutinating anti−red cell IgG antibodies in animals given multiple transfusions.

It has been a generally accepted principle in veterinary medicine that the first transfusion can be given safely without regard to blood typing and crossmatching, whereas subsequent transfusions require a proper match. This is not recommended, however, because it could be dangerous in certain animals (Giger and Akol, 1990; Jain, 1986). It is best to give properly matched blood to females, even the first time, to avoid primary sensitization, which carries a risk of offspring being born that may develop hemolytic disease. In studies from Australia, it was shown that about 50 to 60% of group B cats may experience a severe transfusion reaction, even the first time, when given as little as 1 ml of a 50% suspension of group A red cells. Hemolytic transfusion reactions are rarely seen in the United States because blood group B cats are rare in this country (Table 22–2). In any event, the destruction of erythrocytes by naturally occurring alloantibodies should be avoided by transfusing red cells lacking corresponding antigens. Furthermore, potent red cell antigens on donor red cells can evoke an antibody response within a few days, so that the second transfusion may carry the risk of a hemolytic transfusion reaction by immune-induced antibodies. The intravascular red cell survival in mismatched transfusions in cats is short (minutes to hours), even when given the first time (Giger and Bucheler, 1991).

Autotransfusion avoids the risks of alloimmunization to blood components, transmission of disease, and incompatible transfusion reactions. In addition, the patient itself serves as a ready source of compatible blood. Immediate complications of autotransfusion include intravascular hemolysis, disseminated intravascular coagulation (DIC), microembolism, and sepsis (Williams et al., 1990).

Blood transfusion studies in domestic ferrets have revealed some interesting findings (Manning and Bell, 1990). Blood groups of the type found in humans and other mammals were not detected, either because they did not exist or represented antigen systems too weak to elicit measurable responses. It was suggested that blood transfusion in this species poses little clinical risk, even without crossmatching.

HEMOLYTIC DISEASE OF THE NEWBORN

Hemolytic disease of the newborn, or neonatal isoerythrolysis (NI), is a consequence of maternal alloimmune blood group antibodies gaining access to the circulation of the fetus or newborn and destroying its erythrocytes (Williams et al., 1990; Jain, 1986). The principle involved is that the dam becomes sensitized to "foreign" red cell antigens in one or more of the following ways: (1) from the leakage of fetal red cells through the placenta during pregnancy and at parturition; (2) after immunization with homologous tissue vaccines or vaccines containing blood components; or (3) after injection of incompatible blood or blood products. The dam consequently synthesizes antibodies against such antigens and remains sensitized indefinitely. Mares have been found to produce antibodies to fetal red cells as soon as 56 days postconception. Cows vaccinated with red cell alloantigens may continue to produce alloantibodies for years. Such antibodies, depending on the type of placentation, enter the circulation of the fetus through transplacental passage or are acquired by the newborn after colostrum consumption (Table 22–1). Once in the blood of the fetus or newborn, these antibodies react with specific antigens on the erythrocytes and cause accelerated red cell destruction. Generally, the first offspring is born unaffected but subsequent ones are affected, with the severity increasing with the number of pregnancies involving the same sire or another sire of an identical blood group. Only the newborns carrying the red cell antigens acquired from the sire and not represented on erythrocytes of the dam are at risk. If the dam becomes sensitized through vaccination or blood transfusions, the chances are that the first offspring can be affected.

The disease has been recognized in humans, horses, mules, cattle, pigs, dogs, and cats (Bailey et al., 1988; Cain and Suzuki, 1985; Jain, 1986; Jonsson, 1990; Kahn et al., 1991; Luther et al., 1985; Williams et al., 1990; Zaruby et al., 1992). The natural incidence of the disease varies with the species and may be influenced by the geographic distribution of different blood group factors in a random animal population. The incidence of NI is estimated at 8 to 10% in mules, 0.05 to 1.0% in thoroughbred foals, and sporadic in ponies. NI has been recognized as a problem in calves from cows vaccinated for anaplasmosis or babesiosis. The occurrence and incidence of NI in calves were shown to be directly related to the number of doses of anaplasma vaccine injected and how close they were administered prior to calving. Natural NI is extremely rare in the dog and cat. The disease has been produced experimentally in the pigs, dogs, cattle, horses, cats, and chickens.

Alloimmunization with the Rh antigen causes erythroblastosis fetalis in the human newborn. In the horse, the antigens most often involved in NI include Aa and Qa (Bailey et al., 1988) and rarely Ab, Pa, and Ua (Zaruby et al., 1992). In the pig, the antigens involved are of blood group systems B, E, F, K, and L. In the cow, these have been antigens of the A and F-V systems and, in the dog, antigen A.

Natural antibodies to certain blood groups are found in the serum of some animal species and may appear in the colostrum (Table 22–1). Offspring of such dams, however, are not affected. This is thought to result from the absence of the corresponding antigen on erythrocytes at birth and from the presence of the soluble blood group factor in the gastric juice and plasma of the newborn. The former makes the red cells refractory to the antibody and the latter may neutralize the ingested antibody, first in the stomach and then in the circulation. The problem usually develops when dams produce alloantibodies as an immune response to foreign red cell antigens (see above). Antibodies to Aa and Qa antigens are produced in approximately 1 to 2% of all brood mares and may be associated with NI. Natural antibodies to Ca blood group antigen are found in 10% of the thoroughbred mares and 20% of the standardbred mares, but NI does not develop in foals ingesting the colostrum containing these antibodies (Bailey et al., 1988). Horses can develop transfusion-associated antibodies to red cell antigens Aa, Ae, Db, and Dc, and antibodies to the antigen Aa can persist up to 1 year. The occurrence of NI was avoided by withholding colostrum from two Aa-positive foals born of mares with corresponding alloantibodies in serum and colostrum, and a Db-positive foal remained healthy after nursing the mare with serum antibodies against Db (Wong et al., 1985).

Antibodies in the serum, colostrum, and early milk of the dam and in the serum of the newborn can be detected by the appropriate serologic tests. The colostrum usually contains higher concentrations of the antibody than the serum. Sensitization of erythrocytes of the newborn can be demonstrated by the complement-mediated hemolytic test or by the direct antiglobulin test. The antibody can be eluted from the erythrocytes by heat (50 to 56°C), and is generally of the IgG class.

Animals are generally born healthy but can develop the hemolytic syndrome within a few hours to a few days after the ingestion of colostrum. Affected animals show mild to severe signs typical of hemolytic anemia—weakness, pale mucous membranes, splenomegaly, icterus, hemoglobinemia, and hemoglobinuria. Neutrophils and monocytes with phagocytosed erythrocytes and sideroleukocytes may be found in anemic and icteric foals. Piglets with NI may also have thrombocytopenic purpura and neutropenia. Piglets may also develop neonatal isoimmune (alloimmune) thrombocytopenia from the absorption of colostral antiplatelet antibodies. Similarly, foals may develop neonatal isoimmune neutropenia from the absorption of colostral antineutrophil antibodies. Peracute NI in calves causes death in less than 24 hours; acute NI causes death in 5 to 7 days. Chronically affected calves recover in 3 to 4 weeks, but remain unthrifty and show increased susceptibility to infection such as anaplasmosis (Luther et al., 1985).

The severity of NI depends on the following: (1) the concentration of the antibody in the serum and colostrum of the dam; (2) the amount of antibody entering the serum of the newborn (this depends on the amount of colostrum ingested and on the absorptive capacity of the digestive tract of the young); and (3) the nature of the antigen-antibody reaction. Severely affected animals may die within 24 hours from acute respiratory distress, but death in most untreated patients occurs within 2 to 6 days. Death is attributed to DIC resulting from the activation of the coagulation system by membranes of the lysed red cells. At necropsy, hepatomegaly and splenomegaly may be found, and histopathologic examination reveals degenerative changes in the liver and kidneys. Some animals recover within a few weeks.

Treatment of the affected animal consists of a blood transfusion, given intravenously or intraperitoneally. An exchange transfusion may be given when the red cell values fall below a critical level for the species, but this might not be feasible if adequate facilities are unavailable. A healthy compatible donor is ideal, but difficult to find. Alternatively, thoroughly washed (at least three times with isotonic saline) red cells of the dam may be transfused, with favorable results. Corticosteroids may be given to reduce the immune elimination of red cells.

The possibility of an offspring experiencing the hemolytic disease can be determined by testing the sire's red cells against the dam's serum during pregnancy. If positive results are obtained, foster-feeding the newborn for the first 2 days before allowing it to suckle the dam would prevent development of the hemolytic disease. Thus, NI can be prevented by withholding colostrum because colostrum is the main source of antibodies for the newborn calves and foals. A practical approach for preventing the sensitization of women and the development of hemolytic disease of the newborn involves injecting anti-Rh antibodies to mothers at risk soon after delivery.

LEUKOCYTE ANTIGENS AND ANTIBODIES AND HISTOCOMPATIBILITY ANTIGENS

Numerous leukocyte antigens have been found in humans, and similar results on various animal species are being obtained. These leukocyte antigens include histocompatibility or transplantation antigens, blood group or red cell antigens, and leukocyte-specific antigens. Transplantation antigens may be defined as those antigens on the cells and tissues that, after grafting, induce an immune response in the host, resulting in a rejection phenomenon. Such antigens are found on the leukocytes of humans and many animal species. A few lymphocyte-specific and neutrophil-specific antigens have also been recognized in humans, but these are not considered transplantation antigens. Human leukocytes have been found to contain several blood group factors in minute quantities, but the evidence is equivocal, except for antigens A and B. In animal studies, porcine red cell antigens of systems A, E, G, and N, bovine B-system and J antigens, and ovine B-system and R antigens have been found on the lymphocytes of the respective species. In addition, some human leukocyte antigens are partially or wholly represented on the leukocytes of several animal species.

Leukocyte Antigens and Antibodies in Humans

LEUKOCYTE ANTIGENS

Well-defined human leukocyte (lymphocyte) antigens (HLA) are considered gene products of four separate loci, designated HLA-A, HLA-B, HLA-C, and HLA-D. The first three loci control HLA-A, HLA-B, and HLA-C antigens, respectively, whereas the HLA-D region encompasses genes controlling HLA-D, HLA-DR, HLA-DP, and HLA-DQ antigens. Thus, seven groups of HLA antigens have been recognized so far in humans. HLA-A, HLA-B, and HLA-C antigens are present on most nucleated cells, and antigens of the remaining HLA groups are found primarily on B lymphocytes. HLA-A, HLA-B, and HLA-C antigens are recognized by serologic tests, but HLA-D antigens are determined by the mixed lymphocyte culture or reaction (MLC or MLR). They are also known as serologically defined (SD) and lymphocyte-defined (LD) antigens, respectively. HLA-DR and HLA-DQ antigens are detected by serologic tests using B lymphocytes. Similar antigens have also been found in dogs, pigs, and cattle. HLA-DP antigens are determined by a variant of the MLC test.

HLA loci are situated in close proximity on a small segment of the short arm of chromosome 6. This genetic region is known as the major histocompatibility complex (MHC) and its gene products constitute the major histocompatibility system (MHS). Several minor histocompatibility systems have also been recognized. Observations in humans and animals have indicated that the MHC region also contains immune-response genes and genes for some complement components and select red cell enzymes. These findings form the basis of distinguishing different regions within the MHC in various species. The class I region controls serologically defined antigens of the HLA-A, HLA-B, and HLA-C systems, which are important in transplantation. The class II region controls antigens of the HLA-D system clustered into 4 distinct subregions referred to as DO, DP, DQ, and DR, as well as immune responsiveness to particulate antigens and graft-versus-host reaction. Cloning and sequencing data indicate that the HLA-D regions contains at least 6 α chains and 7 β chains. The class III region, located between the HLA-B and HLA-DR regions, controls the expression of complement components C2, C4, and factor B. Class I and II HLA antigens control T-cell responses.

The antigens at each HLA locus are controlled by mutually exclusive multiple allelomorphic genes. This means that, in a given instance, only one allele is present at each locus on each chromosome of the pair. Therefore, in regard to phenotype, only two antigens from each locus can be present in an individual, and a parent can pass on to a child only one antigen from each locus. For example, with four siblings, each has a 1:4 or 25% probability of being identical to another sibling. This chromosomal combination of genetic determinants from each locus (from one parent) is called a haplotype, and is significant in organ transplantation.

Various human leukocyte antigens form a component of the cell surface membrane with some subcellular location. Highly purified, soluble MHC class I (HLA-A, HLA-B, and HLA-C) antigens are transmembrane glycoproteins (MW, 56,000) composed of two asymmetric polypeptide chains, one larger (MW, 45,000) and the other smaller (MW, 11,000), bound by noncovalent bonds. The larger chain carries the HLA specificity, whereas the smaller chain is a β_2-microglobulin. This structural configuration indicates some homology among antigens of these loci and the IgG molecule. The class II or HLA-D family of antigens similarly has two noncovalently bound chains, a larger chain (MW, 34,000) and a smaller β chain (MW, 29,000), but lack the β_2-microglobulin. The biochemical characterization of some MHS antigens in the dog, pig, and cattle has yielded generally similar results. Soluble forms of class I molecules have been found in sera of mice and horses.

LEUKOCYTE ANTIBODIES

Leukocyte antibodies are almost always acquired by alloimmunization. Acquired isoantibodies to leuko-cytes develop after multiple transfusions, during pregnancy (usually in multiparous females), after immunization with skin grafts or leukocytes, and after organ transplantation. Sera from such individuals have been used for leukocyte typing after adequate absorption to produce a "monospecific" serum. Monoclonal antibodies can be produced and utilized for blood and tissue typing.

The occurrence of natural isoantibodies to leukocytes has not been conclusively demonstrated. Autoantibodies to leukocytes have been found in human patients with connective tissue diseases, cirrhosis, viral infections, leukemia, and drug allergies. Neutropenia or agranulocytosis has been observed in association with such autoantibodies in some cases.

Leukocyte antibodies in vitro inhibit mobility and the phagocytic activity of neutrophils and induce cytopathic changes that lead to leukocytolysis. A febrile reaction and anaphylaxis may develop following an intravenous injection of a potent antileukocyte serum. Marked leukopenia is a consistent finding. These effects of antileukocyte antibodies are not species-specific, because a certain degree of cross-reactivity has been found.

Leukocyte and Histocompatibility Antigens in Animals

Research on leukocyte antigens in animals during the last two decades has discovered several antigenic systems in common domestic animals (Table 22–3). These constitute an MHS, which is generally referred to by an acronym specific for each species. International conferences and workshops are being held to standardize methodology and develop a unified system of nomenclature for the lymphocyte antigens of various animal species. The swine leukocyte antigen (SLA) complex is located on chromosome 7, is linked with the J and C blood group loci, and has 3 class I and 2 class II loci (Varewyck et al., 1990). Significant differences have been found in the frequency of various bovine leukocyte antigens (BLA) in different breeds of cattle (Stear et al., 1988). Similarly, dog lymphocyte antigens (DLA) vary between Beagles and mixed-breed dogs (Bull et al., 1987).

Typing reagents can be obtained from various sources, such as planned immunization (skin grafts and lymphocyte preparations), pregnant females, and colostrum. Lymphocyte cytotoxic antibodies, presumably resulting from transplacental immunization of the fetus, have been found in the sera of parous females of different animal species with a high frequency. Bovine red cell typing reagents have been found to contain antibodies against lymphocyte antigens, but the two groups of antibodies seem to be directed against distinct cellular antigens rather than against antigens in common. Similarly, some equine blood typing reagents may contain antibodies against lymphocytes, and infrequently contain antibodies against neutrophils and platelets. Leukocyte antibodies have been found with increasing frequency in sera of cows

Table 22–3. Major Histocompatibility System (MHS) in Different Animal Species

Species	Term for MHS	Loci or Antigens Defined*
Cattle	BoLA	50 specificities recognized; 2 SD loci and 1 LD locus
Chicken	B	15 SD antigens on 4 loci of classes I through IV
Chimpanzee	ChLA	14 SD antigens on 2 loci; 5 antigens on 1 LD locus
Dog	DLA	15 antigens on 3 SD loci; 9 antigens on 1 LD locus
Goat	GLA	12 SD antigens on 2 loci; 2 class II loci recognized
Guinea pig	GPLA	6 SD antigens on 2 loci; 3 LD antigens on 3 loci; 1 DR antigen
Horse	ELA	19 specificities coded by 1 SD locus; 3 specifics coded by a class II locus
Human	HLA	3 SD loci and 1 LD locus on chromosome 6
Mouse	H-2	Many antigens; 3 SD loci (K, D, L) and 2 LD loci (A, E) on chromosome 17
Rabbit	RLA	About 10 SD antigens on 2 loci; 5 antigens on 1 LD locus
Rat	RT1	13 SD antigens on 2 loci; 12 LD antigens on 2 loci
Rhesus monkey	RhLA	24 SD antigens on 2 SD loci; 1 more SD locus postulated; 1 major LD locus and 1 minor LD locus
Sheep	OLA	12 antigens on 2 SD loci; 1 class II locus recognized
Swine	SLA	30 SD antigens on 3 loci; 6 LD antigens on 2 LD loci

* SD, serologically defined or MHC class I; LD, lymphocyte-defined or MHC class II; DR, D-related antigens demonstrated serologically or class III antigens.

carrying unrelated transferred embryos (Matousek and Riha, 1991). Unlike most species, cats do not appear to develop lymphocyte cytotoxic antibodies in response to pregnancy- or transfusion-mediated antigenic exposure, although some cats have natural lymphocytotoxic antibodies. Cats also show only a relatively weak MLR among unrelated cats of different breeds.

The MHC of cattle is comprised of the BoLA system antigens. It contains a class I locus (BoLA-A) with at least 50 serologically-defined specificities and a class II locus (BoLA-D) with several specificities defined earlier by MLC assay and more recently by serologic and biochemical analyses (Andersson et al., 1986; Bernoco et al., 1991). Some of the BoLA-A specificities may be gene products of a second class I locus, namely BoLA-B (Joosten et al, 1992). The BoLA-D locus contains DN, DO, DQ, DR, and DY subregions, analogous to those described for the human HLA-D locus (Andersson and Rask, 1988; Joosten et al., 1989) and appears to be highly polymorphic as shown by isoelectric focusing and restriction fragment length polymorphism (RFLP) analysis (Bernoco et al., 1991; Vage et al., 1992). Some genes of the BoLA-D locus are closely linked to the bovine MHC Class I locus. A serologic relationship has been found between some antigens of the BoLA-A system and the bovine M blood group

system (Hines and Ross, 1987). Associations of BoLA-A locus antigens with increased susceptibility to polyclonal expansion of bovine leukemia virus-infected B lymphocytes (Lewin et al., 1988) and with increased antibody-dependent neutrophil cytotoxicity and decreased susceptibility to subclinical mastitis (Weigel et al., 1991) have been found.

The DLA system is comprised of 3 serologically-defined loci, designated DLA-A, DLA-B, and DLA-C (Bull et al., 1987) and an MLC-defined system, termed DLA-D (Deeg et al., 1986). The genomic hybridization studies have shown that the DLA-D region has at least 5 α genes and 7 β genes, and RFLP analysis indicated the presence of at least 9 DLA-D types. Nucleic acid sequence analysis further defined 9 distinct alleles belonging to the 3 major allelic groups in the DLA-DRB subregion (Sarmiento et al., 1990). The DLA-B locus codes for the MLC class II antigens on almost all lymphocytes in the dog (Doxiadis et al., 1989). Two monocyte-associated antigens have been recognized in the dog, but their inheritance pattern remains to be established (Krumbacher et al., 1991).

The Fifth International Workshop on equine lymphocyte antigens (ELA) recognized 19 specificities belonging to the ELA-A locus, 3 specificities as gene products of a second ELA locus other than ELA-A, and the possibility of still another locus defined by a specificity (Lazary et al., 1988). It was also apparent that pregnancy immunization produces primarily antibodies to class I antigens, whereas planned alloimmunization of recipients lacking certain ELA-A antigens results in production of antibodies to class I and II antigens as well non-MHC antigens. Biochemical studies subsequently indicated that the above 3 specificities recognize antigens of an equine MHC Class II locus (Hesford et al., 1989). A predisposition of horses for sarcoid tumors was associated with an ELA-linked gene (Brostrom et al., 1988).

The expression of ovine leukocyte antigens (OLA) is controlled by at least 2 distinct class I MHC loci (Gogolin-Ewens et al., 1985). A class II MHC locus with at least 7 α genes and as many as 24 β gene fragments has been defined (Deverson et al., 1991). In the goat, 12 specificities believed to be coded by 2 closely linked MHC class I loci have been reported (Nesse and Ruff, 1989). Biochemical analysis defined 2 goat MHC class II loci, one of which was a DR-like locus with 7 allelic variants (Joosten et al., 1991).

The MHC in the chicken is described under the B blood group system and various MHC antigens are coded by 3 loci, namely B-F, B-G, and B-L (Kline et al., 1988; Toivanen and Vainio, 1987). Class I or B-F antigens are present on most nucleated cells, including the leukocytes and erythrocytes. Different B-F antigens may be found on different cells (T- or B-cells) and their expression may be related to the stage of development (erythrocytes from embryos or adults). Class II or B-L antigens are present on B lymphocytes, monocytes, macrophages, and some stimulated T lymphocytes. Class IV or B-G antigens are found on erythrocytes and their precursors and are unique for the avian species. The existence of class III genes encoding for complement component remains to be confirmed.

Laboratory Determination

Several techniques can be used to detect leukocyte antigens and antibodies. Those commonly used are lymphocyte microcytotoxicity, leukoagglutination, and complement fixation tests. These techniques vary in sensitivity, but the lymphocyte microcytotoxicity test is the basic tissue typing procedure. As mentioned previously, this test detects antigens of the HLA-A, HLA-B, and HLA-C systems, or corresponding antibodies. It also detects HLA-DR and HLA-DQ antigens. HLA-D antigens are detected by the MLR, whereas the HLA-DP antigens are detected by a modification of the MLR called the primed lymphocyte test. The basis of the latter test is that lymphocytes primed to respond to a particular antigen during an initial MLR respond to only that antigen in a secondary MLC. The degree of compatibility between two individuals (histocompatibility matching) without regard to knowledge of their HLA identity can be assessed by the MLR test.

Significance of Histocompatibility or Transplantation Antigens

ABO and HLA-A, HLA-B, and HLA-C antigens are strong transplantation antigens in humans because they are present in many tissues (in differing concentrations), including the skin, kidneys, heart, liver, lungs, leukocytes, and platelets. Antigens of the HLA-D family are found primarily on B lymphocytes and also on macrophages, monocytes, endothelial cells, and activated T cells. They can be induced on tissues normally lacking them by γ-interferon treatment. Soluble HLA antigens are found in plasma and urine. HLA antigens are not found on erythrocytes, although some may be present on reticulocytes. In mice, H-2 antigens are found on red cells.

The significance of histocompatibility antigens is varied. It is becoming increasingly apparent that they play a central role in the immune response through the regulation of T-lymphocyte responses. The HLA system is the most polymorphic system known in humans. Lymphocyte antigens, like red cell antigens, therefore appear to be suitable markers for anthropologic studies and paternity testing. In animals, correlations of these antigens with certain physiologic traits such as body weight and productivity and breeding are being determined.

Histocompatibility antigens are important in various clinical situations in human medicine. It is now accepted that ABO compatibility is a prerequisite for transplantation. The importance of HLA antigens as

the histocompatibility antigens has been demonstrated in many in vitro and in vivo experiments involving skin grafts and kidney, heart, and bone marrow transplants. HLA compatibility significantly improves the chances of graft survival. It has become evident that HLA-B antigens are more important in graft survival than are antigens of the A and C loci. The importance of DLA in organ transplantation has been demonstrated in studies on dogs. In addition to the clinical application of SLA in pigs as experimental models for organ transplantation, it is becoming increasingly apparent that they are also important in the breeding and selection of pigs.

Leukocyte antibodies are considered a cause of most febrile transfusion reactions. Leukocyte antibodies found in the sera of pregnant and multiparous women are formed during pregnancy in response to "foreign" HLA antigens on the fetal cells. Most of these antibodies are of the IgG type and can therefore cross the placental barrier. These antibodies, on rare occasions, have been found to produce cytopenias (e.g., neonatal thrombocytopenia or isoimmune neonatal purpura) because HLA antigens are present on platelets. Long-term platelet transfusions may provoke an immune response to HLA antigens and platelet-specific antigens not present in the recipient. Such antibodies can cause problems in subsequent transfusions; in particular, they can induce a febrile reaction or decreased survival of cells (platelets and leukocytes). Non-HLA antibodies, but not HLA-antibodies, have been found to produce isoimmune neonatal neutropenia. Similarly, leukocyte antibodies have been associated with rare instances of leukopenia in newborns pigs, calves, and foals.

Studies of the relationship of certain HLA antigens to the susceptibility to disease in humans are being undertaken. A particular disease may be associated or linked to certain HLA antigens. In general, more correlations have been found with HLA-D/HLA-DR antigens than with HLA-A and HLA-B antigens. For example, the HLA-B8, DR3 haplotype is associated with many autoimmune diseases and about 90% of patients with ankylosing spondylitis have HLA-B27 antigen, compared to only a 9.4% incidence in controls. Similar disease associations are being investigated in animals.

PLATELET ANTIGENS AND ANTIBODIES

Human platelets, like leukocytes, contain the following: (1) blood group antigens A and B, and possibly others; (2) all currently known HLA-A antigens, most HLA-B antigens, and some HLA-C antigens; and (3) some platelet-specific antigens. Platelet-specific antigens are associated with membrane glycoproteins Ia, Ibα, IIa, IIbα, IIIa, and V (Kunicki and Beardsley, 1989). Some of the antigens of human platelets are also shared by the platelets of animal species, such as the pig, sheep, cattle, and dog (Jain, 1986).

Neonatal and Post-transfusion Purpura in Humans

Isoantibodies reacting with platelets may develop after multiple blood transfusions, pregnancies, leukocyte or platelet injections, or skin or organ grafting. Although the thromboagglutination test can detect some antibodies, the complement fixation test is the method of choice for detecting platelet antigens and antibodies. Transplacental alloimmunization of the mother to fetal platelet antigens or HLA-A antigens has been reported to cause neonatal alloimmune thrombocytopenia and purpura in human newborns (Bussel et al., 1991; Kaplan et al., 1991; Kunicki and Beardsley, 1989). Infants become thrombocytopenic shortly after birth. Neonatal alloimmune amegakaryocytosis has been found to occur in association with thrombocytopenia (Bizzaro and Dianese, 1988). Neonatal thrombocytopenia may also develop in a child born of a mother with autoimmune thrombocytopenia (AITP).

Platelet alloantibodies in humans reduce graft survival and the intravascular life span of platelets carrying the corresponding antigens. Rare cases of what is known as post-transfusion purpura (PTP) have been encountered in humans. In this condition, sensitization to the transfused platelets develops, resulting in the destruction of the platelets (of both the donor and the recipient) and purpura in the sensitized individual. The mechanism involved is not definitively known (Kunicki and Beardsley, 1989). Similar observations about PTP have been made in dogs and pigs (Jain, 1986)

Neonatal Thrombocytopenic Purpura in Pigs

Thrombocytopenic purpura in piglets has been reported to occur as a result of maternal alloimmunization. Agglutinating antibodies against thrombocytes of the piglet and sire can be demonstrated in the serum of the dam. Antibodies in the colostrum have not been detected because of technical difficulties. Sensitization of the sow persists indefinitely, and may affect subsequent litters, even with a different sire. Although a relationship between red cell and platelet antigens has not been established, alloantibodies to certain red cell antigens were found (mainly of the E, but also of the K and L systems) in about 50% of sows having thrombocytopenic litters.

The piglets are generally born healthy, although an occasional piglet may be thrombocytopenic and purpuric at birth. The platelets decrease in number abruptly after 5 to 9 days, reach a nadir at 10 to 13 days, and completely disappear in some piglets at 1 to 2 days before death. The thrombocytopenia results from both platelet destruction and impaired marrow production. Abnormalities in coagulation tests corresponding to a low platelet count may be found. The thrombocytopenia is accompanied by subcutaneous hemorrhage along the ventral abdominal wall and medial aspects of the legs and behind the ears. A concurrent anemia, sometimes accompanied by leukopenia, may develop in some piglets. Death can occur within a few days in severely involved cases or by 2 to 3 weeks of age. Lesions at necropsy are typical of those of hemorrhagic diathesis. The most outstanding finding on histopathologic examination is a complete or almost complete absence of megakaryocytes in the bone marrow. The surviving pigs appear clinically and hematologically normal by 16 weeks of age.

BONE MARROW TRANSPLANTATION

Bone marrow transplantation is now being performed more frequently in humans with various neoplastic or non-neoplastic diseases and inherited hematologic and metabolic diseases. It is the treatment of choice for patients with lethal primary immunodeficiencies, severe aplastic anemia, or congenital aregenerative anemia. It is also beneficial to patients with acute myeloid and lymphoid leukemias, chronic myelogenous leukemia, lymphoma, or other congenital and acquired disorders of hematopoiesis, such as lysosomal storage disorders. Prior to marrow transplantation, patients with malignant diseases may be given total body irradiation and aggressive chemotherapy to destroy as many neoplastic cells as possible. Progress in marrow transplantation in humans has been achieved through a better understanding of histocompatibility antigens, the development of methods to select appropriate donors, achieve adequate immunosuppression, and control infection, the availability of cloned hematopoietic growth factors, and supportive care, such as granulocyte and platelet transfusions (Lasky, 1991; Metcalf, 1989; Sullivan, 1989; Williams et al., 1990). All these factors have contributed to the long-term, disease-free survival of many transplant recipients.

Bone marrow transplantation has been performed in dogs with cyclic hematopoiesis, pyruvate kinase deficiency, and lysosomal storage diseases (Constantopoulos et al., 1989; Gompf et al., 1990; Jain, 1986; Taylor et al., 1989) and as a model for bone marrow transplantation in humans (Greinix et al., 1991; Kolb et al., 1990). Bone marrow transplantation studies performed on 72 cats with lysosomal storage disorders at the Colorado State University Bone Marrow Transplant Laboratory have shown an engraftment rate of 70.6%, with survival being as long as 5 years (Fulton et al., 1990). In another study, successful bone marrow engraftment was achieved in cats by using intensive total body γ-irradiation, with or without the administration of cyclosporin A (Cain et al., 1990). Immune-mediated hemolytic anemia and thrombocytopenia developed as a complication in 1 of 7 cats reported in the latter study.

Bone marrow transplantation in humans has been performed using marrow from syngeneic (genetically identical) or allogeneic (genetically nonidentical) donors or autologous marrow. Autologous marrow is collected from the patient (and kept frozen) prior to ablative cytoreductive therapy. Autotransplantation and transplantations between HLA-identical siblings or identical twins are invariably successful. The chances of finding an ideal unrelated compatible donor are extremely low, because the MHS is highly pleomorphic. Marrow aspirates are dispersed into single-cell suspensions by filtration and infused intravenously. Engraftment usually occurs in about 2 weeks. A successful transplantation results in gradual increases in bone marrow cellularity and blood cell counts. Host resistance is markedly reduced during the early phase, however, because of marrow aplasia induced by intensive preparatory immunosuppressive therapy. An increased frequency of bacterial and fungal infections during this period may require therapy with broad-spectrum antibiotics, antifungal agents, and neutrophil transfusions. The development of severe anemia and thrombocytopenia may require red cell and platelet transfusion, respectively. Other complications include bleeding, immune-mediated hemolysis, endocrine disorders, malignant disease, and disease recurrence.

Major problems with bone marrow transplantation arise from the development of graft-versus-host disease (GVHD), which leads to rejection of the graft when the donor and recipient are genetically different. This has been shown in human studies and in canine and murine models of bone marrow transplantation. The lymphoid cells of an immune-competent host recognize the graft as "nonself" and develop an immunologically destructive reaction against the graft within weeks to months. The destruction of all host lymphocytic tissue by total body X-irradiation or some other immunosuppressive conditioning regimen leads to the acceptance of an allogeneic graft. Unless the donor and recipient are histocompatible, the repopulated donor-type lymphoid cells mount an immune response against the host and cause a GVHD, producing destruction of the host's tissues. Loss of weight, diarrhea, organ dysfunction, interstitial pneumonia, and infection lead to death in those with acute and chronic GVHD. Infections usually involve opportunistic organisms (e.g., Pneumocystis carinii and cytomegalovirus).

The severity of the GVHD increases with a disparity in histocompatibility. Animal experiments have shown that the severity of the GVHD is reduced and survival of the recipient is increased if a donor is matched with the recipient at the MHC. Human patients are matched for antigens of the HLA-A, HLA-B, and HLA-D loci, but complete identity is rarely found. Furthermore, GVHD also occurs in many cases of HLA identity, perhaps indicating nonidentity in yet to be identified HLA antigens, or for reasons unknown. Immunosuppressive agents such as glucocorticoids, cyclosporin, and methotrexate have been used to control GVHD. Newer approaches are being sought to prevent GVHD and prolong graft survival by various means, such as the removal of T lymphocytes including cytotoxic T cells from the donor marrow using immunologic methods (Raff et al., 1988). Treatment of blood with gamma irradiation alone or in combination with heat (45°C

for 45 minutes) prevents transfusion-induced sensitization to minor histocompatibility antigens (Bean et al., 1991). Allogeneic bone marrow transplantation in utero in sheep and monkey fetuses resulted in a long-term postnatal hematopoietic chimerism without the development of a GVH disease or without the use of cytoablative procedures (Zanjani et al., 1991).

AUTOIMMUNE HEMATOLOGIC DISORDERS

Immune-mediated hematologic disorders can be broadly categorized into two groups. One group is comprised of conditions induced by alloantibodies (isoantibodies), which may occur naturally or develop after exposure to alloantigens (isoantigens). These conditions include neonatal isoerythrolysis or hemolytic disease of the newborn, neonatal alloimmune thrombocytopenia, neonatal alloimmune leukopenia, and hemolytic transfusion reactions, and have been discussed in previous sections in this chapter. The other group is comprised of conditions caused by autoantibodies produced against self-antigens at some time during the postnatal period. Examples in this category are autoimmune hemolytic anemia (AIHA), autoimmune thrombocytopenia (AITP), autoimmune neutropenia, and certain drug-induced hemolytic anemias, thrombocytopenias, and leukopenias. Each of these conditions has been reported in humans (Bux and Mueller-Eckhardt, 1992; Collins and Newland, 1992; Engelfriet et al, 1992; Kaplan et al., 1992; Kiefel et al., 1992; Waters, 1992; Williams et al., 1990) and some have been found in animals (Jain, 1986).

Autoimmune Hemolytic Anemia

Autoimmune hemolytic anemia has been reported in the dog, cat, horse and, rarely, in the ox. AIHA is a consequence of red cell destruction mediated by autologous antibodies. Thus, it is characterized by a decreased survival of circulating erythrocytes and the presence of autoantibodies to the red cells. The anemia is usually regenerative—it is accompanied by increased reticulocytosis, polychromasia, normoblastemia in blood, and bone marrow erythroid hyperplasia. Associated findings can include jaundice, hemoglobinemia, hemoglobinuria, an elevated indirect bilirubin level, and an increased fecal stercobilin level, depending on the extent and mode of red cell destruction. The presence of spherocytes (Plate XVI-4; Fig. 22–1) and increased erythrocyte osmotic fragility (Figs. 7–15, 22–2) further indicates an immune-mediated hemolytic process.

Essential for the definitive diagnosis of AIHA is the demonstration of autoantibodies to erythrocytes. The classic procedure used for this purpose is the antiglobulin (Coombs) test (see below). Because of limitations in the sensitivity of the Coombs test, however, red cells coated with extremely low levels of antibody

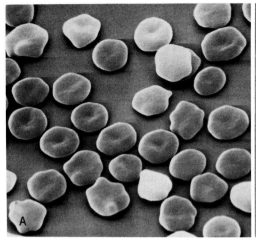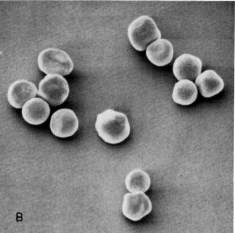

Fig. 22–1. Scanning electron photomicrographs of feline normal biconcave discocytic erythrocytes (A) compared with spherocytes (B) from a cat with autoimmune hemolytic anemia. A few slightly crenated cells are also present in A (× 3600). (From Jain, N.C.: Schalm's Veterinary Hematology. 4th Ed. Philadelphia, Lea & Febiger, 1986, p. 1015.)

(less than 300 to 400 molecules of IgG/cell) or complement (less than 60 to 115 molecules of C3/cell) may escape detection, constituting the so-called Coombs-negative AIHA. Such cases should be investigated using more sensitive methods, such as the enzyme-linked immunosorbent assay (ELISA) and radioimmunoassay procedures (Jones et al., 1992; Porter et al., 1989). With the use of ELISA, it was shown that the degree of hemolysis in primary immune-mediated hemolytic anemia is related to the degree of red cell sensitization, particularly when IgG antibody is involved (Jones et al., 1992).

CLASSIFICATION AND ANTIBODIES INVOLVED

AIHA is generally classified according to its cause and the thermal reactivity of the autoantibody involved. AIHA resulting from antibody formation of unknown cause is considered primary or idiopathic, whereas that having a well-defined disease association is considered secondary or symptomatic. The latter category includes AIHA seen in association with lymphoproliferation disorders, connective tissue diseases (e.g., systemic lupus erythematosus, SLE), viral, bacterial and parasitic infections, certain chronic inflammatory conditions, and therapy with certain drugs. Both primary and secondary AIHA have been found in dogs (Feldman et al, 1985; Jackson and Kruth, 1985; Jones and Gruffydd-Jones, 1991; Jain, 1986; Jones et al,. 1992; Porter and Weisser, 1990; Porter et al., 1989; Tsuchida et al., 1991; Victoria et al., 1990), cats (Jain, 1986), horses (Beck, 1990; Mair et al., 1990; Messer and Arnold, 1991; Sockett et al., 1987; Taylor and Cooke, 1990), and cattle (Fenger et al., 1992; Jain, 1986). Rarely, AIHA and AITP may occur simultaneously; the condition is then called Evans syndrome. In Evans syndrome, different antibodies are directed against platelets and red cells and cellular immunity is probably also abnormal (Wang, 1988).

What provokes individuals to develop antibodies to their own tissue remains unknown. It may involve an interplay of immunologic, genetic, viral, hormonal, and other factors. In the broadest sense, it is hypothesized that this process may involve a change in the antigenicity of red cells or a change in the immune status of the individual (humoral and cellular immunity). Sometimes it can involve the destruction of red cells by cross-reactive antibodies or as innocent bystanders.

Antibodies involved in AIHA are primarily of the IgG and IgM types, often referred to as warm- and cold-reactive antibodies, respectively. The warm-reactive antibody is optimally active at 37°C, whereas the cold-reactive antibody is typically active at 30 to 32°C and below. Most cases of AIHA involve IgG antibody and some involve both IgG and IgM, but IgM alone is rarely found. Occasional cases of AIHA in humans may be associated with IgA. The cold-reactive antibody agglutinates red cells directly (maximally at 0 to 5°C), so it is also called cold agglutinin. Low levels of cold agglutinins may occur naturally in some people, dogs, and horses, and are usually of no clinical concern. AIHA caused by cold agglutinins (cold agglutinin disease), however, has been described in the dog, horse, and sheep. Cold agglutinin disease in humans is less responsive to corticosteroid therapy and splenectomy than the warm-reactive type of AIHA. Rarely IgG may agglutinate red cells at body temperature

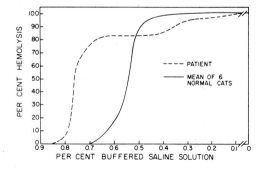

Fig. 22–2. Demonstration of markedly reduced erythrocyte osmotic resistance to hypotonic saline solution in a cat with autoimmune hemolytic anemia. (From Jain, N.C.: Schalm's Veterinary Hematology. 4th Ed. Philadelphia, Lea & Febiger, 1986, p. 1147.)

directly, or it may react with red cells in the cold and induce hemolysis. Overt red cell agglutination in a blood sample can cause errors in the measurement of erythrocyte parameters (e.g., RBC counts, MCHC, and red cell volume distribution) using a multichannel blood analysis system (Porter and Weisser, 1990).

CLINICAL OBSERVATIONS

Reports of AIHA in dogs have indicated that either sex may be affected, with a broad age and breed involvement. Clinical signs generally vary with the rapidity and severity of onset of the AIHA. In most cases, the sudden appearance of a progressive anemia is noted. Anorexia and lethargy are the most common clinical complaints. Increased water intake and emesis are often reported by the dog's owner, followed in several days of weakness, staggering, and collapse. The most prominent physical finding is pale mucous membranes. Jaundice, hepatomegaly, and splenomegaly are frequently present. Frank intravascular hemolysis, although infrequent, is indicated by hemoglobinemia and hemoglobinuria. An increased heart rate with a weak rapid pulse and a low-grade systolic heart murmur may be heard, possibly in conjunction with abnormal electrocardiographic findings associated with prolonged severe anemia. An increased respiratory rate, especially with excitement or exertion, is observed. If thrombocytopenia is present, petechiae, epistaxis, retinal hemorrhages, melena, frank bleeding from the bowel, and hematuria can occur. The body temperature may be elevated, especially if infection is present. Weakness may be moderate to profound. Syncopal episodes may be reported, but are not to be confused with epileptic seizures.

The ambient temperature should be taken into consideration when patients are suspected of having cold agglutinin disease. Skin lesions (cyanosis, necrosis, and gangrene), especially on the nose, pinnae, tail, and toes, may be seen with cold agglutinin disease. These result from obstruction of the microcirculation by agglutinated red cells because of high-titer antibody reactive at temperatures below 30 to 32°C. In a retrospective study of AIHA from Canada, twice as many cases of AIHA were seen in the cooler months, although this could not be related to antibody class or thermal reactivity (Jackson and Kruth, 1985).

The differential diagnosis of AIHA must include and distinguish among other causes of hemolytic disease in the animal being investigated. A Coombs-positive immune-mediated hemolytic anemia, in association with a thrombocytopenia presumed to be immune-mediated, was observed in a 10-year-old quarterhorse filly. Its cause remained undetermined, but treatment with corticosteroids was successful (Sockett et al., 1987).

LABORATORY FINDINGS

Severe intravascular hemolysis is indicated by hemoglobinemia, hemoglobinuria, bilirubinemia (mostly caused by indirect-reacting bilirubin), increased levels of serum lactic dehydrogenase and urine urobilinogen, and decreased levels of serum haptoglobin. Hemoglobinemia and a high icteric index from bilirubinemia are seen in the early stages, when antibody-coated red cells undergo massive destruction in the circulation and in the mononuclear phagocyte system (MPS), respectively. Elevations of the icterus index and urine urobilinogen level are not always present (see Table 11–5), however, because they depend on the degree of hemolysis and functional capability of the organs involved in bilirubin metabolism (e.g., the liver, kidney, and intestine). Serum haptoglobin concentration is elevated in most cases of AIHA in the dog, possibly because of acute phase response to macrophage activation (see Fig. 21–5); extravascular destruction of red cells is the most common cause of anemia in AIHA (Jones and Gruffydd-Jones, 1991).

Blood from patients with cold agglutinin disease undergoes intense autoagglutination on storage at 4°C and usually at room temperature (see Fig. 11–5), but not above 30 to 32°C; the agglutination is reversible at 37°C. Cold agglutination can be distinguished from the rouleau by diluting the sample 1:1 with normal saline solution or by placing the blood vial in the refrigerator (4°C) and then examining the sample. The former procedure disaggregates rouleaux and the latter accentuates cold agglutination. Errors in RBC counts and the MCV are introduced when agglutination is prominent in blood samples (Porter and Weiser, 1990).

The classic erythrocytic response in AIHA is that of a marked regenerative anemia, but a nonregenerative anemia may also occur (Jones and Gruffydd-Jones, 1991). In the stained blood film, a bone marrow response to anemia, manifested by reticulocytosis, polychromasia, and normoblastemia (Table 11–5), is usually evident. Spherocytes are invariably present (Plate XVI-4) and clumps of agglutinated red cells (Plate XVI-5) are generally seen when cold agglutinins are involved. The presence of spherocytes in blood films strongly suggests immune-mediated red cell destruction. The reticulocyte count varies, depending on the duration of illness, degree of response, and severity of the anemia. If erythropoiesis is not impaired, the patient shows an elevated reticulocyte count within 3 to 5 days of an acute hemolytic episode. The bone marrow aspirate reveals a decreased myeloid:erythroid ratio from increased erythropoiesis. The mean corpuscular volume may be elevated, depending on the degree of reticulocytosis. An inadequate reticulocyte response (reticulocytopenia) can indicate the destruction of reticulocytes by autoantibodies against antigens on reticulocytes or antibody-mediated inhibition of erythropoiesis, or it may result from a lack of the specific nutrients needed for intensified erythropoiesis. An IgG inhibiting in vitro proliferation of erythroid colony forming units (CFU-E) was isolated from the sera of 1 out of 3 dogs with direct Coombs test positive and 3 out of 5 dogs with Coombs-negative erythroid aplasia (Weiss, 1985). The reticulocyte response is temporarily inhibited by blood transfusion (Fig. 22–3).

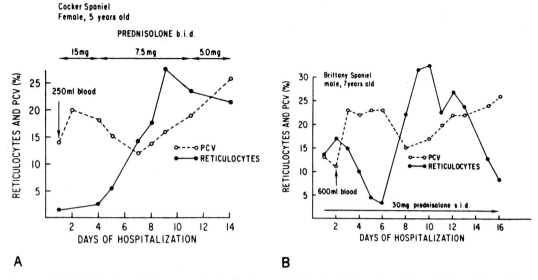

Fig. 22-3. Influence of whole blood transfusion on packed cell volume (PCV) and reticulocyte numbers of dogs with autoimmune hemolytic anemia (AIHA). *A,* A 250-ml transfusion increased the initial PCV of this dog from 14 to 20%, which gradually fell to 12% over the next 4 days. The initial reticulocyte count was 1.6%, but its rapid increase was delayed until after the fifth day. A significant reticulocytosis probably would have occurred early if the transfusion had been withheld. *B,* A 600-ml transfusion in this patient increased the PCV from 11 to 23%, at which level it remained for 4 days. This transfusion dramatically reduced the reticulocyte count from a 17% level to less than 2%, thereby indicating inhibition of reticulocytosis and probably diminished erythropoiesis. A subsequent drop in PCV from 23 to 15% between the sixth and eighth days was associated with a heightened reticulocytosis into the circulation to attain a peak of 31.4% on the tenth day. (From Schalm, O.W.: Autoimmune hemolytic anemia in the dog. Canine Pract., 2:37, 1975.)

The leukocyte count is frequently elevated, with a slight to marked neutrophilia and a left shift. A moderate monocytosis and thrombocytopenia may be present. The plasma protein concentration is generally within the normal range and the fibrinogen concentration may be slightly elevated. The erythrocyte sedimentation rate (ESR) may be elevated or reduced because of the response to the disease process or reticulocytosis, respectively. A biphasic ESR is a common finding when both reticulocytosis and red cell agglutination are present. Erythrocyte osmotic fragility is usually increased and often parallels the degree of spherocytosis in the dog and cat (see Figs. 7–15 and 22–2). The determination of erythrocyte osmotic fragility can provide useful information for diagnosis and monitoring prognosis of immune-mediated hemolytic anemia also in the horse (Taylor and Cooke, 1990).

Coombs' Antiglobulin Test. The serologic diagnosis of AIHA is confirmed by the demonstration of antibodies and/or complement on the red cells and/or in the patient's serum by the Coombs antiglobulin test. Most cases yield a positive direct Coombs test result, although some may be Coombs negative. In the latter instances, other clinical and laboratory results may be used to arrive at a diagnosis of Coombs-negative AHIA. These findings include the presence of hemoglobinemia, autoagglutinated red cells, spherocytes, and a persistently high number of reticulocytes. Sometimes, diagnosis is based on the exclusion of other causes of hemolytic anemia and patient's response to corticosteroid therapy.

The direct Coombs test (DCT) demonstrates the presence of antibody or activated complement com-

ponents on the surface of the patient's red cells. The indirect Coombs test (ICT) reveals the presence of antierythrocyte antibody in the serum or in eluates prepared from the patient's red cells. The principle involved in these tests is that a suspension of the patient's washed red cells (in the DCT) or of normal homologous washed red cells exposed to the patient's serum (in the ICT) is allowed to react with species-specific antiglobulin to induce visible agglutination of the red cells (Fig. 22–4). IgG or complement (C3)-coated red cells do not ordinarily undergo saline agglutination, whereas those coated with IgM do (Fig. 22–5). IgG and C3b, alone or in combination, generally participate in a positive direct Coombs test (Table 22–4). A positive ICT in AIHA is usually accompanied by a positive DCT.

Red cell suspensions for the Coombs' test must be obtained from blood anticoagulated with EDTA, because EDTA is anticomplementary and prevents the in vitro binding of complement to erythrocytes. Enzyme-treated red cells are more susceptible to complement-mediated lysis and yield a higher degree of positivity in the ICT. Titers or scores of a Coombs test may be helpful in following the progress of an individual patient. With cold-reactive antibody, the thermal reactivity of the antibody is more important than the titer in this regard. The use of a polyspecific antiserum containing anti-IgG, anti-IgM, and anti-complement is recommended as a broad-spectrum reagent to diagnose AIHA. Tests with monospecific anti-IgG, anti-IgM, or anti-complement may be performed to ascertain the roles of IgG, IgM, and complement, respectively.

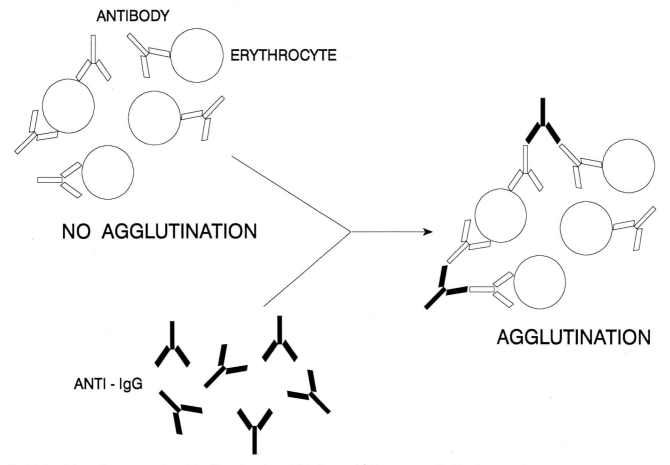

Fig. 22–4. Schematic representation of the direct Coombs antiglobulin test. Erythrocytes coated with only antierythrocyte IgG do not agglutinate, but they undergo agglutination after interaction with a species-specific anti-IgG.

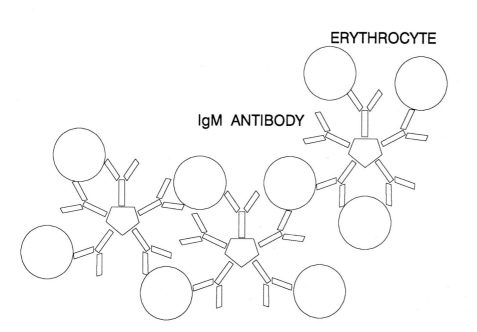

Fig. 22–5. Erythrocytes coated with antierythrocyte IgM (cold agglutinins) undergo spontaneous agglutination, in contrast to cells coated with antierythrocyte IgG (see Fig. 22–4).

Table 22–4. Patterns of Results of Direct Coombs Tests for 32 Canine Patients with Autoimmune Hemolytic Anemia

No. of Cases	% of Total	Reagent*		
		Anti-IgG and Anti-C'3	Anti-IgG	Anti-C'3
16	50	+	+	+
10	31.2	+	+	−
6	18.8	+	−	+
		100%	81.2%	58.8%

From Switzer, J.W., and Jain, N.C.: Autoimmune hemolytic anemia in dogs and cats. Vet. Clin. North Am. [Small Anim. Pract.], 11:405, 1981.

* Percentages of all cases giving positive test results with each reagent.

Interpretation of the Coombs test results requires an understanding of the mechanisms of antibody and complement interactions with the red cells, the circumstances leading to and the types of immune responses, and the response to therapy. Many conditions have been found to yield a positive Coombs test result in dogs and cats, including various neoplastic, infectious, parasitic, inflammatory, and other immune-mediated diseases. A positive DCT is also obtained in patients with hemolytic transfusion reaction and in neonatal isoerythrolysis. Several factors can influence the outcome of an antiglobulin test (Jones et al., 1990). False-negative and false-positive results may be obtained because of errors in sample handling, laboratory manipulations, and modified patient's status as a result of immunosuppressive therapy. In cases of drug-induced AIHA, the offending drug must be incorporated into the test system, or the test could yield negative results.

Cold agglutinating antibody can fix complement at temperatures below 30 to 32°C and can lyse red cells at a pH of 6.5 to 7 in vitro. Because the antibody usually fixes C3 and C4, a positive direct Coombs test with anti-complement reagent is usually obtained. The antibody attachment to the red cells is generally not detected with anti-IgM reagent because the IgM is eluted from the erythrocytes at 37°C in vivo, and possibly also during washing of the red cells in vitro. In contrast, the complement components are irreversibly bound to the red cells. Blood samples used to detect circulating cold antibodies must be collected using a warm syringe and allowed to clot at 37°C, and the serum must be separated as soon as possible to prevent the loss of cold agglutinins by attachment to red cells in vitro.

Other Tests. Other laboratory tests that may be helpful in prognosis and treatment of AIHA include the following: (1) lupus erythematosus (LE) cell and antinuclear antibody (ANA) tests, if SLE is suspected; (2) bone marrow examination, particularly in unresponsive or leukopenic patients; (3) serum biochemical analytes to assess liver and kidney disease; (4) urinalysis for the detection of cystitis or renal disease; (5) stool examination for occult blood and parasites; and (6) blood examination for dirofilariasis. A cardiopulmonary examination for carditis and pulmonary disease is indicated as part of a thorough medical examination.

PATHOGENESIS

Stimulus for Autoantibody Production. The pathogenesis of AIHA involves conditions that lead to the formation of the autoantibody and the associated red cell destruction. The underlying mechanisms for the formation of the autoantibody remain unknown, but two major hypotheses prevail. According to one, a fundamental change occurs in the erythrocyte membrane, resulting in the formation of a new or altered antigen or unmasking a hidden antigen that subsequently stimulates the normal immune system to synthesize antierythrocyte antibodies. The red cell antigen can be modified by such factors as drugs, chemicals, viruses, and bacteria. A defect of the structural composition of the rhesus genome may be involved in the initial development of autoantibody in certain cases of AIHA in humans. Most cold agglutinins in humans are directed against I antigen, but some are directed against i antigen. The cold-reactive, nonagglutinating IgG (Donath-Landsteiner antibody) associated with paroxysmal cold hemoglobinuria in humans is typically specific for the P blood group antigens. IgG eluted from the red cells of human patients with AIHA consists predominantly of a single, totally erythrocyte-absorbable antibody that binds to antigenic determinants on band 3 (Victoria et al., 1990). In a study on 6 dogs with AIHA, several autoantigens were identified by immunoprecipitation with autoantibody and included 29-kD to 100-kD peptides and an antigen with molecular mass identical to band 3 glycoprotein (Barker et al., 1991). Changes in band 4.1 region proteins occurred in a dog between the crisis and remission of AIHA involving IgG and IgA autoantibodies (Tsuchida et al., 1991).

The second theory states that a spontaneous change somehow occurs in the normal immune apparatus, which then recognizes normal erythrocyte antigens as foreign and produces antibodies. This represents the development of forbidden clones of cells and may occur when a generalized hyperactivity of the immune system is present, such as in lymphoma. It is also suspected that patients developing AIHA may be genetically prone to form autoantibodies. The occurrence of AIHA in the NZB/BL hybrid of mice is well known, and certain breeds of dogs have been found to have a higher incidence of immune-mediated hematologic disorders. Imbalances of immunoregulatory mechanisms that involve the T and B lymphocytes concerned with antibody production and cellular immunity may also be associated with the expression of autoimmunity in some cases.

Mechanisms of Red Cell Destruction. Red cell destruction in vivo is a consequence of direct lysis, erythrophagocytosis, or both. Intravascular hemolysis is associated with IgG or IgM antibodies that cause the activation of all complement components (C1 to C9). Intravascular hemolysis is rare but, when observed, is generally proportional to the amount of antibody in circulation, its thermal amplitude and binding to the red cell surface, and the degree of complement activation. A role for T lymphocytes in the cell-mediated lysis of antibody-coated erythrocytes has also been suggested. The destruction of antibody-coated red cells by neutrophils has been demonstrated in vitro, but its in vivo significance remains to be established. The neutrophils and monocytes of dogs with immune-mediated hemolytic anemia given whole blood transfusion may show small to medium (1 to 4 μm in diameter) brownish granules (hemosiderin) that stain positive for iron with Prussian blue stain (Gaunt and Baker, 1986).

Erythrophagocytosis is associated with a relatively low concentration of IgG antibody alone or in combination with the partial activation of complement to C3b on the red cell surface. Complement fixation up to the C3b stage does not cause frank hemolysis, but is sufficient to promote phagocytosis. Macrophages have surface receptors for the Fc region of IgG and for complement components C3b, C3bi, and C4. Therefore, circulating IgG-coated and C3b/C3bi-coated red cells adhere to macrophages during their sojourn through organs rich in the MPS, particularly the spleen and liver. Macrophages exhibit partial or complete phagocytosis of antibody-coated and/or complement-coated red cells. IgG and C3b/C3bi act synergistically in this regard. Partial erythrophagocytosis results in the formation of spherocytes, whereas complete erythrophagocytosis contributes to bilirubinemia (see Fig. 11–4). Erythrocytes sensitized with IgG alone or with IgG and C3b are removed primarily by the spleen, but those coated with C3b resulting from the activation of IgM are removed primarily by the liver. Also, macrophages from AIHA patients may exhibit greater phagocytic activity for red cells compared to macrophages from normal persons. Spherocytes are relatively rigid (less deformable) and their osmotic fragility is greatly increased (see Figs. 7–15 and 22–2) because they have a low surface area-to-content ratio as a result of the increased phagocytic loss of red cell membrane compared to content. Thus, spherocytes are vulnerable to trauma of the microcirculation, particularly in the spleen, and have a short intravascular life span.

THERAPY

The primary goals in treating AIHA are the management of the anemic crisis, inhibition of red cell destruction, and reduction of autoantibody production. Corticosteroids and immunosuppressive drugs such as cyclophosphamide and azathioprine are the mainstay of therapy. A few cases also require plasma exchange or plasmapheresis, thymectomy, treatment with high-dose intravenous γ-globulins (IV IgG), and administration of danazol, a nonvirilizing androgen (Gibson, 1988; Holloway et al., 1990; Kaveri et al., 1991; Williams et al., 1990). Splenectomy has been found beneficial in many cases of AIHA in humans. Intensive care consisting of warmth, oxygen, intravenously administered fluids, and blood transfusion may be required for the most severe cases. Avoidance of cold is essential in dogs with cold agglutinin disease. Early detection and the prompt institution of treatment are important if a terminal anemic crisis is to be prevented. A therapeutic regimen of sufficient length and intensity is required to secure remission and prevent relapse. Long-term or lifetime therapy is often a possibility in these patients. Regular follow-ups are essential to follow progress and monitor possible relapse.

Corticosteroids are the drugs of choice for the treatment of immune-mediated diseases, including AIHA and AITP. Generally, large doses of oral prednisone (2 to 4 mg/kg body weight) are given daily; after a favorable response, the dose is gradually reduced to maintain remission. Corticosteroids appear to reduce the immune-mediated destruction of red cells (or of platelets in AITP) in several ways: (1) suppression of phagocytic activity of the MPS by reduction in the number of Fc receptors on macrophages; (2) reduction of antibody production; (3) increased catabolism of immunoglobulins; and (4) decreased antibody avidity to red cells (or platelets). A positive response to corticosteroid therapy usually occurs within the first 7 days . Dexamethasone was successfully used to treat 4 horses with AIHA (Mair et al., 1990).

Cyclophosphamide (Cytoxan) is a potent antimetabolite that has been successfully used to treat AIHA. The recommended oral dosage is 50 mg/m² body surface area, given daily for 4 consecutive days per week and repeated in weekly cycles until the response is evident. Cyclophosphamide therapy is instituted in patients that fail to show a satisfactory remission with corticosteroids. Its beneficial effect is mediated through a reduction in antibody production. It may be preferable to begin cyclophosphamide therapy at the onset in more severe cases of AIHA. Antibiotics are suggested when infection is present or suspected (as in fever of unknown origin) and when vigorous immunosuppressive therapy is instituted. Hematuria and bacterial cystitis are frequent complications. Azathioprine (Imuran) may be used instead of cyclophosphamide to immunosuppress the patient, and is given in a dosage similar to that for prednisone. Cyclophosphamide and azathioprine therapy should be stopped when adverse reactions, particularly bone marrow suppression, develop. Cyclophosphamide and azathioprine were used to treat a horse with AIHA that was nonresponsive to corticosteroid therapy (Messer and Arnold, 1991).

Heparin may be used to reduce massive red cell destruction and prevent DIC. Although the value of heparin as an anticomplementary agent to treat patients in anemic crisis has been questioned, some impressive results have been documented in certain critical cases with plunging PCV values. The suggested starting dose is 10,000 IU (100 mg) subcutaneously bid or tid, or 100 mg/kg body weight intravenously every 4 to 6 hours. The clotting time should be checked to determine the necessity and size of each subsequent dose. Heparin may inhibit complement-mediated intravascular hemolysis and the formation of clots in the microvasculature through the activation of clotting factors by the membranes of lysed red cells. Some believe that heparin therapy is preferable to the risks of transfusion in dogs and cats with AIHA.

Blood transfusion is recommended only in life-threatening, severe anemic states. The benefit of transfusion therapy must be weighed against the risks involved for the AIHA patient. Transfused cells may be rapidly destroyed by the patient's antibodies and result in an acute or delayed serious transfusion reaction, DIC, thromboembolism, and renal failure. The blood used for transfusion must be crossmatched with the recipient's serum and red cells. The recipient's serum must also be checked for immune antibodies (IgG) to red cells by performing an ICT against donor red cells when multiple transfusions are to be given.

Splenectomy may be indicated in situations of persistent relapse or inadequate response to prolonged corticosteroid and immunosuppressive therapy. Patients exhibiting extravascular hemolysis (primarily resulting from warm-reactive antibodies) and hypersplenism are the most likely candidates. Splenectomy eliminates a major site of red cell destruction and an important site of antibody production. In times, these functions are taken over by similar sites in the body and relapses continue to occur, despite splenectomy. Secondary hemolytic disease caused by haemobartonellosis or babesiasis is a frequent consequence of splenectomy. Splenectomy in 9 canine patients with immune-mediated thrombocytopenia, immune-mediated hemolytic anemia, and Evans syndrome appeared to be useful in the clinical management of the disease processes (Feldman et al., 1985).

Other supportive therapy, such as a nutritious, high-protein diet, folic acid and B-complex vitamins, and other drugs may be given to meet the demands of increased erythropoiesis. Myelostimulatory therapy may prove beneficial in AIHA associated with poorly responsive bone marrow and red cell aplasia. Anabolic steroids may stimulate erythropoiesis through several mechanisms, including the stimulation of erythropoietin production. Recombinant erythropoietin may also be tried in those with inadequate marrow response.

Autoimmune Thrombocytopenia

Autoimmune thrombocytopenia has been recognized as a distinct entity in humans and the dog, cat, and horse. AITP in these species is characterized by the following: (1) clinical signs of thrombocytopenia, such as hemorrhages into the skin and tissues and from body orifices; (2) coagulation defects related to thrombocytopenia, such as prolonged bleeding time and poor clot retraction; (3) hematologic abnormalities, such as severe to moderate thrombocytopenia, blood loss anemia, and signs of increased erythropoiesis; and (4) an absence or decreased number of megakaryocytes in the bone marrow during the early phase and an increased number during the compensatory phase. Megakaryocytes may also show morphologic abnormalities. The serologic diagnosis of AITP involves the demonstration of antiplatelet antibody in the serum or associated with platelets or megakaryocytes.

SPECIES INVOLVED

AITP in Humans. The occurrence of AITP as a distinct clinical entity in humans was long suspected but not clearly established until 1951, when Harrington and co-workers confirmed autoantibody as a cause of idiopathic thrombocytopenia (ITP) in some patients. When the presence of antiplatelet antibody cannot be demonstrated, the diagnosis of AITP or ITP is usually made by excluding other causes of thrombocytopenia. Other causes of thrombocytopenia include disorders of production (e.g., drug therapy or hypoplastic or aplastic marrow), preferential distribution of platelets in the spleen (as in splenomegaly), and increased platelet utilization or destruction (as in DIC or hypersplenism). Characteristic hematologic findings of AITP in humans include thrombocytopenia, reduced platelet survival, and normal or usually increased megakaryocytes in the bone marrow. Dogs with AITP may show normal, increased, or even markedly decreased megakaryocytopoesis. The mean platelet volume is elevated from increased numbers of circulating young platelets (megathrombocytes).

Clinically, AITP may manifest as an acute, chronic, or intermittent disorder. Acute AITP is seen primarily in children. It has an abrupt onset, is often preceded by viral infection, and is usually self-limiting. Spontaneous remission usually occurs within a few weeks to months. Chronic AITP is primarily a disease of adults, and rarely resolves spontaneously. It has a prolonged course and usually has a preferential sex distribution in females, with a female:male ratio of 3:1. Women with chronic AITP may give birth to thrombocytopenic babies because maternal IgG antibody can cross the placenta and react with the fetal platelets. A similar mechanism causes alloimmune thrombocytopenia in neonates, in which the mother produces antibodies to "foreign" antigens on fetal platelets that are acquired from the father and not shared by the mother. Intermittent AITP may occur at any age and is characterized by cycles of thrombocytopenia at intervals of 3 to 6 months or more.

A positive diagnosis of AITP is made by demonstrating antiplatelet antibody in the serum, or by increased levels of platelet-associated IgG (PAIgG), IgM, or both in the absence of sepsis or hypergammaglobulinemia. Positive reactions for antiplatelet antibody, however, may vary greatly. The antiplatelet antibody in chronic AITP appears to react preferentially with antigens on glycoproteins (GPs)—GPIIb, GPIIIa, GPIb, GPV (Hegde, 1992). The significance of PAIgG remains controversial, because platelets store IgG nonspecifically in α granules and release it when stimulated (Handagama et al., 1990). It has been conjectured that as methods for detecting antiplatelet antibody are simplified and improve in sensitivity, an immune-mediated cause of ITP will be increasingly demonstrated.

AITP in Animals. AITP occurs in dogs, cats, and horses, but its frequency in various animal populations remains to be established. The following discussion is based on observations of AITP in these species and in humans.

CLASSIFICATION

AITP may be caused by alloantibodies, autoantibodies, or drug-induced immune mechanisms (von dem Borne and Ouwenhand, 1989). Acquired AITP may be primary or idiopathic, or may be secondary or symptomatic to other diseases. In dogs, secondary AITP is about three times more prevalent than primary AITP, and spontaneous remission may occur in some cases of primary AITP. Secondary AITP in dogs has been seen in association with AIHA, SLE, ehrlichiosis, DIC, multiple myeloma, myelogenous leukemia, lymphoma, solid tumors, severe generalized exfoliative dermatitis, nephropathy, portocaval shunt, possible Cushing's disease, and von Willebrand's disease. AITP in association with SLE has been seen in a cat. Antiplatelet antibody in the serum or increased levels of PAIgG have been found in humans with thrombocytopenia associated with various conditions, including lymphoproliferative and myeloproliferative disorders, SLE, thrombotic thrombocytopenic purpura, bacterial, protozoal and viral infections, tumors, and following therapy with certain drugs.

CLINICAL OBSERVATIONS

In the dog, AITP is about twice as common in females as in males, and may occur without any age or breed preference. The clinical signs of AITP are identical to those of thrombocytopenia in general. Signs of purpura are present in severely thrombocytopenic patients (platelet counts of less than 20,000/μl of blood). Petechiae may be seen in the oral, gingival, nasal, and vaginal mucous membranes. With ecchymoses, they may also be seen on the skin over the abdominal areas, inner aspects of the thighs and forelimbs, and in the ear canal. Bleeding may occur following the slightest trauma, such as during grooming. Epistaxis, melena, hematuria, scleral hemorrhage, and hyphema may occur. Bleeding from the body orifices is more prevalent than tissue hemorrhages, and in some cases no signs of bleeding are seen.

Signs of blood loss anemia may be apparent in patients with significant external hemorrhage. Stress on blood vessels plays an important role in the manifestation of bleeding in the thrombocytopenic state; thus, bleeding episodes are more common in the thrombocytopenic dog than in the thrombocytopenic cat, probably because of differences in their activities (see Chap. 6). Various nonspecific clinical signs such as fever, increased thirst, anorexia, and lethargy may be found in these patients.

HEMATOLOGIC FINDINGS

Dogs and cats with AITP may show similar blood and bone marrow findings. The characteristic finding is thrombocytopenia, with platelet counts usually less than 50,000/μl of blood. A mild to severe blood loss anemia may be indicated by a reduction in both red cell parameters (PCV, hemoglobin, and RBC count) and total plasma protein concentration. Some anemic dogs may present evidence of an increased erythropoietic response, such as polychromasia, reticulocytosis, and macrocytic hypochromic erythrocytes. Nucleated red cells may be found in some cases, particularly when a significant erythrogenic response to anemia is present. The ESR is variable and the icterus index is generally normal. The total and differential leukocyte counts can vary. Leukocytosis, neutrophilia with a slight to moderate left shift, and monocytosis may occur, particularly in dogs briskly responding to anemia. A few dogs may have leukopenia, lymphopenia, or eosinopenia.

Reduced numbers of mature and immature megakaryocytes are generally found in the bone marrow of severely thrombocytopenic dogs. In smears of marrow aspirates from ribs, 70 to 84% mature and 16 to 30% immature megakaryocytes are normally present, with a ratio of 2.35 to 5.25:1. In AITP, the ratio of mature to immature megakaryocytes is usually less than 1 (0.17 to 0.85:1). Morphologic abnormalities are also evident in mature and immature megakaryocytes. In rare cases, the marrow may be devoid of megakaryocytes at the initial examination. The examination of blood films taken during the uncompensated or compensated thrombocytopenic state reveals microthrombocytes and megathrombocytes. The former type of platelet morphology results from the fragmentation of circulating platelets, whereas the latter represents young forms of platelets.

The megakaryocytes of dogs with AITP produce a moderate to strong cytoplasmic immunofluorescence for IgG, in contrast to the negative fluorescence of megakaryocytes from normal dogs or dogs with non-immune-mediated thrombocytopenia. This positive immunofluorescence is reduced or disappears following therapy with corticosteroids and/or immunosuppressive drugs.

DETECTION OF ANTIPLATELET ANTIBODIES

Various tests can detect circulating or platelet-bound antiplatelet antibodies. These methods include detection of antiplatelet antibody in serum by the PF-3 test, a direct immunofluorescence technique to demonstrate antibody associated with megakaryocytes, and methods to detect PAIgG. Observations on canine patients have indicated that the PF-3 technique is less sensitive than the immunofluorescence technique for the detection of megakaryocyte-bound antibody. More sensitive methods include radioimmunoassay, ELISA, and flow cytometry techniques (Thiem et al., 1991; Dhawedkar et al., 1991; Jain et al., 1990a).

Ideally, specimens for the demonstration of antiplatelet antibody should be collected prior to the institution of immunosuppressive therapy, because negative results may be obtained as a result of a therapy-induced reduction in antibody levels. Specimens from some patients recently placed on such a therapy, however, may still yield positive test results. In a few canine patients, an antiplatelet antibody test may remain positive, even when platelet counts have increased to normal levels. Such patients are probably in a compensated thrombocytolytic state—that is, they have a subclinical compensated AITP, in which, increased bone marrow production keeps up with the increased peripheral destruction of platelets. Such patients are probably extremely vulnerable to thrombocytopenia from secondary causes. Serum levels of antiplatelet antibody in humans vary widely and show little or no relationship with platelet counts or clinical response to therapy. In comparison, the amount of PAIgG generally correlates with platelet counts, and has some clinical usefulness.

PATHOGENESIS

Circumstances leading to the formation of autologous antiplatelet antibody have not been fully delineated, except in certain cases of drug-induced thrombocytopenias. In general, the formation of autoantibodies to platelets may involve situations similar to those described for AIHA. These include the following: (1) modification of platelet antigens or unmasking of cryptic platelet antigens so that they are recognized as foreign by the immune system; (2) selective modification of the immune system or the formation of abnormal clones of lymphoid cells, which recognize normal platelet antigens as nonself; and (3) abnormalities of immunoregulatory cells. The formation of cross-reactive antibodies or hapten mechanisms involving platelets in an antibody response may also be involved in the immune destruction of platelets. The spleen and bone marrow are important sites for the production of antiplatelet antibodies. The antiplatelet antibody has specificity for antigens associated with platelets and megakaryocytes, although it may vary in its ability to bind to platelets from different individuals. The autoantibody directed against platelet antigens may be IgG or IgM, but rarely IgA.

Thrombocytopenia is primarily caused by the sequestration and destruction of platelets in the MPS. Macrophages phagocytize antibody- and complement-coated platelets in a similar manner as red cells in AIHA. Fragmented platelets (microthrombocytes) and fragmented red cells have been found, respectively, in the blood of such patients. Platelets heavily coated with antibody are removed by the liver, whereas lightly coated ones are destroyed in the spleen. The complement-mediated lysis of antibody-coated platelets in the circulation may occur to some extent, and contribute to thrombocytopenia.

A reduction in effective megakaryocytopoiesis from the destruction of productive (mature) megakaryocytes in the bone marrow also contributes to thrombocytopenia, particularly in dogs. This thrombocytopenic effect occurs because the platelets and megakaryocytes have common antigens, and the antiplatelet antibody binds to the megakaryocytes.

The purpura associated with thrombocytopenia may result from damage to the vessel wall by antibodies directed against the capillary endothelium, or may result from weakness of the vascular wall, because platelets are necessary for maintaining vascular integrity.

THERAPY

The therapeutic management of AITP is generally similar to that of patients with AIHA. The prognosis is favorable with early diagnosis and prompt initiation of adequate therapeutic measures, particularly in primary AITP. Spontaneous remissions have been noted in a few patients with primary AITP. Long-term therapy is indicated in many cases, because relapses may occur on termination of therapy. The transfusion of fresh platelets (suspended in the donor's plasma) or fresh whole blood may be given to elevate platelet counts immediately, although this is only of temporary benefit. Plasmapheresis may be performed to aid in the treatment of dogs with immune-mediated diseases such as AIHA, AITP, and SLE, but facilities for performing this procedure are not commonly available (Matus et al., 1985a, 1985b). Plasmapheresis is performed to quickly reduce the concentration of circulating immunoglobulins and alleviate the acute effects of autoantibodies.

Corticosteroids are the drugs of choice for the initial therapy of AITP or ITP. Prednisone therapy may be expected to increase platelet counts significantly by the third day of therapy and, in responding dogs, platelet counts may attain normal or even higher levels in 5 to 7 days. In an occasional dog, platelet counts may remain in the range of 100,000 to 200,000/μl, but physical improvement occurs. The mode of action is similar to that for AIHA (see above). In addition, corticosteroids promote the reduction of capillary fragility with the restoration of normal bleeding time. Because of high frequency of relapses, platelet counts must be monitored frequently (weekly to monthly), especially after any reduction in corticosteroid therapy. A decrease in the platelet count may be detected 1 to 4 weeks after the cessation of corticosteroid therapy, and is often evident before the onset of clinical bleeding. Some patients do not respond to corticosteroid therapy; in these, platelet counts remain below 100,000/μl or no real increase in platelet number occurs, even after as long as 2 weeks of therapy.

Cyclophosphamide (Cytoxan) may be given in conjunction with corticosteroid therapy, particularly when a response to the latter drug is not seen within the first 3 to 5 days. Platelet counts may be expected to rise within 5 to 6 days, but in some dogs it can take about 2 weeks. Cyclophosphamide should be withdrawn from the treatment program as soon as possible because of its cytotoxic and immunosuppressive actions. The patient is maintained on corticosteroid therapy after the withdrawal of cyclophosphamide. Azathioprine may be used instead of cyclophosphamide, as in AIHA. It appears to be a cost-effective drug for the treatment of immune-mediated thrombocytopenia in the horse (Humber et al., 1991).

Vincristine (Oncovin) is a valuable drug in the management of ITP (0.2–0.6 mg/m^2 given intravenously at 7–10 day intervals). Its use is generally indicated in cases resistant to corticosteroid administration or to combined corticosteroid and cyclophosphamide therapy. The mode of action is believed to be the direct stimulation of platelet production by megakaryocytes in the bone marrow. Vincristine is also effective in suppressing antibody production. Thrombocytopenic canine patients treated with vincristine may be expected to respond by increasing platelet counts, usually within 3 to 5 days, and sometimes dramatically—counts might exceed 1,000,000/μl of blood within 7 to 10 days. An occasional patient may take longer to respond, require more than one treatment, or require experimental therapy such as administration of allogenous platelets loaded with vincristine (Helfand et al., 1984). No response may be evident in some cases, even after repeated vincristine or immunosuppressive therapy.

Secondary infections are frequently associated with potent immunosuppressive therapy, so any signs of infection must be monitored and periodic urine checks are required. Antibiotic therapy is guided according to the organisms involved and their antibiotic sensitivity.

Splenectomy should be considered in selected cases in which recurrent thrombocytopenia prevails, despite continuous immunosuppressive therapy. In any event, surgery should not be performed until the bleeding is under control. Platelet counts in splenectomized human patients return to normal levels, although antiplatelet antibody may persist in some cases; 20 to 30% of splenectomized patients undergo subsequent relapse. The beneficial effects of splenectomy are attributed to the removal of an important site of platelet pooling and destruction and that of antiplatelet antibody synthesis. Relapses can occur because of the formation of antibodies at other sites, such as the bone marrow and lymph nodes, and the destruction of sensitized platelets by the MPS at sites other than the spleen. Splenectomized individuals are at high risk of infection. The usefulness of splenectomy in dogs and cats with AITP remains to be established, although observations on some canine patients have suggested that it could be beneficial (Feldman et al., 1985).

Drug-Induced Autoimmune Hemolytic Anemia and Thrombocytopenia

Many drugs are implicated in the immunologic destruction of platelets, red cells, and granulocytes in humans (Salama and Mueller-Eckhardt, 1992; Williams et al., 1990). Information about the drug-induced immune-mediated agranulocytosis is scanty compared to thrombocytopenia and hemolytic anemia. Drug-induced thrombocytopenia has been seen in dogs (see Chap. 6). Sensitivity to a drug usually develops after continued therapy and may persist indefinitely after termination of the therapy. The onset of thrombocytopenia is generally rapid, and may be accompanied by a generalized purpura or bleeding. Similarly, a hemolytic anemia may manifest early or may be delayed until the patient has received the offending drug the second time. Discontinuation of the drug results in an increase in the platelet count, usually within 7 to 10 days. The antibodies involved in drug-induced AITP and AIHA are usually IgG, and sometimes IgM. In contrast to classic AITP and AIHA, the antibody in drug-induced cases is demonstrable only in the presence of the drug or its metabolite.

The mechanisms of antibody formation and platelet destruction have been described for quinine, quinidine, and sedormid and, similarly, for penicillin and α-methyldopa, which cause red cell destruction. In certain instances, a drug metabolite, rather than the drug itself, may act as the antigen. Three modes of antibody formation and platelet and red cell destruction have been delineated.

The high-affinity hapten mechanism applies to drugs that bind firmly to proteins, including those on the red cell or platelet membrane. Studies with sedormid showed that the drug, acting as a hapten, conjugated with the circulating platelets and that the drug-platelet complex acted as an antigen to produce specific IgG antibodies. The antibodies reacted with the drug-platelet complex, but not with the platelets alone. Alternatively, the drug may initially bind to a plasma antigen or "carrier" to form a primary antigen. Antibodies formed against such an antigen may react with the drug bound to the platelets and induce destruction. Penicillin is a prime example of a drug that involves a high-affinity hapten-induced mechanism, in which IgG antibody formation leads to red cell destruction. The destruction of platelets and red cells occurs mainly through sequestration by splenic macrophages. Penicillin-induced Coombs-positive hemolytic anemia was diagnosed in a horse (Step et al., 1991).

The ternary complex or low-affinity hapten mechanism, involves drugs with a weak or low affinity for red cells and platelets (e.g., quinidine and quinine). This process was formerly referred to as the immune complex mechanism. The antibody binds by its Fab domain to a compound neoantigen consisting of a loosely attached drug and a blood group antigen on the red cell (e.g., Rh, Kell, Kidd, or I/i antigen) or glycoproteins of platelets (e.g., GPIb, GPIIb-IIIa). This neoantigen is also thought to induce an immune response that results in specific antibody formation. Blood cell destruction mainly occurs through complement activation, and partly by sequestration in the MPS. Red cells in such cases usually yield a positive Coombs test result with anti-complement reagent. Similarly, immune-mediated thrombocytopenia in horses infected with equine infectious anemia virus appeared to involve the deposition of immune complexes (virus-antiviral antibodies) on platelets and the removal of such platelets from the circulation by the Kupffer cells and splenic macrophages (Clabough et al., 1991).

The formation of IgG autoantibodies reactive to red cell or platelet antigens may be induced by several drugs, such as α-methyldopa. The drug complexes with the cell membrane and is believed to induce antibody formation to a native antigen on blood cells. Thus, the antibody does not react with the drug, and its presence is not required for platelet or red cell destruction. The antibody shows specificity for the Rh antigen on the red cells. These red cells are usually Coombs-positive with anti-IgG reagent. Most patients with IgG antibodies do not undergo hemolysis, while many hemolyzing patients may show IgM antibodies on their red cell surface (Murphy and Kelton, 1988).

Autoimmune Neutropenia

Autoimmune neutropenia (AIN) results from the action of an antibody directed against antigens located on the neutrophils (Bux and Mueller-Eckhardt, 1992; Madyastha and Glassman, 1989). In human patients, the antibody is specific for neutrophils, as opposed to HLA antileukocyte antibody. The latter has been implicated in rare cases of allogeneic neonatal neutropenia in children. AIN may occur at any age. Its typical manifestations include fever and recurrent infections associated with neutropenia. Autoantibodies to neutrophils are increasingly detected in human patients with chronic idiopathic neutropenia and in cases of neutropenia secondary to several other diseases, including AIDS. Most patients have IgG antibody, some have both IgG and IgM, and rarely IgA can be found (Madyastha and Glassman, 1989; Robinson et al., 1987). Some of the patients with IgG antineutrophil antibodies may also contain antibodies directed against monocytes.

Antibodies to neutrophils can be detected by several methods, including the leukoagglutination test, direct and indirect immunofluorescence tests, and the nonspecific binding of protein A to the Fc receptors of neutrophil-bound IgG (Chickering et al., 1985a; Jain et al., 1990b; Madyastha and Glassman, 1989). Flow cytometry and ELISA can be used to increase the sensitivity of antibody detection methods. (Dhawedkar et al., 1991; Jain et al., 1991; Robinson et al., 1987). AIN has not been investigated in animals as much as in humans. Rare cases of alloimmune neutropenia have been reported in the pig and horse. A dramatic neutropenia results after the experimental injection of heterologous antibodies in several species, including cattle (Jain et al., 1968) and cats (Chickering et al.,

1985b). Studies in cats have shown that a left shift and toxic changes may occur in the blood. The bone marrow reveals corresponding changes in various pools of myeloid cells, and phagocytized neutrophils are found in marrow macrophages and in Kupffer cells in the liver.

Antineutrophil cytoplasmic autoantibodies (ANCA) specific for constituents of neutrophil primary granules and reactive with monocyte lysosomes have been detected in humans with inflammatory vascular disorders (Gross et al., 1991). Pathogenesis of systemic vasculitis involves ANCA-induced activation, adherence, and degranulation of neutrophils. Toxic oxygen radicals and lysosomal enzymes released from activated neutrophils are capable of causing vascular damage.

LE CELL PHENOMENON AND ANTINUCLEAR ANTIBODIES

The lupus erythematosus (LE) cell is a leukocyte, mainly a neutrophil, that contains a large homogeneous or amorphous reddish-purple cytoplasmic inclusion body of nuclear origin. The LE cell phenomenon was first observed by Hargraves in 1943 in bone marrow preparations of persons with SLE. LE cells are mainly formed in vitro in anticoagulated blood. LE cells may be found in diseases other than SLE, yet continue to serve as an important indicator of SLE.

LE Cell Formation

The formation of LE cells depends on an IgG antibody to deoxyribonucleoprotein (DNP) that binds to the nuclei of injured or nonviable leukocytes. Viable neutrophils phagocytize the opsonized nuclear mass and are designated as the LE cells. Their cytoplasm contains a round homogeneous mass, about the size of a lymphocyte nucleus, that takes the nuclear stain but lacks the normal chromatin pattern of a viable nucleus (Plate XI-3). LE cells must be distinguished from simple nucleophagocytosis (tart cells), in which the phagocytosed nuclear mass retains its normal morphologic features and usually has a darker-staining rim. Although LE cell formation typically involves neutrophils, other cells, including eosinophils, basophils, monocytes, lymphocytes, and even plasma cells, may be involved.

Phagocytosis of the altered nuclear mass leading to LE cell formation occurs only when sufficient IgG anti-DNP antibody is present along with complement. In low concentration, the IgG anti-DNP antibody produces only the nuclear alteration known as extracellular material (ECM) or hematoxylin bodies. IgM anti-DNP antibody does not produce LE cells, even at a high concentration, although ECM is formed. The inability of the IgM anti-DNP antibody to produce LE cells is probably the result of its inability to fix complement, although IgM is normally an excellent complement-fixing antibody. An amorphous ECM may be surrounded by leukocytes, which form a collar of rosette (Plate XIV-12). The rosette alone is not acceptable as evidence of a positive LE test, but it highly suggests the presence of anti-DNP antibodies in the test serum.

In addition to anti-DNP antibodies, the serum of patients with SLE may contain antinuclear antibodies (ANA) against various cellular components, including DNA, histone, nucleolus, and RNA (Mongey and Hess, 1991; Toth and Rebar, 1987). These antibodies can be demonstrated by the indirect immunofluorescence test in which the antibody titer and the pattern of immunofluorescence are recorded. Different patterns of immunofluorescence produced by an ANA in humans include diffuse, peripheral, speckled, and nucleolar patterns. Mixed patterns may occur, and a pattern may change with serum dilution. A homogeneous or diffuse pattern is associated with antibody binding to native DNA or histone and is seen in patients with SLE, drug-related lupus, and rheumatoid arthritis. A peripheral or rim pattern results from antibody binding to DNA and is usually found in acute phase SLE. A speckled or reticulate pattern, associated with binding to acidic, nonhistone, nuclear proteins, is the most common and is found in various rheumatic diseases including SLE and scleroderma. A nucleolar pattern associated with binding to nucleolar RNA, is seen in collagen diseases other than SLE. In general, the LE cell test is more specific but less sensitive for SLE, whereas the ANA test is more sensitive but less specific. Thus, a positive ANA test alone is not diagnostic of SLE; it must be interpreted in conjunction with the clinical findings.

Newer assays, such as ELISA, radioimmunoassay, and immunoprecipitation, provide increased sensitivity for detection of various ANA in SLE and other connective tissue diseases (Mongey and Hess, 1991; Sontheimer et al., 1992). For example, clinical studies in humans have shown that antibodies to double-stranded DNA and Sm (Smith) antigen are highly specific for SLE. Antibodies to single-stranded DNA are not specific for SLE and can be found even in some normal individuals. Antibodies to histones occur chiefly in SLE, drug related lupus, and rheumatoid arthritis.

Canine, Feline, and Equine Systemic Lupus Erythematosus

SLE in dogs, as in humans, involves several body systems, usually affects young females, and often terminates in renal failure. A typical patient with SLE sequentially or simultaneously develops AIHA, thrombocytopenic purpura, and glomerulonephritis. Symmetric polyarthritis, dermatitis or other skin lesions, or thyroiditis may also sometimes occur. Significant relationships have been found among ANA titer and polyarthritis, lymphadenopathy, and anemia or thrombocytopenia (Kass et al., 1985). Dogs having the MHC class I antigen DLA-A7 are at a greater risk of developing SLE, whereas dogs with DLA-A1 and DLA-B5 antigens appear to be at a lesser risk (Teichner et al., 1990). A colony of dogs was developed by mating 2 dogs with SLE (Monier et al., 1988). Antinuclear

Table 22–5. Principal Clinical and Hematologic Signs in Dogs with Positive LE Cell Test

Dog. No.	1	2	3	4	5	6	7	8
Breed*	GSX	Basenji	GS	Cocker	GS	GS	Doberman	GS
Sex	F	F	F	M	M	M	M	M
Age	14 mo	16 mo	2 yr	5½ yr	8 yr	10 yr	9 yr	7 yr
Muscle wasting	+	−	+	+	+	−	−	−
Lameness	+	+	+	+	+	+	+	+
Joint swellings	+	+	+	−	−	−	−	−
Edema of limbs	+	±	−	−	+	+	—	+
Pyrexia	+	+	+	+	−	−	−	+
Heart murmur	−	+	−	+	−	−	−	−
Proteinuria	+	−	−	±	−	4 +	+	+
Lymphadenopathy	−	−	−	+	+	+	−	+
Hyperkeratosis	−	−	−	Nose	Inguinal	−	−	−
PCV (mean, %)	34	37	36	27	51	47	50	40
RBC sed. rate (mean, corrected)	23 +	33 +	1 −	30 +	−	26 +	3 +	12 +
Neutrophila	+	+	+	+	−	+	−	−
Lymphopenia	+	−	−	−	−	−	−	−
Plasma protein (g/dl)	7.7	7.3	7.0	7.2	9.0	8.3	7.8	6.6
Fibrinogen (g/dl)	0.45	0.45	0.30	0.40	0.30	0.42	0.30	0.30
Coombs test	−	2+	−	3 +	−	−	−	−
LE cell test	+	+	+	+	+	+	+	+
Antinuclear antibody test	—	+	−	+	—	−	−	—
Diagnosis	SLE	Polyarthritis	Polyarthritis	Arthritis (SLE)	SLE	Glomerulonephritis	Myopathy	SLE

From Schalm, O.W., and Ling, G.V.: The L.E. cell phenomenon in the dog. Cal. Vet., 24:20, 1980.
* GS, German shepherd; GSX, crossbred, shepherd-type.
† Globulin 5.6 g/dl.
+, present; −, absent or negative test result; —, not tested.

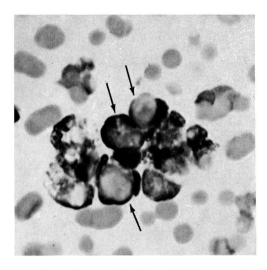

Fig. 22–6. Cluster of neutrophils, three of which are LE cells *(arrows)* from a cat with autoimmune hemolytic anemia. Also shown are two clumps of agglutinated erythrocytes with polychromatophilic erythrocytes included within the clumps (×2250). (From Jain, N.C.: Schalm's Veterinary Hematology. 4th Ed. Philadelphia, Lea & Febiger, 1986, p. 1148.)

antibodies and clinical signs of SLE occurred with increasing frequency in many of the colony dogs compared to the controls.

The diagnosis of SLE is substantiated by positive results for LE cells, ANA, complement-fixing antibodies to DNA-histone complexes, and rheumatoid factor. Multiple serologic abnormalities may be found. In the indirect immunofluorescence test for ANA in the dog, the homogeneous pattern is the most common, speckled and peripheral patterns are detected occasionally, and the nucleolar fluorescence is rare (Murtaugh and Jacobs, 1983). A new antibody, producing a speckled pattern of fluorescence with a 43-kD glycoprotein in the nucleus of mammalian cells, was detected in dogs with SLE (Soulard et al., 1991). In dogs with SLE, anti-double stranded DNA antibodies detected by ELISA or indirect immunofluorescence test are rare, where as anti-histone antibodies are common (Brinet et al., 1988). The pattern of canine SLE antihistone antibodies on immunoblot is different from that in human SLE. Histone fractions most often recognized by the canine antibodies are, by order of frequency, H3, H4, and H2A, but for humans the order is H1, H2B, and H3.

Clinicopathologic findings in dogs with SLE have revealed that hemolytic anemia, thrombocytopenia, and glomerulonephritis may not always be prominent findings. Hematologic changes have varied in other cases of SLE, with primary findings being neutrophilia, hyperfibrinogenemia, and hyperproteinemia, mainly resulting from hypergammaglobulinemia of a polyclonal pattern (Table 22–5). In 8 German Shepherd dogs with a lupus-like syndrome, autoimmune hemolytic anemia or thrombocytopenia was not detected, but anemia, leukopenia, and elevated serum IgG levels were found, probably as a result of chronic inflammatory process (Thoren-Tolling and Ryden, 1991).

Several cases of feline SLE have been reported, with a positive or negative LE cell test and ANA titers ranging from negative to 1:40 (Fig. 22–6). The disease has occurred in association with immune-complex glomerulonephritis, AIHA, or AITP. Guidelines for SLE therapy are similar to those for AIHA and AITP. Anemia in SLE may also result from other mechanisms, such as those associated with anemia of chronic disease and impaired erythropoietin production by diseased kidneys (Lam and Quah, 1990).

SLE was diagnosed in a 2-year-old standardbred filly (Geor et al., 1990). Clinical signs included weight loss, bilateral symmetric alopecia, seborrhea, oral ulceration, and lymphadenopathy. Laboratory abnormalities included a Coombs-positive AIHA and serum ANA. Skin biopsies revealed an immune-mediated skin disease. The filly was euthanized after an unsuccessful glucocorticoid therapy. Membranous glomerulonephritis and fibrous synovitis were prominent necropsy findings.

REFERENCES

Andersson, L., Bohme, J., Rask, L., et al.: Genomic hybridization of bovine class II major histocompatibility genes: 1. Extensive polymorphism of DQα and DQβ genes. Anim. Genet., 17:95, 1986.

Andersson, L. and Rask, L.: Characterization of the MHC region in cattle. The number of DQ genes varies between haplotypes. Immunogenetics, 27:110, 1988.

Andrews, G.A., Chavey, P.S., Smith, J.E., et al.: N-glycolylneuraminic acid and N-acetylneuraminic acid define feline blood group A and B antigens. Blood, 79:2485, 1992.

Auer, L. and Bell, K.: The AB blood group system of cats. Anim. Blood Groups Biochem. Genet., 12:287, 1981.

Bailey, E., Albright, D.G. and Henney, P.J.: Equine neonatal isoerythrolysis: evidence for prevention by maternal antibodies to the Ca blood group antigen. Am. J. Vet. Res., 49:1218, 1988.

Barker, R.M., Gruffydd-Jones, T.J., Stokes, C.R., et al.: Identification of autoantigens in canine autoimmune haemolytic anaemia. Clin. Exp. Immunol., 85:33, 1991.

Bean M.A., Storb, R., Graham, T., et al.: Prevention of transfusion-induced sensitization to minor histocompatibility antigens on DLA-identical canine marrow grafts by gamma irradiation of marrow donor blood. Transplantation, 52:956, 1991.

Beck D.J.: A case of primary autoimmune haemolytic anaemia in a pony. Equine Vet J., 22:292, 1990.

Bernoco, D., Lewin, H.A., Andersson, L., et al.: Joint Report of the Fourth International Bovine Lymphocyte Antigen (BoLA) Workshop. East Lansing, Michigan, USA, 25 August 1990. Anim. Genet., 22:477, 1991.

Bizzaro, N. and Dianese, G.: Neonatal alloimmune amegakaryocytosis. Case report. Vox Sang., 54:112, 1988.

Brinet, A., Fournel, C., Faure, J.R., et al.: Anti-histone antibodies (ELISA and immunoblot) in canine lupus erythematosus. Clin. Exp. Immunol., 74:105, 1988.

Brostrom, H., Fahlbrink, E., Dubath, M.L., et al.: Association between equine leucocyte antigens (ELA) and equine sarcoid tumors in the population of Swedish halfbreds and some of their families. Vet. Immunol. Immunopathol., 19:215, 1988.

Bull, R.W., Vriesendorp, H.M., Cech, R., et al.: Joint report of the third international workshop on canine immunogenetics. II. Analysis of the serological typing of cells. Transplantation, 43: 154, 1987.

Bussel, J., Kaplan, C. and McFarland, J: Recommendations for the evaluation and treatment of neonatal autoimmune and alloimmune thrombocytopenia. The Working Party on Neonatal Immune Thrombocytopenia of the Neonatal Hemostasis Subcommittee of the Scientific and Standardization Committee of the ISTH. Thromb. Haemost., 65:631, 1991.

Butler, M., Andrews, G.A., Smith, J.E., et al.: Thin layer chromatography of erythrocyte membrane glycolipids from type A and type B cats. Comp. Haematol. Int., 1:196, 1991.

Bux, J. and Mueller-Eckhardt, C.: Autoimmune neutropenia. Semin. Hematol., 29:45, 1992.

Cain, G.R. and Suzuki, Y.: Presumptive neonatal isoerythrolysis in cats. J. Am. Vet. Med. Assoc., 187:46, 1985.

Cain, J.L., Cain, G.R., Turrel, J.M., et al.: Clinical and lymphohematologic responses after bone marrow transplantation in sibling and unrelated donor-recipient pairs of cats. Am. J. Vet. Res., 51:839, 1990.

Chickering, W.R., Brown, J., Prasse, K.W., et al.: Effects of heterologous antineutrophil antibody in the cat. Am. J. Vet. Res., 46:1815, 1985b.

Chickering, W.R., Prasse, K.W. and Dawe, D.L.: Development and clinical application of methods for detection of antineutrophil antibody in serum of the cat. Am. J. Vet. Res., 46:1809, 1985a.

Clabough, D.L., Gebhard, D., Flaherty, M.T., et al.: Immunemediated thrombocytopenia in horses infected with equine infectious anemia virus. J. Virol., 65:6242, 1991.

Collins, P.W. and Newland, A.C.: Treatment modalities of autoimmune blood disorders. Semin. Hematol., 29:64, 1992.

Constantopoulos, G., Scott, J.A. and Shull, R.M.: Corneal opacity in canine MPS I. Changes after bone marrow transplantation. Invest. Ophthalmol. Vis. Sci, 30:1802, 1989.

Cotter, S.M.: Clinical transfusion medicine. Adv. Vet. Sci. Comp. Med., 36:187, 1991.

Deeg, H.J., Raff, R.F., Grosse-Wilde, H., et al.: Joint report of the third international workshop on canine immunogenetics.I. Analysis of homozygous typing cells (HTCs). Transplantation, 41:111, 1986.

Deverson, E.V., Wright, H., Watson, S., et al.: Class II major histocompatibility complex genes of the sheep. Anim. Genet., 22:211, 1991.

Dhawedkar, R.G., Jain, N.C., Mount, M.E., et al.: Detection of equine antiplatelet and antineutrophil antibodies by enzymelinked immunosorbent assay. Res. Vet. Sci., 51:292, 1991.

Doxiadis, I., Krumbacher, K., Neefjes, J.J., et al.: Biochemical evidence that the DLA=B locus codes for a class II determinant expressed on all canine peripheral blood lymphocytes. Exp. Clin. Immunogenet., 6:219, 1989.

Ejima, H., Kurokawa, K. and Ikemoto, S.: Feline red blood cell groups by naturally occurring isoantibody. Jpn. J. Vet. Sci., 48:971, 1986.

Engelfriet, C.P., Overbeeke, M.A. and von dem Borne, A.E.: Autoimmune hemolytic anemia. Semin. Hematol., 29:3, 1992.

Eyquem, A., Podliachouk, L. and Milot, P.: Blood groups in chimpanzees, horses, sheep, pigs and other mammals. Ann. NY Acad. Sci., 97:320, 1962.

Feldman, B.F., Handagama, P. and Lubberink, A.A.M.E.: Splenectomy as adjunctive therapy for immune-mediated thrombocytopenia and hemolytic anemia in the dog. J. Am. Vet. Med. Assoc., 187:617, 1985.

Fenger, C.K., Hoffsis, G.F., and Kociba, G.J.: Idiopathic immunemediated hemolytic anemia in a calf. J. Am. Vet. Med. Assoc., 201:97, 1992.

Fulton, R., Gasper, P.W., Thrall, M.A., et al.: Complications associated with bone marrow transplantation in the cat (abstract). Vet. Clin. Pathol., 19:5, 1990.

Gaunt, S.D. and Baker, D.C.: Hemosiderin in leukocytes of dogs with immune-mediated hemolytic anemia. Vet. Clin. Pathol., 15(3):8, 1986.

Geor, R.J., Clark, E.G., Haines, D.M., et al.: Systemic lupus erythematosus in a filly. J. Am. Vet. Med. Assoc., 197:1489, 1990.

Gibson, J.: Autoimmune hemolytic anemia: current concepts. Aust. NZ J. Med., 18:625, 1988.

Giger, U.: Frequency of feline A and B blood types in purebred cats and their clinical significance. Vet. Clin. Path., 19:7, 1990.

Giger, U. and Akol, K.G.: Acute hemolytic transfusion reaction in an Abyssinian cat with blood type Br. J. Vet. Intern. Med., 4:315, 1990.

Giger, U. And Bucheler, J.: Transfusion of type A and type B blood to cats. J. Am. Vet. Med. Assoc., 198:411, 1991.

Giger, U., Bucheler, J. and Patterson, D.F.: Frequency and inheritance of A and B blood types in feline breeds of the United States. J. Hered., 82:15, 1991.

Giger, U., Kilrain, C.G., Filippich, L.J., et al.: Frequencies of feline blood groups in the United States. J. Am. Vet. Med. Assoc., 195:1230, 1989.

Gogolin-Ewens, K.J., Mackay, C.R., Mercer, W.R., et al.: Sheep lymphocyte antigens (OLA). I. Major histocompatibility complex class I molecules. Immunology, 56:717, 1985.

Gompf, R.E., Shull, R.M., Breider, M.A., et al.: Cardiovascular changes after bone marrow transplantation in dogs with mucopolysaccharidosis I. Am. J. Vet. Res., 51:2054, 1990.

Greinix, H.T., Ladiges, W.C., Graham, T.C., et al.: Late failure of autologous marrow grafts in lethally irradiated dogs given anticlass II monoclonal antibody. Blood, 78:2131, 1991.

Gross, W.L., Csernok, E., and Schmitt, W.H.: Antineutrophil cytoplasmic autoantibodies: immunobiological aspects. Klin. Wochenschr., 69:558, 1991.

Handagama, P., Rappolee, D.A., Werb, Z., et al: Platelet alphagranule fibrinogen, albumin, and immunoglobulin G are not synthesized by rat and mouse megakaryocytes. J. Clin. Invest., 86:1364, 1990.

Hegde, U.M.: Platelet antibodies in immune thrombocytopenia. Blood Rev., 6:34, 1992.

Helfand, S.C., Jain, N.C. and Paul, M.: Vincristine-loaded platelet therapy for idiopathic thrombocytopenia in a dog. J. Am. Vet. Med. Assoc., 185:224, 1984.

Hesford, F., Lazary, S., Curty-Hanni, K., et al.: Biochemical evidence that equine leucocyte antigens W13, W22 and W23 present on horse major histocompatibility complex class II molecules. Anim. Genet., 20:415, 1989.

Hines, H.C. and Ross, M.J.: Serological relationships among antigens of the BoLA and the bovine M blood group systems. Anim. Genet., 18:361, 1987.

Holloway, S.A., Meyer, D.J. and Mannella, C.: Prednisolone and danazol for treatment of immune-mediated anemia, thrombocytopenia, and ineffective erythroid regeneration in a dog. J. Am. Vet. Med. Assoc., 197:1045, 1990.

Holmes, R.: Blood groups in cats. J. Physiol., 3:611, 1950.

Humber, K.A., Beech, J., Cudd, T.A., et al.: Azathioprine for treatment of immune-mediated thrombocytopenia in two horses. J. Am. Vet. Med. Assoc., 199:591, 1991.

Hunt, E. and Moore, J.S.: Use of blood and blood products. Vet. Clin. North Am. Food Anim. Pract., 6:133, 1990.

Ikemoto, S., Sakuria, Y. and Fukai, M.: Individual difference within the cat blood group detected by isohemagglutinin. Jpn. J. Vet. Sci., 43:433, 1981.

Jackson, M.L. and Kruth, S.A.: Immune-mediated hemolytic anemia and thrombocytopenia in the dog: A retrospective study of 55 cases diagnosed from 1969 through 1983 at the Western College of Veterinary Medicine. Can. Vet. J., 26:245, 1985.

Jain, N.C.: Schalm's Veterinary Hematology. 4th ed. Philadelphia, Lea & Febiger, 1986, pp. 990–1039.

Jain, N.C., Carroll, E.J. and Schalm, O.W.: Influence of antiserum to bovine leukocytes on circulating leukocytes of the cow. Am. J. Vet. Res., 29:2081, 1968.

Jain, N.C., Dhawedkar, R.G. and Kono, C.S.: Detection of antiplatelet antibody: Comparison of platelet immunofluorescence, agglutination, and immunoinjury tests using rabbit antiequine platelet serum. Vet. Clin. Pathol., 20:23, 1990a.

Jain, N.C., Stott, J.L., Vegad, J.L., et al.: Detection of anti-equine neutrophil antibody by use of flow cytometry. Am. J. Vet. Res., 52:1883, 1991.

Jain, N.C., Vegad, J.L. and Kono, C.S.: Methods for detection of immune-mediated neutropenia in horses, using antineutrophil serum of rabbit origin. Am. J. Vet. Res., 51:1026, 1990b.

Jones, D.R.E. and Gruffydd-Jones, T.J.: The haematological consequences of immune-mediated anaemias in the dog. Comp. Haematol. Int, 1:83, 1991.

Jones, D.R., Gruffydd-Jones, T.J., Stokes, C.R., et al.: Investigation into factors influencing performance of the canine antiglobulin test. Res. Vet. Sci., 48:53, 1990.

Jones, D.R., Gruffydd-Jones, T.J., Stokes, C.R., et al.: Use of a direct enzyme-linked antiglobulin test for laboratory diagnosis of immune-mediated hemolytic anemia in dogs. Am. J. Vet. Res., 53:457, 1992.

Jonsson, N.N., Pullen, C. and Watson, A.D.: Neonatal isoerythrolysis in Himalayan kittens. Aust. Vet. J., 67:416, 1990.

Joosten, I., Ruff, G., Sander M.F., et al.: Biochemical and serological typing of caprine class I and class II products. Anim. Genet., 22, Suppl 1:48, 1991.

Joosten, I., Sanders, M.F., van der Poel, A., et al.: Biochemically defined polymorphism of bovine MHC class II antigens. Immunogenetics, 29:213, 1989.

Joosten, I., Teale, A.J., van der Poel, A., et al.: Biochemical evidence of the expression of two major histocompatibility complex class I genes on bovine peripheral blood mononuclear cells. Anim. Genet., 23:113, 1992.

Kahn, W., Vaala, W. and Palmer, J: [Neonatal isoerythrolysis in newborn foals]. Tierarztl. Prax., 19:521, 1991.

Kaplan, C., Morel-Kopp, M.C., Kroll, H., et al.: HPA-5b (Br(a)) neonatal alloimmune thrombocytopenia: clinical and immunological analysis of 39 cases. Br. J. Haematol., 78:425, 1991.

Kaplan, C., Morinet, F and Cartron, J.: Virus-induced autoimmune thrombocytopenia and neutropenia. Semin. Hematol., 29:24, 1992.

Kass, P.H., Strombeck, D.R., Farver, T.B., et al.: Application of the log-linear model in the prediction of the antinuclear antibody test in th dog. Am. J. Vet. Res., 46:2336, 1985.

Kaveri, S.V., Dietrich, G., Hurez, V., et al.: Intravenous immunoglobulins (IVIg) in the treatment of autoimmune diseases. Clin. Exp. Immunol., 86:192, 1991.

Kiefel, V., Santoso, S. and Mueller-Eckhardt, C.: Serological, biochemical and molecular aspects of platelet autoantigens. Semin. Hematol., 29:26, 1992.

Kline, K., Briles, W.E., Bacon, L., et al.: Characterization of different B-F (MHC Class I) molecules in the chicken. J. Hered., 79:239, 1988.

Kolb, H.J., Losslein, L.K., Beisser, K., et al.: Dose rate and fractionation of total body irradiation in dogs: short and long term effects. Radiother. Oncol., 18, Suppl. 1:51, 1990.

Krumbacher, K., Happel, M. and Grosse-Wilde, H.: Recognition of monocyte-associated antigens in the dog. Tissue Antigens., 37: 21, 1991.

Kunicki, T.J. and Beardsley, D.S.: The alloimmune thrombocytopenias: neonatal alloimmune thrombocytopenic purpura and post-transfusion purpura. Prog. Hemost. Thromb., 9:203, 1989.

Lam, S.K. and Quah, T.C.: Anemia in systemic lupus erythematosus. J. Singapore. Paediatr. Soc., 32:132, 1990.

Lasky, L.C.: The role of the laboratory in marrow manipulation. Arch. Pathol. Lab. Med., 115:293, 1991.

Lazary, S., Antczak, D.F., Bailey, E., et al.: Joint Report of the Fifth International Workshop on Lymphocyte Alloantigens of the Horse. Baton Rouge, Louisiana, 31 October-1 November 1987. Anim. Genet., 19:447, 1988.

Lewin, H.A., Wu, M.C., Stewart, J.A., et al.: Association between BoLA and subclinical bovine leukemia virus infection in a herd of Holstein-Friesian cows. Immunogenetics, 27:338, 1988.

Luther, D.G., Cox, H.U. and Nelson, W.O.: Screening for neonatal isohemolytic anemia in calves. Am. J. Vet. Res., 46:1078, 1985.

Madyastha, P.R. and Glassman, A.B.: Neutrophil antigens and antibodies in the diagnosis of immune neutropenias. Ann. Clin. Lab. Sci., 19:146, 1989.

Mair, T.S., Taylor, F.G. and Hillyer, M.H.: Autoimmune haemolytic anaemia in eight horses. Vet. Rec., 126:51, 1990.

Manning, D.D. and Bell, J.A.: Lack of detectable blood groups in domestic ferrets: Implications for transfusion. J. Am. Vet. Med. Assoc., 197:84, 1990.

Matousek, J. and Riha, J.: Anti-leucocyte antibodies and embryonic mortality in embryo transferred cows. Anim. Genet., 22:245, 1991.

Matus, R.E., Gordon, B.R., Leifer, C.E., et al.: Plasmapheresis in five dogs with systemic immune-mediated disease. J. Am. Vet. Med. Assoc., 187:595, 1985a.

Matus, R.E., Schrader, L.E., Leifer, C.E., et al.: Plasmapheresis as adjuvant therapy for autoimmune hemolytic anemia in two dogs. J. Am. Vet. Med. Assoc., 186:691, 1985b.

Messer, N.T and Arnold, K.: Immune-mediated hemolytic anemia in a horse. J. Am. Vet. Med. Assoc., 198:1415, 1991.

Metcalf, D.: Hemopoietic growth factors and marrow transplantation: An overview. Transplant. Proc., 21:2932, 1989.

Mongey, A.B. and Hess, E.V.: Antinuclear antibodies and disease specificity. Adv. Intern. Med., 36:151, 1991.

Monier, J.C., Fournel, C., Lapras, M., et al.: Systemic lupus erythematosus in a colony of dogs. Am. J. Vet. Res., 49:46, 1988.

Murphy, W.G. and Kelton, J.G.: Methyldopa-induced autoantibodies against red blood cells. Blood Rev., 2:36, 1988.

Murtaugh, R.J. and Jacobs, R.M.: Antinuclear antibody associated with lupus erythematosus in a dog. Vet. Clin. Pathol., 12(3):29, 1983.

Nesse, L.L. and Ruff, G.: A comparison of lymphocyte antigen specificities in Norwegian and Swiss goats. Anim. Genet., 20: 71, 1989.

Nguyen, T.C.: Genetic systems of red cell blood groups in goats. Anim. Genet., 21:233, 1990.

Porter, R.E., Jr., Weiser, M.G. and Callahan, G.N.: Development of an enzyme-linked immunosorbent assay to detect IgG, IgM, and complement (C3) on canine erythrocytes. Am. J. Vet. Res., 50:1365, 1989.

Porter, R.E.J.R. and Weiser, M.G.: Effect of immune-mediated erythrocyte agglutination on analysis of canine blood using a multichannel blood cell counting system. Vet. Clin. Pathol., 19: 45, 1990.

Price, G.S., Armstrong, P.J., McLeod, D.A., et al.: Evaluation of citrate-phosphate-dextrose-adenine as a storage medium for packed canine erythrocyte. J. Vet. Intern. Med., 2:126, 1988.

Raff, R.F., Severns, E., Storb, R., et al.: L-leucyl-L-leucine methyl ester treatment of canine marrow and peripheral blood cells. Inhibition of proliferative responses with maintenance of the capacity for autologous marrow engraftment. Transplantation, 46:655, 1988.

Robinson, J.P., Duque, R.E., Boxer, L.A., et al.: Measurement of antineutrophil antibodies by flow cytometry: simultaneous detection of antibodies against monocytes and lymphocytes. Diagn. Clin. Immunol., 5:163, 1987.

Sako, F., Gasa, S., Makita, A., et al.: Human blood group glycosphingolipids of porcine erythrocytes. Arch. Biochem. Biophys., 278:228, 1990.

Salama, A. and Mueller-Eckhardt, C.: Immune-mediated blood cell dyscrasias related to drugs. Semin. Hematol., 29:54, 1992.

Sarmiento, U.M., Sarmiento, J.I. and Storb, R.: Allelic variation in the DR subregion of the canine major histocompatibility complex. Immunogenetics, 32:13, 1990.

Slappendel, R.J.: Blood transfusions in the dog and cat. Tijdschr. Diergeneeskd., 117. Suppl. 1:16S, 1992.

Smith, J.E., Maheffey, E. and Board, P.: A new storage medium for canine blood. J. Am. Vet. Med. Assoc., 172:701, 1978.

Sockett, D.C., Traub-Dargatz, J., and Weiser, M.G.: Immune-mediated hemolytic anemia and thrombocytopenia in a foal. J. Am. Vet. Med. Assoc., 190:308, 1987.

Sontheimer, R.D., McCauliffe, D.P., Zappi, E., et al.: Antinuclear antibodies: clinical correlations and biologic significance. Adv. Dermatol., 7:3, 1992.

Soulard, M., Barque, J.P., Della Valle, V., et al.: A novel 43-kDa glycoprotein is detected in the nucleus of mammalian cells by autoantibodies from dogs with autoimmune disorders. Exp. Cell Res., 193:59, 1991.

Stear, M.J., Pokorny, T.S., Muggli, N.E., et al.: Breed differences in the distribution of BoLA-A locus antigens in American cattle. Anim. Genet., 19:171, 1988.

Step, D.L., Blue, J.T. and Dill, S.G.: Penicillin-induced hemolytic anemia and acute hepatic failure following treatment of tetanus in a horse. Cornell. Vet, 81:13, 1991.

Stone, E., Badner, D. and Cotter, S.M.: Trends in transfusion medicine in dogs at a veterinary school clinic: 315 cases (1986-1989). J. Am. Vet. Med. Assoc., 200:1000, 1992.

Sullivan, K.M.: Congress review: progress and prospects in bone marrow transplantation. Transplant. Proc., 21:2919, 1989.

Symons, M. and Bell, K.: Expansion of the canine A blood group system. Anim. Genet., 22:227, 1991.

Taylor, F.G. and Cooke, B.J.: Use of erythrocyte fragility profiles for monitoring immune-mediated haemolysis in horses. Res. Vet. Sci., 48:138, 1990.

Taylor, R.M., Stewart, G.J. and Farrow, B.R.: Improvement in the neurologic signs and storage lesions of fucosidosis in dogs given marrow transplants at an early age. Transplant. Proc., 21:3818, 1989.

Teichner, M., Krumbacher, K., Doxiadis, I., et al.: Systemic lupus erythematosus in dogs: association to the major histocompatibility complex class I antigen DLA-A7. Clin. Immunol. Immunopathol., 55:255, 1990.

Thiele, O.W.: Biochemistry of the J blood group substance of cattle. J. Vet. Med. (A), 35:161, 1988.

Thiem, P.A., Abbot, D.L., Moroff, S., et al.: Preliminary findings on the comparison of flow cytometric and solid-phase radio-immunoassay techniques for the detection of serum antiplatelet antibodies in dogs. Vet. Clin . Pathol., 20(1):18, 1991.(Abstract)

Thoren-Tolling, K. and Ryden, L.: Serum auto antibodies and clinical/pathological features in German shepherd dogs with a lupuslike syndrome. Acta Vet. Scand., 32:15, 1991.

Toivanen, P. and Vainio, O.: MHC of the chicken. Anim. Genet., 18, Suppl. 1:3, 1987.

Toth, L.A. and Rebar, A.H.: Measurement of antinuclear antibodies in the dog: A review. Vet. Clin. Pathol., 16:76, 1987.

Tsuchida, S., Usui, R., Muramatsu, U., et al.: Autoantibodies and red blood cell membrane proteins in a case of canine autoimmune hemolytic anemia. J. Vet. Med. Sci., 53:19, 1991.

Vage, D.I., Olsaker, I., Lungaas, F., et al.: High levels of linkage disequilibria between serologically defined class I bovine lymphocyte antigens (BoLA-A) and class II DQB restriction fragment length polymorphism (RFLP) in Norwegian cows. Anim. Genet., 23:125, 1992.

Varewyck, H., Renard, C., Kristensen, B., et al.: Swine lymphocyte alloantigens (SLA) class I serology and genetics in Belgian Landrace and Pietrain breeds. Anim. Genet., 21:59, 1990.

Victoria, E.J., Pierce, S.W., Branks, M.J., et al.: IgG red blood cell autoantibodies in autoimmune hemolytic anemia bind to epitopes on red blood cell membrane band 3 glycoprotein. J. Lab. Clin. Med., 115:74, 1990.

Vlahakes, G.J., Lee, R., Jacobs, E.E., Jr., et al.: Hemodynamic effects and oxygen transport properties of a new blood substitute in a model of a massive blood replacement. J. Thorac. Cardiovasc. Surg., 100:379, 1990.

von dem Borne, A.E. and Ouwehand, W.H.: Immunology of platelet disorders. Baillieres. Clin. Haematol., 2:749, 1989.

Wang, W.C.: Evans syndrome in childhood: pathophysiology, clinical course, and treatment. Am J Pediatr. Hematol. Oncol., 10:330, 1988.

Waters, A.H.: Autoimmune thrombocytopenia: Clinical aspects. Semin. Hematol., 29:18, 1992.

Weigel, K.A., Freeman, A.E., Kehrli, M.E., Jr., et al.: Association of a BoLA-A locus antigen with increased antibody dependent neutrophil cytotoxicity and decreased susceptibility to subclinical mastitis. Anim. Genet., 22, Suppl. 1:43, 1991.

Weiss, D.J.: Antibody-mediated suppression of erythropoiesis in dogs with red blood cell aplasia. Am. J. Vet. Res., 47:2646, 1985.

Wilkerson, M.J., Meyers, K.M., Wardrop, K.J., et al.: Anti-A isoagglutinins in two blood type B cats are IgG and IgM. Vet. Clin. Pathol., 20(1):10, 1991.

Williams, W.J., Beutler, E., Erslev, A.J., Litchman, M.A.: Hematology. 4th ed. New York, McGraw-Hill, 1990, Chaps. 67–70, 86, 143, 164, 165, 171.

Wong, P.L., Nickel, L.S., Bowling, A.T., et al.: Clinical survey of antibodies against red blood cells in horses after homologous blood transfusion. Am. J. Vet. Res., 47:2566, 1985.

Zanjani, E.D., Mackintosh, F.R. and Harrison, M.R.: Hematopoietic chimerism in sheep and nonhuman primates by in utero transplantation of fetal hematopoietic stem cells. Blood cells, 17:349, 1991.

Zaruby, J.F., Hearn, P. and Colling, D.: Neonatal isoerythrolysis in a foal, involving anti-Pa alloantibody. Equine Vet. J., 24:71, 1992.

Index

In this index, page numbers in *italics* designate figures; page numbers followed by the letter "t" designate tables. *See* cross-references designate the synonymous term under which entries may be found. *See also* cross-references designate related topics *or* detailed topic breakdowns.

Dogs
  anemias, 165
    AID, 218
    aplastic/hypoplastic, 215–216
    autoimmune hemolytic, 205t, *206,*
      393
    enzyme deficiency, 195
    evaluation, 4
    hemolytic infectious, 182, 185
    hemorrhagic, 172t
  autoimmune thrombocytopenia, 399
  bacterial infections: leptospirosis, 190
  Basenji, 25t, 195t
  blood volume:body weight, 170t
  bone marrow differential cell counts,
    13t
  collies: cyclic hematopoiesis in silver
    gray, 77–78
  combined immunodeficiency, 372–373
  corticosteroid therapy, *25, 44*
  DIC, 99t
  distemper, 300t, 300–301, *301*
  Doberman Pinschers, 243
  eosinophilia, 249t
  eosinophils, *250*
  ESR values, 33t
  hereditary coagulopathies, 92t
  hyperadrenocorticism (Cushing's
    syndrome), 298t
  icterus index, 50
  Irish setters, 243
  Japanese Shiba, 144
  leukemias
    basophilic and mast cell, 339–340
    lymphoproliferative, 333–336, 334t,
      336t, *365*
    malignant histiocytosis, 339
    myeloproliferative/myelodysplastic,
      336–338, 337t
    radiation-induced, 339
  leukocytic response to disease, 300t
  megakaryocyte abnormalities, *121*
  monocytes, *269*
  normal blood values, 6t, 7t, 20t
  normal WBC differentials, 7t
  parasitic infections
    babeosis, 182
    haemobartonellosis, 185–186, *186*
  physiologic leukocytosis, 42t, 42–43
  plasma protein levels, 51
  platelet disorders, 128, 129–130
  platelet morphology, *106, 107*
  poisoning
    lead, 199
    zinc toxicosis, 200
  polycythemias, 166t
  poodles
    anemia in, 165
    macrocytosis vs. B₁₂ deficiency, 214,
      214
  renal failure, 218t, 218–219
  systemic lupus erythematosus, 403–404
  thrombocytopenia, 126t, *127*
Döhle bodies, 46–47, 240, *244*
Donath-Landsteiner antibody, 396
Donkeys: normal values, 58t
2,3-DPG, 145
Drepanocytes, 148
Drug therapy
  anemias related to, 198–199, 208
    autoimmune hemolytic, 401–402
      Heinz body formation, 32, 144, 153,
        200–202, *202, 203*

  in autoimmune hemolytic anemia, 397–
    398
  in autoimmune thrombocytopenia, 400–
    401
  M:E ratio and, 14
  neutrophil disorders and, 243
  platelet disorders and, 117, 123, 128–
    129
Dysfibrogenemia, 95
Dysplastic changes in leukemia, 314
Dysproteinemias, 96–97
  classification, 361t
  gammopathies, *364,* 364–366, *365*
    Aleutian disease in mink, 368
    benign monoclonal gammopathy, 368
    gastrointestinal disorders, 368–369
    hyperviscosity syndrome, 367
    infection-related, 369–370
    kidney disease, 369
    liver disease, 369
    multiple myeloma, 366
    parasitism, 369
    Waldenström's macroglobulinemia,
      366–367
  quantitative
    albumin, 362
    α- and β-globulins, 363
    fibrinogen, 362–363
    gamma-globulins, 363–364

E
Eccentrocytes, 149
Echinocytes, 149–150
EDTA, 1, 3
Ehrlichia canis, 130
Ehrlichia equi, 130
Ehrlichia phagocytophilia, 131
Ehrlichia platys, 129–130, *130*
Ehrlichia risticii, 130–131
Elephants, 57t
  leukocyte response, *69*
  unique blood features, 68
ELISA test for feline leukemia virus, 320–
  321
Elliptocytes, 150
Elliptocytosis, 193–194
Emaciation in horses, 16t
Endocrine disorders and anemia, 220
Endotoxemia, 48–49, 303
End-stage kidney disease. *See* Renal
  failure
Enzyme deficiency anemias
  congenital erythropoietic porphyria,
    195–196
  phosphofructokinase deficiency, 195
  pyruvate kinase, 194–195, 195t
Eosinopenias, 256–257, 297t
Eosinophilias, 9, 256, 297t
Eosinophilic leukemia
  equine, 345
  feline, 331–332
Eosinophils
  basophil/mast cell interrelationships,
    261, *262*
  in bone marrow, 304
  comparative hematology, 5–6
  disorders
    eosinopenias, 256–257
    eosinophilias, 9, 256, 297t
  functions, 252–253, 253t
    allergic/inflammatory regulation,
      254–255
    parasitical activity, 253–254, *255*

  phagocytosis and bactericidal activity,
    253, *254*
  in tissue injury, 255–256
  maturation, 10
  morphologic abnormalities, 304
  production and release
    eosinopoiesis, 247
    migration in tissues, 249
    regulation, 247–248
  structure and constituents, 248, 249–
    252, *250, 251, 252*
Eperythrozoonosis, 187–188
Epinephrine and physiologic leukocytosis,
  42–44
Erythremic myelosis in cats, 328–329
Erythrocyte antigens, 381–383
Erythrocyte indices, 4
Erythrocytes, 139–140, *141, 142. See also*
  RBC count
  agglutination, 5
  comparative hematology, 5, 63
  2,3-DPG and O₂ affinity, 145
  fusiform in Angora goat, *30, 31*
  in leukemias, 313
  life cycle, 8–9, 34, 145t, 145–147
  membrane, 140–143, *143*
  metabolism, 143–145, *144, 145*
  morphology, 23–27
    abnormal, *32,* 138, 147t, 147–153,
      148–152
      basophilic stippling, *32,* 138
      diseases/conditions associated with,
        153t
      Heinz bodes, *32*
      Rouleau formation, 5, 8
    ESR, 32–33
    Hb types, 34–35
    osmotic fragility, 33–34, *34,* 34t, 146t
    reticulocytes, 28–32
  nomenclature, 134t
  physiology
    age and, 35–36
    altitude and, 36
    breed differences, 36
    fetal blood values, 35
    interrelationships of parameters, 35
    iron requirement in suckling pigs, 38
    sex/parturition/lactation, 36
    splenic influences, 36–37
    training influence in horses, 37–38
Erythrocyte sedimentation rate. *See* ESR
Erythroleukemia in cats, 12, 329t, 329–
  330, 331t
Erythropoiesis, 79–80, *134, 135*
  cellular morphology, 136
  cellular nomenclature, 134t
  effective and ineffective, 135–136
  erythroblastic islands and nurse cells,
    133, *136*
  erythropoietin in, 138–139, *140*
  ferritin and hemosiderin, 134–135
  hemoglobin and, 153–158
  nutrients essential to, 139
  reticulocytes in, 136–138, *138*
ESR
  comparative hematology, 32–33, 33t
  significance, 8
Estrogen toxicity, 128–129
Ethylenediaminetetra-acetic acid (EDTA),
  1, 3
Exercise and blood values in horses, 37–
  38
Exocytosis, 239